Geographical Aspects of Health and Disease in India

Revised and Enlarged Edition

About the Editors

Rais Akhtar is presently Adjunct Professor, International Institute of Health Management and research, New Delhi. Formerly National Fellow and Emeritus Scientist (CSIR), CSRD, Jawaharlal Nehru University, New Delhi, and Visiting Professor Dept. of Geology, AMU, Aligarh. He has taught at the Jawaharlal Nehru University, New Delhi, University of Zambia, Lusaka and The University of Kashmir, Srinagar. He is recipient of a number of international fellowships including Leverhulme Fellowship (University of Liverpool), Henry Chapman Fellowship (University of London), Visiting Fellowship, (University of Sussex), Royal Society Fellowship, University of Oxford and, Visiting Professorship, University of Paris-10. He was Lead Author (1999-2007), on the Inter-governmental Panel on Climate Change, which is the joint winner of Nobel Peace Prize for 2007. Prof. Akhtar received Nobel Memento from IPCC, Geneva. Prof. Akhtar has to his credit 91 research papers and 18 books published from India, United Kingdom, United States, Germany and The Netherlands. Prof. Akhtar's book entitled: Environmental Degradation and Human Health, was published in 2014 by Springer (with A. Malik and E. Grohmann). His book entitled: Climate Change and Human Health Scenario in South and Southeast Asia, was published in 2016 by Springer. Prof. Akhtar's latest book: Climate Change and Air Pollution was published by Springer in 2017 (with Cosimo Palagiano as co-editor). Prof. Rais Akhtar is Member of Expert Group on Climate Change and Human Health of the Ministry of Health and Family Welfare, Government of India.

Andrew Learmonth, (Medical Geographer, born December 17, 1916; died March 16, 2008), who had died aged 91, will be remembered as the first chair of geography at the Australian National University, and as a prominent researcher and teacher of medical geography, who made a significant contribution to our understanding of malaria. But it is for his role as a founder member of the Open University in Britain, and its first professor.

The OU offered the chance to combine a higher education with family and work commitments at any age, which resonated with Andrew's own experience growing up in the depression.

His experiences of organising medical services in tropical conditions and dealing with tropical diseases would form important strands in his later academic work. He displayed an ability as a strategic thinker and a practical organiser, and would have been promoted to quartermaster had his colonel not decided he was "not enough of a scoundrel". In 1945 he applied to read economics at Edinburgh University.

In India, Andrew developed his research interest in the field of malaria. His focus on the environmental and cultural factors involved in its return demonstrated the importance in linking our interaction with our environment to the spread of disease. In 1962, he was appointed the first chair of geography at the Australian National University in Canberra. During his time there, in partnership with his wife Nancy, he produced Regional Landscapes of Australia, Encyclopaedia of Australia, and a revision of OHK Spate's India and Pakistan.

Geographical Aspects of Health and Disease in India

Revised and Enlarged Edition

Editors

Rais Akhtar

Andrew Learmonth

CONCEPT PUBLISHING COMPANY PVT. LTD.

NEW DELHI-110059

ISBN-13: 978-93-86682-22-2 (HB)
ISBN-13: 978-93-86682-23-9 (PB)

Revised and Enlarged Edition 2018

Published and Printed by

Concept
Since 1974

Concept Publishing Company Pvt. Ltd.
A/15-16, Commercial Block, Mohan Garden
New Delhi-110059 (India)
T: 25351460, 25351794, *F*: 091-11-25357109
E: publishing@conceptpub.com, W: www.conceptpub.com

Cataloging in Publication Data—Courtesy: D.K. Agencies (P) Ltd. <docinfo@dkagencies.com>

Rais Akhtar, Andrew Learmonth. — Revised and enlarged edition.
Geographical aspects of health and disease in India/editors,
pages cm
Includes bibliographical references and index.
ISBN 9789386682222 (HB)
ISBN 9789386682239 (PB)

1. Medical geography—India. 2. Nutrition surveys—India. 3. Social medicine—India. 4. Health service areas—India. 5. Medical geography—South Asia. 6. India—Statistics, Medical. I. Akhtar, Rais, 1946- editor. II. Learmonth, A. T. A. (Andrew Thomas Amos), 1916- editor.

LCC RA911.G46 2018 DDC 614.4254 23

Preface

Medical geography utilizes the concepts and techniques of geography to investigate health-related issues. It employs spatial analysis, the study of the distribution of discrete variables or indicators. The analysis of the "areal or spatial patterns of disease and health care provisions" may often based on mapping of various indicators of disease and health care provisions. Such maps using GIS techniques are utilized as analytical tool to understand the environmental framework of the occurrence of disease, and to break-up a disease process into separate components which may be employed in explanation. It is obvious that the medical geography has to delve into wide range of medical and biological literature, extending beyond the normal limits of geographical study and stepping into the fields such as medical ecology and epidemiology. Although the subject of medical geography is widely developed in developed countries, there is now a growing interest in this field along with climate and its impacts on human health in developing countries, including India.

Besides disease ecology, medical geography focuses on health care planning, ever since Swedish geographer S. Godlund, utilized geographical techniques in the location of regional hospitals in Sweden in 1962. Health care dimension of medical geography relates to the spatial analysis of population-based measures of access, health care delivery patterns, and resource allocation. These issues are particularly relevant to policy-makers, health services researchers, and planners. Thus, the aim of the present volume is two folds. First, it aims at throwing light on the present status of research in medical geography in India and understanding the geomedical processes in different geographical regions. Secondly to stimulate as much as possible researches, to explore new dimensions and wider horizon in this field of medical geography.

In order to obtain a systematic knowledge of the studies of medical geography in India, the chapters included in this book have been grouped into five parts.

Part I contains chapters on introductory, methodological, and on South and Southeast Asian perspectives. Rais Akhtar and Nilofar Izhar (1) have traced the origin and development of medical geography in India and highlight the present scenario of medical geography in the country. Andrew Learmonth's chapter (2) on reflections on the regional geography of disease in late colonial South Asia highlights both progress and problems in the development of medical geography since independence. A.K. Dutt and H.M. Dutta (3) summarise the disease dynamics in South and Southeast Asia in general and with particular reference to India.

M.J. Joshi and C.D. Deshpande (4) discuss the pattern of disease distribution and ecology in Southern Asia, with special reference to Indian sub-continent. They have spatially analyzed a number of infective and communicable diseases and found out that the distribution of disease follows a well-defined pattern. A group of diseases which occur in the Western region are rare in the Eastern region and *vice versa*. The borderland between these two regions in respect of disease ecology corresponds with ecological watershed. A.K. Tewari in his chapter (5) on the geomedical method and its application in the study of medical geography of Rajasthan, generates a good discussion on the methodology to be adopted in regional geomedical studies.

Part II comprises case studies in disease ecology at both macro- and micro-levels, some covering India as a whole and others concentrate at district, regional and state units.

M.K. Dutta (6) examines ecology and diffusion of cholera in India. Rais Akhtar and A.T.A. Learmonth (7) concern with the resurgence of malaria in India during 1965-76. This chapter highlights various factors which led to malaria resurgence and also identified areas which were affected by the disease since 1965.

Rais Akhtar (8) asserts that historical medical geography is a fascinating area of research which highlights the pattern of environmental conditions, people's adjustment with the environment and the occurrence of health problems as a result of man's interaction with the environment. The chapter discusses the environment and cholera outbreaks in Kashmir during nineteenth century.

In chapter 9 Rakesh Arya and Abdul Qayum utilize GIS based spatial distribution analysis and locate malarial hotspots and suggest serious governmental spatial based interference for its effective cure and prevention. Rais Akhtar (10) looks into the distribution and intensity of various cancers types in India, and Mohammad Shafi (11) measures the levels of food production efficiency in terms of caloric requirements in India. Rais Akhtar (12) examines the food insecurity in selected villages in the valley of Kashmir with the objective to analyse various drivers of food insecurity in the region, and identify coping strategies by people when faced with shocks. In chapter 13, B. Hyma and A. Ramesh discuss the spatial distribution and trends of cholera incidence in Tamil Nadu. In chapter 14 Rais Akhtar focuses on the geoecology of goiter zonation in the Kumaon region of Uttarakhand and G.M. Rather and T.A. Kanth (15) address geomedical perspective of Iodine and Thyroid problem in North Kashmir Himalayas.

Part III comprises chapters which focus on socio-economic and cultural dimensions of disease and health care. L.S. Fonaroff and A. Fonaroff (16) throw light on the cultural factors influencing health conditions of rural population in a village in northern India. A. Ramesh and B. Hyma (17) study the practical aspects of traditional Indian medicine and are primarily concerned with the distribution and socio-economic characteristics of the practitioners, rather than theoretical and developmental ideals. S.M. Bhardwaj (18) in his chapter takes note of attitude towards different systems of medicine in four villages in Punjab. Such a study is unique in importance as it helps understand beliefs which people have in different systems of medicine, and such an understanding may be useful in holistic health care planning. In chapter 19, Nilofar Izhar focuses on medical pluralism in India and asserts that in India different traditional medical systems existed not only in the historical perspective, but still these traditional medical systems are practiced in different regions of the country.

Part IV contains chapters which deals with health care. Rais Akhtar and Nilofar Izhar (20) identify inequalities in the distribution of health care facilities in India. B.N. Mukherjee's chapter 21 focuses upon formulation of health hazard index to be adopted in micro-regional health planning. Ishtiaq A. Mayer and his colleagues (22) examine regional disparities in the health care delivery in the state of Jammu & Kashmir.

Rais Akhtar (23) highlights on India's medical education, doctors' behavious, lopsided health care pattern with expenditure primarily concentrated on sophisticated facilities in urban areas, and variation in per capita expenditure on health in different states. The provision of a doctor is the most important component of health care facilities. However, there is not only maldistribution of doctors in the country, but it is questionable, as author asserts if establishment of more medical colleges in the country can benefit the country itself. The chapter asserts that India is the largest exporter of doctors, but large number of our own health care centres located in rural and in accessible areas lack sufficient doctors.

Part V contains chapters which deals with contemporary issues in medical geography.

Shyamoli Sen and Nitasha Malhotra (24) explore the spatio-temporal variation of air pollution in Delhi with focus on respiratory diseases. Anita Bhargawa and Anuradha Banerjee (25) highlight gynaecological morbidity which is a neglected health issue among married women in Western India.

Nitasha Malhotra in her chapter 26 describes the geoecology of cataract blindness in India, and M. Ganga Raju and colleagues in chapter 27 investigate the incidence of kidney diseases in Kaviti and Kanchili Mandals in Srikakulum district of Andhra Pradesh State.

There are sufficient evidences that El Niño affects the occurrence and distribution of vector-borne diseases including malaria and cholera. R. Akhtar in chapter 28 discusses the association of El Niño, climate change and human health scenario in general with particular reference to India, and Carsten Butsch (29) explains the urban health transition in India. The chapter tries to shed some light on the urban transitions currently taking place in India and the way in which these transitions affect human health. Air Pollution is an important human disaster and is causing havoc globally, particularly in developing countries. Hem Dholakia (30) asserts that for India addressing the emerging health risks of outdoor air pollution requires an integrated policy approach across all sectors and sustained effort over time.

In chapter 31, Rais Akhtar asserts the association between CO_2 emission and socio-economic development in developing countries with special reference to India. Chapter 32 highlights the conclusion and future research directions in medical geography.

New Delhi

Editors

Acknowledgements

The Editors wish to acknowledge with thanks for the permission of the editors/authors to reprint chapters which were first published in journals.

Social Science and Medicine; Geo-Journal, The Rajasthan Medical Journal; Geographical Review of India; Pacific Viewpoints; Proceedings: 21st International Geographical Congress; International Journal of Environmental Studies; The Indian Geographical Journal; Journal of IIuman Evolution; The Geographer; Regional Studies; Annals, National Association of Geographers, India (NAGI); Current Science; Indian Journal of History of Science; Manohar Publisher; and *Royal Academy of Overseas Sciences, Brussels.*

We are grateful to Shri Ashok K. Mittal, Managing Director of Concept Publishing Company Pvt. Ltd. for fruitful suggestions and cooperation in the publications of this book.

Editors

Contents

PART II
Disease Ecology

PART III
Socio-cultural Aspects and Health

PART IV
Health Care

PART V
Contemporary Issues

List of Contributors

A. Fonaroff, formerly Public Health Officer, The World Bank, Washington D.C., U.S.A.

Prof. A. Ramesh, formerly Professor of Geography, University of Madras, Chennai, India.

Prof. A.K. Dutt, Professor Emeritus, University of Akron, Akron, Akron, U.S.A.

Dr. A.K. Tewari, formerly Professor of Geography, University of Jodhpur, Jodhpur, India.

Prof. A.T.A. Learmonth, formerly Professor Emeritus, Faculty of Social Sciences, The Open University, Milton Keynes, U.K.

Anita Bhargava is a Doctorate in Population Studies from Jawaharlal Nehru University. She has completed her Masters of Philosophy from the same university. Her knowledge witness's commendable research experience in health sector particularly reproductive health issues of women. She has worked in many projects and published enriched research articles and continues to render her experiences and skills in research.
Email: *annubps@gmail.*

Prof. Anuradha Banerjee is, currently, Professor at Jawaharlal Nehru University, New Delhi, India. Her thrust areas of research are population issues including urbanisation and urban environment, maternal and child health, reproductive health, and others. She has numerous published research articles, edited and published books and had carried out many national and international projects. Email: *banerjee.anb@gmai1.com*

Dr. B. Hema Malini, is an UGC Emeritus fellow in the Department of Geography, Andhra University, Visakhapatnam, India. She has 38 years of research and teaching experience in the field of Climatology and Medical Geography. She has published 95 research papers and guided 16 Ph.Ds and 8 M.Phils. Participated in number of conferences in India and abroad. Andhra University has conferred "Best Researcher award and Deccan Geographical Society" conferred "Best Geography Teacher award" to her. So far conducted 6 major research Projects and at present conducting one UGC Major Research Project on "Weather Extremes". Email: *bhmalini@yahoo.com*

Dr. B. Hyma, formerly Associate Professor of Geography, University of Waterloo, Waterloo, Canada.

Prof. B.N. Mukherjee, formerly Professor of Regional Planning, Indian Statistical Institute, Kolkata, India.

Prof. C.D. Deshpande, formerly Professor of Geography, University of Bombay, Mumbai, India.

Dr. Carsten Butsch was trained in Geography and urban planning at the University of Bonn (2000-2006). He received his Ph.D. from the University of Cologne for his research on access to health care in Pune, India, Currently he is working as senior researcher on Indian migration to Germany, urban transformations in India and migrants' health in Germany and India. Email: *butsche@uni-koeln.de*

Dr. Demudu G., got his Post-graduate as well as Ph.D. degrees from Department of Geography, Andhra University. He received Ph.D. in the year 2015. He has published twelve research papers so far in National/International journals. At present, working as Post-Doctoral fellow funded by University Grants Commission. Email: *demuduug@mail.com*

Dr. G.M. Rather is Sr. Assistant Professor in the department of Geography and Regional Development, University of Kashmir and has been teaching geography at P.G. level for the last twenty years. He is guiding research scholars in the medical geography. He has more than forty research papers to his credit. He has attended a number of seminars, conferences and workshops throughout the country and has contributed a number of research papers both in the national and international journals.
Email: *gmrather@rediffmail.com*

Dr. Ganga Raju, M. is Rajiv Gandhi National Fellow/UGC from 2012-March 2017, in the Department of Geography, Andhra University, Visakhapatnam. He has received his Post-graduate as well as Doctorate degrees in July 2017. So far published five papers in Geography journals.
Email: *mallarapugangarajuyahoo.com*

Prof. H.M. Dutta, Formerly Professor of Biological Sciences, Kent State University, Kent, U.S.A.

Dr. Hem H. Dholakia is a Senior Research Associate with the Council of Energy, Environment and Water. His research addresses the linkages between energy, environment human health and public policy in India. His previous work experience covers a mélange of clinical patient care; product development with healthcare startups and research. Hem holds a PhD from the Indian Institute of Management (Ahmedabad); Master's in Exercise Science from University of Brighton (UK) and Bachelor's in Physiotherapy from Seth G.S. Medical.
Email: *hem.dholakia@ceew.in*

Prof. Ishtiaq A. Mayer, Professor of Medical Geography, has more than 35 research papers and published 4 books, and other book chapters on various themes of Geography. He is reviewer of some of the prestigious international journals like Environmental Monitoring and Assessment-Springer and others. Prof. Mayer is also member of policy-making bodies such as Coordinator, Students exchange programme between University of Malaya, Malaysia and Kashmir University. He has served as Chairman of the Department of Geography and Regional Development, University of Kashmir, Srinagar (J & K) from 2014-17. He is member of the evaluation committee for DST package for state colleges. He is life member of some of the eight premier journals of Geography in India. Email: *ishimayer@gmail.com*

Dr. Kakani Nageswara Rao is an ICSSR Senior Fellow in the Department of Geo-Engineering, Andhra University, Visakhapatnam, India. He has more than three decades of teaching and research experience in the fields of morphology and evolution of landforms, land use/land cover analyses, the impact of human activities on the coastal/delta environments, coastal zone management, and geospatial technologies. He has published more than 75 research papers, guided 16 doctoral theses, carried out 14 research projects and visited several countries like USA, Japan, Thailand, Vietnam, and China on research assignments. His current research involves geospatial analysis of the socio-economic impact of aquaculture along the east coast of India. Email: *nrkakani@yahoo.com*

Prof. L.S. Fonaroff, Formerly Professor of Geography, University of Maryland, College Park, U.S.A.

Dr. Lalitha, K., did her post-graduation and Doctorate degrees from the Department of Geography, She has received Ph.D. in the year 2017. She has published three research papers.
Email: *lalitha132@yahoo.com*

Prof. M. Shafi, Formerly Professor of Geography and Pro-Vice-Chancellor, Aligarh Muslim University, Aligarh, India.

Dr. M.J. Joshi, formerly Hon. Surgeon, B.J. Medical College, Pune, India.

Dr. M.K. Dutta, Department of Health, Winnipeg, Ontario, Canada.

Dr. Mohd. Sabar, M.Phil., Ph.D., NET is presently working as teacher in School Education Department, J & K.

Dr. Nilofar Izhar, Senior Research Fellow, ICSSR, Department of Community Medicine, Aligarh Muslim University, Aligarh, India.

Dr. Nitasha Malhotra, is an Associate Professor in Kamala Nehru College, University of Delhi. She is M.A., M.Phil. and Ph.D. in Geography from Delhi School of Economics, University of Delhi. She is a Medical Geographer and has written on "Disease Ecology of Cataract Disease and the Environment". She is also well known in the field of climatology and holds an experience of teaching climatology for the last 15 years or so. Besides teaching, she has also supervised Ph.D. dissertations, Her areas of interest include medical geography, climatology and urban issues.

Prof. Rais Akhtar, Adjunct Professor, IIHMR, New Delhi and formerly Professor of Geography, Kashmir University, Kashmir, Srinagar, J & K.

Dr. Raja Rao, G., at present working as an Assistant Professor, in the Department of Geology, Andhra University, Visakhapatnam. He has received his Post-graduate degrees in Geography as well as in Geology subjects from Andhra University. He got his doctoral degree in Geography in the year 2008. He has published eight research papers.

Prof. S.M. Bhardwaj, Formerly Professor of Geography, Kent State University, Kent, U.S.A.

Sheraz Ahmad Lone, M.A Geography, M.Phil., NET is presently perusing Ph.D. from Department of Geography and Regional Development, University of Kashmir, J & K.
Email: *sheraz7geog@mail.com*

Dr. Shyamoli Sen, M.A., M.Phil. and Ph.D. in Geography from Delhi School of Economics, University of Delhi, Delhi. She has worked in numerous research projects with reputed national and international government as well as non-governmental organizations. Her areas of interest primarily include issues relating to health and disease in urban areas, in particular, metropolitan cities besides Climatology and environmental geography. She has also written a book titled "Air Pollution and Respiratory Diseases in Delhi" which was published recently. For the last few years, she has been teaching in various colleges of University of Delhi.

Prof. T.A. Kanth, is a senior professor in the University of Kashmir, J & K. He is well known geomorphologist, academician and researcher of high repute. He has guided a number of scholars in the university. He is very much interested to teaching and research and has always given preference to academics over any other assignment. He has a number of research publications to his credit.
Email: *tasawoork@yahoo. com*

Dr. Tamminaidu G., did his post-graduation and Doctorate degrees from the Department of Geography, Andhra University, Visakhapatnam. He received his doctorate degree in the year 2008. He has worked as Post-Doctoral fellow of ICSSR from 2013 to 2015, in the Department of Geography, Andhra University. He has published eight research papers so far. Email: *tammi_geo@yahoo.co.in*

Dr. Visweswara Reddy B. got his Post-graduate degree from S.V. University, Tirupati and M.Tech. and Ph.D. degrees from Geo-Engineering Department of Andhra University, Visakhapatnam. He has received his Ph.D. degree in the year 2013. He has eleven research publications. At present, he is working as an Assistant Professor in the Department of Civil Engineering of Aditya Institute of Technology and Management, Tekkali, Andhra Pradesh.
Email: *bvreddy7gmail.com*

PART I
Introductory

1
Medical Geography in India: An Introduction

Rais Akhtar and *Nilofar Izhar*

Medical geography is generally defined as the branch of Human Geography concerned with the geographic aspects of health (status) and health care (systems). It seeks, along with sister disciplines such as Medical Anthropology, Medical Sociology and Health Economics, as well as epidemiology, zoology, botany, parasitology, meteorology, geology, urban planning, environmental engineering, and biostatistics, to broaden our understanding of the various factors which affect the health of population. According to Meade and Earickson, medical geography draws on the concepts and uses the techniques of all these disciplines and adds spatial and ecological perspectives (Meade and Earickson, 2000, and Meade, 2010). The idea that place and location can influence health is a very old and familiar concept in Western medicine. As far back as the time of Hippocrates, physicians have observed that certain diseases seem to occur in some places and not others, or the intensity of some diseases is region specific. People have also been aware of the process of disease diffusion across geographic regions for centuries. Attempts to understand why certain diseases seem to only occur in certain places and not others has led to new insights into the nature of disease itself.

In a classic study undertaken in 1854, Dr. John Snow demonstrated the utility of mapping disease outbreaks to gain insights as to their cause. Snow mapped the distribution of cholera cases in Soho, London during an epidemic. He discovered that the highest density of cases occurred in households which used the public pump on Broad street as their water source. Snow suspected that infected water from the pump was the cause. He instructed the authorities to remove the handle to the pump, making it unusable, the number of new cholera cases promptly declined. Later at the end of 19th century, Sanitary Reports of British India, contain maps of cholera distribution in the subcontinent. In early twientieth century S.R. Christopher and J.A. Sinton produced a map of Malaria in India. These were very good examples of the use of geographical techniques by medical experts.

According to John Giggs, the relevant area for research in medical geography can be expressed in a simple health system model which comprises three interacting elements, namely :

1. The spatial patterning of ill health and mortality.
2. The spatial patterning of the physical and human environmental characteristics which adversely affect man's state of health.
3. The spatial patterning and use of the main elements of the health care delivery systems developed to combat diseases and the environmental hazards which affect man's health.

According to Giggs, the above model provides useful framework for a review of the main foci of spatial research into health problems at the intra-urban level/intra-regional level (Giggs, 1979). However, according to Hunter, the contributions of medical geography in preventive medicine and health care services should not be viewed as separate, independent entities, but rather they should be seen as complementary to, and tandem with, those of the basic and applied medical and health sciences (Hunter, 1988). Most research in medical geography during 1980s and 1990s revolves around these ideas both in developed and developing countries.

With the passages of time, and continuing process of adoption of modern techniques in medical geography, both the conceptual and methodological foundation of the current concerns in medical geography reflects a shift and is more devoted with the 'rational development', and testing of theories that explain and predict the spatial distribution of diseases and health care and location of various socio-economic, cultural and political characteristics in a region, which are responsible for a given ecology of diseases and health care delivery.

Studies of spatial variation in health and clustering of illness or deaths have also been made from different perspective, based on research using GIS and spatial modelling. These continue to extend our understanding of variations and clustering in space and time of the incidence and prevalence of disease, thus contributing to the knowledge of the spatial epidemiology of diseases in relation to social and environmental risk factors (Asthana *et al.*, 2002).

Progress in Medical Geography (1950-2000)

1950s

- Mapping of diseases and ecological explanations

1960s

- Analytical studies : Disease diffusion studies

1970s

- Health care geography : Location and accessibility analysis of health care resources, i.e. physicians and hospitals/health centres.

1980s

- Health care planning model : Health care behaviour, geography of traditional medical systems; Epidemiological transition, geography of mental health.

1990s

- Health effects of global, national and local environmental change, climate change and health, impact of urbanization on health in developing societies, Geography of AIDs.
- Natural and human induced disasters, including environmental toxicology, the consequences of socio-economic change with special reference to economic rises and structural adjustment impacts on health and health care. Development and disease (examples : dams and malaria) schistosomiasis incidence and irrigation and malaria

2000-2014

- In addition to themes above, more emphasis was placed on the utilization of techniques in medical geography such as remote sensing, GIS and other methods of spatial analysis which are becoming available as separate software modules or are embedded in GIS.

According to Mei-Po Kwan, "It is now widely recognized that geographic variations in health behaviours and outcomes cannot be explained exclusively in terms of the characteristics of individuals, as specific characteristics of place or neighbourhoods (e.g. collective efficacy) also exert significant influence on health (Kwan, 2012).

- *Alzheimer's disease* : Spatial distribution at birth place; regional assessment of elderly disability; Ageing and regional inequalities in health and health care; Geography of survival after surgery for colorectal cancer [geography of survival manifests itself more through where are treated than through area (deprivation) effects or relative location].
- Geographies of disabilities, obesity and ageing and climate change and ageing population.
- Migration and human health variation in time and space.
- Complementary therapies and the informal sector of health care.
- Spatial inequalities in health and health care and role of 'place'.
- Spatial disparities in health outcomes.
- Urban health *v/s* rural health, concentration of urban population, influence of cities and associated processes, including demographic changes (notably migration) and changing patterns of way of life (genre devie).
- Development and health.
- Globalization and its impact on health and health care processes operating at the global scale include environmental change, demographic shifts, diffusion of diseases, international trends in health care reforms, impact of policies of international organizations such as International Monetary Fund (IMF) as health policies in developing countries.

It is evident from the above that idiographic tradition in medical geography continued to be important up to 1980s and early 1990s, then began the entry of quantitative revolution particularly GIS in the subject. While in geography in general welfare/radical/humanistic perspective began finding roots, medical geography became more a technique pushing the spirit subject in the background. The saying 'servant became master' became more pertinent in medical geography. Research themes such as below reveal the trend of medical geography by some medical geographers:

1. GIS be made to sing and dance to an epidemiological time.
2. What's the point ? Exploring the spatial epidemiology of Motor Neurone Disease in part of North-West England.
3. Testing for clustering of health events within a geographical information system framework.
4. Spatial point process modelling in GIS environment.
5. The relative utility of the central postcode.
6. Spatial point pattern analysis and its application in geographical epidemiology.
7. Interactive spatial data analysis in medical geography.
8. Spatial process modelling of cancer data within a geographical information systems framework.

A paper published in 2000 by Gatrell focuses on the complexity theory with particular emphasis given to relations and networks, non-linearity, emergence, and hybrids. Gatrell further emphasies that complexity theory potentially has much to say to those interested in research on health inequalities, spatial diffusion, emerging and resurgent infections, and risk (Gatrell, 2000).

In 2007, Sui, a geographer, published a paper on GIS and Medical Geography that presents a comprehensive review of the reciprocal interaction between the two and calls for a new synergy between both fields in future research and education efforts (Sui, 2007). Rosenberg and Wilson placed more emphasis on linking research to policy and activism and the creation of a more inclusive medical geography. Focusing on issues such as HIV/AIDS, health and the environment and vulnerable populations such as elderly and immigrant women, medical geography is increasingly contributing to public policy at various geographic scales (Rosenberg and Wilson, 2005).

A New Shift : Impact of Latest Technological Revolution

There has been a shift in paradigm in medical geography from 1950s to present pattern of research. Medical geography had witnessed the 'quantitative revolution' and the use of models, and GIS. All these, I believe, are methods and techniques, means, not the end. Geography is the study of the interplay between nature and nature with its varied forces, between nature and man, between man and man, in the given framework of a terrain and its environmental cover. On the question of declining spirit of geography in researches being carried out by many geographers, it has rightly been observed, the geographer has to make 'sorties' into allied disciplines, and to absorb new techniques and that while doing so, he must know how to get back to his moorings, and not to get lost. I prefer a more humanistic perspective of geography by focusing on Man-Man (rather man *vs.* man) theme to Man-Nature. Two major themes for research in the beginning of 21st century may be considered :

1. How do the people try to live in an environment that is inimical to them both in rural and urban areas? i.e. floods, earthquakes, Tsunami, snowstorms, damaged wetlands, cyclones and famines. The urban poor living on the brink of ill drained streams and earning their modicum of sustenance under the harsh and indifferent urban society around them. Besides the impact of urban stress as a result of globalization with focus on increased intensity of mental illnesses. Why not study them and galvanize social and political awakening to ameliorate their health conditions.
2. The second theme of study is the health and health care inequalities between regions. It is important to know how these inequalities could be reduced by proper deployment of resources— natural and human in each region. Today modern technology and the process of globalization are aggravating the inequalities between regions just as it does in the case of individuals.

Similar ideas were expressed by John Hunter when he elaborated that geography, as a humanistic science, examines relationships between people and their environment. In medical geography focus confines upon those interactions and relationships that bear specifically upon human health (Hunter, 1988). Commenting on geographic method, John Hunter opined that our main tool is spatial analysis, best represented by the basic map that shows distributional patterns of selected phenomena. These can be random or non-random, dynamic or statistic. Maps of health related phenomena with their accompanying associative analyses, which are suggested by emerging spatial patterns, lead us toward better conjoint questions of what? where? when ? why ? and how ? appropriately examined in a full context of population environment interrelationships—bring insight and strategy to the struggle for better health (Hunter, 1988 : 117).

This is the holistic spirit of medical geography as elaborated by John Hunter.

Medical Geography in India

There has been considerable progress in medical geography in India in terms of M.Phils., Ph.Ds., award of research projects by University Grants Commission, Department of Science and Technology (DST) Government of India, and Indian Council of Social Science Research (ICSSR) and research publications particularly during the period 2007-2013. A number of M.Phil. and Ph.D. theses were submitted in medical geography in various universities. Sharmishtha Das submitted her Ph.D. on Maternal and Child Health Care Services in West Bengal (2009), Shweta Kumari on Health Seeking Behaviour and Reproductive Rights of Antenatal Women in Delhi (2010), and Chandramallika Biswas on Knowledge Attitude Practices and Sexual Behaviour of Urban Educated Youth:A Case Study of Kolkata (2011), at the Jawaharlal Nehru University, New Delhi. Several M.Phil. dissertations were also submitted in medical geography at the Jawaharlal Nehru University. Ph.D. researches in progress on identification and spatial analysis of groundwater vulnerability zones of Murshidabad district, West Bengal, and on Assessment of human health in the neighbourhood of chemical and petro-chemical industries in Vadodara city, at M.S.University Vadodara in 2009. Hina Khan was awarded Ph.D. in 2008 on Women's Health in Urban Srinagar, Jammu & Kashmir from the University of Kashmir, Srinagar. M. Sabar was awarded Ph.D. in 2015, on: Geographical Distribution of Diseases on the Basis of Regional Disparities in Socio-economic Parameters of Jammu Division, J&K State, by the University of Kashmir, Srinagar, J&K.

Research Projects

A number of research projects in medical geography were awarded by various agencies including University Grants Commission and the Indian Council of Social Science Research, during the period 2007-2013. Researchers in the Department of Geography, M.S. University, Vadodara were awarded research projects to Rolee Kanchan on: Geographical perspective of child health care (ICSSR), Ecology of infectious disease in Vadodara district (UGC), Status of health of women in tribal belt of Vadodara district (UGC), Waste disposal, environment and health in Nandesari (GIDC), Women, health and rural development (UGC), Arsenic in ground water in West Bengal UGC), and on A micro-level study of environmental aspects in Golden Corridor of Gujarat (ICSSR). Rais Akhtar has completed a UGC sponsored project: Urban medical geography of Jammu & Kashmir in 2007. Rais Akhtar was awarded a Project (as Co-Principal Investigator) on climate change and health, by the Department of Science & Technology, Government of India in 2013.

Publication of Books

During 2007-2015 several books were published in the field of medical geography. R.P. Misra's seminal book "Geography of Health: A Treatise on Geography of Health" published by Concept, in 2007 deals with wide ranging themes from history of medicine, evolution of medical geography, heredity and health, natural and cultural environment and health, health policy and planning and medical nemesis. The book is based on the information obtained from the WHO, UNDP, Ministry of Health and Family Welfare, Government of India. Rais Akhtar and Nilofar Izhar published their book "Global Medical Geography" (2010) in honour of Yola Verhasselt—A prominent Belgian Medical Geographer who chaired medical geography commission of International Geographical Union during 1988-2002. The book deals global scenario in medical geography, including case studies on India. Philosophical, methodological and empirical studies in disease ecology and health care have been included. The origin of the term medical geography by Frank Barrett, Medical geography: Has J.M. May borrowed M. Sorre's 1933 concept of pathogenic complexes?, Quality of life: The essence of the geography of health, Diversity in the geography of natural-endemic diseases, GIS, spatial epidemiology and health care planning, Muslim or Greek? Past and present of Yunani medicine in the Deccan, and health status of women in rural areas of Kashmir valley, are some of important chapters in this book.

Rais Akhtar's book on "Regional Planning for Health Care System in Jammu and Kashmir" was published by Concept in 2009 focuses on the spatial pattern of health care delivery system and pinpoints regional inequalities for future health care planning.

In 2010, Springer has published a book "Malaria in South Asia:

Eradication and Resurgence during the second half of the Twentieth Century" and was edited by Rais Akhtar, A.K. Dutt and Vandana Wadhwa. The book contains couple of chapters on geography of malaria in India with focus on urban malaria in the country. Abdul Malik, Elisabeth Grohmann, and Rais Akhtar edited a book entitled "Environmental Deterioration and Human Health" published by Springer in 2014. The book discusses the natural and anthropogenic determinants of the environment and their impact on human health.

Publication of Papers

With growing research interest in medical geography among researchers in India, a number of papers have been published in Indian and International journals during the period 2007-2013. These papers cover both disease ecology and health care perspectives. Besides impact of climate change on human health has become an important theme globally as well as in India.

Climate Change and Human Health

Rais Akhtar's paper on Health and climate in Kashmir, was published in the Tiempo: A Bulletin on Climate and Development (London) (Akhtar, 2007) investigate the influence of geographical factors on the occurrence of health problems in the mountainous areas of Kashmir. Another paper by Rais Akhtar entitled: Climate change and health and heat wave mortality in India was published in Global Environmental Research (Akhtar, 2007). As one of the lead authors on the Human Health chapter of the Intergovernmental Panel on Climate Change (IPCC), Rais Akhtar contributed in the 4th Assessment of the IPCC which was published in 2007 (IPCC, 2007). In a joint study with A.K. Dutt, H.M. Dutta and M.McVay, Rais Akhtar examined the outbreak of plague in Surat and its diffusion patterns (Dutt *et al.*, 2007).

In 2008, Sari Kovats and Rais Akhtar published his research on impact of climate change on urban health scenario in Asian cities including Indian cities, in Environment and Urbanization (Kovats and Akhtar, 2008).

Impact of El Niño on health hazards have been studied globally by a number of scholars. Rais Akhtar's paper entitled: El Niño-related health hazards in India was published in 2010 in the Current Science.

The paper examines rainfall and temperature related health hazards, including heat wave mortality pattern in the country (Akhtar, 2010) In the context of CO_2 emission policy in developing countries, Rais Akhtar published his paper on CO_2 emission reduction and the emerging socio-economic development in developing countries:A case study of India, originally presented at the conference on the Developing Countries Facing Global Warming : A post-Kyoto Assessment, held in Brussels in 2009 (Akhtar, 2010). Recently, a review paper by Rais Akhtar, on the impact of climate change on human health, was published in the book: Health, Environment and Sustainable Development (Akhtar, 2012).

Disease Ecology

Anuradha Banerjee and C.Biswas's study on regional dimensions of HIV/AIDS in India is a landmark research which focuses on the status of HIV/AIDS in West Bengal in general and Kolkata in particular, and to identify the issues and challenges regarding HIV/AIDS among youth and the role played by Government and non-governmental organizations. (Banerjee and Biswas, 2007). In a comparative study of vulnerability of HIV/AIDS in South Africa and India, Jayati Ghosh and Bentley Olson assert that poverty, illiteracy, absence of health care for the marginalized, use of recreational drugs, and economic and social subordination of women trigger the spread of HIV/AIDS (Ghosh & Olson, 2007). Rajeshwari took up the aspect of sanitation situation in relation to disease pattern in Haryana (2008), and also tested the theory of demographic transition in the state (2009). Rajeshwari has also studied the nutritional aspects of children and women in rural Haryana (2011).With focus on tribal areas, V.K. Baraik examined the nutritional status of tribal children in Jharkhand (2008) and in association with S. Sinha, described the developmental perspective in relation to nutritional status in Jharkhand (2010). Rolee Kanchan in her studies focused on the excess arsenic content in groundwater and health implications in Nadia district of West Bengal (2009). Rather and colleagues assessed the impact of urban waste on the quality of river Jhelum, leading to the incidence of waterborne diseases (Rather *et al.,* 2010). Madhusree Mazumdar highlights the Healthy City Project in the context of improving environmental hygiene for health promotion in Mirzapur, Uttar Pradesh (Mazumdar, 2007). With reference to cultural factors, A.K. Chakravarti focuses on cultural dimensions of diet and protein malnutrition in India (2007), and Nitasha Malhotra Surinder Aggarwal examined different kinds of blindness and describe the geo-ecology of blindness in India (Malhotra and Aggarwal, 2007). Regional geomedical studies have become very important in health care planning. Preeti Tewari studied geoecology of Kali river basin, and concluded that long-term solution to the health problems in the region lay in its socio-economic development (Tewari, 2007). Giri and colleagues describe the spatial patterns of tuberculosis in Varanasi District (Giri *et al.*, 2010). Ishtiaq Mayer focuses on the association between health and socio-economic status of people living on water bodies in Srinagar city, Kashmir (Mayer, 2011).

Health Care and Gender Studies

Anuradha Banerjee and S. Das analysed the Utilization of Maternal and child health care services (MCH) and its impact on infant mortality in India with special reference to West Bengal (2006). Rais Akhtar examined the inequalities in the availability and utilization of doctors in India. He argues that although India is the largest exporter of medical manpower including doctors, but our large number of health centres and hospitals, especially in rural and hilly areas function without doctors (2008).

It has rightly been said that while the phenomenon of women's inequality is universal, its magnitude and severity vary from country to country and within a country, from community to community and within a community too. In her paper on academic and health status of women in Aligarh Muslim University Nilofar Izhar (2012) focuses on the scenario of gender disparity among highly educated/intellectual group. V.K. Baraik and P.M. Kulkarni describes the health status and access to health care services disparities among social groups in India (2006) M.B. Singh and Shivabali Singh assessed the availability of health care facilities and their utilization pattern in Mirzapur district of Uttar Pradesh (Singh and Singh, 2007). R.B. Bhagat assessed health and family welfare services that are provided at Primary Health Centres and Sub-Centres and clients' views of the availability and delivery of these services in selected districts of Uttar Pradesh (Bhagat, 2012). Singh and colleagues discuss impact assessment and analysis of health care facilities in Varanasi city (Singh, 2012). Singh and

Baba focus on health implications of poor housing in Srinagar city (Singh and Baba, 2015).

History of Medicine

Research in history of medicine does not attract many geographers. Rais Akhtar studied the diffusion of cholera in the valley of Kashmir during late nineteenth century, and asserted that the outbreaks of cholera in Kashmir was the result of disease diffusion wave that spread from Bengal to Central Asia (2008). Recently Royal Society of Medicine Journal: Journal of Medical Biography, published an article by Rais Akhtar highlighting the contribution of Dr. Arthur Neve in the disease ravaged valley of Kashmir during late nineteenth and early twentieth centuries (Akhtar, 2011). Exploring a rich trove of literature in the form of letters and poetry of the great Urdu poet Mirza Ghalib, Nilofar Izhar and Rais Akhtar reveal dimensions of social and medical geography in the latter half of nineteenth century. Ghalib was witness to the last days of the crumbling Mughal Empire and the consolidation of the British Empire after the historic revolt of 1857. The socio-cultural, political, environmental and even health and health care situations prevalent at Ghalib's time have been unveiled through the use of literary geography (Izhar and Akhtar, 2012).

References

Akhtar, R. (2007), Health and Climate in Kashmir, Tiempo, *A Bulletin on Climate and Development* (London), Issue, 63, April, pp. 19-21.

Akhtar, R. (2007), Climate Change and Health and Heat Wave Mortality in India, *Global Environmental Research* (Japan), 11, 1, pp. 51-57.

Akhtar, R. and Rather, G.M. (2007), Lifestyle Change and Cardiovascular Diseases in Srinagar City, In B. Thakur *et al.,* (eds.), *City, Society and Planning*, New Delhi: Concept Publishing Co., pp. 206-220.

Akhtar, R., *et al.,* (2007), Human Health, Climate Change, 2007, Report of the Inter-governmental Panel on Climate Change (IPCC), Cambridge University Press, (As Lead Author, Chapter 8 on Human Health).

Akhtar, R. (2007), Changing Disease Ecology of Leh District : Contemporary Scenario and Historical Perspective, *Punjab Geographer*, Vol. 3, October, pp. 39-44.

Akhtar, R. (2008), Environment and Cholera in Kashmir During Nineteenth Century, *Indian Journal of History of Science,* Vol. 43, No. 2, 2008, pp. 211-230.

Akhtar, R. and I.A. Mayer (2008), Disease Ecology of Ladakh Himalayan Region, *Annals of National Association of Geographers*, India, Vol. 28, No. 2, pp. 40-48.

Akhtar, R. (2009), Why should we Produce more Doctors?: Socio-economic and Political Framework of a Doctor in India, In Alain Vaguet (Ed.), *Indian Health Landscapes under Globalization*, New Delhi: Manohar, pp. 207-220.

Akhtar, R. (2010), El Niño-related Health Hazards in India, *Current Science*, Vol. 98, No. 2, pp. 144-147.

Akhtar, R. (2010), CO_2 Emission Reduction and the Emerging Socio-economic Development in Developing Countries: A Case of India, In De Dapper, M., Swinne, D. and Ozer, P. (Eds.), *Developing Countries Facing Global Warming : A Post Kyoto Assessment,* Royal Academy of Overseas Sciences, Brussels, pp. 15-26.

Akhtar, R. (2011), Arthur Neve and a Mission Hospital in Srinagar, Kashmir, *Journal of Medical Biography*, Royal Society of Medicine, Vol. 19, No. 4, pp. 53-64.

Akhtar, R. (2012), Impact of Climate Change on Human Health, In N. Audinarayana *et al.,* (eds.), *Health Environment and Sustainable Development: Perspectives and Issues,* New Delhi : Global Research Publications, pp. 221-232.

Asthana, S., Curtis, S., Duncun, C. and Gould, M. (2002), Themes in British Health Geography at the End of the Century : A Review of Published Research 1998-2000, *Social Science & Medicine*, Vol. 55, pp. 167-173.

Banerjee, A. and Biswas, C. (2007), Regional Dimensions of HIV/AIDS in India: An Emerging Concern, *Geographical Review of India*, Vol. 69, No. 1.

Banerjee, A. and Das, S. (2006), Regional Analysis of MCH Service and its Impact on Infant Mortality in India: A Case Study of West Bengal, *Geographical Review of India*, Vol. 68, No. 1, pp. 89-111.

Baraik, V.K. and Kulkarni, P.M. (2006), Health Status and Access to Health Care Services: Disparities among Social Groups in India, Working Paper Series, Vol. 1, No. 4, New Delhi : IIDS.

Baraik, V.K. (2008), Nutritional Status of Tribal Children in Jharkhand, *Journal of Development and Management Studies*, Vol. 6, No. 1, pp. 2753-2772.

Baraik, V.K. and Sinha, S. (2010), Development and Morbidity Prevalence in Jharkhand: Special Reference to Tribal Population, *Jharkhand Journal of Social Development*, Vol. 2, Nos. 1 & 2, pp. 15-31.

Barrett, F. (2000), *Disease and Geography : The History of the Idea*, Toranto, New York University.

Bhagat, R.B. (2012), Health Infrastructure and Health Care Services in Uttar Pradesh, In A.K. Dutt *et al.,* (eds.), *Facets of Social Geography: International and Indian Perspectives*, New Delhi : Cambridge University Press, pp. 455-473.

Chakravarti, A.K. (2007), Cultural Dimensions of Diet and Disease in India, In B. Thakur *et al.,* (eds.), *City, Society and Planning*, New Delhi : Concept Publishing Company, pp. 141-161.

Dutt, A.K. Akhtar, R., Dutta, H.M. and M. McVay (2007), From Black Death to Surat Plague of 1994: A Quantum Leap in Medical Science Development, In A.K. Dutt *et al.,* (eds.), *Exploration in Applied Geography*, New Delhi: Prentice-Hall of India.

Gatrell, A.C. (2005), Complexity Theory and Geographies of Health : A Critical Assessment, *Social Science and Medicine*, June, Vol. 60, No. 12, pp. 2661-2671.

Ghosh, J. and Olson, B. (2007), Vulnerability of HIV/AIDS in South Africa and India, In B. Thakur *et al.,* (eds.), *City, Society and Planning*, New Delhi : Concept Publishing Company, pp. 162-180.

Giggs, J.A. (1979), Human Health Problems in Urban Areas, In D.T. Herbert and D.M. Smith (eds.), *Social Problems and the City*, Oxford: Oxford University Press, pp. 85-115.

Giri, A.K., Srivastava, G.N. and Mishra, A.P. (2010), Spatial Distribution of Tuberculosis Disease in Varanasi District: A Case Study in Health Geography, *National Geographical Journal of India* (NGSI), Vol. 56, Pt. 2, pp. 53-64.

Hunter, J. (1988), Geography and Public Health, In Earth 1988 : Changing Geographic Perspectives, *National Geographic Society*, Washington, DC., pp. 116-17.

Izhar, N. (2012), Status of Women in Aligarh Muslim University, In A.K. Dutt *et al.* (eds.), *Facets of Social Geography: International and Indian Perspectives*, New Delhi, Cambridge University Press, pp. 475-482.

Izhar, N. and Akhtar, R. (2012), Writings of Mirza Ghalib: A Study in Literary Geography, In A.K. Dutt *et al.,* (eds.), *Facets of Social Geography: International and National Perspectives*, New Delhi : Cambridge University Press, pp. 574-587.

Kanchan, R. (2009), Arsenic Contaminated Ground Water : Human Health Catastrophe in Nadia District, India, *Asia-Pacific Journal of Social Sciences*, Vol. 1, No. 2, pp. 123-143.

Kovats, S. and Akhtar, R. (2008), Climate, Climate Change and Human Health in Asian Cities, *Environment and Urbanization*, Vol. 20, No. 1, pp. 165-174.

Malhotra, N. and Aggarwal, S. (2007), Geo-ecology of Blindness in India, In B. Thakur *et al.,* (eds.), *City, Society and Planning*, New Delhi: Concept Publishing Company, pp. 221-252.

Kwan, Mei-Po (2012), Introduction: Geographies of Health Special Issue, *Annals of Association of American Geographers*, Vol. 102, No. 5, pp. 891-92.

Mayer, I. (2011), Health and Socio-economic Status of People Living on Water Bodies in Srinagar City, Kashmir, India, *Malaysian Journal of Tropical Geography*, Vol. 39, Nos. 1 & 2, pp. 43-50.

Mazumdar, M. (2007), Improving Environmental Hygiene for Health Promotion: The Healthy City Project of Mirzapur, U.P., In B. Thakur *et al.,* (eds.), *City, Society and Planning*, New Delhi: Concept Publishing Company, pp. 113-140.

Meade, M.S. and Earickson, R.J. (2000), *Medical Geography*, New York: The Guilford Press, p. 6.

Meade, M.S. (2010), *Medical Geography*, New York: The Guilford Press.

Rajeshwari (2008), Sanitation Situation and Disease Pattern in Haryana: A Spatial Analysis, *Demography India*, Vol. 37, No. 1, pp. 79-94.

Rajeshwari (2009), Demographic Transition in Haryana: A Spatio-temporal Analysis, *Population Geography*, Vol. 31, Nos. 1 & 2.

Rajeshwari (2011), Women Nutrition and its Correlates in Rural Haryana, *Punjab Geographer*, Vol. 7, pp. 32-45.

Rather, G.M., Bhat, M.S., and Kanth, T.A. (2010), Impact of Urban Waste of Srinagar City on the Quality of Water of River Jhelum, *International Journal of Lakes and Rivers*, Vol. 3, No. 1, pp. 17-24.

Singh, A.L. and Baba, S.A. (2015), Health Implications of Poor Housing Conditions in Srinagar City, *Annals*, *NAGI,* Vol. 35, No. 1, pp. 11-25.

Singh, S.N., Giri A. K., and Mishra, A.P. (2012), Impact Assessment and Analysis of Health Care Facilities in Varanasi City: A Geographical Perspective; *Eastern Geographer*, Vol. XVIII, No. 1, pp. 41-48.

Sui, D.Z. (2007), Geographic Information Systems and Medical Geography: Toward a New Synergy, *Geography Compass*, Vol. 1, Issue 3, pp. 556-582.

Tewari, P. (2007), Disease Ecology in the Kali River Basin, In B. Thakur *et al.*, (eds.), *City, Society and Planning*, New Delhi: Concept Publishing Company, pp. 253-276.

2

Reflections on the Regional Geography of Disease in Late Colonial South Asia

A.T.A. Learmonth

Mainly based on the admittedly inaccurate but analysable health records of the former British India, and on the contemporary literature, the present writer made a study of the medical geography of the late-colonial period 1921-40, to fill in gaps and assist in understanding disease patterns and relationships of mainland South Asia. Between the great mountain arcs of the north-west and north-east and east, and the warm waters of the Indian Ocean lies a compact landmass of about 4.5 million km^2, stretching some 2500 kilometres north-south and about the same distance east-west. The terrain varies from mountain tundra to tropical desert and sub-equatorial rainforest, from alluvial plains and deltas to great swathes of lava flows and black sticky soils, and almost African rolling plateaus of granite and gneiss, their skyline broken by ridges of older, often metalliferous schists, the roots of ancient mountain systems exposed by periods long even on geological time-scales. Upon these lands, many of them over-cultivated, eroded, exhausted, lived then some 400 million people; now there are almost 700 millions. Humid South Asia, with over 100 cm. mean annual rainfall, generally more reliable as well as wetter than the remainder of the subcontinent, includes ricelands, especially on alluvial and deltaic plains, as well as a good many areas of maize and millet cultivation, and small areas growing tropical tubers like tapioca in the extreme south-west. Semi-arid and arid South Asia

Social Science and Medicine, Reprinted from 14, 271-276, 1981.

includes the wide tracts of winter wheat, complemented by irrigated summer rice, and summer rain-fed maize and millets (sorghum, pennisetum and eleusine are all locally dominant). Everywhere cattle are used for draught and dairy purposes, but not for meat in Hindu India, with buffaloes in wetter area. Dairy produce is esteemed but rare in poor diets.

The study of the late-colonial period should give a valuable benchmark survey for comparison with post-independence perspectives at various points. The independent countries have rightly discarded the inaccuracy of old data, but registration and health services have not yet evolved to the point where overall coverage, as distinct from limited surveys, can be contemplated.

My original analysis for the inter-war period consisted mainly of a series of maps similar to Figs. 2.1 and 2.2. They are designed to distinguish by the heavier shadings the administrative districts with

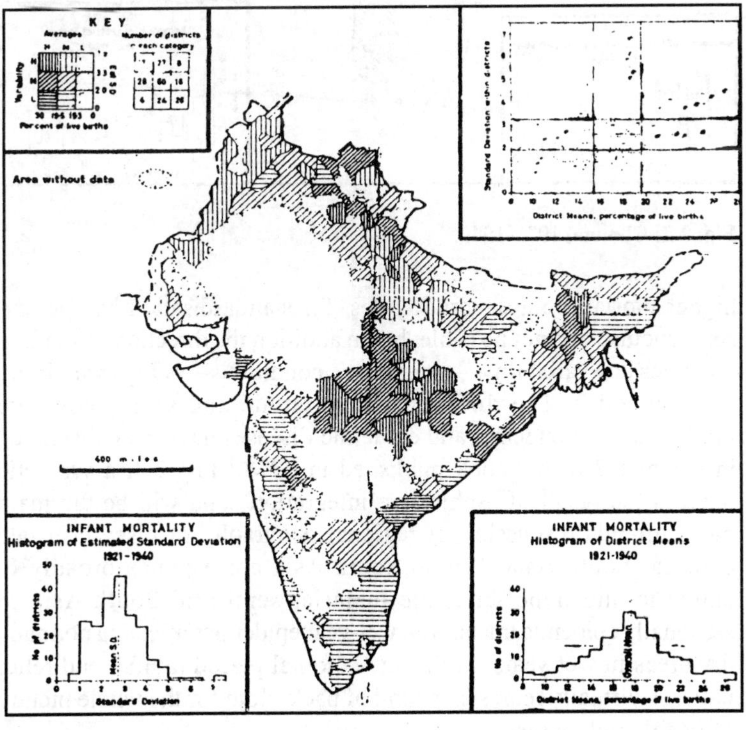

Fig. 2.1: Infant Mortality, 1921-1940.

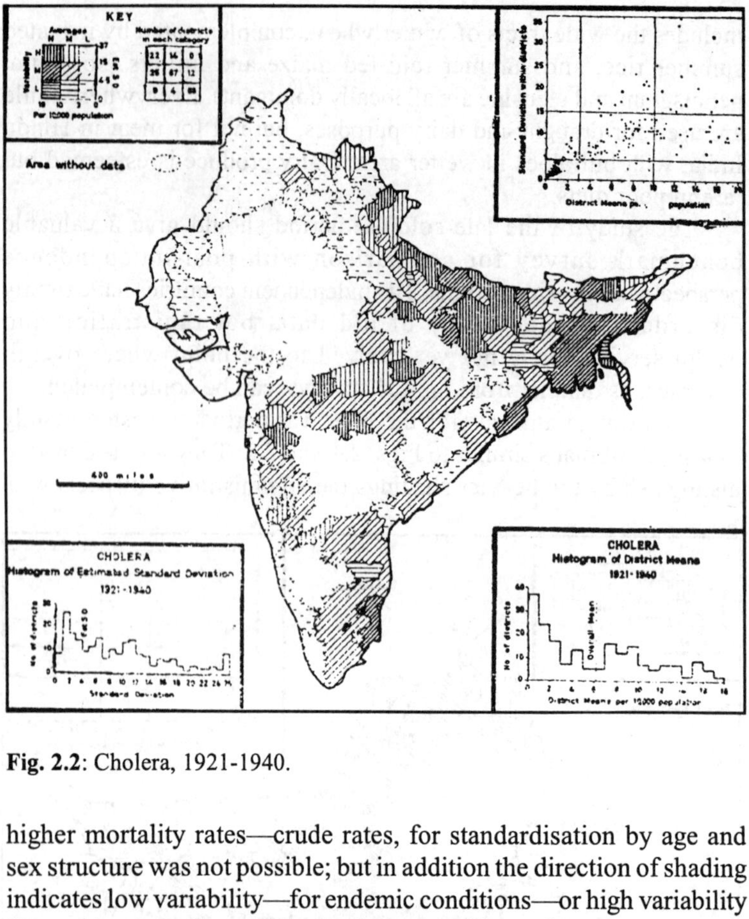

Fig. 2.2: Cholera, 1921-1940.

higher mortality rates—crude rates, for standardisation by age and sex structure was not possible; but in addition the direction of shading indicates low variability—for endemic conditions—or high variability for epidemics. The different demographic and socio-economic implications of endemic and epidemic diseases have been discussed in Chapter 2 of my book published in 1978.[1] Fig. 2.3, a synthetic map, is the result of "subjective integration" and will be the main basis for this discussion of regional geography of disease in late colonial South Asia. Humid South Asia corresponds broadly to endemic and hyper-endemic malaria, semi-arid South Asia to seasonally epidemic tracts, with wet-year epidemics affecting normally dry areas in wet years. In the late-colonial period rainfall and relief patterns virtually represent a kind of back-cloth for the whole picture of health and disease.

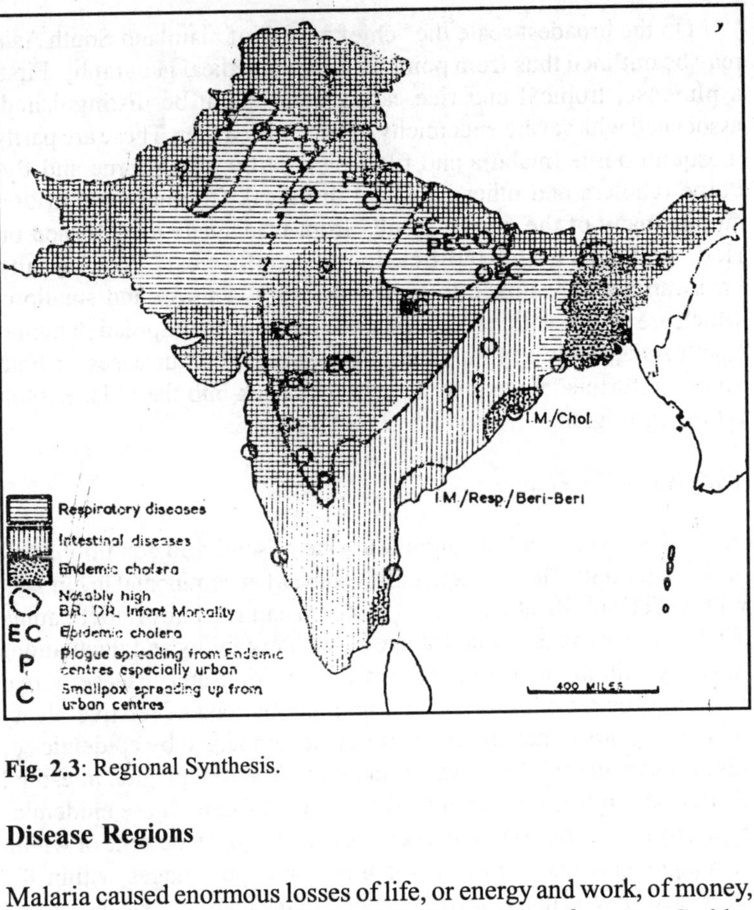

Fig. 2.3: Regional Synthesis.

Disease Regions

Malaria caused enormous losses of life, or energy and work, of money, and estimated costs showed astronomical figures.[2] Arthur Geddes showed that in some regions, it was a major cause of what he called population "stagnation", through increasing abortions as well as infant and child mortality; he chose the term stagnation not "stability" to reflect what he considered to be an unhealthy and deplorable form of population control.[3] Epidemics also certainly affected demographic trends and social and economic life, for instance the great regional epidemic in Punjab of 1912. There were other epidemic diseases. Cholera, plague and smallpox were occasionally almost as devastating as famines.

Writing in the *Indian Geographical Journal* for 1958[4], my retrospect over my findings read as follows :

On the broadest scale the "chief zones" of mainland South Asia may be outlined thus from point of view of medical geography, First, a pluviose, tropical and rice-eating zone might be distinguished, associated with severe endemicity of several diseases. These are partly mosquito borne (malaria and filariasis), partly water-borne and fly-borne (cholera and other intestinal diseases). Chronic malnutrition among many of the people results from inadequate diets, based on rice, or on rice-and-tapioca in the south-west. Poverty and backwardness are linked to such diseases as leprosy and smallpox which are severe in this zone. Yaws seems to be widespread in humid South Asia, while syphilis and gonorrhoea, urban diseases of both zones, unfortunately extend their impact back into the villages with returning migrants.

The Semi-arid Zone

In contrast, one might distinguish a zone of semi-arid conditions and variable rainfall. The northern half is somewhat continental in climate, with millet and wheat-eating; the southern half is mainly millet-eating. This great zone is associated above all with instability and fluctuations in its conditions of economy, health, nutrition and disease. Great variations occur in harvests, bringing alternations of relative plenty with lean years or actual famine, often accompanied by epidemics of disease spread by insects, water and man. Malaria, plague, intestinal disease and influenza may all strike in this fashion. These epidemics typically spread from endemic centres either outside the zone or within it. Plague spreads from urban centres or large villages within the zone, and beyond that from the enzootic of the marmots, etc. in Central Asia, while malaria is maintained in wet and forested hill and hill-foot tracts within the zone. Cholera, however, usually spreads into the zone from its endemic homes in eastern deltaic India. In the northern half of this zone, universal diseases such as pneumonia, measles and influenza are probably more important in the cool season, especially during a famine.

The Himalayan Zone

The few Himalayan districts afford glimpses of a far from favourable picture, but with a depressing complex of low standards of material life and health, poor nutrition, liability to severe epidemics of cholera, to endemic or epidemic malaria, and to diseases of poverty, backwardness and ignorance like leprosy and osteomalacia.

Some Relevant Disease Aspects

Still conceptualizing on the broadest scale, one should overlay upon this outline one disease which is certainly of great present and potential importance—tuberculosis. The profoundly unsatisfactory conditions under which most towns folk live are vital in the maintenance and spread of tuberculosis. They play a similar and important role in the natural history of other diseases such as smallpox, and in places plague, during the period studied.

One should also consider an interesting possibility, that the intestinal diseases may be even more important in peninsular India as a substratum to the paramount problem of malaria than in the northern plain, presumably because of different conditions of the water-table.

Within these great zones, there are, of course, regional differences of the utmost significance. To consider only the plain-lands of north-eastern India, fundamentally different problems are found in the mature delta of West Bengal, whose population is in the state termed "stagnation", in the active delta of East Bengal (now Bangladesh) with its high natural increase in population until 1943 and in the colonisation tract of the Assam Valley.

Population Disequlibrium

Regional differences in health and demographic trends may be considered in ecological terms, as evidence of differing stages of adjustment of equilibrium between groups of men and their environment. In a subcontinent in which the greater proportion of the people still largely depend on the food they produce themselves from the land, there is still much justification for this point of view. One view of the unfavourable extremes of population stagnation and recurrent crises might be that they represent different varieties of Malthusian checks on population growth; and that they therefore represent a state of "unstable equilibrium" or of oscillation, more or less violent according to climatic, and biotic complexes involved. On this view, if disequilibrium has arisen, it is because of a number of new factors. Thus during the later British period, major famines were prevented save during the stress of war, and many outbreaks of epidemic disease were checked which might have spread as pandemics. Craft-workers were ousted by competition from large-scale manufacturing industries in Britain, India and elsewhere, and this had driven yet more people back to the land. Cash cropping has been increased.

All these new factors had operated with few major steps—except the great irrigation schemes—either to increase the amount and flow of food supplies through increase in cultivated areas or in yields, or to pave the way to a higher standard of living, a more even balance between agriculture and industry, and a new state of equilibrium, given the more or less limited natural resources of the land.

The present review of the medical literature and statistics leads the writer to lend some support to such a view. Western medicine, and its many devoted servants in India, both European and Indian, have accomplished great work especially by acquiring basic knowledge, notably of pathogens and nutritional diseases. They have prevented the spread of many epidemics and have saved many lives and much individual suffering. Yet though the literature has been written mainly by doctors trained in curative rather than in preventive medicine, it reiterates the theme of interlocking vicious circles—poverty, backward agriculture and malnutrition, ignorance, poor environmental hygiene and disease. Here, it might be argued that from any practical point of view geographical studies of these problems must be futile, since man cannot alter the regional differences of climate. Conversely, social and economic elements are factors very largely common to the whole subcontinent.[5]

So, much for the late colonial period of the study. Since then there have been almost 30 years of independence, several 5-Year Plans in India and comparable efforts in Pakistan, several wars between the two countries, brief but damaging both directly and in diversion of funds from development to defence, and after much terrible civil war in Pakistan and the intervention of the Indian forces, there was the birth of Bangladesh in 1972. India had been very sensitive about Chinese pressure on the northernfrontier, Especially, what she regarded as invasion in Ladakh, again with the effect of diverting funds, manpower and energy from development to military ends. Still there has been much industrial development and a slight rise in per capita incomes in India and Pakistan, despite rapidly rising population—it is too soon to expect much improvement in strife-torn

Bangladesh. It is sometimes said that India's rich are getting richer and the poor poorer, a reflection of the tendency in the world as a whole between rich and poor countries. It seems to be nearer the truth that many rich people get richer, while the poor tend to become a little less poor. Except for the most vulnerable groups, there seems to be a slow rise in standards of material living, even if *relative* deprivation compared with the rich is increasing and is felt to be so by at least some of the relatively deprived.

Declining death rates and rising population

On the health front let us take the largest component, India, as an example. Death rates declined from about 30 per thousand in 1951 to about 18-19 by 1971; and infant mortality from over 20 per cent of live births to about 15, still a very high figure; birth rates have remained about 30 per thousand rising slightly 1951-1961 and falling slightly 1961-1971. Family Planning measures may have had marginally more impact than had been expected by pessimistic or even realistic forecasts. Population increase, however, has gone up from about 1.2 per cent per annum to about 2.2 per cent per annum 1951-61 and 2.5 per cent per annum 1961- 1971. While urbanization was high following the large population migrations of the period of partition and independence in 1947 rising by 41 per cent 1941-51, the increase 1951-61 was markedly lower at about 25 per cent, and the increase 1961-71 was of the same order. Though this increase is regarded as disappointing in a sense—it is only about the same as the national growth rate—it is also true that many towns and cities including the largest ones have their housing and social provision overwhelmed and that until national development and probably industrialisation in towns are proceeding faster more rapid rate urbanization will simply compound the miseries of present patterns for many people. The street dweller of Calcutta, while an extreme case, in a city subject to repeated streams of refugees in the decades since independence, and little enough to cope, these hapless people do make the point that urban migrations where the push factor predominates are apt to produce conditions of terrible squalor for many of the migrants, i.e., where people are pushed out from their villages by poverty there rather than attracted by job opportunities in the towns. (Recent research suggests that the push factor is easily exaggerated, but evidence is conflicting, probably because India is so large and complex that different conditions do maintain in different parts.)

Malaria Control

Returning to Fig. 2.3 and consideration of South Asia in general, how has the regional health picture changed? Malaria has been controlled, indeed by 1966, it appeared that the disease had been eradicated; as noted earlier, spraying was stopped in order to reduce the build-up of resistance to the residual insecticides in the anopheline population. Malarial control has been a factor in the population explosion in South Asia, though only one factor· in an age of 5-Year Plans and many successful projects in economic development, public and private. Locally malaria eradication has certainly done what was always hoped; it released local energies for land reclamation and other productive enterprise. I have been in spice-garden villages in western Karnataka (formerly Mysore) where gardens abandoned because of malaria and population decline were being brought back into cultivation, and in countless villages new irrigation wells are dug. In the high plateau part of the Deccan lava flow country I have seen new small fields being carved out from the jungle—unfortunately in very marginal land, since all the fertile and easily tilled land had long since been taken up. But there is no doubt that locally there have been positive responses to freedom from malaria and increased population.

Comparing the modern map of malaria vector species with figures of the paper written by Dutt, Akhtar and Dutta[6] *Anopheles stephensi,* the early adaptor to urban cisterns, etc. had extended its territory into south-eastern India, and urban malaria may be of increased importance. Several previously minor vector species have become more important in north-eastern India. The resurgence, early map interpretation suggests, may follow classic patterns, formerly, hyperendemic zones leading the way, while in wet years in arid and semi-arid tracts the disease sweeps out in epidemic form. However, there are notable blanks in the malaria maps so far: West Bengal, formerly hyperendemic, Kerala in south-western India which formerly had hyperendemic conditions along the edge of the Western Ghats. Fortunately, the milder *vivax* malaria predominated, and surveillance facilities were immensely greater than say in the late colonial period, so that mortality is so far comparatively light. *Falciparum* malaria does however extend in a belt across middle India, parts of which fortunately are comparatively lightly populated. The areas of mosquitoes resistant to particular insecticides are fairly well known and mapped by the National Institute of Communicable Diseases.

Malaria and Population Explosion

Since spraying did cease as soon as possible in order to minimise the build-up of anopheline immunity to insecticides, it should be possible to control the present resurgence of millions of malaria probably by simultaneously attacking the disease cycle at several points, with regional variations according to the different ecologies involved .... While malaria control has been accompanied by many other social and economic developments, the varying regional pattern in differing rates of population increase is suggestive that removal of malaria's inhibiting effect on fertility and of its role in late infant and child mortality has been a major element in the "population explosion" in South Asia.

Plague, Cholera, Smallpox and Other Diseases

The great epidemic diseases of plague, cholera and smallpox have long attracted great attention by health authorities and by the public inside and outside South Asia. Plague has virtually disappeared, but cholera still could be a serious problem at times.

Cholera

The Bengal delta remained a world endemic home of cholera, and if a wet year and severe floods, or especially if war and unrest were added as in 1971-72, the disease was ready to add to the miseries of the victims and especially of refugees subject to stress and poor diet and living conditions. On the other hand, the great pandemic of recent years of El Tor cholera is named from part Celebes or Sulawesi in Indonesia, where the particular strain of the vibrio was first recorded; and while it has found a congenial home in the Bengal delta, many other parts of the world have been involved in its spread, including resorts in Spain and Morocco and in U.S.S.R. on the Black Sea. Again the severity of the disease seems to be decreasing, even in low-lying hollows in the delta near Calcutta or in the dreadful, insanitary slums or *bustees* of the city. Again, the authorities have been very successful in control measures, not least in respect of the great gathering of pilgrims at the periodic festivals like the Jagganath (so-called Juggernaut) festival of sunrise at Puri on the Orissa coast, or Haridwar where the sacred Ganga leaves the Himalaya, or Allahabad or Prayag, a sacred confluence of rivers. Inoculation against cholera is possible but short-lived as most air travellers now know, but is used along with sanitation control and surveillance along pilgrim routes with impressive results.

Smallpox

Lastly smallpox has been patiently and systematically tackled using vaccination campaigns, not necessarily an easy matter when victims would traditionally be regarded as claimed by a particular goddess of death or of swellings (varying regionally across India); this is part of a world eradication campaign regarded as successful all-over the world and certainly in India a reward of a thousand rupees was offered in the mid-seventies to anyone who can produce a case of smallpox. Now, the disease has not only been eradicated from India, but also from the world.

Tuberculosis

So much for the three most dreaded epidemic diseases of the late-colonial period. A major campaign against tuberculosis has also been mounted with international help, but as elsewhere its effects are capable of different interpretations, and it seems likely that this is one of many diseases where economic development is the ultimate answer, permitting early diagnosis and immunization campaigns among the young. However, a major advance must be recorded in wedding advanced technology to *domiciliary* and not institutional treatment, care and surveillance, along lines realistic under present Indian conditions.

Bronchial Diseases

Bronchitis and pneumonia remain important causes of illness, loss of efficiency and distress, and of death, especially among the underprivileged in the cooler northern half of the subcontinent. Yaws remains difficult to control—surprisingly so far a country so largely cleared for agriculture and in which the wearing of a considerable covering of clothes is normal except when men are engaged in very hard work in the fields. The dysenteries still cause much illness, lassitude, inefficiency and misery, and so far there is no *deus ex machina* as in malarial control, or even a way of effective control as with cholera where outbreaks can be pinpointed and controlled; again economic development seems to be needed to break the grip of this and other intestinal diseases, causing high infant mortality among other evils. But as these diseases become less important, as already in some areas and some socio-economic classes, infant and child mortalities are falling and the expectation of life at birth is already comparable to that in Britain earlier this century.

Poverty, Modern Technology and Prospects

Protein-calorie malnutrition, as elsewhere in the Third World, is severe especially in young children, and infections like measles and gastro-enteritis add to its impact, mainly in underprivileged groups likc landless labourers and their families. When confronted with this kind of hard core problem there invariably seems to be only one answer: that all-round economic development and rising standards of living and housing and feeding must somehow be obtained. Despite all the problems of the 5-year and other plans, and all the inefficiencies of nationalised enterprises in South Asia, as elsewhere, it seems that somehow this sort of planning must be made to succeed—though not necessarily aping the high technology Western pattern. In the India of 1977, there are many signs of successful economic development: the rich farmers, the busy towns and tractor repair shops of Punjab and Haryana, the successful industrial expansion, often of small-to-medium sized enterprises, the growing exports of industrial items including machinery to the Middle East and elsewhere, the successes in international competition of both private and public sector industry and again of advisory and consultancy services, the considerable inflow of foreign exchange from emigrants to the U.K., Canada, U.S.A., the Middle East and elsewhere. There are problems of distribution of wealth and of the benefits of economic development, and problem areas in both town and country. But it is now much less visionary, much more credible, to look forward to an India in which the health problems of an underdeveloped country will recede; with luck and foresight, some of the problems of developed countries may be avoided.

Notes

1. Learmonth, A., *Patterns of Disease and Hunger,* Chap. 2, David and Charles, Newton Abbot (1978), Endemic Diseases Tend to Cause Severe Illness and Many Deaths Among Young Children and Old People while Epidemic Diseases Tend to be Spread more evenly Across the Age Groups; the latter therefore have direct impact on the main economic producers, to cause orphaning of young children and so on.
2. Sinton, I.A. (1935-36), What Malaria Costs India. *Rec, Malar, Surv. India,* 6, 223 and 413.
3. Geddes, A. (1942), The Population of India: Variability in Change as a Regional Demographic Index, *Geog. Rev.,* 32, 562.
4. Learmonth, A.T.A. (1958), Medical Geography in Indo-Pakistan: A Study of Twenty Years' Data for the Former British India, *Ind. Geogr. J.,* 33, 1.
5. *Ibid.*
6. Dutt, A.K., Akhtar, R. and Dutta H.M. (1980), Malaria in India with particular reference to two West Central States, *Soc. Sci. and Med.,* 14, 322.

3
Disease Dynamics in South and South-East Asia
With Special Reference to India

A.K. Dutt and *H.M. Dutta*

The prevalent tropical and equatorial climatic conditions of South and South-east Asia give rise to disease occurrences, especially thc tropical diseases and parasite infestations associated with hot, humid and dry, variable temperature environments. Disease pools before 500 B.C. were more or less confined to relatively isolated areas or "disease islands" owing to the infrequency of interregional contacts between peoples. In the centuries between 500 B.C. and A.D. 1200 separated population groups came into greater contact and the "disease islands" disintegrated giving rise to a "confluence of the civilized disease pools" in Eurasia.[1] In ensuing centuries with the advent of increased sea-trade and large scale conquests, relatively isolated diseases began to disseminate throughout the world at a rapid rate.

Plague, indigenous to India, was reported in Egypt as early as A.D. 542. It has been postulated that plague was transported to the European steppe by Central Asian invaders during the Middle Ages. The steppe is the indestructible habitat of the rodent that carries the plague bacillus, *Yersina pestis.* Plague eventually spread outward from the steppe over the rest of the continent. This was the 'Black Death' (1347-1350) of Europe in which one-third of its population perished. Spread of the plague is, thus an earlier example of disease diffusion and intensified confluence of Eurasian disease pools.

Following the establishment of extensive intercontinental trade links (especially after Columbus discovered the New World in 1492, and Vasco da Gama discovered the Asia-European trade route *via* the Cape of Good Hope in 1498) most diseases entered a "world reservoir". Diseases were carried from one pool to the other by the traders, soldiers, administrators, migrants, missionaries and other travellers on a world-wide basis. The diseases that were either unknown or relatively less prevalent in India became endemic to the country and Indian and Asian diseases were transported elsewhere. South and South-east Asia eventually became part of the world reservoir and most diseases found in other disease island or pools spread to South and South-east Asia. Owing to massive intercontinental contacts, cholera (caused by the agent *Vibrio cholerae)* spread from its Indian habitat to Europe and USA in virulent epidemic form in the 19th century. The symptoms of cholera are severe diarrhoea and electrolyte depletion. Prior to the 19th century cholera was unknown outside India.[2] Smallpox (*Poxvirus variola*), characterized by massive viremia with high fever, severe headache and photophobia followed by skin eruption, was described as early as the 2nd century A.D. The deadly disease diffused from its native Asian home to Europe and North Africa specially in the Middle Ages; and was carried by African slaves to the West Indies in the sixteenth century.[3] "Smallpox occurred in epidemic form less frequently in, North America until 1752" when the disease afflicted 39 per cent of Boston inhabitants killing 30 per cent of those afflicted.[4]

Some diseases inflict greater morbidity in particular regions because of the dominance of certain conditions that give rise to an intra-regional ecological synthesis, which is the most favourable breeding ground for a disease or diseases. Such a synthesis requires a specific combination of multiple conditions related to the cultural, economic and physical aspects of a region. Endemic *kala-azar* (Visceral Leishmaniasis with human reservoir) in the region consisting of north-east India, Bangladesh and parts of Burma is a typical example of the formation of such an ecological synthesis.

Disease occurrence or non-occurrence are dependent upon a systematic integration of three factors: causative, preventive and curative. Figure 3.1 explains the interplay of these factors as they are applicable to India in particular. These factors are the keys to an understanding of disease dynamics in India.

Causative Factors

Among the ecological conditions that can be associated with high incidences of particular diseases in South and South-east Asian realms are physiography, amount of rainfall and rainfall intensity during monsoon months, close proximity of habitats to forests and increasing pollution of the environment (Fig. 3.1). Learmonth and Mukerji refer to winter's association with cough and cold.[5] Aiken *et al.* associate the tropics and a higher relative humidity with the dengue fever, an acute and febrile infectious disease, caused by a virus carried by the Aedes mosquito.[6] Smallpox is classically associated with squalor and overcrowding.[7] Though cholera is mainly associated with the tropical and sub-tropical summer, it can occur all the year round. Lower standards of living and inadequate public health and sanitary facilities are the chief causes of cholera epidemics.

Cultural lifestyles and habitats both encourage as well as discourage diseases. Lack of education and health consciousness cause many diseases which otherwise may be prevented. The Hindu

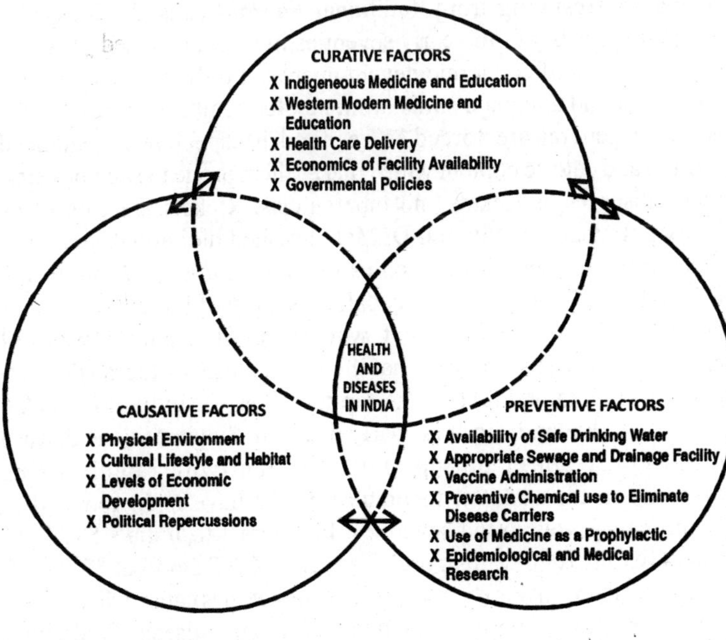

Fig. 3.1: Disease Dynamics in India.

way of staying clean by bathing everyday and washing the hands and mouth before and after meals is an aspect of traditional lifestyle. While believing that one stays clean by bathing in the same tank or river where people dispose of pollutants, the bather actually becomes infected by water-borne diseases such as typhoid caused by *Salmonella typhi,* amoebiasis caused by *Endamoeba histolytica* and cholera. Mukerji refers to such practices with reference to his study area of a north Indian micro-region: the Chandigarh Duns.[8] Dutt, *et al.* point out the association of rice cultivation and malaria.[9] Malaria occurrences in a micro-region of south India has also been correlated with the man-made environmental changes, dwelling types and socio-economic activities of the people.[10] Avoidance of meat and fish from one's diet, usually known as vegetarianism, is common among a large segment of the Hindu population. Such a practice, if not supplanted by milk intake, leads to protein deficiency and malnutrition. Learmonth and Akhtar, and Chakravarti have explored the disease relationships concerning such deficiency.[11] As a matter of fact, even many well-to-do families might suffer from such deficiencies because of dietary habits. Reluctance of women to be vaccinated by male vaccinators (resulting from traditional *Purdah)* caused widespread smallpox mortality in the early seventies in rural areas of Patna.[12]

Low levels of economic development not only limit a country's ability to spend adequate sums of money for health facilities but the people in general are forced to eat food irrespective of balanced nutrition and caloric content which makes them prone to such poverty-related diseases as rickets and tuberculosis. Rickets are caused by dietary deficiency of Vitamin D. Malnourished individuals are more susceptible to tuberculosis bacillus (*M. tuberculosis, M. bovis* and others). In 1977, per capita daily caloric supply of India was only 91 per cent of the total requirement, whereas, in Singapore, it was 134 per cent.[13] It is not surprising that the tuberculosis of the respiratory system has remained among the top ten killers in India, Sri Lanka, Burma and Thailand, since the early fifties. In Singapore, the disease ranked either 5th or 6th up until 1965, but with rapidly rising prosperity in the country, tubercular deaths have been reduced to insignificant levels in the seventies. In contrast to India's $180 per capita GNP in 1978, Singapore's per capita GNP stood at $3,290.[14]

Political upheavals or repercussions sometimes caused dislocation of food and water supply bringing about related disease epidemics. The man-made Bengal famine of 1943 killed five million people including deaths resulting from diseases of malnutrition and decreased body resistance. The 1943 famine occurred while India was still ruled by the British, who diverted railway wagons from civil grain movement to military movement on the Burma front. Learmonth refers to the occasional influx of refugees from East Pakistan (now Bangladesh) to Calcutta and the resultant overburdening of municipal sanitation facilities which led to the emergence of cholera.[15]

The process of modernization in the South and South-east Asian realms leads to greater use of harmful chemicals, poison-emitting internal combustion engines and polluting factory chimneys, bringing with it respiratory and carcinogenic diseases. In Bombay alone, 15 tons of carbon monoxide are emitted everyday into the air by automobiles. In Calcutta, the industrial furnaces and commonly used domestic cooking ovens throw 250 tons of particulate matter into the air daily.[16] Armstrong attributes the increasing occurrences of cancer in South-east Asia to the above factors.[17] Akhtar, however, points out that regional patterns of cancer in India are related to food habits, socio-economic levels and cultural environment.[18]

Preventive Factors

It is said that an ounce of prevention is worth a pound of cure. Disease can be prevented by providing a basic infrastructure which: (i) supplies safe drinking water, efficient sewage and drainage facilities; (ii) administers necessary vaccines and serums; and (iii) uses relatively harmless chemicals to eliminate invertebrate disease carriers. Moreover, strong epidemiological and medical research can be used to locate the focal points of the disease origin and diffusion thus facilitating the development of a strategy to prevent the disease from occurring in new areas. In 1973, three out of the five countries where smallpox had not yet been eradicated were in South Asia (India, Pakistan and Bangladesh). Malaria, a disease transmitted by the *Anopheles* mosquito, can be eradicated among humans, some researchers believe, only when a vaccine is discovered that provides immunity from the bite of an infected mosquito.[19] Preventive mass inoculation before summer season and at the religious fair and provision for safe filtered domestic water supply in many cities have drastically lessened cholera epidemics in India. The experience of Calcutta is typical of preventive steps in controlling cholera. Cholera was endemic to Calcutta. Even in the last century, it was a serious problem in the city. No wonder Kipling had designated the city with an ill-fated title, "Cholera capital of the World". The basic agent for cholera transmission in the city was eliminated in the sixties when unfiltered water used for street cleaning and fire prevention was disinfected by chlorination on the advice of World Health Organization (WHO) experts. This action along with mass inoculation and cleaning of the slums (*bustees*) led to freeing the city from cholera endemicity.

The WHO supported large-scale malaria control programmes have been implemented in most malarious countries. Insecticides have been widely used in the control of malaria in India. India has been actively involved in control programmes for three decades and by 1965 it had almost "eradicated" malaria, but a resurgence occurred because of the lack of persistent surveillance on the part of the government. On the whole, limited success has been achieved all-over South and South-east Asia. Singapore, however, is an exception. It has eradicated malaria .

A scientific understanding of epidemiology is essential in the prevention of diseases. Meade suggests a measure to examine epidemiological transition in the South-east Asian countries.[20] Such a measure would help determine the health plan strategy of a nation. Real prevention can only be achieved through concerted government actions. Governments must have the ability to finance programmes and an understanding of the situation. Siddiqi explains the health policy impact for Pakistan and affirms that the health care facilities reveal serious inadequacies in terms of planning, lack of capital and disregard for socio-cultural factors.[21]

Curative Factors

South and South-east Asia have indigenous medical systems, but modern westernized medical technology and education have brought about better results in curing and preventing diseases. India has 100 medical colleges based on western systems. Advanced research institutes in India include the Indian Council of Medical Research, the National Institute of Communicable Diseases (Delhi), the National Institute of Nutrition (Hyderabad), the Virus Research Centre (Pune), the Haffkine Institute (Bombay) and the Central Research Institute (Kasauli) for vaccines. The existence of modern medical science in South and South-east Asia is an advantage which the European and Anglo-American countries lacked in their earlier stages of development in the 18th and 19th centuries. Modern medical systems throughout South and South-east Asia have recourse to serums and vaccines; antibiotics and other advanced curative medicines. New medical diagnostic tools as well as new techniques such as radiation treatment, surgical transplants of human organs and micro-surgery are now available in South and South-east Asia. These medical developments have reduced death rates in South and South-east Asia, particularly in relation to specific diseases, such as, cholera, typhoid, malaria, tuberculosis, and several other infectious diseases. The post-Second World War "population explosion" in India is partly a result of large scale administration of curative and preventive medicines, which caused the crude death rate to fall drastically by 33.3 per cent during 1960-78, whereas, the crude birth rate registered a decline of only 18.6 per cent.[22]

Health-care delivery systems exist in South and South-east Asia both in the public and private sectors, but there are obvious inadequacies. Siddiqi and Rahman have described these systems in both sectors.[23] Rahman particularly emphasizes the existence of an indigenous system in Pakistan and India, *Unani,* which uses local herbs to cure diseases based on symptoms of the disease. The *Unani* system originated in Greece and diffused into South Asia especially after Alexander the Great conquered the north-western part of India in 326 B.C. *Ayurvedic* medicine, based on *Yajur-Veda* (700 B.C.) formalized by the 2nd century A.D. through the efforts of *Charaka, Susruta* and *Vagbhatta*, is another native system prevalent in India. *Ayurvedic* and *Unani* systems obtained official government support after India's independence. There are over ninety *Ayurvedic* and ten *Unani* government financed under-graduate colleges in India; two graduate Ayurvedic universities, Gujarat Ayurvedic University at Jamnagar and the Post-graduate Training and Research Institute at Varanasi, are particularly significant.

In spite of the availability of the advanced medical technology in India, it is the rich who take advantage of it most because they have the money to make use of the private practitioners or hospitals. The poor depend on crowded public clinics and hospitals or on folk medicine of various kinds. At the international level, the more affluent countries, like Singapore, have better health care facilities because their governments and their people can afford them. The poorer countries like India can afford only limited facilities; this is one of the reasons why malaria has been eradicated from all developed countries of the world and there is perhaps a moral in the fact that malaria seems to have disappeared from England as a result of social and economic development and certainly not as a result of specific campaigns against the disease. Though old age diseases rank among the top causes of death in all the countries of the South and the South-east Asia, Singapore partly reflects the disease syndrome of the economically advanced countries where leading causes of death are neoplasm, influenza, bronchitis and hypertension. In the less economically advanced countries like India, the Philippines, Thailand, Burma and Sri Lanka, deaths from neoplasms are probably occurring with greater frequency owing to modernization and longer life expectancy but pneumonia, tuberculosis, gastric diseases and infant diseases are still the leading causes of death.

There is also a rural-urban differential in health care availability. Siddiqi and Rahman point out that the public has better access to health care facilities in urban areas than in rural areas of Pakistan.[24] Conditions in India are similar to those in Pakistan. Specialized health care facilities tend not to locate in the rural areas. Most private practitioners trained in western medicine prefer to practice in urban areas leaving the rural areas to quacks and outdated *Unani, Ayurvedic* and homoeopathic doctors.

In general, the budget allocations of governments determine, both preventive and curative aspects of health care. A WHO publication states that the recent budget increases of the governments of South and South-east Asia for combatting malaria resurgence are expected to cause a decline in malaria morbidity.[25] In long-run, the improvements in the health of the people of South and South-east Asia will be realized in proportion to financial allocations for health care systems.

Conclusion

Health planning and epidemiological studies must be based on a tripartite relationship involving the cause, cure and prevention of diseases. When the cause of a disease is ascertained, its occurrence can be minimized or prevented by taking preventive measures. Similarly, when a disease occurs curative measures may be taken. Many diseases occur irrespective of preventive measures and many are incurable; in both of those circumstances reassessment of causes becomes essential.

The level of economic development has a far-reaching effect on health and diseases. Parasitic, infectious and poverty related diseases will continue to be significant in South and South-east Asia as long as this area has low levels of economic development. With an improved economy, the disease association will change and life expectancy will be increased. Causative factors with the exception of the physical environment can be controlled. Basic infrastructure facilities and technical know-how for curative and preventive measures are already available in India.

With adequate financing, upgrading and expansion of facilities, and the extensive use of modern scientific methods and medicines, morbidity and mortality can be minimized and a healthy labour force can be generated for sustained productivity.

Notes

1. McNeill, W.H. (1976), *Plagues and Peoples,* New York: Anchore Press Doubleday, pp. 77-148.
2. Cluff, L.E. (1975), Cholera (Asiatic Cholera), In *Textbook of Medicine* Vol. 1, (Edited by P.B. Beeson and W. McDermott), Philadelphia: W.B. Saunders, p. 374.
3. Kempe, C.H., Variola and Vaccine. In *Textbook of Medicine, Ibid.,* p. 206.
4. *Ibid.*
5. Learmonth, A.T.A. (1980), Reflections of Regional Geography of Disease in Late Colonial South Asia, 271-276, and Mukerji, A.B. Disease Ecology of Small Cul-de-sac: Chandigarh Dun, pp. 331-336, In *Social Science and Medicine,* Special Issue: *Contemporary Perspectives on Medical Geography of South and South-East Asia*, (Edited by Dutt, A.K.). 14D.
6. Aiken, S.R. Frost, D.B. and Leigh, C.H., Dengue Haemorrhagic Fever and Rainfall in Penisular Malaysia: Some Suggested Relationships, in Dutt, A.K:. (ed.) *op. cit.,* pp. 307-316.
7. Learmonth, A.T.A. (1958), Medical Geography in Indo-Pakistan: A Survey of Twenty Years' data for the former British India, *Indian Geographical Journal,* 33, 1-59.
8. Mukerji, A.B., *op. cit.*
9. Dutt, A.K., Akhtar, R., and Dutta, H.M. Malaria in India with Particular Reference to Two West-central States, in Dutt, A.K. (ed.) *op. cit.,* 317-330.
10. Hyma, B. and Ramesh, A., The Reappearance of Malaria in Sathanur Reservoir and Environs: Tamil Nadu, India, in Dutt, A.K. (ed.) *op. cit.,* pp. 337-336.
11. Chakravarti, A.K. (1982), Diet and Disease: Some Aspects of Food Use in India, pp. 301-323. Learmonth, A.T.A. and Akhtar, R. Cultural Patterns

and Health and Disease in India, pp. 287-299. In *India: Cultural Patterns and Processes* (Edited by Noble, A.G and Dutt, A.K.), Boulder, Colorado: Westview Press.

12. Singh, S. and Dutta, H.M. (1981), Smallpox Patterns and its Correlates, *Geo Journal,* 5, 77-78.
13. *World Development Report 1980,* 152-153, New York: Oxford University Press.
14. *Ibid.,* pp. 110-111.
15. Learmonth, A.T.A., *op. cit.*
16. Dutt, A.K. (1983), Cities of South Asia. In *Cities of the World* (Edited by Brunn, S.D. and Williams, J.F.) New York: Harper & Row, 325-368.
17. Armstrong, R.W. Geographical Aspect of Cancer Incidence in South-East Asia. In Dutt, A.K. (ed.) *op. cit.,* pp. 299-106.
18. Akhtar, R. (1978), Geography of Cancer in India. *Medicine Biologie Environnement,* July-December, pp. 20-30.
19. Dutta, H.M. and Dutt, A.K. (1978), Malarial Ecology: A Global Perspective, *Social Science and Medicine,* 12, 69-86; Dutta, H.M., Dutt, A.K. and Vishnukumari (1979), Resurgence of Malaria in Tamil Nadu, *Social Science and Medicine,* 13D, 191-196.
20. Meade, M.S., Potential Years of Life Lost in Countries of South-East Asia, In Dutt, A.K. (ed.) *op. cit.,* pp. 277-282.
21. Siddiqi, A.H., Health Care Resources and Public Policy in Pakistan. In Dutt, A.K. (ed.) *op. cit.,* pp. 291-298.
22. Rahman, M., Urban and Rural Medical System in Pakistan, in Dutt, A.K. (ed.) *op. cit.,* pp. 283-290.
23. World Development Report, 1980, *op. cit.*
24. Rahman, M., *op. cit.*
25. Noguer, A. Wernsdorfer, W. and Kouznetsou, R. (1971), The Malaria Situation in 1970 : *W.H.O. Chronicle,* 25, 502.

4

The Pattern of Disease Distribution and Ecology in Southern Asia

With Special Reference to the Indian Subcontinent

M.J. Joshi and *C.D. Deshpande*

The ecological factors which are favourable to the growth and transmission of an infective agent often produce an arcal distribution pattern. The relationship of ecology to the distribution characteristics of infective and communicable diseases has been studied and well outlined on a global basis.[1] Small individual regions, however, have several distinctive ecological factors and broad generalization on a global basis overlook important details of regional eco-biological relationship. Southern Asia is one such part of the world, where the tropical and sub-tropical location and the typical monsoonal rainfall regimes produce an ecological framework which gives rise to a disease pattern that merits a closer study.

The present study aims at analysing the distribution of some of the commonly prevalent diseases in South Asia and correlating its pattern with the prevalent bio-climatological framework.

Distribution of Diseases

The distribution of some of the diseases in Southern Asia reveals some very interesting features.

Leishmaniasis is caused by the protozoan parasite belonging to the genus *Leishmania.* This disease occurs in two forms *viz.*, the cutaneous and the visceral.

The cutaneous form is transmitted by a sandfly *Phlebotomus papatasii* and is perpetuated by the dogs and rodents, who act as primary hosts. It is reported from the Dead Sea area of Israel.[2] It is endemic in Lebanon, Jordan, Saudi Arabia, Southern and Central regions of Iraq.[3] Several foci are known in Iran where the disease is widely distributed in the North Eastern Province of Khorassan, adjoining Afghanistan[4] In Afghanistan itself, several outbreaks have been reported, the last one with a report of 377 cases being in 1967 in Kabul. In Pakistan, it is reported in the North West Frontier Province, Baluchistan and Punjab.[5] In India, Cutaneous leishmaniasis is reported from the Punjab, Haryana, Northern Rajasthan and Delhi. Cutaneous leishmaniasis does not occur further east than longitude 80° E.[6]

Visceral leishmaniasis on the other hand, is a true anthroponosis caused by *L. donovani* and maintained only between man and the sandfly *P. argentipes* in the Indian sub-zone, commonly known as *kala-azar*. It is endemic in eastern Uttar Pradesh, Bihar, West Bengal, Bangladesh, some parts of Nepal and Assam and along the eastern coast in Orissa, Andhra Pradesh and Tamil Nadu.[7] This disease is limited by the mountain ranges that separate Assam from Burma and is not found in the countries of South-East Asia.[8] This form of Visceral leishmaniasis occurs where the soil is alluvial and rain considerable. Characteristically, it comes in periodic outbreaks, once every 15-20 years—the last one being in 1955-56. Recently, *kala-azar* is again reported in various parts of India.[9]

It is interesting to note that the cutaneous form exists in the drier western region, while the visceral form is found only in wet eastern region. Both the forms co-exist only in the adjacent regions of Kashmir, Punjab and Uttar Pradesh.[10]

Virus Diseases (Trachoma and Smallpox)

Trachoma has been regarded as a virus disease, so the authors' discussion of smallpox and trachoma as two virus diseases has been left as written some years ago. However, the pathogen of trachoma *Chlamydia trachomatis* is now classed in the *Bedsonia,* very small bacteria including also C. *psittaci,* the organism causing psittacosis, or parrot's disease. And smallpox has been eradicated from the world some years ago. (*Editors' note*)

Trachoma is very widely prevalent in the South-west Asia. Some 99,071 cases were reported in various provinces of Iran during the year 1969-70.[11] Afghanistan also registers high incidence and it is assumed that more than 30 per cent of the population is attacked by trachoma, at least once in their lifetime.[12] Trachoma is widespread in Pakistan.[13] The incidence is high in Punjab, Rajasthan and in Aligarh district of Uttar Pradesh. Whereas trachoma constitutes 85 per cent of all cases involving ocular pathology in Afghanistan, it represents only 20 per cent of those in Burma.[14] The distribution is less widespread in the moist regions towards the South and East. For example in Sri Lanka and Nepal it does not assume any major threat to public health. The ecological factors of dry climate and heat make the distribution of this dust borne infection more in the Western than in the Eastern part of Southern Asia.

Smallpox on the other hand, showed wider distribution throughout the Indian subcontinent South and though the disease is now eradicated, during 1968, India, Indonesia and Pakistan recorded over 80 per cent of the world's total smallpox cases.[15] Smallpox shows a cyclical sharp increase every 5-7 years.[16] The Western limit of this disease in the last epidemic was Pakistan and Afghanistan, and the disease was not significantly reported in Iran and in countries to its west.

In contrast to the distribution of trachoma, smallpox is found mainly in the Eastern part of Southern Asia. The main ecological factors involved in this disease, are related to the man and the virus. The majority of cases occurred during winter and early spring, with a peak incidence in April and May.[17]

Non-Venereal Syphilis

Bejal, a form of non-venereal syphilis is essentially a disease of warm and dry climates. This disease is reported in two forms in Southern Asia. Bejal has a limited distribution. It is prevalent in the nomadic Bedouin tribes of Syria, Saudi Arabia, Iraq and Iran.[18] In Iran, it is reported in the western region namely Ahwaz and Kharaghan and in the Bahookalat, Zabol and Dasht-E-Zouzan in the eastern region.[19]

Yaws, on the other hand, is found in humid and warm climates, where the annual rainfall is at least 125 cms and the mean annual temperature is between 70° F and 80° F.[20] It was very widely prevalent in Sri Lanka, where nearly 3000 cases were reported every year.[21] Now, yaws has been practically eradicated from Sri Lanka.[22] The disease probably spread from Sri Lanka to the Indian subcontinent. It is reported widely from South India. In a place like Coimbatore,

129 cases were reported in one year.[23] It is also reported from the Mirzapur district of Uttar Pradesh,[24] Bastar district of Madhya Pradesh and adjacent area of Maharashtra, Andhra Pradesh and Orissa.[25] The control measures in these districts have effectively brought the prevalence rate from 5.36 to 1.44 per cent.[26] The disease is also reported from Chittagong Hills in Bangladesh and Assam. Surveys carried out in Malaysia, Thailand and Indonesia showed even higher prevalence rates ranging from 13 to 56.8 per cent.[27] The areas involved in the distribution of yaws are generally inhabited by tribal people with poor knowledge of personal hygiene. The disease tends to spread in the community, through direct personal contact.

It is thus noticeable that the two forms of non-venereal syphilis have two distinct areas of distribution, Bejal in the dry Western region and Yaws is more frequent in the wet Eastern region.

> It is possible that yaws-bejal-pinta, endemic syphilis, and venereal syphilis represent specialised adaptations treponemal organisms, possibly strains of the single species *T. Pallidum,* to both climate—vegetation belts on the continental scale and to the micro-climates of say rainforest on one hand and desert scrub on the other—but also to the micro-climates of say folds in the human skin. If so, behavioural patterns of individuals and societies are clearly involved—working or recreational patterns in relation to thorny vegetation, clothed or bare skin, sexual behaviour and so on. See, for instance, A. Cockburn, 1963, *The Evolution and Eradication of Infectious Disease,* London: O.U.P.
>
> (*Editors' note*)

Guinea Worms and Filarial Infection

Two forms of nematodes belonging to the order spirurides have special significance to Southern Asia. They are the *Dracunculus medinensis,* giving rise to guinea worm disease and *Wuchereria bancrofti* and *Brugia malayi* giving rise to filariasis.

The guinea worm cycle operates thus: a gravid female worm in a human being moves to a part often exposed to water such as a leg; an ulcer forms over the head of the worm, the uterus is protruded from the ulcer on contact with water, and active embryo worms discharged into the water. Some are swallowed by cyclops water snails, developing in its body into infective forms which, swallowed by people, move from the intestine into the tissues, mature, mate and so again to the gravid female stage.

Guinea worm disease is extensively reported from India.[28] The highest incidence is reported in Rajasthan and in some areas of Uttar Pradesh, Maharashtra, Orissa, Andhra Pradesh, and Tamil Nadu. It is widely prevalent in Pakistan in Dera-Ghazikhan, Muzaffargarh and Mianwali districts of N.W. Frontier Province and the Tharparkar district of Sind.[29] In Afghanistan, the disease is reported in the environs of Balkh.[30] Further eastwards, the disease is reported from Iran adjoining the Persian Gulf. In Bandar Abbas, for example, an infection rate of 1.2 per cent has been reported. On the other hand, the disease is infrequently found in Kashmir, Himachal Pradesh and the eastern part of Southern Asia, such as Bihar, West Bengal, Bangladesh and Assam. The disease is reported from areas of relatively poor rainfall, where water needs are met with from the stagnant open ponds and stepwells.

One of the many filarial worms, *Wuchereria bancrofti* causing bancroftian filariasis is transmitted by the mosquito *Culex fatigans,* which requires atmospheric temperature of about 80° F and humidity above 60 per cent.[31] These conditions are prevalent in the eastern parts of Southern Asia, where filariasis is widely reported. It is also found in Burma[32] and in Bangladesh with the highest incidence in Dinajpur district.[33] In India, filariasis is reported from all States along the eastern coast, *viz.* West Bengal, Orissa, Andhra Pradesh and Tamil Nadu and from Bihar and Eastern Uttar Pradesh.[34] The western coastal area also receives heavy rains and as a result, this disease is found widely prevalent in coastal Kerala.[35] Further north, filariasis is reported from the part of Saurashtra and Surat district of Gujarat and a few foci around Bombay.[36]

Although a few carriers of filariasis are reported from non-endemic areas such as the western part of Deccan plateau, Rajasthan, Haryana, Punjab and the western parts of Uttar Pradesh and Madhya Pradesh[37], clinical disease is rare in these regions. Pakistan is free from this disease. Wolfe and Aslamkhan[38] were unable to find evidence of filariasis in Karachi, in spite of extensive migrations from the erstwhile East Pakistan. Filariasis is unknown in Afghanistan[39] and apart from Turkey, no country in the south-west Asia is known to harbour this disease.

Hydatid Disease

This is caused by a tapeworm of dogs and some wild animals: eggs in (mainly) dog faeces pollute pastures grazed by sheep; people become infected by handling polluted grass or dogs, or by eating infected animals.

Contrary to the belief of some Western authors[40], Hydatid disease is frequently reported in Southern Asia, and shows a very interesting distribution. The disease is rare in south-east Asia. Hardly three cases have been reported so far from Malaysia.[41] In India, the disease is more frequently reported in the States of Tamil Nadu[42], Andhra Pradesh[43], Maharashtra[44], Gujarat[45], Madhya Pradesh[46] and Punjab. A few cases are also reported from Himachal Pradesh and West Bengal, though it is generally uncommon in Uttar Pradesh, Orissa and Assam. Some 80 cases were reported from Multan district in Pakistan. In Afghanistan, hydatidosis is an impôrtant parasitic infection.[47] The disease is widespread in the south-west Asia. A number of cases were reported from Tehran and Shiraz, the majority of them coming from the western part of Iran. The disease is also reported from Iraq.[48] Perhaps, the highest incidence of this disease is found in Lebanon, especially in Beirut and its environs.[49] The distribution of human hydatidosis is directly correlated with prevalence in the animal kingdom. The animal infection is not only reported in sheep, but also in goats and sambhar from Ceylon (now Sri Lanka)[50], buffalos in India[51] and camels in Iran.

Anthrax

People become infected through handling infected animals, meat of animal products such as hides, hair bristles etc. and so it tends to be an occupational disease of farmers, tanners, butchers, and housewives who become infected through abrasions in the skin.

Caused by *Bacillus anthracis,* this disease is widely prevalent throughout Southern Asia in zoonotic form in cattle, sheep and goats. The distribution of human anthrax shows some interesting features. It is reported from almost all the countries of south-west Asia. During the years 1969-70, 1226 cases of anthrax were reported from various provinces in Iran.[52] Eastwards of Iran, the disease shows progressively diminishing incidence. Twenty five hospital cases were reported from Afghanistan during 1962-63.[53] An outbreak of cutaneous anthrax was reported in 1962 in Jhang district of Pakistan with a report of 36 cases.[54] Human anthrax is almost unknown in India. Three cases were reported from Punjab and one case of intestinal anthrax was reported by Rao, *et al.*[55] Anthrax has been reported in the eastern part of south and south-east Asia with 8 cases from Burma in 1964, 17 cases from Ceylon (now Sri Lanka) in 1968, and 25 cases from Thailand in 1966.[56]

Schistosomiasis

Schistosomiasis or bilharzia is caused by several species of a flukeworm which uses people and certain water-snails as alternative host—the snail becoming infected by a larval stage discharged from the human bladder, and after development in the snail a later larval stage may penetrate the skin of people while wading or bathing in infected water; after development to adult flukes in the human body mating and discharge of eggs takes place in the portal or liver area, then entering the bladder and continuing the cycle.

Central Africa constitutes the most important single zone of prevalence of this disease. In south-west Asia, the disease is reported from the former Aden protectorate, several areas of Saudi Arabia, Lebanon, Syria and Iraq.[57] In Iran, the disease is reported from the south-western province of Khuzestan. Eastwards of this focus, schistosomiasis is rarely reported. A small pocket is reported in a village Gimvi in the Ratnagiri district on the western coast of India[58] and more recently another one from the Lohager village in the Raipur district of Madhya Pradesh.[59] In any case, these foci are strictly localised and do not offer any serious health problem in India.

It will thus be seen that as with anthrax, the distribution of schistosomiasis shows a progressive decline from the regions of south-west Asia towards the Indian subcontinent.

The distribution of diseases studied so far concern those that are infective and parasitic in origin. The epidemiology of some of the non-communicable disorders also shows an interesting distribution pattern in the Southern Asia. The calculous disease of the renal tract and pancreas will serve as an example.

Calculus Disease of the Renal Tract and Pancreas

The high incidence of renal stones in the north-west and central parts of India has been described by several workers. High incidence of stones is reported[60] from the relatively dry plateau of central

Maharashtra in Ahmednagar district. While analysing 9481 cases from Poona, Joshi, *et al.*[61] found 333 cases of renal stones in three years between 1968 and 1970. Some 176 cases of urinary calculi were seen in north Gujarat by Shah and Julundhwala.[62] Some 150 cases of bladder stones alone were seen in Jamnagar district of Saurashtra.[63] Urinary stones are also common in Rajasthan. High incidence of stones is reported from Gwalior[64], Kanpur[65], New Delhi[66], Chandigarh[67], Amritsar[68], and Kashmir[69] in northern India. High incidence of stones is reported from Pakistan as well as from Afghanistan.[70] In a retrospective study of 2113 operated cases from Iran, Hedayat, *et al.*[71] found that the majority of them lived in dry areas adjacent to the central province and relatively few came from southern Iran.

On the other hand, renal stones are uncommon in south India. For example, they are rare in Kerala.[72] Incidence of stone disease is generally low in south-east Asia except in the Ubol province in the north-east of Thailand.[73] It is thus noticeable that the distribution of calculus disease is mainly restricted to the dry and hot western regions of southern Asia.

Calculus disease of the pancreas on the other hand, shows interesting distribution in contrast to that of urinary stones. Chronic calculus pancreatitis seen in some of the tropical countries differs in several respects from similar disease seen in the Western countries. The disease mainly affects patients under 40 years of age in the absence of biliary disease and alcoholism. It has a very high prevalence in Kerala.[74] In five years between 1961 and 1965, calculus pancreatitis was noted in 135 cases accounting for 0.145 per cent of total hospital admissions in Trivandrum.[75] Similar cases have been reported from Madras, central Maharashtra[76] and Gujarat.[77] The disease is also found in Sri Lanka.[78] In northern India, this form of pancreatitis is very rare. Not a single case of this disease is reported from Pakistan and the countries of south-west Asia. Though not equal in frequency to renal stones, this peculiar form of primary calculus pancreatitis in contrast to urinary stones is reported more often from the southern part of the Indian subcontinent than the northern one.

Geographical Background

The southern part of the Asian continent extends from Turkey, Syria and Saudi Arabia, in the west, to Vietnam, Malaysia, Indonesia and

Philippines in the east. This region is bounded in the north by the Himalayan mountain ranges and their extensions and in the south by the Indian Ocean. Southern Asia comprises three parts *viz.* south-west Asia, the Indian subcontinent (also called south Asia) and south-east Asia. Whereas the entire region of south-west Asia lies in the sub-tropical zone north of the Tropic of Cancer, half of the Indian sub-continent and almost all of south-east Asia lie within the true tropical zone.

The ecology of this region is mainly dominated by the Tropical Monsoon climate, which gives rise to a well defined rainy season from June to September. Some areas in the Indian subcontinent and South-East Asia receive additional rain from the retreating Monsoons from November to January. The south-west Monsoons produce heavy precipitation of rain in the eastern half of the southern Asia including southern and eastern parts of the Indian subcontinent. In the western half on the other hand, the existence of the tropical high pressure belt, the configuration of the land mass and the movement of air masses produce conditions which permit only the scantiest rainfall or no rain at all.

Accordingly, the regional distribution of monsoonal rainfall significantly, though unequally, divides southern Asia into two parts, the western region with very scanty rainfall and the larger eastern region having copious rainfall. The borderland, which divides southern Asia into these regions can broadly be identified as a belt of land lying between the 75 and 100 cm isohyets. This borderland lies in the Indian subcontinent (Fig. 4.1) and effectively demarcates the ecological watershed separating the dry western region from the wet eastern region. It will be seen that, from the ecological viewpoint, central Maharashtra, part of Gujarat and Rajasthan of India, together with Pakistan, Afghanistan and all countries of south-west Asia, constitute a single region with comparable environmental features. The eastern region similarly constitutes a homogeneous ecological region consisting of southern and eastern parts of the Indian sub-continent and the whole of south-east Asia. The mountain relief and rivers somewhat alter conditions locally, but the broader picture is not materially changed.

Availability of water has influenced the flora and fauna of this region as also the density of human population. Abundance of rain in the eastern region favours cultivation, of rice, a staple diet of this region. The western zone mainly produces wheat while central zone

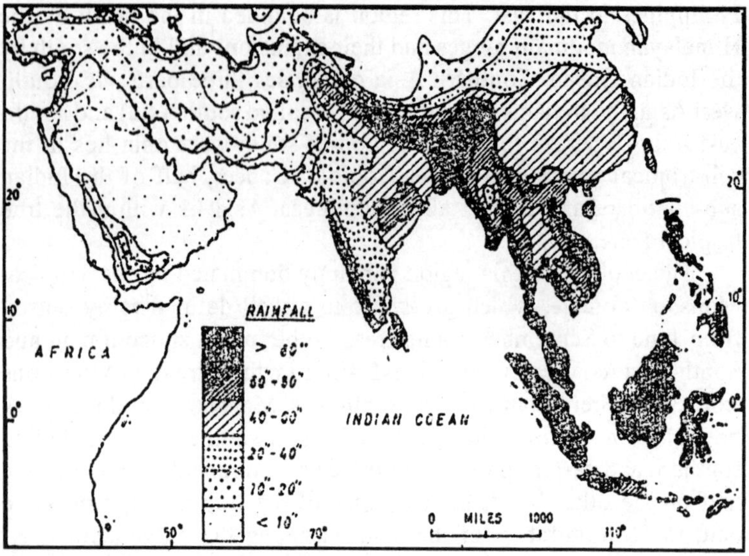

Fig. 4.1 : Distribution of Rainfall in Southern Asia.

produces mainly millets. Population density of the eastern region is considerably higher than that in the western region. This is highlighted in the two contrasting regions of Pakistan and Bangladesh whose population is seven times more than that of Pakistan. The dietary pattern has considerable significance in incidence of disease.

As regards the fauna, the sheep and camel are reared particularly in the western region. The eastern region, with its wet climate has favoured certain vectors like *C. fatigans, P. argentipes* etc. transmitting various parasitic diseases.

The hot and arid climate of south-west Asia has not only influenced the geography but also its history. Most of the invasions by the Mughal, Afghan and Iranian emperors took place by land routes towards the Indus Valley and then onwards towards the fertile Gangetic plains. This has resulted in the admixture of south-west Asian races with those of Pakistan and northern India. Southern India was comparatively less affected by these invasions. In the east and south of the ecological watershed one meets with the Dravidian races in the south and the Mongoloid races are seen in the eastern parts, which are anthropologically different from the north Indian Caucasian races.

Discussion

The present study thus reveals that the distribution of diseases throughout the Southern Asia follows a well defined pattern which is largely related to its ecological features. The monsoonal rainfall divides Southern Asia into two parts: the dry and hot western region and the wet eastern region. The ecological watershed which runs through India not only represents the boundary zone of these two regions but also tends to demarcate the distribution of some of the diseases found on either side.[79]

Climatic factors greatly influence the breeding of certain vectors, which in turn, determine the distribution of some of the diseases. The best example is found in the case of leishmaniasis. While having similar underlying pathogenic organisms, the cutaneous form is prevalent in the western side of the watershed whereas the visceral one is found in the eastern region. The bio-climatological factors favourable for the breeding of the sandflies which transmit these two forms of disease are found as characteristic in the respective zones, *viz.* the dry climate for the sandfly *P. papatasii* for transmission of cutaneous leishmaniasis in the western zone and the wet climate and the alluvial soil for *P. argentipes* for transmission of visceral leishmaniasis in the eastern zone.[80] These two forms seldom co-exist except the ecological watershed in some parts of Uttar Pradesh.[81]

The two virus diseases, *viz.* trachoma and smallpox show a similar pattern of distribution. Trachoma constitutes one of the major health problems in the south-west Asia. Smallpox on the other hand, was more widely seen in the Indian subcontinent and in the south-east Asia while it did not significantly affect the countries of the south-west Asia.

Another disease which shows the influence of climate on its distribution is endemic syphilis in the form of yaws caused by spirochetes. The disease is reported in the southern and the eastern parts of the Indian subcontinent, Indonesia and Malaysia. This disease is not reported in the dry western region and its place is taken by a rather infrequently, reported disease known as 'Bejal'.

Filariasis which is caused by *W. bancrofti* and *B. Malayi* is found extensively on the eastern side of the ecological watershed. The high rainfall and other climatic factors are favourable for the mosquito

C. fatigans. This is an important public health problem in several countries of south-east Asia. On the other hand, south-west Asia and the north-western part of India, are virtually free from this disease.

Guinea worm disease, which is caused by *D. medinesis* is found in places where the rainfall is scanty and people have to depend on the water supply from the stagnant ponds and wells. It is found essentially to the west of the ecological watershed, though several areas in the dry west zone are free from the disease, presumably because of more hygienic methods of water usage in these areas.

The distribution of hydatid disease is largely governed by the availability of the intermediate host, *viz.*, the sheep, buffalos, and camels. These animals are mainly found in the areas on the western side of the ecological watershed. The distribution of hydatid disease therefore, is mainly found in south-west Asia, the adjacent half of India and the disease is very seldom reported from south-east Asian countries.

Certain diseases which are widely prevalent in Western and Southern Asia seem to have a progressively decreasing incidence towards the regions of south-east Asia, and are seldom found beyond the limits of the ecological watershed. This is well illustrated by progressively diminishing incidence of schistosomiasis and anthrax from the west towards the east (Fig. 4.2).

It must be remembered that the distribution pattern of a large number of communicable disorders considerably alters from year to year. The control measures in various countries for example, further limit their distribution in direct proportion to the intensity of such eradication programmes. An example of such alteration can be seen in the distribution of malaria, which affects practically every country in Southern Asia but varies from year to year.[82] Cholera is another such disease, which involves different areas of the world at different times. In the year 1970, for example, cholera extended up to the Red Sea and even to the west coast of Central Africa.[83] In any case, the classical endemic home of activity for cholera lies in Bangladesh and West Bengal and Assam in India, which lie on the eastern side of the ecological watershed from where the disease exerts a diminishing influence towards the west (Fig. 4.2), where however severe epidemics of cholera—as distinct from endemic conditions—have been common at least until recent decades.

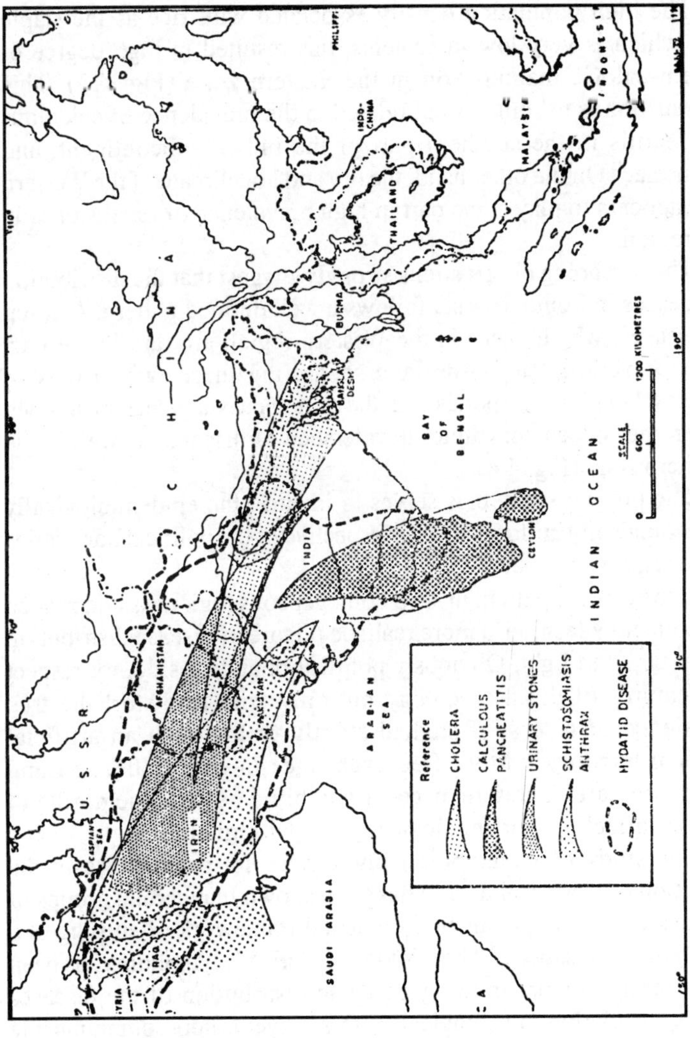

Fig. 4.2: Regional Gradients of Disease Incidence in Southern Asia.

Apart from the distribution of the infective and parasitic disorders, the distribution of certain other diseases also seems to conform to this watershed of ecology.

The high population density associated with rice as the staple diet, which is very low in proteins, has resulted in high degree of protein-calorie malnutrition in the Eastern zone (Fig. 4.3). This malnutrition is to some extent related to the prevalence of calculous pancreatitis in the southern part of the Indian subcontinent, and Indonesia.[84] On the other hand, the dry and hot climate of the Western zone appears to play some part in high prevalence of renal stones in that region.

The foregoing observations strongly suggest that the distribution of diseases in Southern Asia follows a well defined pattern. A group of diseases, which occur in the Western region are rare in the East and *vice versa*. The borderland separating these two groups of diseases, largely corresponds with the ecological watershed mentioned earlier and indeed constitutes a watershed of diseases as well in the Southern Asia (Fig. 4.4).

The present study thus serves to identify the epidemiologically and ecologically uniform areas, irrespective of the political boundaries of the region.

If the disease pattern in such homogeneous regions is undertaken in a collective fashion, a more realistic picture of disease distribution would come to light. Obviously political boundaries do not respect the features of disease ecology but only tend to distort the true prevalence of disease if studied strictly within such an artificial political territory.[85] More free exchanges in data collection and information are, therefore, necessary to bring out the true profile of diseases affecting epidemiologically similar regions.

The study of geographic pathology is not an exercise in the collection of statistical data. It has been shown that certain groups of diseases co-existing in an environmental framework often suggest a clue to their causation.[86] The etiology of Burkitt's lymphoma has been a pioneering attempt in the geographic distribution of the diseases and its correlation to ecological factors. Several non-communicable disorders like peptic ulcer, ulcerative colitis, osteoarthritis of the hip, have an entirely different pattern of distribution in Southern Asia. The clue to the causation of these diseases and to their qualitative and quantitative variations may well be found in the detailed study of the environmental factors, in ecologically similar geographic areas.

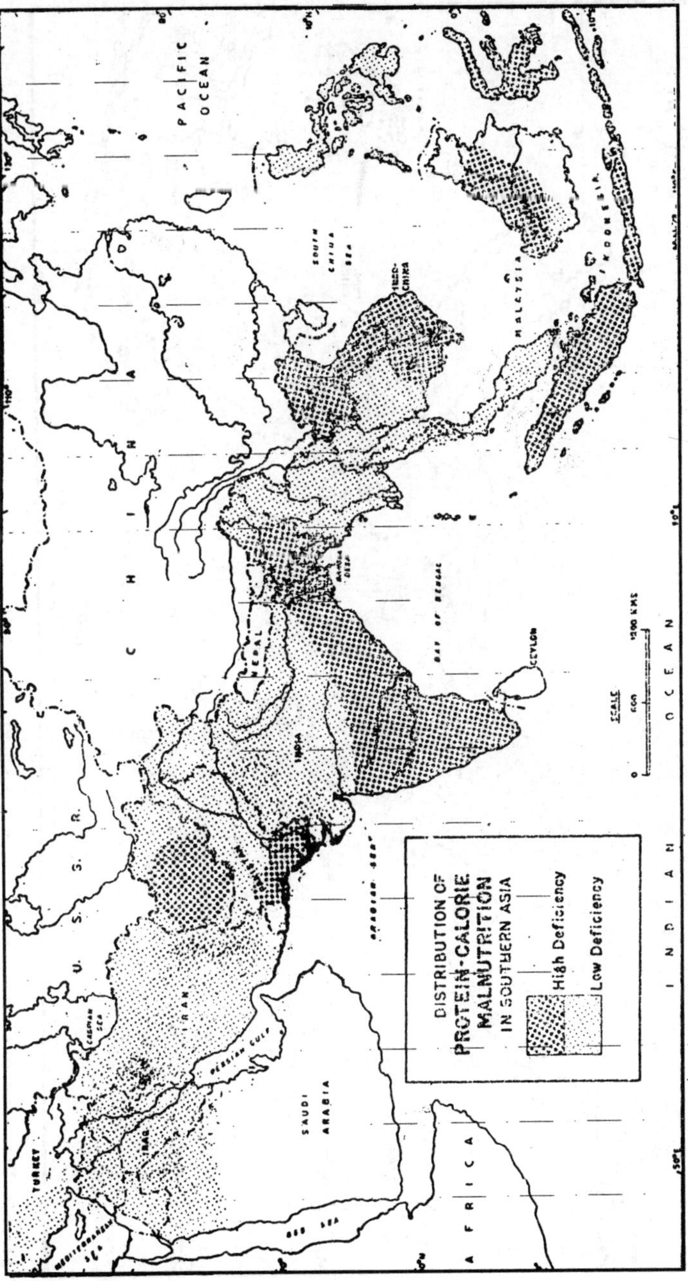

Fig. 4.3: Distribution of Protein-calorie Malnutrition in Southern Asia

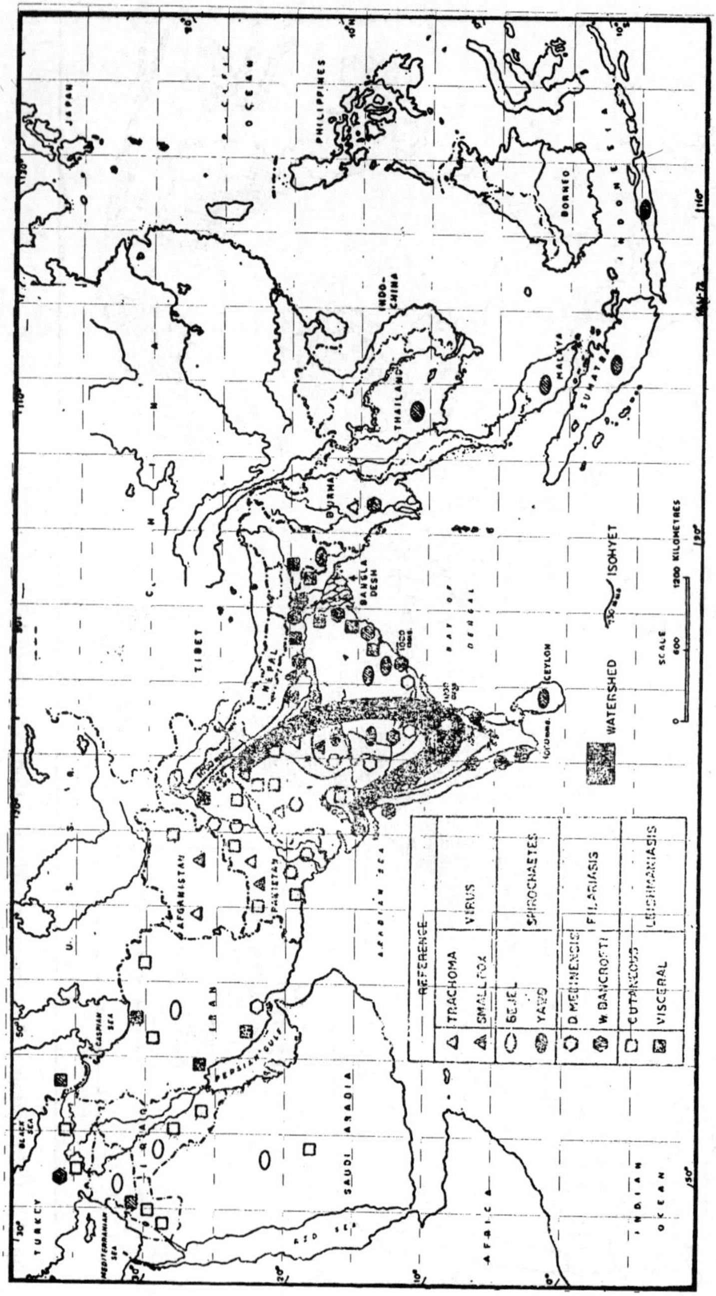

Fig. 4.4: Watershed of Diseases and Ecology in Southern Asia.

Conclusion

The present study is based on the available data regarding the disease distribution and the ecological features in Southern Asia. The ecology of this region is essentially controlled by monsoonal regime of rains in addition to the other features such as the geographic relief and rivers.

The Monsoons divide Southern Asia into two parts, *viz.*, a relatively dry western zone and the wet eastern zone. This division coincides in India roughly with the zone of 75-100 cms. rainfall isohyets.

The disease patterns of the countries in the dry west zone, from Turkey up to about the central India have striking similarities. Similarly, the countries on the eastern side of the Indian Watershed up to south-east Asian countries share a similar disease pattern. The incidence of hydatid disease, stone disease of the renal tract, trachoma, and cutaneous leishmaniasis is remarkably frequently found together in the regions on the western side of the ecological watershed while the diseases such as filariasis, cholera, visceral leishmaniasis, smallpox (now eradicated—Editors) and protein-calorie malnutrition are mainly found on its eastern side.

The peculiarities and features both of ecology and disease are discussed and a watershed separating the two groups of diseases in Southern Asia is outlined.

Notes

1. Rodenwaldt, E. and Jusatz, H.J. (1952-61), *Welt Seuchen Atlas* (World Atlas of Epidemic Diseases, 1-3, 129 maps, Hamburg: Falk Verlag.
2. Haim, S. Hirshomitz, B. and Mahler, D. (1966), A Plastic Surgery Approach in the Treatment of Ulcerative Cutaneous Leishmaniasis, *Israel J. Med. Sci.,* 2,4, 468-471.
3. Tropical Health, (1962), *Report on Study of Needs and Resources,* Publication 996, National Academy of Sciences.
4. Nadim, A.R. and Eagih, M.A. (1969), Epidemiology of cutaneous leishmaniasis in Iran, B. Khirassan Part III, Human Infection, *Bulletin de la Societé Pathlogie Exotique,* 64, 4, 710.
5. Bellezia, J.A. (1957), Survey of Health and Sanitation in Pakistan, *International Co-operation and Administration,* Washington, p. 118. Quoted in *Tropical Health: Report on Study of Needs and Resources,* Publication 996, National Academy of Sciences, p. 113, 1962.

6. Lysenko, A. Ja. (1971), Distribution of leishmaniasis in the Old World, *Bull. World Health Organization,* 44, 515.
7. *Ibid.*
8. Tropical Health, *op. cit.*
9. Editorial, Filarial Problem in Burma, *Burma Med. J.,* 15, 1960.
10. Rodenwaldt, E. and Jusatz, H.J. *op. cit.*
11. School of Public Health and Institute of Public Health and Research, *Geographical Pathology of Iran,* Publication No. 1802, Tehran, 1970.
12. Fischer, L. (1968), *Afghanistan,* Geomedical Monograph Series, Edited by H.J. Jusatz, Heidelberg Academy of Sciences, New York: Springer Verlag.
13. Awan, A.H. (1969), Communicable Diseases Control: Present Status in West Pakistan, *Pakistan J. Med. Res.,* 2, 91.
14. Tropical Health, *op. cit.*
15. W.H.O. Smallpox Eradication: The First Significant Result, *W.H.O. Chronicle,* 23, 10, 465, 1969.
16. W.H.O. A Decade of Smallpox, *W.H.O. Chronicle,* 22, 4, 134, 1968.
17. May, J.M. (1961), *Studies in Disease Ecology,* Vol. 2, *Studies in Medical Geography*, New York: Hafner.
18. Hudson, E.H. (1958), *Non-venereal Syphilis: A Sociological and Medical Study of Bejal,* Edinburgh: E. & S. Livingstone Ltd.
19. School of Public Health and Institute of Public Health and Research, *op. cit.*
20. Tropical Health, *op. cit.*
21. Cestellani, A. and Chalmers, A.J. (1919), *Manual of Tropical Medicine,* Third Edition, London: Tindall & Cox.
22. Pereira, E.D. and Ratnatunga, G.S. (1965), History of Venereal Disease Control in Ceylon, *Brit. J. Venereal Dis.,* 41, 97.
23. Ayyangar, M.C.R. (1965), Some Observations on the Epidemiology and Manifestations of Yaws, *J. Indian Med. Assn.,* 44, 190.
24. Taneja, B.L. (1967), Yaws Incidence and Epidemiology: Study in Dedhi tehsil of Distt. Mirzapur, U.P., India, *J. Trop. Med. Hyg.,* 70, 9, 215.
25. Saxena, V.B. and Prasad, B.G. (1963), An Epidemiological Study of Yaws in Madhya Pradesh: Histological and Geographical, *Indian J. Med. Res.,* 51, 768.
26. *Ibid.*
27. Tropical Health, *op. cit* .
28. Patnaik, K.C. and Kapoor, P.M. (1967), Incidence and Endemicity of Guineaworm in India, *Indian J. Med. Res.,* 55, 11, 1231. Bildhaiya, G.S., Marwah, S.M. and Patidar, S.R. (1969), An Epidemiological Assesssment of Dracontiasis, *J. Indian Med. Assn.,* 52, 2, 67. Reddy, C.R.R.M., Narasaih, I.L. and Parvathi, G. (1969), Epidemiological Studies on Guinea Worm Infection, *Bull. World Health Orgn.,* 40, 521.
29. Ansari, A.R. and Nasir, A.S. (1963-64), A Survey of Guinea Worm Disease in the Sindh Desert (Tharparkar Distt.) of West Pakistan, *Pakistan J. Health,* 13, 152.
30. Fischer, L., *op. cit.*

31. May, J.M., *op. cit.*
32. Editorial, Filarial Problem in Burma, *op. cit.*
33. Wolfe, M.S. and Aslamkhan, M. (1968), Ecology of Filariasis in East Pakistan, *Abstracts and Review,* 8th International Congress of Tropical Medicine and Malaria.
34. I.C.M.R., 1967. *Report of the Assessment Committee on the National Filaria Control Programme, India,* New Delhi: Indian Council of Medical Research.
35. Joseph, G. and Prasad, B.G. (1967), An Epidemiological Study of Filariasis in the Coastal Belt of Kerala State, *Indian Journal Medical Research,* 55, 1259.
36. Basu, P.C., Rao, V.N. and Pattanayak, S. (1967), *Filariasis in Greater Bombay: Results of a Rapid Survey Conducted in June,1965.* Delhi: National Institute of Communicable Diseases.
37. Rao, C.K., Russel, S. and Das, M. (1976), Filariasis Problem in Non-endemic States—India, *J. Comm. Dis.,* 8, 3, 221.
38. Wolfe, M.S. and Aslamkhan, M. (1969), Filariasis Survey in Karachi, *Trans. R. Soc. Trop. Med. Hyg.*, 63, 147.
39. Fischer, L., *op. cit.*
40. May, J.M., *op. cit.*
41. Kutty, K.M., Krishna, M. and Nambiar, B. (1970), A Case of Pulmonary Hydatid Disease, *Med. J. Malaya,* 24, 4, 302.
42. Devdasan, C. (1974), Hydatid Disease in India, *Acta Trop.,* 31, 4, 378.
43. Reddy, C.R.R.M., Narasaih, I.L. and Parvathi, G., *op. cit.*
44. Bhandarkar, L.D. and Talwalkar, G.V. (1973), Hydatid Disease: A Report of 35 Cases, *Indian J. Med. Sci.,* 27, 11, 849.
45. Upadhyaya, G.H., Rai, P. and Shah, P.K. (1974), Clinical Study of Hydatid Disease in Jamnagar, *J. Indian Med, Assoc.,* 63, 213.
46. Gupta, J.C., Nagrath, C.L. and Salgia, K.M. (1966), Hydatid Disease in Man, *J. Indian Med. Assoc.,* 46, 649.
47. Fischer, L., *op. cit.*
48. Talib, H. (1968), Some Surgical Aspects of Hydatid Disease in Iraq, *Brit. J. Surg.,* 55, 8, 576.
49. Schwabe, C.W. and Daoud, K.A. (1961), Epidemiology of Echinococcosis in the Middle East, I. Human Infection in Lebanon 1949 to 1959, *Amer. J. Trop. Med. Hyg.,*10, 374.
50. Paramanathan, C.D. and Dissanaike, A.S. (1961), Sylvatic Hydatid Infection in Ceylon, *Trans. R. Soc. Trop. Med. Hyg.,* 55, 483.
51. Rao, B.V. (1968), Certain Biological and Epidemiological Consideration of Hydatidosis in India with Special Reference to Buffalo Material, *Bull. Ind. Soc. Med. Com. Dis.,* 3-4, 257.
52. School of Public Health and Institute of Public Health and Research, *op. cit.*
53. Fischer, L., *op. cit.*
54. Khan, M.A. and Ahmad, N. (1962-63), Outbreak of cutaneous anthrax in Jhang Dist. (West Pakistan) in 1962, *Pakistan J. Health,* 12, 76.
55. Rao, B.V., *op. cit.*

56. W.H.O., 1970. *Summary of Vital Health Statistics,* New Delhi: W.H.O. Regional Office, South-East Asia Region.
57. Tropical Health, *op. cit*.
58. Dave, P.J. and Dhage, K.R. (1958), Resurvey and Present Status of the Endemic Focus of schistosomiasis, *Indian J. Med. Res.,* 46, 546.
59. Shrivastava, K.K. and Arora, M.M. (1969), Schistosoma haematobium infection in Lohager, a Village in Raipur District of M.P., *Indian J. Med. Res.,* 57, 11, 2016.
60. Anderson, D.A.; Sriramchari, S. and Khandagale, M.K. (1963), Investigation into Relationship between Bladder Stones and Malnutrition, *Indian J. Med. Sciences,* 17, 617.
61. Joshi, M.J.; Karnik, S.M. and Purohit, G.G. (1975), The Pattern of Surgical Disorders in Poona, *J. Indian Med, Assoc.,* 65, 3, 70. Shah, H.S.; Kanvinde, M.S.; Shukla, B.K. and Mehta, K.N. (1969), Hydatid Disease : A Comparative Review of its Incidence in Ahmedabad with that in other Parts of India, *Indian J. Med, Sci.,* 23, 380.
62. Shah, R.C. and Julundhwala, J.M. (1959), Urinary Calculi in North Gujarat, *J. Indian Med. Assoc.,* 32, 11, 440.
63. Shah, K.K. and Mehta, R.C. (1966), Suprapubic Cystolithotomy in Children, *J. Indian Med. Assoc.,* 47, 11, 554.
64. Rao Balakrishna, B.N., Gupta, H.N. and Ranganker, G.V. (1964), Chemical Composition of Urinary Calculi, *J. Indian Med, Assoc.,* 43, 9, 469.
65. Das, P. (1960), Some Clinical Observations on Urinary Calculi, *J. Indian Med. Assoc.,* 34, 2, 51.
66. Chawla, S. and Gadekar, N.G. (1961), Distribution of Renal Stones in calyces, *J. Indian Med. Assoc.,* 37, 7, 347.
67. Thind, S.K. and Nath, R. (1969), Chemical Analysis of Urinary Calculous in Chandigarh Area, *Indian J. Med. Res.,* 57, 1790.
68. Sachdeva, Y. and Maria, S.K.S. (1966), Partial nephrectomy in calculus Disease, *Indian J. Surg.,* 28, 3, 161.
69. Kaul, S. and Verma, S.L. (1967), Oxalate Contents of Foods Commonly used in Kashmir, *Indian J. Med., Res.,* 55, 274.
70. Fischer, L., *op. cit.*
71. Hedayat, S.H.; Amirshahy, P. Moatamed, K. and Pazeshkan, M. (1970), Urinary lithiasis in Iran: A Retrospective Study based on 2114 operations, *Trop. Geogr., Med.,* 22, 416.
72. Adenwalia, H.S., Menon, P.U., Joseph, A. and Mangrola, P.P. (1965), Multiple Urinary Calculi in Man Aged 59 years, *Indian J. Surg.,* 27, 97.
73. Halstead, S.B. (1961), Bladder Stone in Thailand: A Review of the Problem, *J. Trop. Med. Hyg.,* 10, 918.
74. Geeverghese, P.J. (1968), *Pancreatic Diabetes, A Clinico-pathologic Study of Growth Onset Diabetes with Pancreatic Calculi,* Bombay: Popular Prakashan.
75. Abraham, P.A. (1969), Pancreatic lithiasis, *Indian J. Surg.,* 31, 6, 588.
76. Joshi, M.J. (1972), Tropical form of Primary Calculous Pancreatitis, *Pahalvi Med. J.,* 3, 250.

77. Shah, M.M.; Vyas, B.K. and Smell, W.P. (1969), Chronic Relapsing Pancreatitis, *Indian J. Surg.*, 31, 3, 274.
78. Rajsuriya, K.; Thenabadu, P.N. and Munasinghe, D.R. (1970), Pancreatic Calcification in Ceylon with Special Reference to its Etiology, *Ceylon Med. J.*, 15, 1, 11.
79. Joshi, M.J. (1983), *Surgical Diseases in the Tropics,* New Delhi: MacMillan Co.
80. Sivaramakrishnaiyah, K and Ramanathan, R. (1967), Studies on the Effect of Climate on Leishmaniasis in India, *Indian J. Med. Res.*, 55, 11, 1159.
81. Rodenwaldt, E. and Jusatz, H.J., *op. cit.*
82. W.H.O. Malaria Eradication in 1970, *W.H.O. Chronicle,* 25, 11, 498, 1971.
83. W.H.O. Epidemiological and Statistical Information: Cholera in 1970, *W.H.O. Chronicle,* 25, 11, 509, 1971.
84. Zuidema, P.J. (1959), Cirrhosis and Disseminated Calcification of the Pancreas in Patients with Malnutrition, *Trop. Gegr. Med.*, 11, 70.
85. Burkitt, D.P. and Hutt, M.S.R. (1966), An Approach to Geographical Pathology in Developing Countries, *International Pathology,* 7, 1.
86. Burkitt, D.P. (1970), Relationship as a Clue to Causation (Personal Communication).

5
Geomedical Method with Illustration in the Study of Rajasthan

A.K. Tewari

Geomedical Method

The geomedical method consists of public health studies in varied areal complexes. The geographers' contribution in this field is by way of graphic and numeric analysis of spatial variations and associations of endemic and epidemic diseases. The causative factors of human maladies become self-evident when correlated with the elements of environment. The concrete relationship between areas of contaminated water and incidence of cholera in London was established only after the publication of Dr. John Snow's cholera map of 1849. The possible cause-effect relationship of complex environment can be expressed by mortality and morbidity indices.[1] This yields a unique philosophy of ecological synthesis of public health information. This is what we call Medical Geography. Its aim is three-fold—firstly, to analyse data concerning the incidence of disease, secondly, to map them in a form suitable for correlation and testing and finally, the testing of data through theoretical models to assess whether the pattern has some relationship with other spatial factors and to decide on the relevance of such spatial association.[2]

Health is not merely a diseaseless body but a state of complete physical, mental and social harmony of man.[3] All those factors manifest in our surroundings, our food, genes and material well-being

Reprinted after having been edited, from *The Rajasthan Medical Journal,* 12, 181-190, 1973.

are more important than the pathological factors. J.M. May has truly identified the environmental and pathological factors as 'geogens' and 'pathogens' respectively. Study of geogens in the dimensions of space and time is known as geomedical study.[4] Such studies in micro-regional level constitute an important part of cultural geography in Britain, Germany, France, Sweden, U.S.A. and U.S.S.R. German geographers have undertaken several such studies (medizinische lánderkunde) in developing countries of Asia and Africa.[5]

Scheme of Geomedical Study

In the last two decades medical geography has been subjected to such a great strain that geographers have either divorced this aspect of their discipline or have substantially changed their technique to be fit the needs of medical professionals. The present-day quantitative revolution has come as a saviour to our traditional concepts. Now, it is easier to analyse and interpret varied environmental conditions by the use of numerical and statistical methods. The spatial interaction of regional hospitals and their service areas are depicted by hospital tributary area maps.[6]

Similarly, studies in spatial diffusion have become common in medical geography. Spread of systematic control of bovine tuberculosis in Sweden is an example of diffusion of innovation.[7] The planning for possible location of new hospitals is based on simulation of hourly travel zone maps and population distribution.

Obviously, the statistical technique requires a myriad of data and their computerization is quite unpracticable under condition of paucity of accurate and complete medical health statistics. It will be seen in this chapter that Jusatz's method of regional geomedical study is more suitable for developing countries.[8] In this chapter, the complex ecological conditions of Rajasthan have been examined under four categories: the geo-factor, human factor, environmental sanitation and the disease incidence. In Table 5.1 various schemes of geo-medical studies are given.

The first task of a medical geographer is to analyse all factors of physical environment (climate, soils, water resources and so on) together with their influence on man and his activities. The type and amount of our nutritional needs depend, to a great extent, on the productivity of soil and overall resources of a region. Poor food supply means poor health, malnutrition and more susceptibility to malady.

Table 5.1: Schemes of Geo-medical Study of an Area

Maximilien Sorre 1943	*Wilhelm Rimpau 1945*	*Willy Hellpach 1955-65*	*Helmut J. Jusatz 1968-1970*
I. Relation between physical environment and man	I. Geochoros: Physical conditions of environment	I. Toponosogram : Disease linked to certain type of climate and landscape.	I. Geo-factor: Analysis of the influence of physical environment on man, animal and plant.
II. Living part of the environment and the nutrition of man	II. Biochoros : Population, its customs and changes	II. (a) Genosogram: Genetic Diseases. (b) Ethno-nosogram: Ethnic-diseases. (c) Socionoso-gram: Disease linked to social structure,	II. Strandort-biologie (Environmental biology)-men, his ways of life and traditions.
III. Man and his fight with the biological environment (pathogenic complexes)	III. Nosochoros : Spectrum of disease.	III. Nosogram: Spectrum of diseases.	III. Environmental pathology: Incidence of disease and environmental sanitation.

Source: Classification by the Author of the Chapter.

The next step is to describe and correlate the human factors of socio-economic origin which modify the geo-medical panorama. Certain races are immune to certain diseases whereas certain diseases occur to the people of particular sex and age group. This aspect of medical geography is known as environmental biology (Strandort-biologie). The factors of heredity may be conveniently included in this group of discussion. All these correlations, no doubt, are not always correct until empirical evidences are achieved by proofs of causation.

Finally, the human responses of both individual and community are taken into account by means of which the people protect themselves from the dangerous influence of environment. This is known as environmental sanitation and pathology. In India, such studies are of recent origin although its rudimentary beginning may be traced as far back as the days of Vedic culture.[9] The state of Rajasthan has been selected for the application of this method with a view to identify interregional geo-medical conditions in arid, semi-arid and sub-humid environments.

Geofactors

Primary Factors

The complex problems of medical geography are the consequence of geographical factors, particularly the nature of climate and soil. Lying largely within the arid and semi-arid belt of India the state of Rajasthan exhibits sharp regional variations (Fig. 5.1A) in climate and land use potentialities. It covers an area of 3,42,272 sq km within which climate varies from tropical sub-humid in the southern hilly region to an extremely dry zone of Jaisalmer-Barmer desert. Dry climate and general paucity of fresh water resources are the primary geographical factors responsible for the infection and dissemination of disease vectors in Rajasthan.

Climatic aridity on the one hand, serves as a natural check through desiccation of pathogens, yet on the other hand causes greater infection of wind-borne diseases of eyes and lungs, accentuation of dehydration and loss of body fluids. The deficiency of these elements in human body causes early ageing and greying. The quantity of dust and sand particles is so high in the air that hardly anyone can escape from respiratory diseases. The incidence of respiratory disease in Rajasthan is one of the highest (Table 5.4) as compared to its

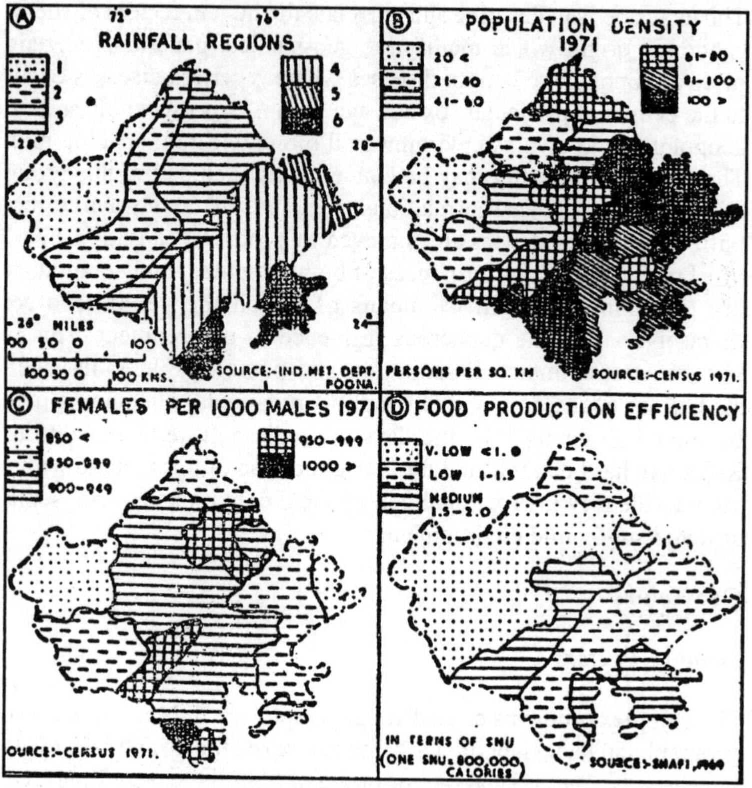

Fig. 5.1: A, B, C, D: 1—*Arid, Rainfall below 200 mm*

1—Arid, Rainfall below 200 mm, Variability above 50 per cent.
2—Semi-arid, Rainfall 200-500 mm, Variability above 50 per cent.
3—Moderately arid, Rainfall 200-500 mm, Variability 50-35 per cent.
4—Transitional zone, Rainfall 500-800 mm, Variability 50-30 per cent.
5—Moderately sub-humid, Rainfall 500-800 mm, Variability 35-20 per cent.
6—Sub-humid, Rainfall 800-1200 mm, Variability 35-20 per cent.

population (more than 1 per 1,00,000 of population mortality rate). The higher intake of fats—in the form of *ghee* and *tila* oil—is an environmental necessity to meet the challenge of dryness. The direct effect of thermal stress and strains can be noted in the internal physiological process of the human body and its performance. Even the tall and slender constitution of the people of western Rajasthan appears to be an anatomical adjustment to hot desertic conditions.

Secondary Factor

Climate manifests the water condition and floral and faunal associations of a region. Consequently, fresh water resources are meagre in the greater part of Rajasthan. People depend mainly upon water stored in tanks and reservoirs or a few wells with scanty inflow feeding. These reservoirs are usually contaminated and provided natural habitat for several types of cyclops harbouring parasitic diseases. Scarcity of water also causes insanitary living and unhygienic habits. On the eastern and southern parts of Rajasthan both surface and groundwater conditions are better, yet the unhygienic habits of the rural folk makes them victims of parasitic diseases. The endemic zone of guinea worm (dracunculiasis) in Rajasthan is an expression of population dependence on contaminated groundwater resources.[10]

Apart from the contamination of ground water, the quality of aquifers also poses several ecological problems. Many minerals and salts accumulated in the closed aquifers during the geological past, render the groundwater heavy and brackish. There are vague yet definite associations between iodine deficiency and goitre, and fluorine excesses and softening of bones. Around the village of Ranigaon (Tahsil Parbatsar, District Nagaur) in Rajasthan, there is a belt of more than 300 sq. km. where fluorine content in groundwater is more than 10 p.p.m. with a result that 20 per cent of its estimated population of 25,000 are suffering from skeletal fluorosis. Similarly, around village Sagaria (District Sirohi) about 4000 people inhabiting an area of 80 sq. km. are virtually crippled due to fluorosis. From time immemorial, the intake of fluorine-rich water has deformed these people and spoiled their teeth and jaws. These areas abound in hunchbacks with mottled enamel. The samples of groundwater have revealed the presence of soluble fluorides of calcium, sodium and potassium in these areas. Strangely, fluorine in drinking water has an inverse relationship to the incidence of caries in a community. Mottled teeth are strongly resistant to dental decay because the fluoride deposited on the enamel lowers the solubility of calcium tissues to acids.

Tertiary Factors

Apart from the climate and water conditions of a region, the floral and faunal composition is also an important determinant of the occurrence and prevalence of diseases. The gerbille (mouse) of Indian desert is a great public health hazard. Apart from causing damage to crops and property, it carries germs of bubonic plague and typhus. Fortunately, plague is unknown in Rajasthan for the last several decades. But the damage to crops and animal feed is of such a great dimension that rodents can snatch away more than half of our nutritional reserves. Incidentally, the gerbille population is highest at the time of famines. The religious sanctity and superstitions have complicated this problem in Rajasthan. In the Karni Devi Temple (near Bikaner) rats are fed and protected for the last 500 years. Sparrows and crows are other agents of dissemination of pathogens.

Human Factors

Nutritional Factor

Among human factors affecting the occurrence and endemicity of diseases, the man, his heredity (genes), mode of living, socio-economic status and movements are most important. Although the density of population in Rajasthan (Fig. 5.1B) is not high (75 per sq. km.) yet the carrying capacity of soil is so low that the agricultural production can hardly match the nutritional requirement of people. Agriculture in the eastern region and agriculture-*cum*-pastoralism in the western region are the mainstay of the economy. The main items of the diet of the people are *bajra,* and wheat—among the carbohydrates and starch, *moth* and *mung* among the legumes, onions and potatoes (also starchy) among the roots and vegetables, and *ghee* (clarified butter) and *til* oil among the fats and vitamin-A. It will be seen from Table 5.2 that the diet of average people in Rajasthan is amazingly deficient in proteins and vitamins.

The human body under Indian conditions requires a minimum intake of 2000 calories a day which amounts to a farm production equivalent to 8,00,000 calories per acre in a year, taking into account a loss of 10 per cent in extracting and cooking. This unit is known as the standard nutrition unit (S.N.U.). In Rajasthan, the food production efficiency is very low (Fig. 5.1D). The total S.N.U. is hardly 26,50,00,000.[11] In terms of the present population of 25,70,00,000 (Census, 1971) the per capita S.N.U. is less than a unit in the major part of the state (Table 5.2). This leads to under-nutrition, to take a section of society particularly the farm labourers

Table 5.2: Percentage of Caloric Intake in an Average Diet of Rajasthani (Based on Sample Survey in Jodhpur District 1971)

Items	*Per cent of Calories*	*Remarks*
Cereals	69	Carbohydrate, starch
Legumes	10	Proteins, carbohydrate
Ghee and oils	8	Fats and vitamin-A
Milk (including condensed milk—Khoa or Mawa)	6	Fats and proteins
Sugar and liquor	3	Glucose
Meat, eggs and pork	1.5	Proteins
Roots, vegetables, fruits	1	Starch, minerals, vitamins
Others	1.5	Variable

Apart from undernutrition, the actual intakes of protein, minerals and vitamins are far from satisfactory. Malnutrition is a serious problem of Rajasthan. The absence of fruits and vegetables in the normal diet of people is a potent cause of several deficiency diseases such as dental decay, grey hair, wrinkled faces, baldness, bladder stones and lack of initiative. The incidence of malnutrition in Rajasthan is more than 5 per 1000. The medical registers testify to the fact that more than 2,00,000 people have been reported suffering from diseases caused by vitamin, protein and iron deficiencies. Moreover, the regional variations in agricultural production warrant further hardships to the people who have witnessed repeated famines.

Complex Demographic Factor

The other human factor worthy of notice in the context of medical geography is the percentage of literacy and distribution of tribal and nomadic groups who constitute a sizeable part of the population. Literacy in Rajasthan is far below the national level particularly in the western section of the state (Fig. 5.2A). Nomadism is a dryland response to arid climate and has become an important trait of life in western areas. Most nomadic groups are associated with parasitic and venereal diseases. Their frequent movement during drought years disseminates these diseases to the sedentary peoples of Rajasthan and neighbouring states.

Similarly, the tribal population and their unhygienic ways have determined the geo-medical structure of the rural folk. They serve as the carriers and intermediate hosts of helminthic diseases, guinea worm and syphilis. Perhaps next to Africa the highest tribal population

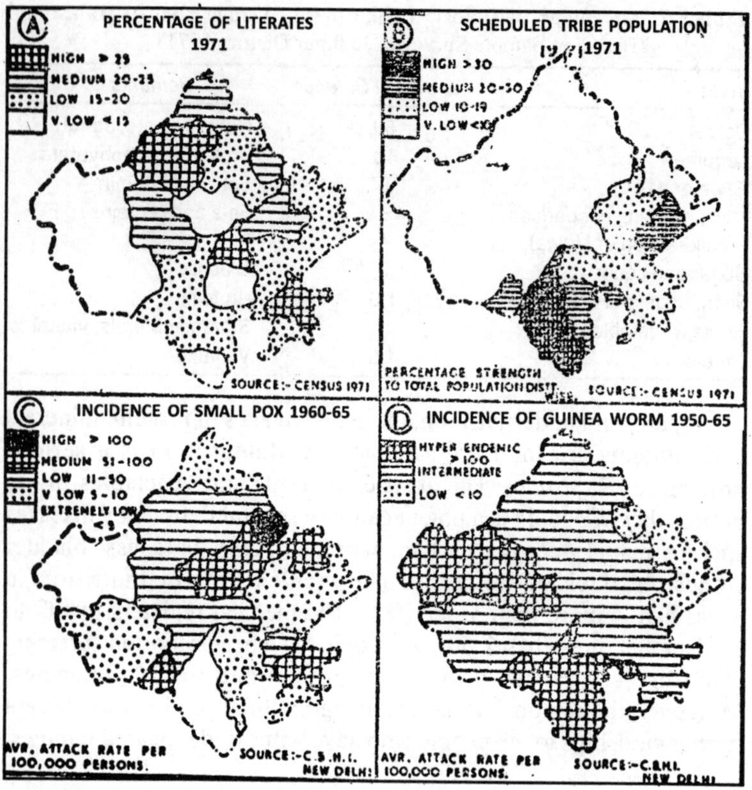

Fig. 5.2: A, B, C, D : *Literacy Distribution in Rajasthan, 1971.*

A. Percentage of Literates, 1971.
B. Scheduled Tribe Population, 1971.
C. Incidence of Small Pox 1960-65.
D. Incidence of Guinea Worm 1950-65.

of the world is to be found in India. Rajasthan is one of the important sanctuaries of tribal population accounting for 11 per cent people as tribals. Among more than 20 tribal groups, Minas (50%), Bhils, (40%) and Garasia (2%) constitute 92 per cent of the tribal population of Rajasthan. The tribal belt of Rajasthan runs from Sirohi (Fig. 5.2B) through Udaipur, Dungarpur, Chittorgarh, Banswara and Bundi to Tonk, Kota, Jaipur and Sawai Madhopur. Conspicuously, this is also an hyper endemic zone of guinea worm disease in Rajasthan (Fig. 5.2D).

The human factors as a whole are conveniently grouped as socio-economic status of the people which determine the type and amount of nutritional intake, form of dwelling and clothing, and degree of education. The economists call these factors standard of living. The per capita income of Rajasthan is hardly ₹ 240 and it varies from ₹ 370 for Ganganagar to ₹ 175 for Barmer.[12] People suffering from poverty are bound to suffer from malnutrition and disease.[13] Further hardships are added by their illiteracy, unhygienic traditions, superstitions and widespread fears to visit hospitals of modern medicine.

Environmental Sanitation

The environmental sanitation includes municipal amenities such as supply of filtered water and sewage and refuse disposal as well as the public health and medical facilities. Owing to the low rate of urbanisation and overall backwardness of the state, the public health facilities are far from satisfactory. The physical layout of villages and small towns does not favour sanitation. There are only 149 towns in Rajasthan, only 16.5 per cent of state population where filtered water and sewage facilities are available. Out of these towns only 6 towns (Ajmer, Bikaner, Jaipur, Jodhpur, Kota and Udaipur) are of the category of class-I cities and four (Alwar, Beawar, Ganganagar and Sikar) of class-II types, where municipal amenities are tolerably good. The total expenditure on public lighting and water supply in Rajasthan is only ₹ 25,000,000 (about Re 1 per capita) and on drainage, conservancy and sanitation is only ₹ 6,000,000 (about Re 0.36 per capita). In rural areas, there is practically no facility for filtered water and disposal of refuse and sewage. Narrow lanes function as drainage channels and adjoining fields as lavatories. Men and their pets usually share the same roof and drink water from common ponds. It will be seen that the diseases of zoonosis types are due to this type of living. The greater incidence of guinea worm, tape worm, ring worm, 'cow-pox' and skin disorders are the direct reflection of inadequate social hygiene.

Medical and Health Facilities

Although the per capita investment in medical and health is a bit higher than the all-India average, yet the medical and health facilities

* *Editors' note*: During the resurgence of malaria since 1965, however there is some though disputed incidence of stable malaria in western Rajasthan.

are far from satisfactory in Rajasthan. Rajasthan is fortunate enough to be situated out of the hyper-endemic zones of malaria*, cholera and other humid tropical diseases which sway our subcontinent. The per capita expenditure on public health is only ₹ 2.6 per annum. The average number of indoor and outdoor patients treated every year in Rajasthan (modern medicine) is 6,20,000 and 14,000,000 respectively. This also includes the patients who have visited hospitals and dispensaries for more than one time. There are 90 specialist doctors, 1800 Civil Assistant Surgeons and 2000 *Vaidya* and *Hakims* in Government hospitals. Fig. 5.3A gives a synoptic idea of the Government medical institutions in Rajasthan. Table 5.3 shows the distribution of in-patient beds in Rajasthan. The doctor-population ratio is between 1:1600 to 1:20,000 in different districts of Rajasthan.

Hospital Tributary Areas

It will be seen from the analysis of Fig. 5.4 that there are eight regional centres of medical facilities in Rajasthan out of which five are coupled with medical colleges. Alwar and Beawar, though they are bigger cities as compared to Bharatpur yet the number of patients is not high in these hospitals because the patients prefer to go to Delhi and Jaipur in the case of the former and to Ajmer in the case of the latter. The identification of these regional centres is based on the number of specialist doctors, in-patient bed capacity, number of patients and overall facilities in these hospitals. The serious cases reported to the district hospitals are usually referred to these institutions and the people prefer to go to them instead of getting treatment at their immediate locality. The hospital tributary areas by rail and roads have been shown by isochrones or lines of equal time distance. The heavy lines enclose the presumed region for each hospital, based on minimum travel time.

The maximum transit time from the residence of the patient to a regional hospital is more than 12 hours in the western parts of Jaisalmer and Bikaner districts. These are the sand dune stricken areas without any road and automobile service. The camel is the only mode of transport. From the areal point of view Jodhpur commands the largest hospital tributary area. The medical register of M.G. Hospital, Jodhpur, shows that patients (mostly of accidents and chronic diseases) from Tanot and Kishangarh (deep in the Thar desert near Indo-Pak border) have been treated or died at Jodhpur. Ajmer and Jaipur rank at the top in serving the highest number of patients.

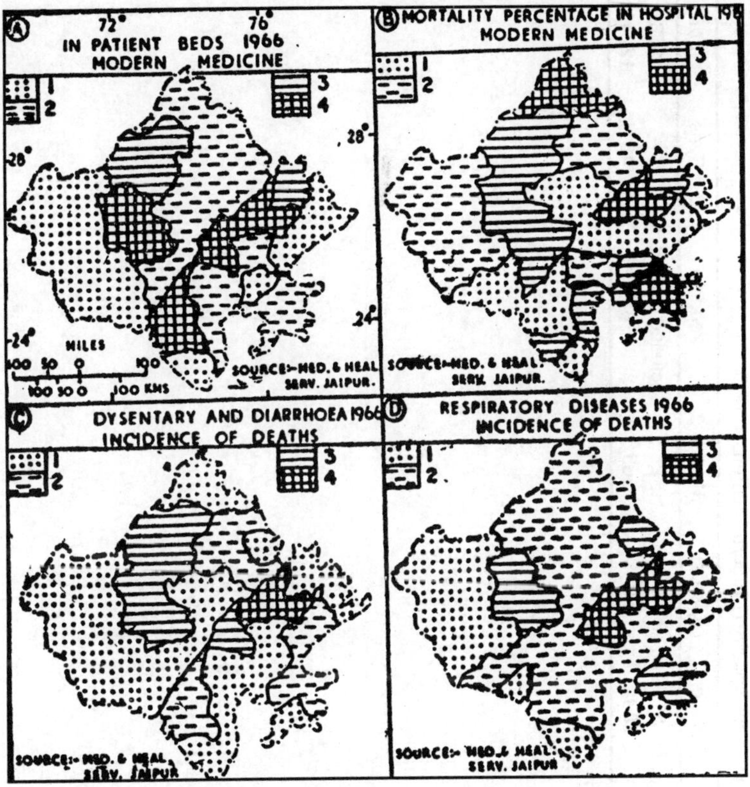

Fig. 5.3: A, B, C, D : *Medical Facilities and Incidence of Diseases.*

A—1. Very poor facilities below 200 beds in one district;
 2. Poor, 200-500 beds in one district;
 3. Medium 500-1000 beds in one district;
 4. Good facilities, 1000-2000 beds in one district.

B—1. Very low, below 1 per cent to total patients treated.
 2. Low 1-2 per cent;
 3. Medium 2-3 per cent;
 4. High 3-3.6 per cent to total patients treated.

C—1. Very low, 3-25 in a year per district;
 2. Low 25-100;
 3. Medium 100-500:
 4. High 500-600 in a year per district.

D—1. Very low, 9-15 in a year per district;
 2. Low 25-100;
 3. Medium 100-500;
 4. High. 500-550 in a year per district.

Table 5.3: State Public Hospitals and their in-patient Bed Capacity (Modern Medicine)

Institution	*General*	*Maternity*	*T.B.*	*Isolation*	*Leperosy*	*Mental*	*Venerial*	*Eyes*	*Total*
Numbers	298	4	21	2	2	2	Included in general	—	368
Beds	8066	1478	1482	289	95	305	45	481	12241

Source: Medical and Meal Survey, Jaipur, Rajasthan.

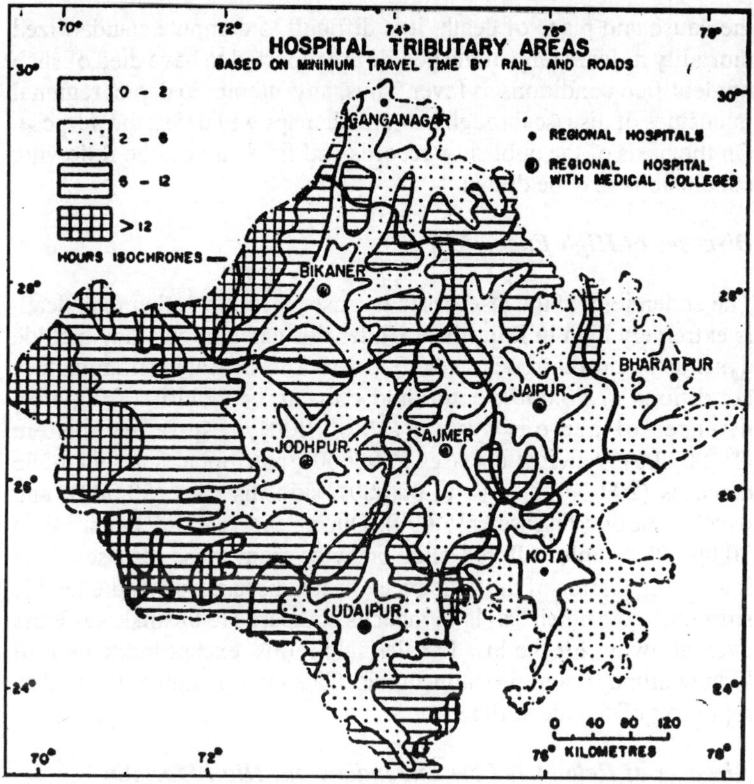

Fig. 5.4: Hospital Tributary Areas: Based on Minimum Travel Time by Rail and Roads.

Source: Rajasthan State Roadways and Railway Map of India.

Disease Incidence

The medical statistics published by the Rajasthan Medical and Health Department are most misleading, for they include only those cases which are reported in the state hospitals and dispensaries. A majority of patients in rural areas are neither attended by physicians nor reach the clinical stage of sickness. This results in an evident concentration of incidence of diseases in urban areas where medical institutions are located. Moreover, the medical and diagnostic practices vary from hospital to hospital and registration of actual causes of mortality or morbidity is unreliable. In the absence of death certificates indicating the cause and place of death, it is difficult to compute standardized mortality ratios. Many of the people are reported to have died of such unidentified conditions as fever. Thus, any attempt to depict regional intensities of disease through choropleth maps will defeat the purpose. On the basis of the published records and field survey, the following conclusions may be drawn.

Diseases of High Endemicity

The endemicity of the diseases that cause morbidity rather than death is extremely high in Rajasthan. Under this category we may include dysentery and diarrhoea (8,00,000 cases in a year), inflammatory conditions (7,50,000), acute and chronic bronchitis (7,00,000), diseases of nervous system (10,00,000), respiratory system (10,00,000), venereal diseases (3,00000), nutritional and metabolic diseases (20,00,000), eye (1,00,000), skin diseases (50,000), and psychoneurotic diseases (15,000). During the year 1971 more than 20,00,000 people suffered once or twice from these diseases. One interesting feature of the incidence of such diseases is that the female sufferers were much less in number as compared to the male sufferers even allowing for the low female/male ratios, except in the case of kidney ailments and psychoneurosis. This may be due to the under-reporting of female sufferers.

Diseases of Relatively Low Endemicity but High Mortality

Such diseases as those called great killers of tropical lands are few in Rajasthan. Cholera, smallpox, malaria and plague are almost non-existent in the western region of the state (Table 5.4). The isohyet of 66 mm may be considered as the geo-medical boundary for the epidemics in Rajasthan. In the year 1971, the percentage of deaths to total indoor patients in the hospitals of Rajasthan was only 1.3, which is much below the all-India average. Accidents, injuries and suicides cause more mortality in the age group of 14-45 than disease itself. Human sacrifice is also common in the tribal belt of Rajasthan*. The incidence of cancer in Rajasthan is highly variable. Between 1960 and 1971 about 20,000 to 90,000 (malignant neoplasm) cases have been reported from Rajasthan but the mortality rate in the state

* The editors wonder if female infanticide has somehow become confused with human sacrifice as such, and if either of these practices survive in 1985 on the scale suggested in the text.

hospitals is hardly more than 10 a year. It may be possible that the patients who reached the serious stage of this ailment may have either died at home or at other nursing centres outside Rajasthan. Table 5.4 shows causes of mortality as reported from state medical and other institutions (average of 1961-1971).[14]

Table 5.4: Diseases of low Endemicity and High Mortality

Causes of mortality	*Male*	*Female*	*Total*
Fevers (Other than Malaria)	4000	1000	5000
Respiratory Diseases	2000	600	2600
Dysentery and Diarrhoea	1000	400	1400
Heart Diseases	400	130	530
T.B.	230	150	380
Smallpox	200	100	300
Malaria	13	2	15
Cancer	7	3	10
Infant Mortality	2000	1800	3800
Injuries, Suicides and so on	2000	450	2450
Causes not Known	5	10	15

Zoonoses and other Parasitic Diseases

Several diseases harboured by animals and man are common in the rural areas of Rajasthan. Helminthic diseases (hookworm and roundworm) and dracunculiasis (guinea worm) may be included in this category. The occurrence of hookworm is highest in Jodhpur, Bikaner and Jaisalmer because of the higher density of cattle and livestock population in these areas. The maximum levels of round worm cases are recorded in the sub-humid eastern districts of Rajasthan such as Bharatpur, Sawai Madhopur, Ajmer, and Jaipur. The endemic zone of guinea worm is situated in southern Rajasthan where the step-wells and ponds are the only source of drinking water. These water reservoirs are easily contaminated by the infected people and animals. In the districts of Udaipur, Dungarpur, Banswara, Bhilwara, Chittorgarh and Jodhpur more than 70 per cent of the adults, especially males suffer from this disease during the rainy season.

Notes

1. Howe, G.M. (1970), *National Atlas of Disease Mortality in the United Kingdom,* London: Nelson.

2. McGlashan, N.D. (1972), *Medical Geography: Techniques and Field Studies,* London: Methuen.
3. W.H.O. *International Classification of Disease,* Vol. 1, Geneva, 1965 *W.H.O. Weekly Epidemic Record,* No. 18, Geneva, 1972.
4. May, J.M. (1950), Medical Geography: Its Methods and Objectives, *Geographical Review,* 40, 10-41.
5. Jusatz, H.J. (1968), Methods for Compilation of Regional Geo-medical Study, Paper presented at the *21st International Geographical Congress, Commission on Medical Geography,* New Delhi. Geo-medical Monographs on *Libya* by H. Kanter (1967), *Afghanistan* by L. Fischer (1968), *Kuwait* by G.E. French and A.G. Hill (1971), and *Ethiopia* by K.F. Schaller and W. Kuls (1972). These Monographs were edited by H.J. Jusatz and published by the Heidelberg Academy of Sciences, Berlin: Springer-Verlag.
6. Godlund, S. (1961), *Population, Regional Hospitals, Transport Facilities and Regions,* Lund Studies in Geography, Series B. Human Geography, No. 21.
7. Hàgerstrand, T. (1967), *Innovation Diffusion as a Spatial Process,* Chicago: Chicago University Press.
8. Jusatz, H.J., *op. cit.*
9. Misra, R.P. (1970), *Medical Geography of India,* New Delhi: National Book Trust.
10. Tewari, A.K. (1970), Incidence and Ecology of Guinea Worm Disease in Rajasthan, *Deccan Geographer,* 8, 1-14.
11. Shafi, M. (1969), Can India Support Five Times Her Population? *Science Today,* 3, 21-27.
12. N.C.A.E.R. (1963), *Techno-economic Survey of Rajasthan,* New Delhi.
13. Kariel, H.G. and Kariel, P.E. (1972), *Exploration in Social Geography,* Philippines: Addison Werley Pub. Co. Inc.,
14. Directorate of Medical and Health Services, Rajasthan, Jaipur, Data compiled for 1960-71.

PART II
Disease Ecology

6

The Diffusion and Ecology of Cholera in India

M.K. Dutta

Cholera, a water-borne infectious disease, is believed to have existed in India since the beginning of recorded history.[1] It was endemic only in parts of India, and the first great spread of an epidemic occurred in the years 1817 to 1819. During this period, it became the scourge of Monsoon Asia being spread by shipping eastwards of China and Japan. It further moved up to the shores of the Mediterranean through Mesopotamia and up to the east coast of Africa across the Indian Ocean. This period of expansion was followed by the pandemics of 1826-1837, 1842-1862, 1865-1875, and 1879-1911, and, thereafter, it was stopped by quarantine. Later, it broke out in Europe in 1923 and in Egypt in 1947. But today cholera is back to its pre-1817 endemic area where it breaks out at intervals.[2]* Undoubtedly, several ecological factors allow the development of the disease in this area. The prime objective of this study is to shed light on the factors involved in its incidence in limited areas in the endemic form and in scattered areas in the form of epidemics and to focus on its diffusion over space.

Endemic Areas

In studying the incidence of cholera from 1900 to 1945, Swaroop

---

Reprinted after having been edited, from *Geographical Review of India*, 35, 243-262, 1973.

* This discussion is not designed to include the spread of El Tor cholera since 1961—see Jusatz, H.J. Cholera, in G.M. Howe (Ed.) *A World Geography of Human Diseases*, London: Academic Press, 1977.

and Pollitzer distinguished between areas where the disease never died out completely and those where it was absent during several weeks and months. They believed that the prime centres of cholera endemicity "lie at and around the confluence of the Hooghly, Rupnarayan and Damodar rivers"[3], and the important endemic centres are limited to six areas which are mentioned here in order of importance: (i) districts of Burdwan, Midnapore, Hooghly, Howrah, Calcutta, 24-Parganas, constituting the western part of the Ganga delta; (ii) districts of Balasore, Cuttack, Puri in the Mahanadi delta; (iii) districts of Bhagalpur, Monghyr, Gaya, Patna, Muzaffarpur, Ballia, Azamgarh, Gorakhpur, Basti, Ghazipur, Varanasi, Shahabad in the middle Ganga plain; (iv) districts of Darrang, Kamrup, Goalpara in the lower Brahmaputra Valley; (v) districts of Tanjavur, Tiruchirapalli, South Arcot in the Ponnaiyar-Kaveri delta; and (vi) districts of Krishna, West Godavari, Guntur in the Krishna-Godavari delta (Fig. 6.1).

Common factors to all these endemic areas are that they are situated in close relation to surface-water systems, that they are densely populated, and that they lie at an altitude hardly exceeding 500 metres above the sea-level.

Epidemic Cholera and Periodicity

Although endemic areas spread over parts of several States of India, it is believed that Indian epidemic cholera originates from the Bengal delta and shows a seasonal incidence.[4] Cholera has been found to occur here during the period of September to November, and reaches its peak in late December or early January. It then travels westward, and the epidemic sweeps through Bihar and Uttar Pradesh where it remains latent when the winter starts. But it starts moving again in March or April, and extends in two directions. It proceeds easily up to the Punjab in the north-west where it reaches between July and September. This extension from West Bengal through Uttar Pradesh to the Punjab is known as the "northern epidemic highway". Another branch, called the "southern epidemic highway", carried cholera through Madhya Pradesh to the States of South India between August and November. According to the records available, cholera epidemics have mostly followed these general routes. It is a matter of surprise that the disease has never followed any route along the eastern coast to reach Madras and any short route to reach Bombay. The reason

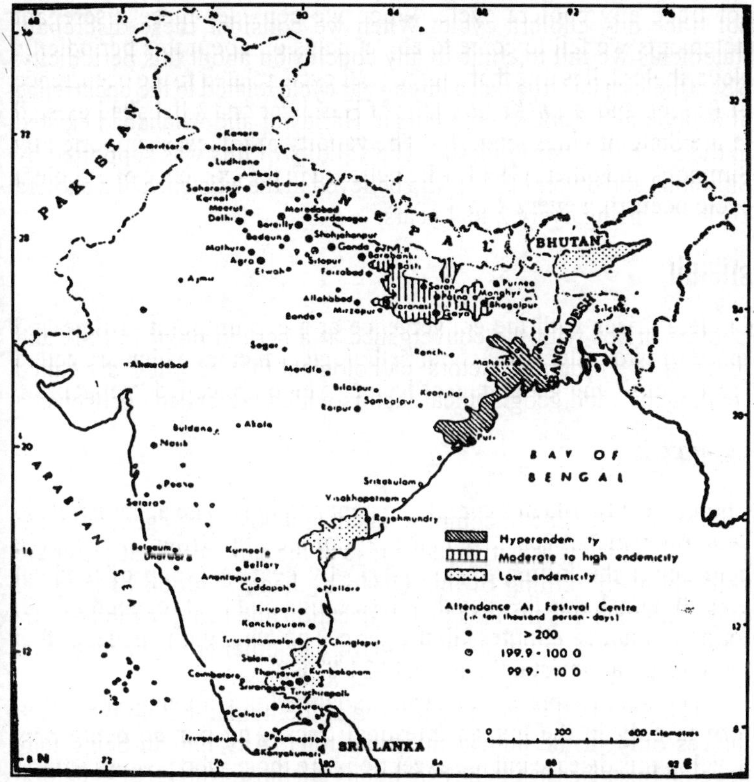

Fig. 6.1: Endemic Areas and Festival Centres Related to Cholera Diffusion.

may be that cholera has always been checked by the sparsely inhabited areas of the northern and north-eastern parts of the Deccan plateau as well as by the absence of any perennial river flowing latitudinally.

Cholera might exhibit features of a long-term periodicity which was propounded by yearly observers.[5] H.W. Bellew, in 1884, produced statistics for every province of India relating to the period 1862-1881 to prove that cholera occurred in three yearly periods, and it tends to run a definite course of revival, decline, and subsidence in the successive year of each cycle. In 1925, J.H. Russell found evidences of a six-year cycle in the State of Madras for a period of 25 years, and believed that an immunity developing in the survivors from cholera attacks accounted for the periodicity of the outbreaks. But Rogers comparing cholera epidemics for about half a century in India could not trace any cholera cycle. When we consider these discrepant statements we fail to come to any conclusion about this periodicity. Nevertheless, it is true that a three-year cycle related to the occurrence of *Kumbh* and *Ardh-Kumbh* fairs at Haridwar and Allahabad existed in the State of Uttar Pradesh". The validity of this was supported by Simmons and others (1944) who believed in the existence of a cholera cycle occurring every 2 to 4 years.[7]

Stimuli

Cholera arises with the convergence at a certain point in time and space of two orders of factors: pathological factors which are called "pathogens" and geographical factors which are called "geogens."[8]

Pathogens

Cholera is a two-factor complex: agent and host. The agent is *Vibrio cholerae* which is sensitive to the rays of the sun. Different views are held about the killing of this *vibrio* by heat. A group of medical practitioners holds the idea that desiccation and heat (beyond 56° C) for more than 15 minutes kill the germ. The other group believes that the *Vibrio* can resist cold even at –31.8° C.[9]

The host to this *Vibrio cholerae* is the human being; the *vibrio* thrives only in the human intestinal tract. Any human being may develop this disease but the exceptions are those who possess natural immunity, those who have acquired immunity after inoculation, and those who have been attacked with the disease within the last few years. People belonging to the last category grow an immunity which probably endures for a couple of years.

As a rule, cholera is transmitted through the oral introduction of the causative organism. Ingestion of water which has been contaminated with human feces and which contains *Vibro cholerae* in a viable state develops this disease. Under favourable conditions, flies too can carry the infectious feces to food. What follows after a man swallows the *Vibrio* depends on whether the juice of the stomach is high or low in hydrochloric acid. If the acid content is low, the vibrio proceeds to the intestine in which it generates quantities of endotoxins. Contrarily, the *Vibrio* is killed if the hydrochloric acid content is high. People who take curds or fresh lime juice regularly contain high quantities of this acid in their stomach, and thus acquire immunity.[10]

Geogens

The geographical factors consist of both (a) physical and (b) cultural environments. The physical environment that causes cholera in India can be studied under the headings: climate, water, and soil, and the cultural environment under the titles: pilgrimages and miscellaneous habits.

Physical environment

Climate: Reports of early observers[11] like James L. Bryden and W.R. Cornish indicated the existence of a close relationship between rainfall and spread of cholera in India. But it was Rogers who first made a large-scale study on this subject, and explored the correlation between the climatic factors and cholera in India. He found that rainfall alone did not account for the seasonal distribution of disease, because the latter was at its minimum during the south-west monsoon in Assam and the lower parts of Bengal delta, but at its maximum during the same season in other parts of the country such as the Punjab.

The mean temperature showed a closer relationship to the incidence of cholera since the disease was at its minimum during the winter season in the Punjab, the then United and Central Provinces, and the Deccan area of Bombay. But this was not true of lower Bengal. Further, the relative humidity also failed to be a good reason for the occurrence of cholera since in the Punjab, for example the latter was almost as high in the minimum cholera months of December to February as in the maximum ones of the rainy season. So, Rogers could rely only upon the absolute humidity, and plotted the seasonal cholera mortality and the data for absolute humidity on maps of India. He then pointed out that the incidence of the disease rises successively with the rise of absolute humidity to over 10 mm of vapour pressure. This is found to be true when the mortality rate is very low in most parts of the country as the 10 mm line runs very close to the littorals during the period of December to February. But from March onwards, with the rise of heat and humidity, the 10 mm line moves north-westward, and its position is taken by 20 mm line. This results in an increase of mortality which reaches its maximum in July and August. It is at this time of the year that cholera attains its peak in the whole of India except Assam and the deltaic parts of West Bengal. Then, as the 10 mm line starts retreating from a small area in the extreme north-western part of India in October, the mortality rate declines. But this decline is accompanied by a great rise in Assam and lower parts of West Bengal where in November absolute humidity is still over 11 mm. This relationship of absolute humidity to the incidence of cholera was confirmed by Banerjea[12] who made a study on the occurrence of cholera in the then United Provinces.

Water: In India rivers, their tributaries, and *nullahs,* and both open shallow wells and tube-wells are significant from the point of water-supply in rural areas. Open shallow wells yield water that is inferior to tube-well water in bacteriological quality. Besides these rivers and wells, tanks and ponds play an important role in the dissemination of cholera in different parts of the country, especially in West Bengal because of their large concentration. Contamination of water in all these sources of water-supply will be discussed in detail under the heading of : miscellaneous habits.

Soil: The nature of soil is also an important factor in the development of cholera. In the first place, it allows the seepage of water mingled with *Vibrio cholerae* which ultimately contaminates the water of ponds and wells by its horizontal movement. Secondly, the intensity of cholera is related to the nature of the soil. Sea in her study of the distribution of cholera at the *thana* (police district) level, based on 1949 to 1956 mortality data, came to the conclusion that the *thanas* having high cholera mortality occupy the new alluvial soil which is alkaline in nature and contains 15 to 50 per cent of silt and 15 to 75 per cent of clay.[13] Accordingly, most of the *thanas* of the districts of Howrah and 24-Parganas of West Bengal have a high intensity of cholera. In contrast, no death was recorded from cholera during the period under study in different *thanas* of the districts of Darjeeling, Jalpaiguri, and Coochbehar which are rich in acidic soil.

Cultural Environment

Pilgrimages: Pathologically man is tied to his culture. Religious gatherings have been notorious, specially for spreading epidemics of cholera in India. Besides pilgrims, a large number of people such as hawkers, vendors of varieties of articles, professional beggars, lepers, and *sadhus* move from one centre to another, and are almost permanently in motion. Most of the people who congregate in the holy places from far and wide are ignorant, poor, and undernourished villagers. These characteristics associated with other difficulties in providing adequate sanitary arrangements and hygienic food and water supplies for such huge assemblies brought about optimal conditions for the generation and diffusion of cholera in the past.[14]

A study of the *Kumbh* fairs is instructive. These are by far the largest fairs in India attended by several millions of people in a few days. These are held at Haridwar and Allahabad alternatively every sixth year. There is an *Ardh-Kumbh* at either place in between two *Kumbhs*. Obviously, there is a major pilgrimage every third year at either of the two places. The graph (Fig. 6.2) shows that most of the peak years of cholera during the period of 1879 to 1951 coincided with the years in which these fairs were held. But a further explanation of the graph is necessary with a view to understanding the real situation of the incidence of the disease. In a later paper, Rogers modified his absolute humidity theory of the twenties, and proved statistically that

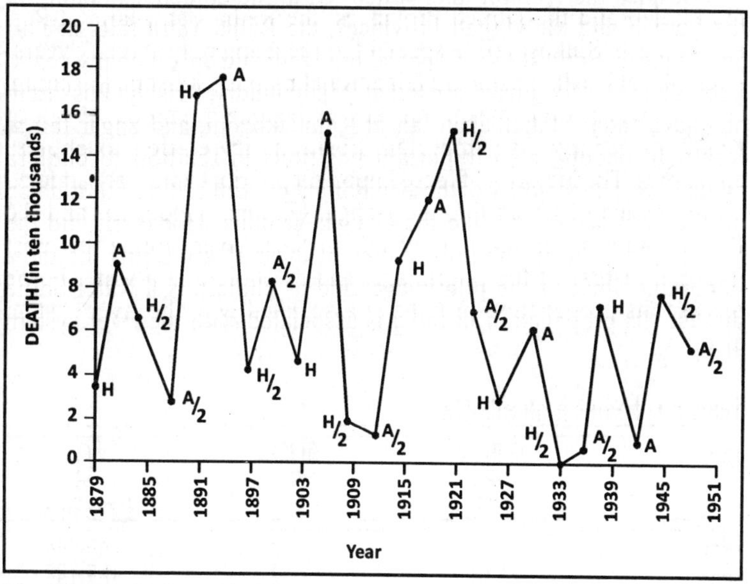

Fig. 6.2: Deaths from Cholera in U.P.

A—Allahabad *Kumbh*
A/2—Allahabad *Ardh-Kumbh*
H—Haridwar *Kumbh*
H/2—Haridwar *Ardh-Kumbh*

the annual variations in the occurrence of cholera in India are due to the "climatic conditions, together with the effects of the larger pilgrimages."[15] It is true that the high cholera mortality of 1882, 1891, and 1894 in the province were due to the facts that these years not only witnessed the *Kumbh* fairs but also deficiency of monsoon rains in the preceding years. But his explanation is not true for the high mortality of 1906 and 1918. Both 1905 and 1907 recorded normal rainfall, but it was the deficiency of the same in those two particular years that created such high mortality. On the other hand, as normal rainfall was recorded by the rest of the peak years, the spread of infection was not so severe as in other years just mentioned above. It might be concluded, therefore, that the shortage of rainfall not only in the preceding year, as postulated by Rogers, but also in a particular year has direct bearing upon the incidence of cholera.

A comparative study of the incidence of cholera before, at, and after the *Kumbh* fairs at Hardwar held during the said period can be made from Table 6.1.

Besides the Kumbh fairs which led to the epidemics mainly in the Punjab and the United Provinces, the Ratha Yatra fairs at Puri and Mahesh, Sinhast fair (a special fair recurring only at many years' intervals) at Nasik, Puskaram fair at Rajahmundry, Krishna Puskaram at Vijayawada, Mahamakan fair at Kumbakonam, and Sagar fair at Kakdwip occupy also important positions in relation to cholera epidemics. The majority of these important pilgrim centres are situated on the banks of rivers like the Ganga, Yamuna, Godavari, and the Kaveri. As a dip in the holy waters of these rivers forms the most important ritual of the pilgrimage, and as cholera is a water-borne disease, its propagation in India is associated with the river system also.

Table 6.1: Deaths from Cholera

Year	*January to March*	*At the fair*	*April to December*
1879	—	—	35,892
1891	3,910	3	165,103
1903	353	11	46,806
1915	515	302	89,973
1927	98	26	28,135
1938	474	337	70,148
1950	193	14	6,035

Source: B. Gopal (1951), "Compulsory preventive inoculation as a measure of control of cholera in fairs", *The Indian Medical Gazette,* Public Health Section, November, p. 511.

There are two types of festival centres in India: perennial festival centres which have special religious sanctity, and periodic centres which are important for special functions. Both these kinds of festivals attract people from far and wide, and thus become the foci of cholera epidemics.

Swaroop and Raman studied the magnitude of important fairs and festivals in terms of "person-days" of attendance as obtained by multiplying the estimated average attendance of people with the total number of days upon which each fair was held (Fig. 6.1).[16] They found that the persistence of cholera depends on the time of the year at which a gathering took place; if the festivals were held during the seasons favourable to the propagation of the disease they led to cholera epidemics.

The range of the spread of infection is dependent on the limit and sphere of travel of pilgrims, and both the places of congregation and the nodal points along the lines of communications are spots of danger. This becomes evident from a study of spatial diffusion of the disease in 1817-19 (Fig. 6.3) and the 1875-77 (Fig. 6.4) epidemics. Almost a regular pattern of the propagation of cholera over the country has been represented in Fig. 6.3. In both cases, the usual increase of cholera occurred over the deltaic parts of the then Bengal in the last parts of 1817 and 1875 respectively. During the cold season, however, it subsided over Bihar and eastern parts of the then United Provinces and stopped to fan out. But it burst out and created epidemics at Allahabad in early March of 1818 and late February of 1875. From this focus, it spread along the routes of travel into the north-western and central parts of the country. The 1817-19 epidemic passed into the whole of the peninsular India, and reached Ceylon (present Sri Lanka) in the long-run. Contrarily, the 1875-77 epidemic invaded Central India both from the Allahabad and the Nasik pilgrim centres. An offshoot of the latter continued south to the Malabar coast. South India was also attacked by two currents of infection radiating from Ceylon. One of these currents first reached the district of Tirunelveli and proceeded northward through Madurai and Tiruchirapalli while the other hit the port of Nagapattnam first and then, moved to the north through Tiruchirapalli to meet the streams of cholera coming from the Bombay Deccan. It is interesting to note from the figures that the spatial diffusion of cholera was not rapid due to the absence of or immature transportation system, that is, it was not comprehensive by modern standards.

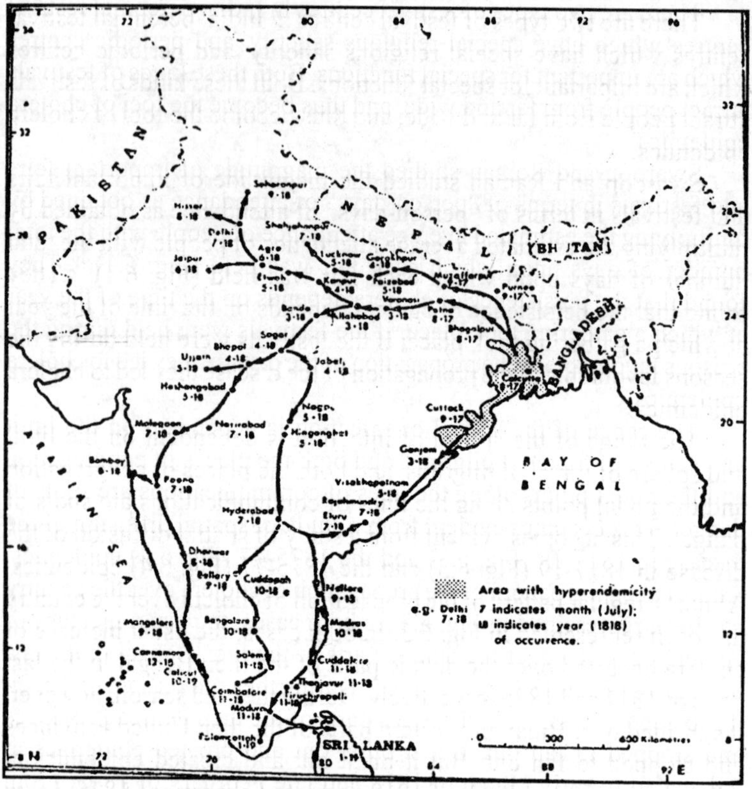

Fig. 6.3: Spatial Diffusion of Cholera in 1817-1819 Epidemic.

N.B. : The present political borders and names were not valid at the time of the epidemic diffusion shown in the map—*Editors.*

Miscellaneous Habits: The way people pollute water bodies and use their water, exercise an influence upon the outbreak of cholera. The continuous contamination of a river or a pond is caused by bathing and washing of infected clothes and materials in it. Regular entry of trash from town or village into the river and washing of dirt and filth from the town surface into the river by heavy rain are responsible for the gross pollution of river water. Further, as cremation is mostly practised in India and the charred remains are thrown in rivers, the river water gets contaminated. The well water is polluted by the dirt coming through its open top and by buckets and ropes which are used for lifting water. In West Bengal, there are a large number of

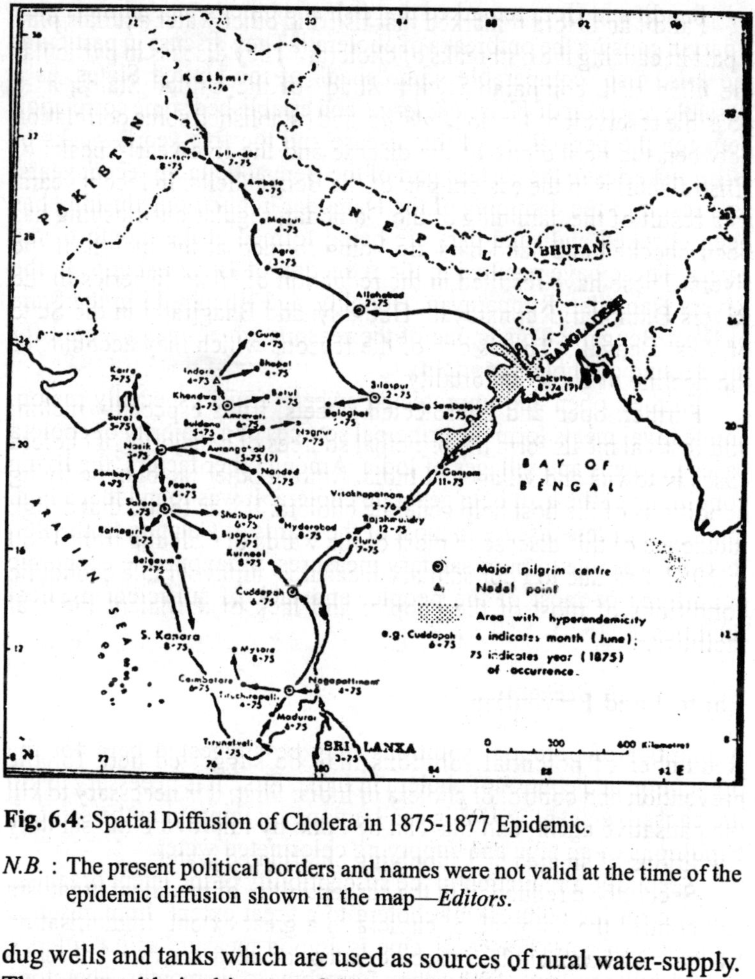

Fig. 6.4: Spatial Diffusion of Cholera in 1875-1877 Epidemic.

N.B. : The present political borders and names were not valid at the time of the epidemic diffusion shown in the map—*Editors*.

dug wells and tanks which are used as sources of rural water-supply. The water-table in this part of the country is found at a very shallow depth. Dyer and others detected that the borehole latrine, characteristic of this region, pollute the ground-water and water of tanks and wells.[17] Foods and milk are always open to contamination. They sometimes become the dangerous carriers of *Vibrio cholerae*. Articles like vegetables and fruits are often cleaned by water which is already polluted. Obviously, these things, if consumed without cooking, cause cholera. Apart from the question of deliberate adulteration, a certain amount of polluted water used for cleaning and rinsing utensils gains access to milk and makes it contaminated.

Pandit and Hora remarked that fish and other water animals play a part in causing the outbreaks of cholera.[18] They discuss in particular the *hilsa* fish, comparable with "shad" of the United States, as a possible reservoir of *Vibrio cholerae,* and established some correlation between the periodicity of the disease and the five-yearly peaks of *Hilsa* fisheries in the eastern part of the Bengal delta. In recent years, as a result of the damming of the Damodar, regular out-flushing has been checked and sand-bars are being formed at the mouth of the rivers. These have resulted in the reduction of *Hilsa* fisheries in the Rivers Damodar, Rupnarayan, Hooghly, and Bhagirathi in the State of West Bengal.[19] This is one of the reasons which may account for the decline of cholera mortality.

Further, open and unprotected sweets, fruits especially melon, and festival meals form the principal sources of a majority of cholera cases in towns and villages of India. Among other factors, the living conditions of the host help generate cholera. It was found that a high incidence of this disease in most of the wards of Calcutta from 1960 to 1963 was due to poor sanitary measures, unfavourable economic conditions of most of the people, and lack of sufficient medical facilities.[20]

Control and Prevention

A number of potential solutions may be suggested here for the prevention and control of cholera in India. First, it is necessary to kill the causative agent, and this can be done by improving the sanitary conditions of an area and supplying chlorinated water.

Secondly, a reduction in the susceptibility of the latent organism can control the outbreak of cholera to a great extent. Immunisation by means of anti-cholera vaccine is a good measure as it confers a considerable amount of protection from three to six months. Therefore, it is difficult to prevent the recurrence of the disease without subjecting the people to yearly re-vaccination. But in many places cholera is mostly imported. If vaccination prior to the departure for attending a fair or festival is made compulsory, the importation of cholera can be checked.

In Uttar Pradesh, compulsory inoculation was enforced in 1945 on the occasion of the *Ardh-Kumbh* fair at Haridwar, Barriers were created at different nodal points along the pilgrim routes to Haridwar, and uninoculated persons were not allowed to enter the area within a radius of 10 miles from the fair. Arrangements were also made for the isolation and treatment of the infected persons proceeding to or returning from the fair. As a result of all these measures cholera did not break out either on the spot or outside. This was an unprecedented incident in the history of this colossal gathering.[21] Since then compulsory inoculation has been enforced in different States of India as a prerequisite for entry into the major fairs.

The results obtained then and during the following years upto 1961 reveal that the compulsory immunisation of the pilgrims in place of voluntary vaccination was a successful method of controlling the outbreak of cholera.[22] The control of this disease also calls for a reduction in the contact between the causative agent and the host. This can be accomplished by improving the cultural habits which include the ways in which water is used, clothes are washed, foods are prepared and taken, and people live.

Conclusion

In India, endemicity of cholera is found well below the 500-metre line where the population is dense, the surface-water system is elaborate, and humidity is always high. But cholera in the epidemic form is confined to certain areas which are not humid. As the germ of the disease is orally introduced to the human stomach, the cultural and religious habits of human groups influence its spatial distribution.

Cholera can be eradicated by killing the causative agent, by reducing the susceptibility of the potential host, and by minimising the contact between the agent and the host. But for a country, like India, where most of the people are illiterate, poor and undernourished, these are not feasible propositions. Hence, community education is necessary, and it is to be designed in such a way that it can combat the outbreak of cholera. The enforcement of isolation, quarantine, protection of water, food, and milk supplies, and so on depend upon the public understanding and the acceptance of the responsibility. In fact, a properly educated community does not need any enforcement of regulation for the control of cholera or any other infectious disease. Education is, therefore, essential for the promotion of any programme of control on a permanent basis. This further needs bands of properly trained personnel who would help a community to improve its health, and learn to think like the people of that community. "Before asking a group of people to assume new health habits, it is wise to ascertain the existing habits, how these habits are linked to one another, what functions they perform and what they mean to those who practice them".[23]

Notes

1. Shattuck, G.C. (1951), *Diseases of the Tropics,* pp. 314 and 318; New York: Appleton-Century-Crafts, Inc.
2. May, J.M. (1958), *The Ecology of Human Disease,* pp. 36 and 48, New York: MD Publications, Inc.
3. Swaroop, S. and Pollitzer, R. (1952), World Distribution of Cholera Endemicity, *Epidemiological and Vital Statistical Report,* W.H.O. 5, 569-589, cited by J.M. May. *Ibid.,* p. 54.
4. Rogers, Sir L. (1926), The Conditions Influencing the Incidence and Spread of Cholera in India, *Proceedings of the Royal Society of Medical Epidemiology,* Section 19, 60-91.
5. *Ibid.*
6. Gopal, B. (1951), Compulsory Preventive Inoculation as a Measure of Control of Cholera in Fairs, *The Indian Medical Gazette,* Public Health Section, 510-511.
7. Simmons, J.S., *et al.* (1944), *Global Epidemiology—A Geography of Disease and Sanitation,* p. 119, J.B. Lippincott, Philadelphia, Vol. 1.
8. May, J.M. (1950), Medical Geography: Its Methods and Objectives, *Geographical Review,* 40, 9-10.
9. *Ibid.*
10. Shattuck, G.C., *op. cit.*
11. Rogers, Sir L., *op. cit.*
12. Banerjea, A.C. (1951), Notes on Cholera in the United Provinces, *Indian Journal of Medical Research,* 39, 17-21.
13. Sen, U. (1957), Distribution of Cholera on the Soil of West Bengal, *Geographical Review of India,* 19, 45-46.
14. Swaroop, S. and Raman, M.A. (1951), Endemicity of Cholera in Relation to Fairs and Festivals in India, *Indian Journal of Medical Research,* 39, 42-49.
15. Rogers, Sir L. (1944), Cholera Incidence in India in Relation to Rainfall, Absolute Humidity and Pilgrimages: Inoculation of Pilgrims as a Preventive Measures, *Transactions of the Royal Society of Tropical Medicine and Hygiene,* 38,76.
16. Swaroop, S. and Raman, M.A., *op. cit,*
17. Dyer, B.R.; Bhaskaran, T.R. and Chandra Sekhar, C. (1945), Investigations of Ground-water Pollution, Part III, Ground-water Pollution in West Bengal, India, *Indian Journal of Medical Research,* 33, 62.

18. Pandit, C.G. and Hora, S.L. (1951), The Probable Role of Hilsa Fish in Maintaining Cholera Endemicity in India, *Indian Journal of Medical Research,* 5, 342-356.
19. Saha, K.C. (1970), *Fisheries of West Bengal,* p. 52, Alipur: West Bengal Government Press.
20. Basu, R. (1969), Cholera in Calcutta—A Case Study of Medical Geography, *Geographical Review of India,* 31, 3, See also Banerjee, B. and Hazra, Jayati (1974), *Geo-Ecology of Cholera in West Bangal : A Story in Medical Geograhy,* Calcutta: K.P. Bagchi & Co.
21. Gopal, B., *op. cit.*
22. Banks, A.L. (1967), Religious Fairs and Festivals in India, *Lancet,* January, 162-163, 1961, cited by Spate, O.H.K. and Learmonth, A.T.A., *India and Pakistan,* p. 141, London: Methuen.
23. Paul, B.D. (ed.), (1970), *Health, Culture and Community,* p. 1, Russel Sage Foundation, New York, 1955, cited by Wilson, R.N., *The Sociology of Health: An Introduction,* p. 104, New York: Random House.

7
Resurgence of Malaria in India, 1965-76

Rais Akhtar and *A.T.A. Learmonth*

Introduction

At the time of Indian Independence in 1947 it was estimated that she had some 75 million malaria sufferers with 8,00,000 deaths a year. A national programme to control malaria was started in 1953, converted to the National Malaria Eradication Programme in 1958. While the campaigns were varied to meet regional differences within a large and diverse country, house-spraying with residual insecticides was the essential tool. Vector mosquitoes were mainly house-haunting species, the modest degree of public co-operation needed was achievable and achieved, and it was comparatively easy to recruit staff amply intelligent, educated and conscientious to fill the different grades of post. A rapid fall in morbidity and mortality was achieved, and by 1965 eradication seemed to be almost within grasp, for there were estimated to be only 1,00,000 active cases and no deaths in that year. However, at what now appears to have been a crucial stage the campaign faltered owing to a complex of reasons, and a resurgence began in 1966 and numbers of cases rose, fairly, rapidly and steadily, to over five million recorded in 1975 and 1976. While mortality is difficult to establish, it certainly had increased also while so far insignificant compared with the situation before the campaigns began (Table 7.1 and Fig. 7.1).[1]

Reprinted after having been edited from *Geo Journal, 1,* 69-80, 1977.

Table 7.1: Malaria Incidence in India 1965-76

Year	*Total Malaria Cases*	*Deaths*
1965	1,00,185	—
1966	1,48,136	—
1967	2,78,621	—
1968	2,74,881	—
1969	3,48,647	—
1970	6,94,647	—
1971	13,23,118	—
1972	13,62,806	—
1973	19,34,485	—
1974	31,67,658	3
1975	51,66,142	99
1976	50,82,467	19

Source: National Malaria Eradication Programme, Delhi.

The Causes Viewed Historically

While the control and later the eradication campaigns involved much investment by independent India, there were also significant inputs from international aid programmes notably by the USA. These inputs were crucial especially in ensuring the flow of imports of the vital residual insecticides, DDT, dieldrin and later compounds. Aid for the programmes ceased in 1965.

While the authors cannot pretend to offer an authoritative history of the resurgence to date, the reports of the National Institute of Communicable Disease do set out some major factors.[2]

From 1965 onwards there was a period of interruption or severe delays in the flow of these supplies. The main reason officially given for the initial delays is the closure of the Suez Canal owing to the Middle East war of 1965 and continuing tension there. However, there seem to have followed a series of interacting factors: the mid-60s included several years of crop failure over important areas of the country followed by food imports using scarce foreign exchange; and this probably combined with a feeling that the malaria problem was all but conquered, so that there was probably some loss of urgency even in circles close to the anti-malaria campaigns.

So, with malaria control almost achieved, crucial and damaging delays occurred in the allotment of foreign exchange to import insecticides and the sense of urgency seems to have been lost through

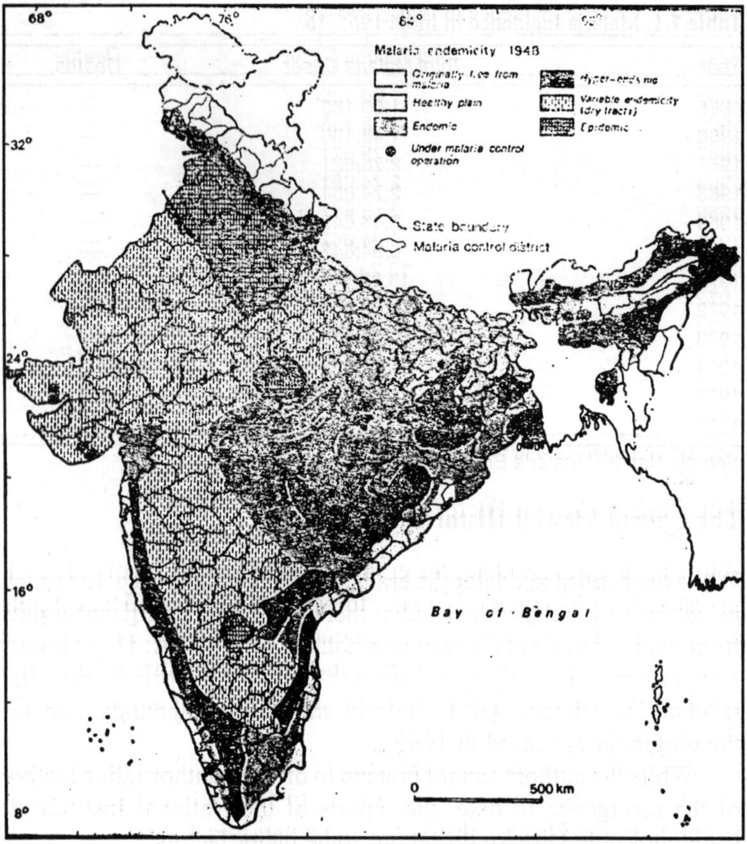

Fig. 7.1: Malaria Endemicity 1948, after Malaria Survey of India.

the complacence on the parts of individual citizens and of Government, central and state, civil servant and politician alike. The Institute continued to point out the dangers, but with insufficient force to prevail in the existing circumstances. It seems likely that the sense of complacency may have caused some surveillance workers to be less zealous in seeking out the comparatively few malaria cases in the mid-60s and in taking blood-films; under-registration may well have affected our data base, so that the increase since 1965 while real, may be from a higher figure than Table 7.1 suggests. However, the resurgence began and gathered force. On the other hand, the machinery for the maintenance and surveillance phases of the campaign was not disbanded, and it continued to work. While there may be unfilled posts here and there, there is machinery still in existence; there is, for example, a worker for roughly 8000/10000 population over much of the country, whose duty is to seek out areas where there may be outbreaks of malaria and to take blood samples for microscopic examination in search of *Plasmodium*. Now, that the resurgence is being taken seriously at home and abroad, it should not be too difficult to re-establish a substantial degree of control of the disease, though the target of eradication may have to be abandoned. And the ratio of surveillance staff to population may have to be increased in areas experiencing sharp resurgence.

Some Feature of the Resurgence—The Vector

On the whole, the area distribution pattern of the main vector species of the late 1940s, as portrayed in Fig. 7.2 seems to have been re-

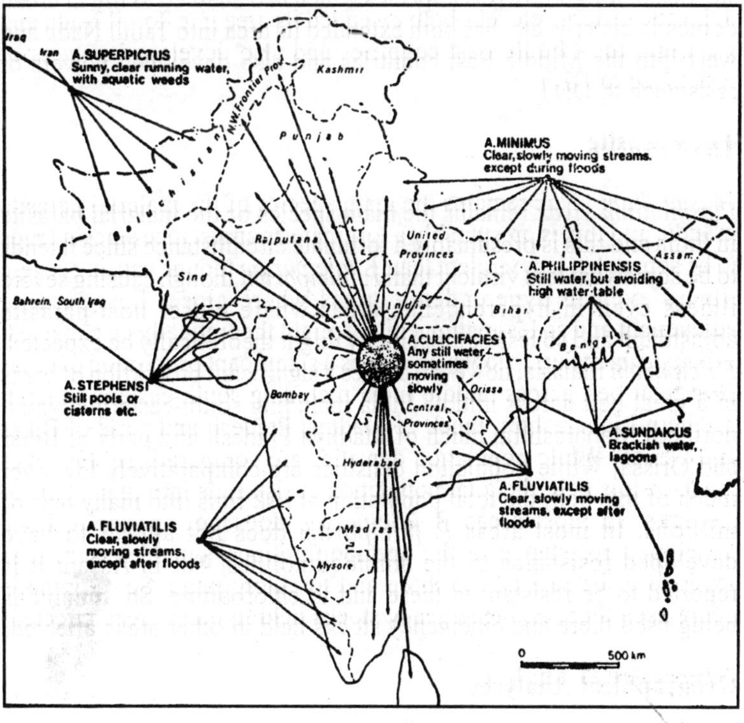

Fig. 7.2: Principal Vectors of Pre-independence India, C. 1945 after G. Covell in M.F. Boyd (Editor) *Malariology*, 1949.

established.[3, 4] In particular *Anopheles culicifacies* is again a core and dominant vector, with its ability to adapt to breeding in water-bodies of all shapes and sizes and all degrees of permanence over a couple of weeks or so. Resistance to DDT is reported over wide areas of the country. Of the stream-breeding jungle species, resistance is reported in *A. fluviatilis* in Maharashtra and Karnataka, while in Assam and the hill states of the north-east *A. minimus* as a main vector is at least complemented by *A. balabacensis* and other species.[5]

The exophilous habits of these two vectors are regarded as a major cause of the persistence of endemicity in substantial pockets of forest and jungle country in Assam and the north-east of the country. *A. culicifacies,* the main vector of the Indian heartland, is now reported to be developing resistance to DDT and HCH in both town and country. In some parts of the country, mud plastering or lime washing of interior walls has proved a serious obstacle to housespraying. *A. stephensi,* long-known as a species which had adapted to life in urban domestic cisterns etc. has both extended its area into Tamil Nadu and west into the Middle East countries and also developed powers of resistance to DDT.

The Parasite

Plasmodium vivax remains the main species of the malarial parasite in India and this is presumably a fortunate circumstance since it tends to be somewhat less virulent than *P. falciparum* though causing severe illness even in hyperendemic areas where closer host-parasite adjustment and so less pathogenicity might theoretically be expected. *Falciparum* malaria, however, causes a significant proportion of cases in a great belt across middle India including south-eastern Gujarat, northern Maharashtra, much of Madhya Pradesh and parts of Bihar and Orissa. While population densities are comparatively low over much of this belt, the total population at risk runs into many tens of millions. In most areas *P. falciparum* does not appear to have developed resistance to the aminoquinolines, but in Assam it is reported to be resistant to these and to chloroquine. So, quinine is being used there and emergency stocks held in other areas affected.

Geographical Analyses

The authors are attempting to complement the historical material from official reports and other sources by geographical analyses based on mapping of the annual parasite index for malaria control units (the rate per thousand population of cases detected by malaria control workers); they will exhibit maps for each year since the resurgence began by choropleths based on the control units. These maps have been drawn for the years 1965 to 1976 inclusive; rainfall anomaly maps for the years) 1969 to 1976 of the Indian Meteorological Department have been brought into the analyses so far (1965 to 1968 inclusive being preparation in the hope of throwing light on the crucial early years of the resurgence). Only first *visual* analyses have been carried out to date, and Figs. 7.3, 7.4 and 7.6 are included in this paper as samples of the malaria mapping, Figs. 7.5 and 7.7 as examples of the rainfall anomaly maps. The level of annual parasite index is

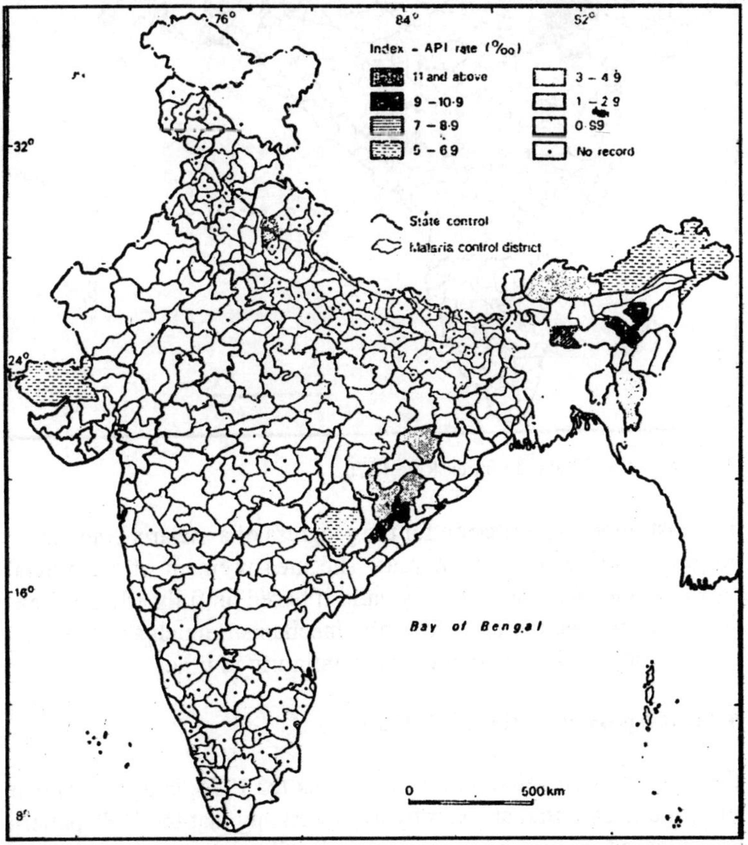

Fig. 7.3 : Annual Parasite Index Rate 1965.

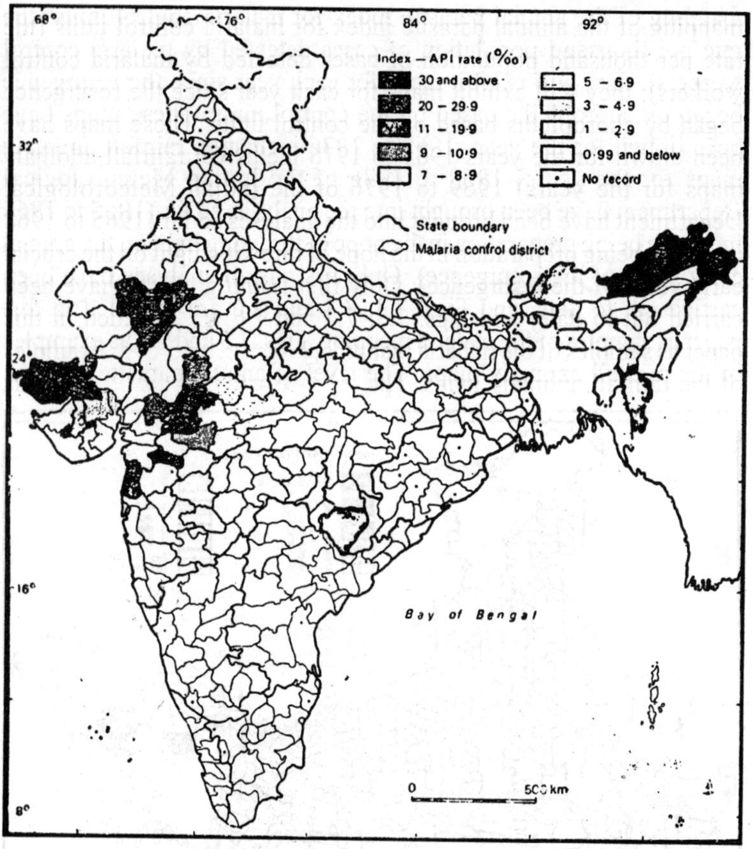

Fig. 7.4: Annual Parasite Index Rate 1970.

the most important criterion for the progress of a malaria eradication programme after its second year. The measurement of the annual parasite index is, however, only valid if based on fully efficient case detection, that is, the case detection mechanism much achieve total geographic coverage and adequate continuity in time.

A First Analysis of the 1975 Map

The first map available for API rates was for 1975, and Rais Akhtar has conducted a first analysis by hypothesising that the 1975 pattern is explained in turn by a particular distribution map : geological formations (no clear relationship); normal rainfall (no clear

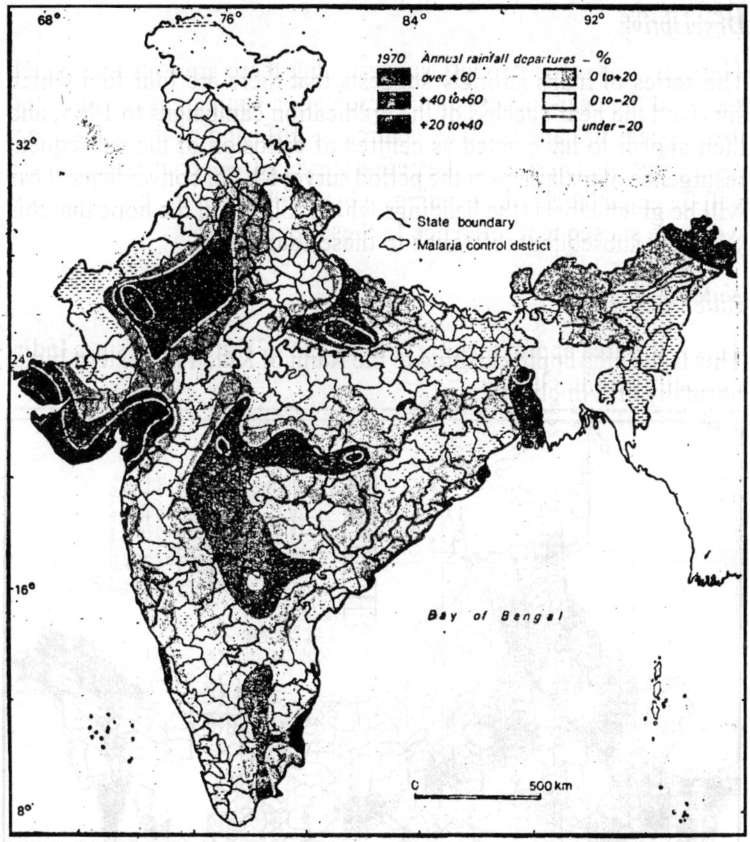

Fig. 7.5: Rainfall Anomaly Map 1970 by Courtesy of Meteorological Department, Government of India.

relationship); percentage departure of 1975 rainfall from the normal (no clear relationship); population density (negative relationship, that is densely populated areas tend to have little or no malaria); irrigation intensity (some inverse relationship is suggested: areas of high proportions intensively irrigated tend to have low malaria incidence); intensity of cropping (again inverse relationships are suggested, low intensity is linked with high malaria, high intensity with low malaria). The three strong but inverse relationships, population density, irrigation intensity, and cropping intensity, are of course liable to be related to each other, but as an interim finding to be treated with due caution, these suggested correlations are of interest.

Descriptive

The series of maps strongly suggests that there are four foci which survived the near-success of the eradication campaigns to 1965, and then appear to have acted as centres of diffusion of the subsequent resurgence of malaria over the period surveyed. For convenience these will be given labels (the headings which follow) in the hope that this will ease subsequent reference to these four areas:

Kutch Saltmarsh

This is the area approximating to the Rann of Kutch in western India, normally arid in climate.

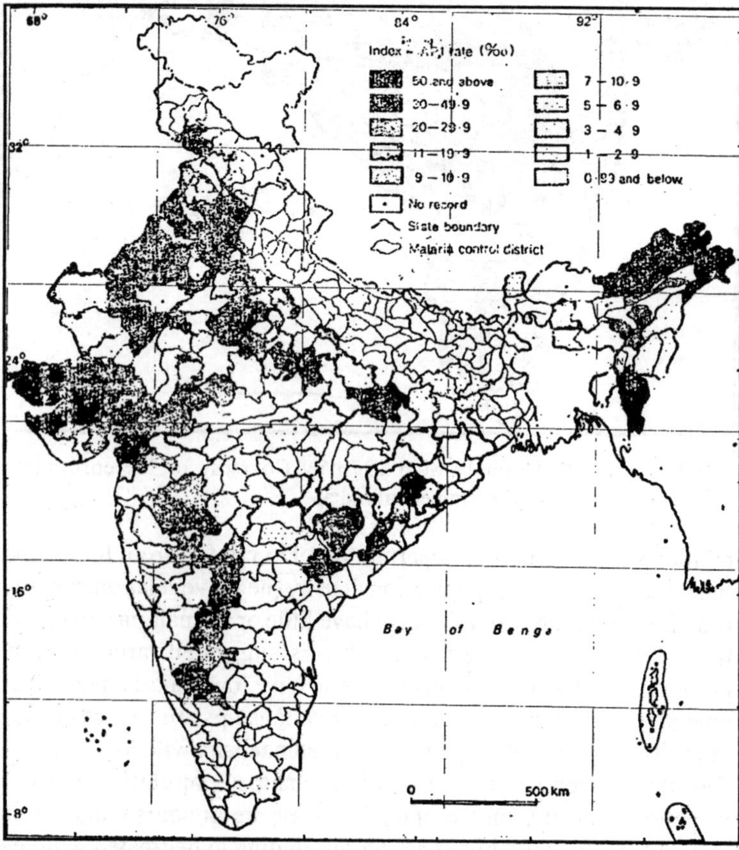

Fig. 7.6: Annual Parasite Index Rate 1976.

Madhya hill-forests (Madhya, central)

These comprise hilly and comparatively wet forested bill tracts, largely tribal territory, mainly in Madhya Pradesh.

Orissa Hill-forests

These are somewhat similar tracts in Orissa State in eastern India.

Assam Hill-forests

This is something of a misnomer, for these extend beyond Assam

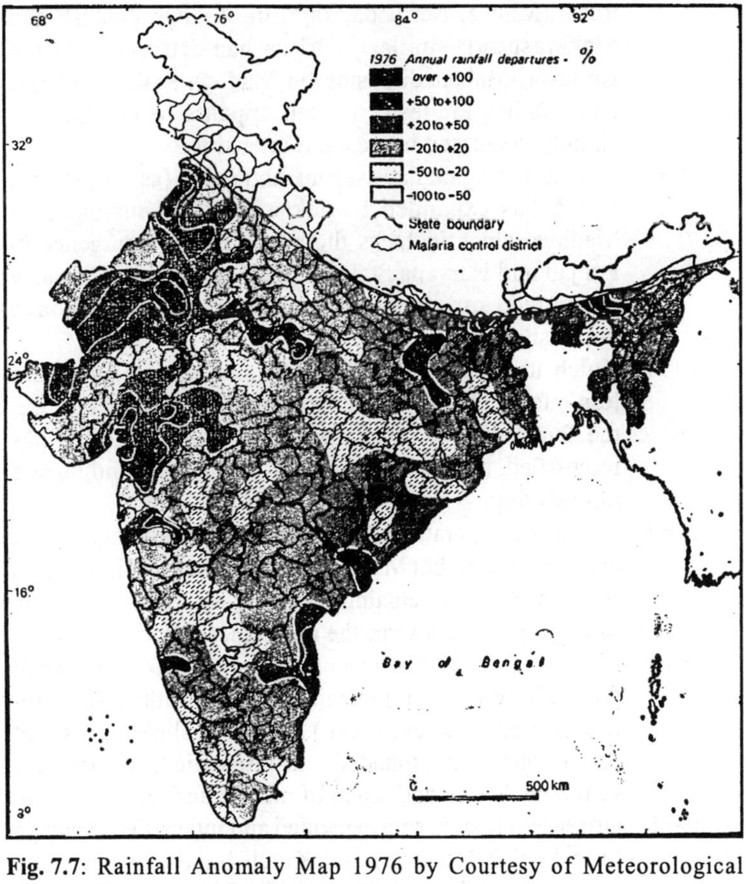

Fig. 7.7: Rainfall Anomaly Map 1976 by Courtesy of Meteorological Department, Government of India.

into other states in north-eastern India; considerable areas are much wetter than in the Madhya or Orissa hill-forests.

Assuming that these four areas are significant centres of diffusion, some of the main trends in diffusion may be summarised for the 12-year period:

1965 API rates are comparatively low in Madhya hill-forests, but moderate in Kutch saltmarsh, and in the Orissa and Assam hill-forests.

1966 Kutch has expanded to cover much of the Kathiawad low plateau (Gujarat state); Madhya has apparently diffused malaria into intermediate plateau and middle riverine tracts (Malwa, Narmada, Tapti in Madhya Pradesh and Maharashtra); similarly Orissa has diffused into the Godavari-Mahanadi basins (in Madhya Pradesh, Orissa and Andhra Pradesh). Assam appears to be static or slightly decreased in area and intensity.

1967 Assam may again have shrunk and paled (as it were) but Kutch has expanded to link up with diffusion from Madhya which includes the beginning of resurgence in Punjab and Haryana States to the North. Orissa has also expanded, and areas with little or no malaria have diminished.

1968 Kutch itself has intensified, but surrounding tracts are less intense. Madhya has shrunk and is less intense, but the Punjab-Haryana malaria has expanded. Orissa has intensified, and the Assam tracts is again expanding and intensifying.

1969 Kutch is comparatively stable, and Orissa slightly shrunk and less intense, but Madhya has expanded and intensified (Punjab-Haryana remaining stable), as has Assam. Only Madhya has a wet year, the rest rather dry to very dry.

1970 Kutch has strongly intensified and linked up with intensifying westward expansion from Madhya (Punjab-Haryana has also expanded). Orissa is slightly less, but Assam has both expanded and intensified. A fairly wet year over Assam and much of middle and western India.

1971 Orissa is stable, Assam expanded and intensified. Madhya (and Punjab-Haryana) and Kutch have expanded and intensified to link up as a marked epidemic in very much of all western India, and there is a sharp increase in the central peninsula much farther south (near Mysore city in central Karnataka State). A dry year in Kutch but wet over much of northern India.

1972 The picture is broadly similar, with a little less coverage and intensity in western India. (It is a drier year there.)

1973 Both Orissa and Assam expand and intensify. The linked areas in western India expand and intensify in places. (It is a wet year there.)

1974 There is a general expansion linking up of the epidemic areas, with local intensification, except in much of the Ganga (Ganges) plains and much of the far south of peninsular India. (It is a wet year in the south-central peninsula, but a drier one in much of western India.)

1975 The patterns are fairly stable areally but intensifying in many areas. (It is a wet year over much of India.)

1976 The broad pattern is similar, parts of the Ganga plains and much (though less than previously) of the far south of the peninsula remaining comparatively free from malaria. (It is again a wet year in many areas.)

Some Interim Thoughts of a more Analytical Nature

We must again emphasize that rigorous and quantitative analyses have not yet been attempted though we hope to undertake such procedures—though the API maps and the rainfall anomaly maps themselves are of course the best quantitative material available. The following discussion is therefore based on visual inspection of the maps put before the seminar, on discussion in the Jawaharlal Nehru University in New Delhi in the period November 1976 to February 1977 when the two authors were able to work together, and some correspondence since then.

The first step is to group together the endemic and hyper-endemic areas of Fig. 7.1 roughly corresponding with humid and perhumid India familiar from maps of mean annual isohyets or from more sophisticated climatic maps, and similarly the variable endemic and epidemic areas roughly equating with arid and semi-arid India. In this hypothesis our basic assumption is that the malaria cycle may be in resurgence because of several interacting factors, and that these interactions may differ as between humid and arid India.

First to discuss the resistant foci of endemicity in 1965 (Fig. 7.3) and 1966: these are dominantly in wet to very wet forested hill country, and may well represent in microcosm the problems of exophily in the vector species encountered on a much larger scale throughout the equatorial rainforest zones of the world, including the survival of exophilous strains of the local species. This applies to the Madhya Pradesh, Orissa and Assam hill-forest tracts. As happens in many environments from the Mediterranean to the equatorial rain-forests, there may be a change in relative importance of vector species in the event of anopheline resurgence after a spray campaign, and here *Anopheles balabacensis* has assumed a new importance along with *A. minimus* in the Assam hill-forest area; both are now recorded as exophilous and resistant to insecticides. Kutch saltmarsh area, however, is different. In 1948, it was classed as an area of variable endemicity of dry tracts, but we may provisionally suppose that in its own way the Rann of Kutch represents difficult terrain, perhaps tackled relatively late during the attempt at eradication in the decade 1956-65, and probably with mud plastering of house walls as a particular difficulty in applying house spraying techniques. In contrast with the other residual foci in hill-forest tracts, with exophilous mosquitoes, the main vector in Kutch is *A. stephensi,* closely adapted of domestic including urban environments.

Second, to attempt a generalisation from say the last three years of our period, 1974-76 (only Fig. 7.6 for 1976 is reproduced here).

Within the endemic-hyperendemic tract of 1948, spread widely across south-western, south-eastern and middle and eastern India, densely populated and intensively cultivated coastal Kerala (south-west), Tamil Nadu (south-east) and West Bengal (north-east) are at least so far comparatively little affected by the resurgence. However, this may be because malaria has not yet spread to them from some centre or centres of diffusion. Considerable areas of high malaria in 1974-76 in southern and western Maharashtra, western Karnataka, inland Tamil Nadu and much of Madhya Pradesh, Orissa, Bihar and the north-eastern states correspond with formerly hyperendemic tracts and it may be that the resurgence will tend to extend to assume a greater resemblance to the 1948 patterns.[6]

With variable endemic and epidemic tracts in 1948 (perhaps more easily comprehended as epidemic and severely epidemic tracts?) are found many of the high and very high rates on the 1974-76 maps. The immediate association is with comparatively dry areas of the country. Comparison with the 1975 rainfall, which proved inconclusive when the whole country was considered, may prove much more meaningful if one postulates different causal factors in humid and semi-arid India. It does seem very suggestive indeed that high 1975 and 1976 rainfall in normally semi-arid or even arid areas was related to high malaria incidence in these years. In the command area of Rajasthan canal, however, it is possible that the high malaria incidence may be related to new irrigation, a familiar phenomenon in the Punjab canal colonies in Sind and in the Visvesvaraya canal tract in Karnataka some decades ago and again from 1971 onwards in our maps. The suggestion that intensive irrigation and intensive cropping are related to low malaria rates in 1975 is interesting, and it will be important to test this further as more data become available. On earlier experience, it seems unlikely that even intensive and well-organised irrigation would protect the population from malaria, but it may be that anti-malaria organisation and discipline are better in just such areas nowadays.

Whilc the maps do not discriminate between rural and urban incidence, it is important to consider any evidence about this from them and from other sources. As one would expect the general impression is of an overwhelmingly rural incidence, now as in the past. However, some areas of important urban populations in western Maharashtra, Gujarat and Punjab are showing high or very high incidence. Moreover, *Anopheles stephensi,* known to have adapted closely to urban existence for 50 years or more, has both extended its range and also developed resistance to important insecticides. Rapid urbanization in areas of considerable economic development, including those mentioned, is accompanied by a good deal of the spontaneous shanty-town development which is now regarded as performing crucial functions in the urbanization process and yet represents substantial health risks. Much urban waste water tends to accumulate, especially of course in the rainy season and notably in wet years in normally dry tracts—the very conditions which maintained over much of western and northern India in 1975 and 1976. While culicine filarial vector mosquitoes are likely to be more tolerant of organic pollution in such waste water than *Anopheles,* it seems clear that malaria as an urban disease has to be taken seriously. A study of Tamil Nadu on more intimate scale than this countrywide survey offers some confirmation of this[7] as does some bitter personal experience of the senior author of this paper. Detailed studies of small areas on large scale maps are required and some may already be in prospect.

Summary and Tentative Conclusions

The eradication campaign faltered, for historical reasons some of which are tentatively suggested above and which would be worthy of fuller study as an important part of recent medical history; it is one of those historical topics so intertwined with political and social history that an interdisciplinary approach would be fruitful—if the necessary documents could be made accessible, in India and perhaps in international organisations and subscribing government archives too.

Once the campaign faltered malaria seems to have diffused from the four foci suggested, the Kutch saltmarsh area and the hill-forest tracts of Madhya Pradesh, Orissa and Assam. The role of wet years in areas normally arid, semi-arid or only moderately humid seems crucial in the diffusion process, and if the gaps in the rainfall anomaly maps can be filled we shall try to provide a more rigorous analysis of this relationship. Some humid and perhumid areas of high agricultural development, and dense or very dense rural populations, and one or two areas of considerable industrial and urban development like Greater Calcutta and nearby towns, seem so far to be happily little affected by the diffusion of malaria, even though as late as 1948 some including much of West Bengal were hyperendemic areas. It remains to be established by detailed studies if these areas are better prepared in some way—natural immunity must have faded especially in the considerable proportion of young people who have been born since malaria eradication was almost within grasp; or are they so far comparatively fortunate through some chances of the diffusion pattern?

Urban malaria, and one might say *Anopheles stephensi* malaria, is probably more widespread and more significant as an important public health problem than in former times. Once more the need for detailed local studies is clear.

It is important to re-read the introductory paragraph of this chapter. The fifty-fold increase from 1,00,000 to 5 million cases represent a sharp resurgence but the 5 million cases of 1975 and 1976, and few score of recorded deaths, still represent a remarkable achievement as compared with the 75 million cases and 8,00,000 deaths a year at the time of Independence. If complacence did indeed play a part in the crucial years of resurgence in the late 1960s, it is unlikely to continue today in medical circles. One can only hope that those engaged in the malaria eradication programme will take the issue seriously. Studies of the economic, educational and demographic impact of the resurgence may help them to do so.

Acknowledgements

Acknowledgements are gratefully made to the National Malaria Eradication Programme (NMEP), Delhi, for data on Annual Parasite Index and other archival material and to the Indian Meteorological Department for rainfall anomaly maps. Cartography is by John Hunt of the Open University.

Notes

1. Christophers, S.R. and Sinton, J.A. (1926), A malaria map of India, *Indian J. Med. Res.,* 14, 173-78, see also Learmonth 1957, 1958.
2. Dhir, S.L. (1970), Resistance to Insecticides in Malaria Vectors, In: *National Malaria Eradication Programme: Retrospect and Prospect,* National Malaria Eradication Programme, p. 17, May, Delhi.
3. Covell, G. (1949), Map of Principal Vectors of Malaria in India, In: *Malariology,* Vols. I and II, Boyd M.F., (ed.) Philadelphia and London, (see also Learmonth 1957, 1958).
4. Learmonth, A.T.A. (1957), Some Contrasts in the Regional Geography of Malaria in India and Pakistan, *Trans. Inst. British Geog.,* 23, 37-57.
5. Bruce-Chwatt, L.J. (1970), Global Review of Malaria Control and Eradication by Attack on the Vector, *Miscellaneous Publications of the Entomological Society of America,* 7, 1, 7-27.
6. Learmonth, A.T.A. (1958), Medical Geography in Indo-Pakistan: A Study of Twenty Years' Data for the Former British India, *Indian Geog.* J., 33, 1-59.
7. Hyma, B. and Ramesh, A. (1976), Malaria Incidence in Tamil Nadu, India, paper to Medical Geography Symposium, *23rd International Geographical Congress,* Moscow.

8

Environment and Cholera in Kashmir

During Nineteenth Century

Rais Akhtar

Introduction

Sudden outbreaks of cholera in Kashmir during 1850-1892 have been described by many writers and physicians working in Kashmir during that period as indigenous due to insanitary conditions prevailing in Kashmir. It is the contention of this chapter that although insanitary conditions were responsible for the spread of the disease, the cholera was brought to Kashmir as a result of population mobility between Kashmir and Punjab, and was the result of a pandemic wave. This is confirmed with the data and information available on the cholera outbreaks in other parts of the Indian-subcontinent, Europe and the United States. The chapter also examines the cholera ecology in Kashmir during nineteenth century.

Historical Medical Geography is a fascinating area of research which highlights the pattern of environmental conditions, people's adjustment with the environment and the occurrence of health problems as a result of man's interaction with the environment.

The outbreak of cholera and its diffusion in Kashmir in the 19th century was more or less considered a local epidemic with its origin in Kashmir and in the neighbouring Punjab. However, the examination of data and other source material on the outbreak and diffusion of cholera at the global scale in general and India in particular, reveal that cholera smouldering in an environmental hearth in the Gangetic delta of Bengal, erupted in four epidemic waves in the 19th century, which caused sudden and widespread mortality throughout the world.

North America was stricken three times. In Europe, the spectre of advancing death, fuelled by word of mouth reports, created an advance wave of panic, heightened by total public ignorance of cholera's aetiology. The eventual discovery that cholera is a water-borne infection was made during the cholera epidemic in London in 1854 by Dr. John Snow. According to J.M. Hunter, "With the widespread adoption of steam boats and the improvement of shipping lanes, global waves of the so-called Indian cholera spread even more quickly. The North American pandemics of 1832, 1848, and 1866 variously entered the seaports of Quebec, New York, and New Orleans and spread along river valleys and waterways. The disease passed through Buffalo, the Great lakes, Detroit River, Chicago and principally along the Mississippi River cholera was even carried west in the California gold rush. Later, the geographical pattern of spread of the disease in North America began to change as towns and railroads were constructed" (Hunter, 1888). A study carried out by G.F. Pyle showed that the 1866 epidemic was strongly influenced by the urban hierarchy, and was also related to distance from the eastern seaboard. Thus, a regular, geographically predictable relationship was observable in the spread of the disease (Pyle, 1979).

The above discussion throws light on two important aspects:

1. To study the cholera ecology in Kashmir; and
2. To test the hypothesis that cholera was not indigenous to Kashmir and was part of the process of cholera outbreak and diffusion globally; since cholera occurred in Kashmir, and northern Indian subcontinent, Europe including the United Kingdom and the USA more or less at the same time.

Geo-ecology of Cholera in Kashmir

Physical Factor

The valley of Kashmir with its clayey loamy soils, nestles in the young folded mountain ranges of the Himalayas. The water in the Kashmir valley is an extraordinary paradox. Considering the total run-off, area of water-bodies and length of water courses, the valley has no match in the Himalayas. In fact, its water features are the principal components in its scenic beauty. The geomorphic character of the valley is however, such that the distribution of water resources is extremely uneven—a situation which renders vast stretches of land totally or partially out of use either due to excess of water or its deficiency. Water is most plentiful in the low lying parts of the valley, which remain literally deluged, while the adjoining Karewa uplands suffer from aridity imposed by its chronic deficiency. The consequence is that the valley presents the anomalous case of scarcity in the midst of plenty. The rivers carry large volumes of water which they cannot possibly contain as their channels get increasingly choked with silt, making floods a recurrent phenomenon with disastrous consequences on agriculture and on health simultaneously. It was this phenomenon of water scarcity in the midst of plenty as a result of particular geomorphological pattern that used to cause famine in the valley (Raza, *et al.*, 1978). When famine is combined with cholera as was the case during 1877-79, it caused havoc among the people of Kashmir. Another aspect of geomorphic characteristics of the valley is the pattern of soil distribution. Writing in early 1890s, Walter Lawrence who was then Settlement Commissioner noted, "it is a curious fact, which I noticed in my tours, that villages on the Karewa plateaus seemed free from cholera, and that the disease was most rampant in the alluvial parts of the valley" (Lawrence, 1895). An examination of geo-ecology of cholera reveals among other factors that, apart from man (as both pathogens and geogens), there are environmental factors which facilitate the survival and spread of cholera. Such geographical factors include : annual temperatures of around 37° C and prolonged dry spells. Moisture is another important factor which favours the outbreaks of cholera. Cholera vibrios thrive best in warm alkaline media (with pH value between 9 and 9.6) while acidic media inhibit their growth and survival. The Karewa soils[1], however, are normal with a pH value of around 7.5 and therefore not acidic. However, the Karewa soils are devoid of vegetal cover and are deficient in organic matter. The moisture-retaining capacity of the soil is poor as the upper layer has a high sand content (Raza, *et al.*, 1978). The characteristics of soils may explain the statement of Walter Lawrence regarding the absence of cholera in the villages on the Karewa soils of Kashmir Valley.[2]

Poor Socio-Economic and Insanitary Conditions

A Report dated 10th December, 1861 from the Deputy Commissioner on special Duty at Kashmir, to Secretary to Government of Punjab, is testimony of the poor economic conditions of the people in Kashmir. The report states, "The people in Kashmir are wretchedly poor, and in any other country their state would be almost one of starvation and famines…." (Report, 1861). Under such socio-economic circumstances, people were not able to maintain a hygienic environment. Dr. William Elmslie, who arrived in Srinagar as a missionary doctor in 1865, described in his letters the unhygienic practices of the people which resulted in the widespread incidence of skin diseases. He writes, "But there are other things in Kashmir which most terribly detract from its pleasure as a place of residence. The dirt is beyond description. Who can tell what Kashmir smells are? Not the odour of roses, such as one has expected to fill the air; but oh! such, that the dirtiest of London courts is sweeter than the cleanest of Kashmir villages. The clothes, too, of the people are filthy; not that the filth shows much, for all their garments are of grey wool, which is a most perfect concealer of dirt; but not a few of their diseases are the result of their uncleanliness, and how often I have almost shrunk away from them, as, in my dispensary, while I have been examining a patient. I have seen the lice crawling on his clothes and his fleas skipping over to me. Of course, if you can avoid all intercourse with the natives, then dirt is not much a continual source of annoyance, but to us it was a daily trouble" (Elmslie, 1875). Similar views regarding insanitary conditions, in Srinagar were expressed by Irene Petrie who was very perturbed when she wrote, "Srinagar, with its water-ways, palaces, bridges and graceful fair skinned inhabitants, suggests Venice, though Venice much dilapidated. But from Venice there are no such views as one may see on a clear autumn day. It is perhaps the dirtiest city in the world, and most of the houses look as if they could not survive the next flood or earthquake" (Wilson, 1900). Irene Petrie pleaded that people should be taught practically that cleanliness is next to godliness.

Most writers on Kashmir agreed to the fact that cholera outbreak was the result of "poor sanitary conditions". The centre and nursery of cholera in Kashmir is the foul and squalid capital Srinagar, but if it is once established there it soon spreads to the dirty towns and villages (Lawrence, 1895 : 219). Besides crowding was another serious problem. Nearly 1, 18, 960 people live in 22,448 houses with a density of 5 persons per house. The houses were "built irregularly and without any method, on narrow tortuous paths. Ventilation in the town is therefore very imperfect. Few houses have latrines, and small lanes and alleys are used as such…. There is no drainage. Slush, filth and ordure are washed by storm water into the river and Nalla Mar which supply the city with drinking water. On account of absence of snow in winter and rains in spring, and river was dry and low and the bed of the Nalla Mar canal was converted into a string of cesspools. People were immersed in a polluted atmosphere caused by the products of putrefactive and fermentable water accumulated in houses and numerous narrow lanes, passes, nooks and crevices which intersect the town. This produced an epidemic constitution in the people fitted for the reception and fostering of cholera-germs" (Lawrence, 1895 : 36).

Riverine Environment

The riverine environment, too, contributes to a greater extent towards cholera outbreak. The riverine environment was significant, in Kashmir in the 19th century. Most of the localities lined the Jhelum River for a length of about 5 kilometres, and the town extended less than a kilometre, with Habba Kadal locality as most densely populated area, with the river as the main source of drinking water. Drew compared the river Jhelum with the Thames, and wrote a vivid account of the layout of Srinagar. "It is (Jhelum) the chief artery of traffic; it is of much more importance as a thoroughfare than any of the streets; indeed there are one or two streets, and those but short ones, that have anything like a continuous traffic, while the river is always with boats" (Drew, 1875). About the riverine environment Drew further noted, "A few canals traverse the interior of the town; one of them is wide, and is overlooked by some of the best of the houses. One is narrow, passing through some of the poorest parts, low dwellings crowd on it that, albeit they are well peopled, seem to be on the point of falling.... A third canal leads from the upper part of the city to the gate of the lake, and shows along its winding course groves of plane-trees on the banks that make a beautiful combination with the smooth waters at their feet and the mountains that rise behind them" (Drew, 1875 : 185). Dr. William Elmslie, who arrived in Kashmir as a medical missionary, wrote about the outbreak of cholera in this riverine locality of Habba Kadal in 1867, "On 20th June, cholera has broken out in the city. The worst was in Habba Kadal" (Elmslie, 1875). Superstitious beliefs were a hindrance in controlling the spread of cholera. Writing about 1872 cholera outbreak, C.L. Tyndale Biscoe, who was an educational missionary, noted, "The flood was followed by an epidemic of cholera, in which it was difficult for the English medical missionaries to help as they wished, because the people, believing their sickness to be judgement from God, trusted chiefly to charms to be swallowed in water. These were pieces of paper, written by the priests and bought from them on which the name of ALLAH, or of some Mohammedan saints, or, in case of Hindus, of some god or goddess, was inscribed. The people continued drinking infected water all the same, and consequently cholera stalked through the land unchecked, claiming its thousands of victims" (Biscoe, 1921).

Movement of Population, Opening of Jhelum Route, and Troop Movement

With the commencement of Sikh rule in 1819, contact between Kashmir and Punjab began especially when Kashmir faced famine and there was acute shortage of food in the valley leading to a large scale migration to Punjab which contained several foci of cholera in north-western India. According to Lawrence, "a number of Kashmiris fled to Punjab as a result of famine in 1831. Sikh governor of Kashmir imported grains and eggs from Punjab and restored some measure of prosperity to the villagers who had lost their grain seed and fowls in the awful famine" (Lawrence, 1895 : 200). However, the Sikh governor, considered sympathetic to Kashmiris, was murdered and the turmoil brought about by Bombas followed by raids by both Bombas and Kukas, Maharaja Gulab Singh, the Dogra[3] ruler of Jummu region took over the rule of Kashmir in 1846. This has further intensified the contacts between Kashmir with the cholera-prone region of Jammu, south of Kashmir. Travel between Srinagar and Jammu, especially the Maharaja's camp, brought cholera from Jammu. Dr. A. Mitra, who wrote Medical and Surgical Practices in Kashmir (1890), opined, "Cholera is not endemic in Kashmir, but visits it often in virulent epidemic form. The last epidemic was in 1880 during which nearly 10,000 persons died from cholera. The disease travelled with the Maharaja's camp from Jummu to Srinagar, where the first case was observed on 6th April. Day by day, the number of cases began to increase till on the 15th of May 250 persons were attacked in Srinagar alone" (Mitra, 1889). Describing the horror of 1888 cholera outbreak, Mitra noted, "Its ravages extended to all parts of the valley. The scene of death and desolation during the summer of 1888 was one that will not soon pass away from living memory. The country was gay, magnificent arrangements were being made for a fitting reception of the Earl Dufferin. The Maharaja and suite arrived earlier than usual to loyally welcome the Viceroy. Suddenly, the disease epidemic came, the Viceregal visit was abandoned and everybody became panic-stricken. The Maharaja and suite and the Resident remained in Srinagar but no doubt in great trepidation" (Mitra, 1889 : 11).

The intensity of cholera occurrence increased in Kashmir from around 1890 when the road between Punjab and Baramulla in Kashmir was thrown open. Lawrence wrote in grave fear, "Now that Srinagar is joined to India by a road, there is a two fold necessity for sanitary reform. For if cholera becomes endemic, the Punjab and the great military cantonment of Rawalpindi will always be threatened, while on the other hand, the occurrence of an epidemic in India is sure to be followed by cholera in Kashmir, for cholera like trade, travels by roads. Before the road from Baramulla to the Punjab was opened cholera might occur in India while Kashmir was healthy, and whereas there were twelve epidemics of cholera in the Punjab between 1867 and 1890, there were only five outbreaks in Kashmir during the same period. Now, it is almost certain that if cholera reaches the Punjab it will find its way along the crowded road and the narrow valley to Srinagar" (Lawrence, 1895 : 219).

It is interesting to note that a report on 1862 Punjab cholera prepared by J.B. Scriven made similar observations. The report noted, "The route of the cholera was particularly well marked in the year 1861, in which it was regularly traced along the grand trunk road, from Delhi to Lahore. This year (1862), likewise it appears to have transmitted in two lines, one on the east and the other on the west of Punjab leaving the immediate country free" (Report, 1861).

Dr. Elmslie's Account

Dr. Elmslie narrated his experiences of cholera outbreak of 1867. He put forward his theory that the Maharaja's sepoys who went to Hardwar (a religious centre in northern India), brought cholera infection, "just as the hostility and opposition of the local government of Kashmir had reached a climax cholera broke out amongst his Highness's troops. It appears that some sepoys who had got leave to go and wash in the Ganges at Hardwar, had returned to their regiment at Srinagar, and brought the seeds of cholera with them. At any rate, those sepoys had scarcely arrived, when that awful pestilence broke out and began to carry off many. Everything was done to prevent the spread of the disease, but it at last invaded the city: and the British Resident deemed it necessary for the safety of the European visitors, to institute a Cordon Sanitaire round the European quarters. As my dispensary is situated there, I was compelled to put a stop to my work for a time.... The poor people of the city are sadly neglected, even by those who ought to take some care of them" (Elmslie, 1875 : 195-96).

As Part of Pandemic

Having studied the geoecology of cholera in Kashmir in the nineteenth century, it is worthwhile to throw light on the pandemics of cholera. F.G. Clemow in his book: *The Geography of Disease* (1903), opined that "the pandemics of cholera have always started from India" (Clemow, 1903). Cholera, smouldering in an environmental heart in the lower Ganges valley, erupted in four epidemic waves in the nineteenth century, which caused sudden and widespread mortality throughout the world. North America was stricken three times. In Europe the spectre of advancing death, fuelled by word of mouth reports, created an advance wave of panic, heightened by total public ignorance of cholera' aetiology (Hunter, 1988 : 117).

Diffusion of cholera from Bengal to Kashmir

F.N. Macnamara, whose book on *Climate and Medical Topography*, was published in 1880, provided the most scientific account on cholera diffusion in northern India (Macnamara, 1880). Based on the analysis of data obtained from the book by Macnamara, the study reveals that cholera outbreaks occur in Bengal during February and March, move through northern India to Punjab and north-west Provinces, where its outbreaks are generally reported in the months of August and September. Because of Kashmir's connection with Punjab, cholera moved to the valley and occur normally during winter months, November-January as mentioned earlier. The analysis of data for the period 1865-76 for Bengal, and 1870-76 for Punjab and north-west Provinces reveals the following pattern of cholera outbreak in northern part of Indian subcontinent (Table 8.1).

Table 8.1: Cholera Out-break Pattern in Bengal, Punjab and North-West Provinces (19th Century)

Province	*Total cases (Average Annual)*	*Outbreak Occurred*
Bengal (1865-76)	4657	February-March
Punjab (1870-76)	3019	August-September
N.W. Provinces (1870-76)	21,960	August-September
Kashmir (1870-76)	Several thousands	December-January
(1888)	10,000	May-August
(1892)	18,000	May-August

It is evident from Table 8.1 that the intensity of cholera generally increased as it moved westwards fron Bengal to N.W. Provinces. In Kashmir, cholera outbreaks were reported both in summer as well as winter. Cholera outbreak in Bengal in February or a little later during slight spring rains, moved to northern India and became epidemic till monsoon winds bring humidity, if not actual rainfalls (Macnamara, 1880 : 112).

It is interesting to note that cholera broke out in Kashmir during both a snow-free winter as well as a winter period which experienced heavy snowfall. In the Gazetteer of Kashmir and Ladak, Bates stated that "in 1857 cholera struck to the valley, strange to say, throughout the winter, when the snow was up to a man's neck" (Bates, 1890). Contrary to this Lawrence wrote in 1895 that "on account of absence of snow in winter and rains in spring, the river was dry and low and the bed of the Nala Mar Canal was converted into a string of cesspools.... This produced an epidemic constitution in the people fitted for the reception and fostering of cholera-germs" (Lawrence, 1895 : 36). Thus, it may be concluded that the outbreak of cholera in Kashmir was result of the pandemic wave and not the local environmental conditions, as cholera broke out both during snow free and heavy snow periods.

Cholera Ecology Model

Table 8.2 provides an insight of the ecological conditions which favour cholera outbreaks in Kashmir. It reveals that not only the physical factors but socio-economic and cultural factors especially mobility of population between Kashmir and cholera foci region of Punjab play a significant role in the outbreak and the diffusion of cholera.

Table 8.2: Cholera Ecology Model in Kashmir (1850-1900 AD)

(a) Physical Factors Rains	+ Estuarine Environment + Prolonged Dry Spells
	+ Sluggishly Flowing Water + Alkaline soils
(b) Socio-Economic and Cultural Factors Unhygienic Living Conditions	
	+ Contaminated Drinking Water
	+ Defecation in the Lanes
	+ Growing contact with Punjab (migration) at the Commecement of Sikh rule followed by Dogra rule
	+ Famine
	+ Incoming of Troops from Cholera Foci Areas

Table 8.3 depicts the pattern of cholera diffusion model based on the movement of cholera from Bengal to Punjab and North-West Provinces. From Punjab, one wave of cholera diffusion moved to the valley of Kashmir, mainly via the Jhelum route and the other wave of cholera reached Peshawar (Fig. 8.1). Besides, diffusion of cholera into Kashmir, also took place via the Central Asian route, possibly via Kabul. It is pertinent to mention that there were intense trade links between Kashmir and Afghanistan; a number of Afghanis were in the service of the Maharaja of Kashmir (Kabul, 1882, 1885).

Table 8.3: Diffusion Model of Cholera in Kashmir (During 19th Century)

Calcutta (Ganga Delta)	Delhi	Jhelum
Jullundhar	Jhelum	Peshawar
Lahore	Srinagar	
	Srinagar	
Lahore	Ambala	
Ambala	Jumbo	Srinagar

Table 8.4 also reveals that cholera outbreaks in Kashmir were not isolated events but part of the pandemic wave spread throughout the world in general and the Indian subcontinent in particular. For example cholera occurred in Kashmir in 1845, and three years later it broke out in the USA and continued until 1850. Outbreak of cholera was reported in London in 1854, in Kashmir 1857-58; in Murree hill station in Pakistan in 1858, and in Nepal during 1857-58.

Rodenwaldt and Jusatz have published a *World Atlas of Epidemic Diseases*, in three volumes during 1952-61, which includes a map of worldwide diffusion of cholera (Fig. 8.2) during the period 1863-68.

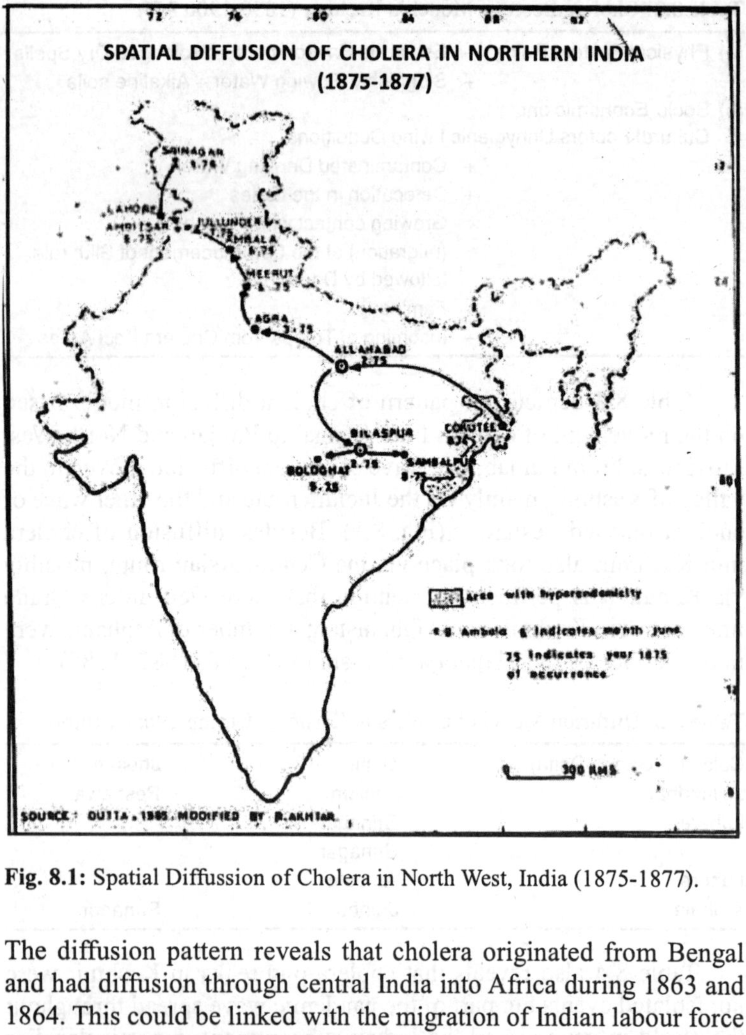

Fig. 8.1: Spatial Diffussion of Cholera in North West, India (1875-1877).

The diffusion pattern reveals that cholera originated from Bengal and had diffusion through central India into Africa during 1863 and 1864. This could be linked with the migration of Indian labour force to British colonies in Africa in the nineteenth century. From Africa it reached the Middle East in 1865 and towards Central Asian countries where cholera outbreak continued to occur up to 1872. In view of the intense contacts between Central Asian countries and Kashmir, cholera arrived in Kashmir in 1867. According to G.F. Pyle (1979), the disease also "diffused southward through the Malay Peninsula and into the East Indies by 1865. Another track was into China. During the period 1865 to 1867, the cholera spread into Europe and Russia, as well as

Table 8.4: Outbreak of Cholera during 1845-67*

Kashmir	*Murree*	*Punjab*	*N.W. Provinces*
1845	1858	1861	1862
1857-58			
1867			

Northern India	*Central India*	*Rajasthan/Rajpootana*
1867	1864	1856
	1866	1866
	1869	1869

UK	*USA*	*Nepal*
1854	1848-50	1857-58
1866-67	1866	

* Based on the table produced by Bellew, 1867 and 1879 were years of severe outbreak of cholera in Kashmir and in the Indian subcontinent. Similarly, 1874 and 1877 were cholera free years in both these regions (Bellew, 1885).

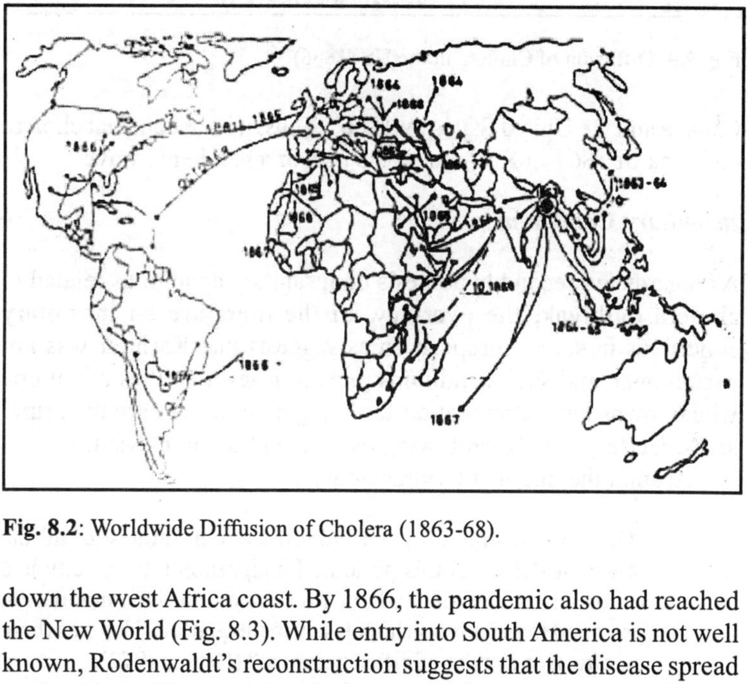

Fig. 8.2: Worldwide Diffusion of Cholera (1863-68).

down the west Africa coast. By 1866, the pandemic also had reached the New World (Fig. 8.3). While entry into South America is not well known, Rodenwaldt's reconstruction suggests that the disease spread up the Rio La Plata and into the interior of the southern part of South America. Cholera spread rapidly to the Antiles in 1865 and reached

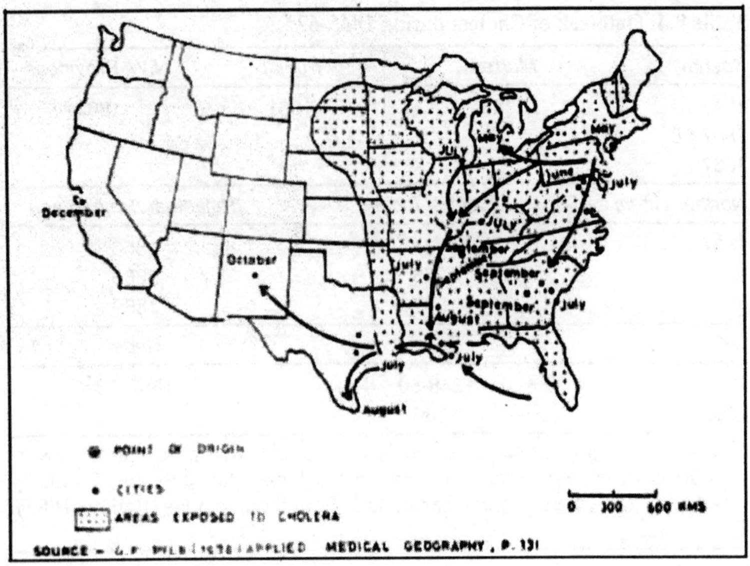

Fig. 8.3: Diffusion of Cholera in the US (1866).

Canada and the United States by 1866". Thus, it is evident that cholera outbreak of 1867 in Kashmir was a part of a pandemic wave.

Insanitary Conditions

As regards the second hypothesis on insanitary conditions related to cholera outbreak, the overview of the literature on insanitary conditions in some European cities suggests that Kashmir was not exceptional, and such conditions prevail in several cities of Europe where towns have a reputation for being more unsanitary than rural areas. (Jeffery, 1988). Following two examples are relevant:

Around the middle of 19th century,

> "Glasgow was possibly the filthiest and unhealthiest of all the towns of Britain at this period...Immigration into the city had occurred on a scale without precedent and accommodation provided to meet it was hopelessly inadequate.... Nor was there an effective system of refuse removal" (Howe, 1972).

About the city of Exeter in England, Dr. Shapter writes:

> "The adequate water supply combined with deficiency of drainage, is so self-sufficient evidence, ... dwellings occupied by from five to fifteen families hudled together in dirty rooms with every offensive accompaniment; slaughter houses in the Butcher Row: with their put rid heaps of offal; of pigs in large numbers kept throughout the city.....poultry kept in confined cellars and outhouses, of dung heaps everywhere...." (Howe, 1972 : 181-82).

The above quotations are comparable to the account of insanitary conditions in Kashmir as described by Irene Petrie and Walter Lawrence. Thus, insanitary conditions prevailing during the latter half of 19th century were not exceptional in the context of Kashmir only, and there was hardly any sanitary improvement in Kashmir until 1892, when the severest outbreak of cholera occurred. The question arises as how to explain the outbreak of cholera in certain years. Mobility of population between Kashmir and Punjab and later with Jammu region could be the main source of infection and subsequent diffusion of cholera in Kashmir. It is also evident from the above discussion that cholera outbreak occurred simultaneously in several other towns and cities of Indian subcontinent as well as in other parts of the world including Europe and the USA.

Meteorological Evidences and Outbreak of Cholera

Regarding the sudden outbreak of cholera in Kashmir, the opinion of J. Fayrer, a medical climatologist needs consideration. Fayrer who wrote books on, *The Natural History and Epidemiology* (1888), and *Preservation of Health in India* (1894) was a prolific writer on medical climatology, had worked in India with the Indian Medical Service. Fayrer preferred atmospheric theory against water borne theory (then generally accepted by the British Medical Professionals a result of Dr. John Snow's work on Cholera in London in 1854). Fayrer noted that the suddenness and virulence of certain outbreaks of cholera are remarkable, and seem to point to some factor apart from contagion or local insanitary conditions. Rather, the evidence seemed to point to changing meteorological conditions:

> "At Kurrachee, in 1866...there was a sudden change in the atmosphere, the wind veered from south-west to north-east, and a thick lurid cloud darkened the air. Later in the evening, cholera

> appeared in thirteen corps of the troops stationed there," (Fayrer, 1888).

Karachi was also affected by sudden cholera outbreak two decades earlier. According to Sanitary Report of 1869, Cholera broke out in Karachi in 1846, and resulted in the death of 438 European soldiers out of 3345, and 199 Native soldiers out of 3045. The Sanitary Report states,

> "It was in the evening of 14th June that Karrachi was struck. The epidemic occurred before Dr. Snow's theory was announced, and it is interesting to observe that among the many hypotheses that were advanced to explain its suddenness, its virulence, and its very partial distribution, no mention whatever is made of the state of water supply. No one appears to entertained the smallest suspicion that the virus could have been disseminated through that medium" (Report on Sanitary Administration, 1876).

It would not be out of context to mention that it seems Dr. John Snow's theory on cholera was quite well known by medical personnel working in Jammu, Kashmir and Ladakh regions during later half of nineteenth century. Caley, a British surgeon who worked at Leh dispensary of Jammu & Kashmir published a paper in 1868 in Indian Medical Gazattee, referred cholera as poison of the disease. It must be mentioned here that in 1849 John Snow published a small pamphlet entitled, "On the mode of communication of cholera", in which he proposed that "cholera poison" reproduced in the human body and was spread through the contamination of food and water. Thus, it seems Caley was aware of the John Snow's work.

In the absence of detailed meteorological data, it is not possible to test the theory of meteorological explanation in the outbreak of cholera in Kashmir. However, two statements, cited earlier that of Dr. Elmslie and Dr. Mitra do give some idea of sudden atmospheric change in relation to cholera outbreak. On an earlier occasion in 1862, Maharaja was held up in Jammu and could not move to Srinagar as a result of cholera outbreak. "In May-June cholera raged with such virulence in Jummu, that the Maharaja delayed his departure for Cashmere till it abated… at the end of July—the season of periodical rains" (Elmslie, 1875 : 195-96).

During the 1867 outbreak, it seems rains were deficient until August 2, when Dr. Elmslie wrote that the city of Srinagar experienced a great storm of wind and rain for about an hour and prayed, "May good result from this". It rained heavily in the coming few weeks, and according to Dr. Elmslie, the cholera seems to lie on the wane (Elmslie, 1875 : 195-96).

However, the analysis of temperature and rainfall data for 1892, the year of the severest outbreak of cholera, reveals that spring rains failed in that year, but the summer rains were in excess, as a result of very high mean maximum temperature during the months of July, August and September 1892. According to annual Administration Report, drier weather than usual during April to May followed by torrential rain, could be the reason for the severe outbreak of cholera in 1892.

Impact of Sanitary Measures

After the 1892 cholera outbreak in Kashmir, efforts were made towards improvement in sanitary conditions. These have brought desired results. According to the Annual Administration Report of 1895-96, the sanitation conditions in the city of Srinagar have improved considerably. "Roads and drains have been made, a supply of pure water has been started and conservancy is systematically and methodically done." Dr. A. Mitra who was also Administrator, Srinagar Municipality during the 1892 cholera outbreak, says, "These measures of public sanitation are having their influence on the habits of the people, and thus the cause of both public and private hygiene is improving with rapid strides.The opprobrium now resting on Srinagar, as a filthy city, and on its inhabitants, as a filthy people, will, I confidently hope, be a thing of the past at no distant date. Never, perhaps in the history of sanitation so quickly and so effectively have sanitary improvements been done as in Srinagar, in spite of financial and other local difficulties" (AAR, 1892).

Describing the horror of 1892 cholera outbreak, Rev. Tyndale Biscoe who arrived in Kashmir in 1890 and started a missionary school, commended the assistance of school boys who rendered valuable services. He writes, "I was very much gratified that at the commencement of the cholera about six boys came and offered their services to help look after the sick. Now, the Kashmiris were in deadly terror of it, and one of these boys who offered to help died of it (such a dear fellow)" (Biscoe, 1892). Dr. E.F. Neve ,who was missionary doctor in the valley discussed the religious-cultural aspect of people's behaviour at the time of the 1892 cholera outbreak. People had faith in the power of shrines. According to Neve, "And even the common people placed the most implicit trust in the protecting power of the shrines. In village after village, where the cholera did not come, the people ascribe their escape to the influence of the village *Ziarat* (shrines) and the offerings which they make. The love of shrines and relics is deeply imbued in the heart of superstitious man" (Neve, 1892).

Politics of Health

Although a critical discussion on the politics of health during the nineteenth century Kashmir is not the objective of the paper, a side reference in this regard will not be out of context. Having discussed the scenario with Mark Harrison (Personal Communication, 1999), I am firm in my opinion that there could be a political motives for portraying Srinagar as filthy, for example. It is a fact that public health was seen as part of the British, "civilising mission", and that it was intimately connected to Imperial ideology pertaining to maximum resource exploitation. Imperial policy of cholera control was not based on a humanistic perspective, but as a result of economic reasons. To prove this point, I quote Lawrence, "I have stated above that if the disease is once established in the congenial filth of Srinagar it soon spreads to the villages, causing heavy mortality among the revenue-paying cultivators of the state, and just as I urge that, even in the interests of the land revenue alone, it is politic to prevent famine, and utter disorganization and financial ruin which attend on famines, so do I urge that it is financially wise to clean Srinagar, and to remove the present danger of cholera" (Lawrence, 1895 : 219). This is a clear evidence that the efforts made by the government to control/eradicate cholera was aimed at to minimize loss of land revenue, other than welfare perspective.

Paradoxically, severe outbreak of cholera occurred even in the Military Cantonment of Lahore, which is considered cleaner than civil areas. According to Bellew, "out of the force comprising 2452 men, women, and children, 880 were attacked with cholera, and 535 died in the space of little more than a month…cholera hardly existed outside cantonments of the troops, and that, while our soldiers were dying by hundreds, the city close by, with its 90, 000 people, remained almost entirely free from the disease" (Bellew, 1885 : 1).

The above examples clearly reveal that political and economic motives were behind the formulation and adoption of sanitary policies.

Conclusion

It is evident from the discussion that though insanitary conditions prevailed in Kashmir throughout the last century, the outbreak of cholera was confined to certain periods of time. The duration of cholera prevalence also varied from one month in 1827 to 13 months during 1875-76. Mortality figures due to cholera also varied from couple of thousands in 1867 to 18,000 in the 1892 outbreak. The study clearly shows that cholera was not indigenous to Kashmir, but was part of pandemic wave with a focus in the Bengal delta, sweeping across the Indian subcontinent and diffusing to Central Asian countries, Europe, Africa and the United States. The study also argued that cholera diffused to Kashmir both via Punjab, i.e. Jhelum River route, as well as *via* Central Asian route including *via* Kabul. The study reveals that after 1892 cholera outbreak, strict sanitary measures and vaccination campaign started, resulting in the decline of a cholera incidence in Kashmir. Similar sanitary measures and vaccination campaigns were also launched in other parts of Indian subcontinent leading to the decline of cholera cases. Finally, the study does highlight the significance of meteorological conditions in the outbreak of cholera in 1892, i.e. the drier weather during April to May followed by heavy rain and high temperature during summer months could possibly be the cause of cholera outbreaks. There are also indications of the relationship between the designation of Srinagar as filthy city and introduction of cholera control measures to enable the fulfilment of Imperial policies of resource exploitation.

Acknowledgements

I am grateful to The Wellcome Trust for providing Travel Grant for consulting research material in Libraries in London. I am also thankful to Dr. Mark Harrison of Director, Wellcome Institute of the History of Medicine, Oxford, for his critical comments. I am also thankful to the Reviewers of the chapter.

Notes

1. On the border of the plain valley of alluvium occur extensive elevated plateaus of alluvial or lacusterine material which occupy a great portion of the valley.

2. Lawrence's stress on the alluvial plains as a source of cholera may have been influenced by the 'sub-soil water' theory of the German Max von Pattenkofer, which was upheld by the British in India against Koch's bacilliary/water-borne (I.M.S. Officers ridicule Koch's findings, *Indian Medical Gazette*, 19, 1884, p. 14).
3. Dogra is the name given to the region around Jammu, and is said to be derived from a word meaning the 'two lakes', as the original home of the Dogra people was cradled between the lakes of Siroensar and Mansar. From Jammu stretching east along the plains of the Punjab the region is Dogra; and all who live in that tract are known as Dogras.

References

A. Mitra (1889), *Medical and Surgical Practices in Kashmir* (1889), Lahore, 1890, p. 9.

Ashley Carus Wilson (1900), *Missionary to Kashmir: Irene Petrie*, Reprinted by Delhi: Swati Publication, 1993, pp. 112-113.

C.E. Bates (1890), *A Gazetteer of Kahmir*, Reprinted in 1980 by New Delhi: Light and Life Publishers, p. 463.

C.E. Tyndale Biscoe (1892), *Letter from Kashmir*, Extract from the Annual Letters, October, Archives, University of Birmingham.

C.E. Tyndale Biscoe (1921), *Thomas Russell Wade: A Pioneer in Kashmir*, London: Church Missionary Society, p. 7.

E.F. Neve (1892), *Letter from Kashmir*, Extracts from Annual Letters, November 9, Archives University of Birmingham.

F. Drew (1875), *The Jummoo and Kashmir Territories: A Geographical Account*, London, p. 181.

F.G Clemow (1903), *The Geography of Disease*, Cambridge Geographical Series, Cambridge, p. 93.

F.N. Macnamara (1880), Climate *and Medical Topography in Their Relation to the Disease Distribution of the Himalayan and Sub-Himalayan Districts of British India*, London: Longmans Green & Co.

G.F. Pyle (1979), *Applied Medical Geography*, Washington, DC.: V.H. Winston & Sons, p. 129.

G.M. Howe (1972), *Man, Environment and Disease in Britain*, London: Penguine Books, pp.178-79.

H.W. Bellew (1885), *The History of Cholera in India from 1862 to 1881*, London: Trubner & Co. Ludgate Hill, p. 502.

J&K Government, *Annual Administration Report*, Jammu: Government of Jammu & Kashmir, 1892.

J.C. Fayrer (1888), *The Natural History and Epidemiology of Cholera*, London, pp. 52-53; Also see, J.C. Fayrer (1894), *Preservation of Health in India*, London.

J.M. Hunter (1988), *Geography and Public Health*, In Earth '88: Changing Geographic Perspective, Proceedings of the Centennial Symposium, Washington, DC: National Geographic Society, pp. 117-18.

M. Raza, A. Ahmad and A. Mohammad (1978), *Valley of Kashmir*, New Delhi: Vikas, pp. 82-85 4. Raza *et al.*, p. 116.

National Archives, Delhi, *Kabul Residents who are in the Pay and Employment of Cashmere*, Report, August, 1875, pp. 82-86, Delhi: (National Archives) Also see: *Arrival of Certain Afghan Refugees at Srinagar*, August, 1882, 1885, secret file, Delhi: (National Archives).

Personal Communication (1999), with Mark Harrison, Director, Wellcome Unit for the History of Medicine, Oxford: University of Oxford.

R. Jeffery (1988), *The Politics of Health in India*, Berkeley: University of California Press, p. 40.

Report from Dy. Commissioner on Special Duty at Cashmere to Government of Punjab, dated 10th December, 1861.

Report from Dy. Commissioner on Special Duty as Cashmere to Government of Punjab, dated 10th December, 1999.

Report on the Sanitary Administration of the Punjab (1869), Lahore: Government Press, 1876, p. 112.

W.J. Elmslie (1875), *Seedtime in Kashmir: A Memoir of William Jackson Elmslie*, London James Street, Edited by Mrs. Elmslie.

W.R. Lawrence (1895), *The Valley of Kashmir*, London: Henry Frowde, p. 36.

9

Geographical Aspects of Malaria Study using Geographic Tools

A GIS-based Spatial Distribution Analysis

Rakesh Arya and *Abdul Qayum*

Background

Malaria endemic zones are predominant in the poorest tropical regions of the world, especially in continental Africa and South-Asia.[1] This has underlined our responsibility and exhaustive efforts towards finding cure for the disease. Current drugs for malaria include quinine and artemisinin, whose origin can be traced from natural resources and were traditionally used Chinese medication prior to the global dissemination.[2] Bio-prospecting, can involve the systematic screening of natural compounds for anti-plasmodic activity and discovery from traditional knowledge system (TKS). India is among one of the richest bio-diverse regions of the world, equipped with enough potential for discovery of anti-plasmodic plants and has a huge traditional and cultural legacy. The need is to integrate various spheres of drug discovery and to bring them under one roof to achieve the target of producing effective malaria drug.[3]

The excessive increase in mosquito borne diseases has been reported in the recent past. It is primarily because of the development of drug resistance in previously contained disease and discovery of novel diseases. Various other reasons including indiscriminate use of pesticides, excessive deforestation and demographic shifts are responsible for snowballing of millennium epidemic.[4] Malaria is a major health problem in the tropical, subtropical world and especially to the world which are socio-economically backward. In India, 89 per cent population resides in malaria endemic regions and it is a major public health problem in most part of the country.[1]

Malaria is a culprit that has victimized almost half of the modern civilization and it has become endemic across more than 100 countries.[5] Malaria is a major public health problem in India, 40 million people are suffering from this single celled *Plasmodium*, a protozoan parasite and more than 1.5 million confirmed cases are reported annually by NVBDCP, New Delhi of which 40-50 per cent is due to *Plasmodium falciparum* (Pf). However, in the study area it is only due to *Plasmodium vivax* as Pf count was found to be zero.[6] Malaria can be considered as poor man's disease and hence it requires focused planning both at the level of government and at the community. In the *Terai* region of Eastern UP, the spreading of vector borne diseases becomes uncontrolled especially during rainy seasons. In recent studies, chloroquine-resistant *P. falciparum* malaria has been observed with increasing frequency across the country though it was effective for treating nearly all cases of malaria in the past. *P. falciparum* has become drug resistant. The continued treatment of such cases with chloroquine is probably one of the factors responsible for increased proportion of *P. falciparum* cases relative to *P. Vivax*.[7]

Malaria control action plans are dying out due to improper implementation, inadequate surveillance and lack of geo-referenced information to pinpoint the trouble spots for timely preventive actions.[8] The present work emphasizes the analysing of the malaria epidemic situation and attaches various dimensions of socio-economic situations, epidemiological circumstances and geographic conditions to develop an integrated map based on the application of GIS (Fig. 9.2). GIS has been widely accepted as a mapping device for anti-malarial plants to develop geo-referenced attributes of all such plants with anti-plasmodic actions.[9] Studies have already been done for geographic association with malaria prevalence and have established that a positive correlation for malaria exists with proximity to water bodies.[10] In Huang-Huai, China it was found that 74 per cent of malaria cases were located within 60 m of water bodies and the risk rate among the people living there was significantly higher than elsewhere.[11]

The socio-economic data, as well as quantitative and qualitative information on health facilities, have spatial basis and can be integrated.[4] GIS mapping has already been done for the study area at

PHC/CHC level but the aim here was to extend this up to the villages. Socio-economic and physico-chemical factors could also be important causes of malaria endemicity in the study region. The data in this work have been acquired from Landsat Thematic Mapper, from Census India 2011 and epidemiological data were collected from district malaria offices (DMO).

The objective of the current study was to develop socio-economic and climatic factors, geographical parameters, and clinical-data based GIS-integrated databank. The work is union of twelve parameters, of which socio-economic (workforce participation, population, child population and literacy), geographical/environmental and climatic features (settlement, forest cover, water body, rainfall, relative humidity and temperature) and epidemiology (API and number of slides collected and examined) are the three major dimensions (Figs. 9.2 and 9.3). It includes finding a list of all those villages/pockets which are later called as malarial hotspots, where preferential allotments of government anti-malarial policies are required, which is GIS-integrated output based on the factors directly affecting malaria dynamics. These maps will help the authorities in reducing malarial risk in the area and hotspots will help in devising and designing strategic malaria control measures.

Methods

Study Area

It lies in the north-eastern corner of India's most populous state, Uttar Pradesh, and comprises a large stretch lying to the north of River Rapti, which is a tributary of the Gandak River, and by River Rohini on the northern side, which is also its major source of water. It has total area of 5808 sq. km. (2.39% of the state). This land is home to the population nearly equivalent to that in countries such as, Greece, Portugal, and Sweden etc., with average density around 1074 per sq. km. and is home to more than 6.23 million.[12] The region is classified as a vector-borne diseases sensitive zone especially for Japanese Encephalitis and malaria.[13]

The area comprises two eastern Uttar Pradesh (UP) districts of Kushinagar (26°39' N to 27°15' N, 83°38' E to 84°15' E and altitude 75 m) and of Maharajganj (26°59' N to 27°19' N, 83°09' E to 83°45' E and at average altitude of 66 m) (Fig. 9.1).

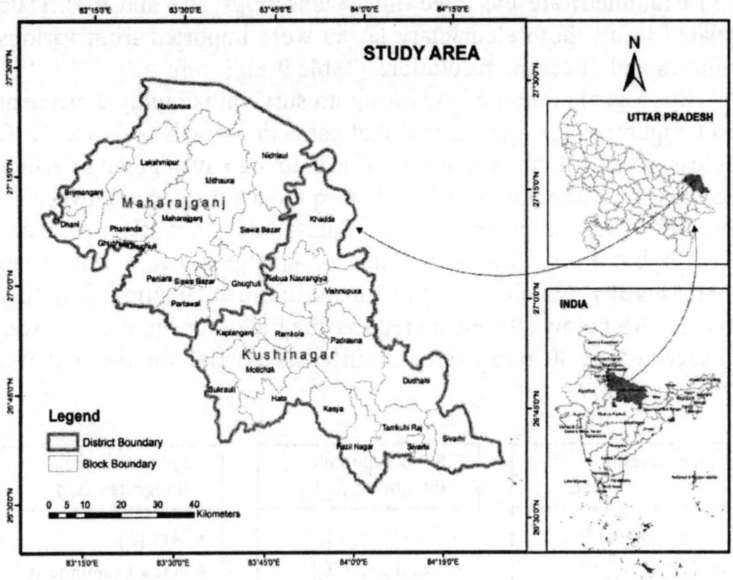

Fig. 9.1: Location of Study Area.

Materials Malarial Hotspot Mapping

Data Resolution and Source

Table 9.1: Data Resolution and Data Sources

Sl. No.	*Data Type*	*Resolution/acquisition (Source)*
1.	Data Validation	GPS Readings (by Garmin e-trex GPS)
2.	Geographical	30 meter (Landsat OLI)
3.	Epidemiology	PHC/CHC wise (DMO, 2012-13)
4.	Socio-economic	Block level (Census of India 2011)
5.	Climatic	0.5×0.5 degree gridded (CRU, UK 2013)

Layers in GIS Integrated Mapping

The work is an amalgamation of twelve parameters, of which socio-economic [Workforce participation (WFP), population, child population and literacy], geographical/climatic/environmental features (settlement, forest cover, water body, rainfall, relative humidity and temperature) and epidemiology (API and number of slides collected and examined) are the three dimensions (Figs. 9.2 and 9.3). Data related to all these elementary layers were imported from various sources and at certain resolutions (Table 9.1).

Sporogenic duration and mosquito survival is highly dependent on temperature. It was claimed that parasitic growth ceases at 16°C or less.[14] Temperatures above 32° C lead to high throughput of vector population. Temperature-induced mosquito deaths occur between 40 and 42° C depending on species.[15] Rainfall does not affect parasites directly but it provides the medium for aquatic mosquito stages and increases Rh, which is crucial for mosquito incubation. Monthly average Rh below 60 per cent reduces the life of mosquitoes.[16] It was observed that 80 mm average rainfall is crucial for the malarial transmission.[17]

Geographic Integrated (L_{15})	Socio-economic Integrated (L_{14})	Epidemology Integrated (L_{13})
• Settlement (L_7) • Forest (L_8) • Water Bodies (L_9) • Relative Humidity (L_{10}) • Rainfall (L_{11}) • Temperature (L_{12})	• Work Force (L_3) • Population (L_4) • Child Population (L_5) • Literacy (L_{10})	• API (L_1) • Slide Examined (L_2)

Fig. 9.2: Layers in GIS Integrated Mapping.

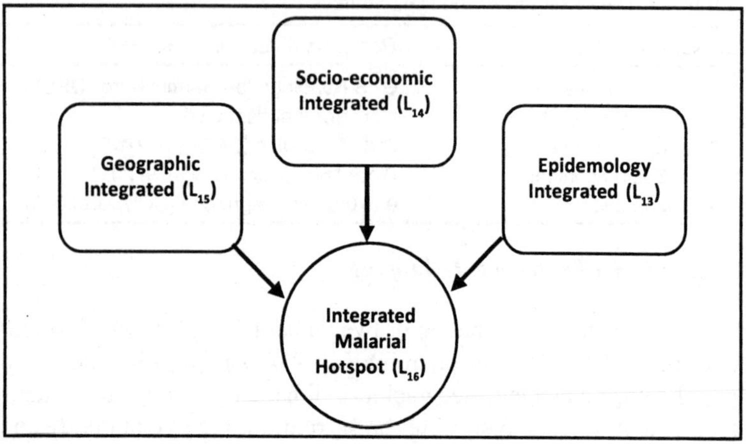

Fig. 9.3: Layers Integration for Hotspot Mapping.

This study could be useful in providing basic knowledge of malaria risk factors and to focus control measures on vulnerable populations alone, thus enabling optimal utilization of resources available, which is essential for developing countries with poor socio-economic indicators. Malarial mapping enables easy update of information and effortless accessibility of geo-referenced data to policy-makers to produce cost-effective measures for malaria control in endemic regions. The success of such control measures mainly depends on the precise identification and geographical reconnaissance of malarial hotspots. Malaria risks maps are a convenient tool for discussing targeted and cost-effective control measures with government authorities. GIS enables the generation of revised maps as soon as new data are available.

Demographic and Socio-economic Data

The data was collected based on the recent census[12] and economics and statistics division, Government of Uttar Pradesh, India. Various factors such as general population, child population, income per capita, total household, number of workers (male-female), population living below poverty line, etc., were taken into consideration and added as new fields to the spatial databank of the study area in ArcGIS 10.1 environment to generate layers for general population and workforce participation.

Socio-economics

Socio-economic and demographic data are collected based on recent Census 2011 and Economics and Statistics Division, Government of Uttar Pradesh, India. Various factors such as population, income per capita, total household, number of workers, population living below poverty line, etc. (Table 9.1) are taken into consideration and added as new fields to the spatial databank of the area in ArcGIS 10 environment to generate socio-economic indicator layers for population, child population, WFP and literacy.

Medical Data

Epidemiological indices API = (total positive cases for infection/ population size) × 1,000 and SPR = (total positive cases/total slides examined) × 100[28], are obtained for Kushinagar and Maharajganj and have been plotted to study monthly variation of API for year 2013. On a monthly basis, malaria incidence in terms of positive cases of *P. vivax* and *P. falciparum* and number of slides examined and collected was obtained from DMO for years 2012 and 2013 at PHC and CHC level. A spatial databank was created in ArcGIS 10.1 using geo-referenced data of study area obtained through satellite imagery. IDW spatial analysis was conducted on clinical data to develop epidemiology layers including API and number of slides collected and examined layer during year 2013.

Geographical Features and Climatic Data

For geographic boundaries, Survey of India (SOI) topographic maps and census atlas containing study area was needed. The features conducive for malarial mosquito proliferation, such as water bodies[11], annual rainfall[14, 17], relative humidity[16, 18], forest cover[17], temperature[14, 15, 19] and settlements[20], were collected for the study area using Landsat OLI satellite imagery technique, while the climatic data was obtained from the CRU 2013, UK.

GIS Mapping Methodology

Methodology was standardised using the following steps:

- *Scanning study area map*: At the scale of 1:50,000 SOI topographic maps containing study area was scanned to bring map data to a GIS connected computer. Big scales were preferred to reduce probability of error in geo-referencing. Feature resolution resembles more closely to the real-world features on a map of large scale and resolution diminishes with decreasing map scale.[21]
- *Geo-Referencing*: The map needs to be referenced to connect it with geographical co-ordinates (Latitude-Longitude) and every image unit (pixel) in the scanned image is defined in a new dimension. For geo-referencing, we search for crossing of lat-long in the scanned map and create a point on it using function "Add Control Points". Actual lat-long co-ordinates for a minimum of three points are input that the study area is completely included. A fourth point uses the automatically

calculated co-ordinate compared with the manual entry to generate root mean square (RMS) error. The values were adjusted to reduce RMS error to ~ 1 per cent and the entire scanned map thereafter auto geo-referenced.

- *Digitization*: It is the process of converting analog into digital information. It includes creation of vector digital database from raster by creating point, line and polygon objects. It is essentially done for spatial analysis of the data in GIS. If digitization is properly done, it will give lat-long for each point on the geo-referenced image on clicking on each point.
- *Attributes for boundaries/blocks*: Non-spatial information such as boundary name, name of blocks, PHCs, CHCs etc. were added as attributes in the digitized spatial map.
- *PHCs/CHCs identification*: It was not virtually possible to reach all health centrEs of the study area and therefore, to get their co-ordinates high resolution satellite imagery data was analyzed and created co-ordinates were verified by the expert from the same region and also with the nearby permanent geographical features present. Later, these co-ordinates were brought on the GIS platform.
- *Data extraction*: The latest data was acquired from Landsat OLI (US databases), commonly known as Landsat 8, while epidemiological data was collected from respective district malaria offices.
- GIS environment was used over these information sets to develop maps for both geographical features and API maps and analysis was done using *overlay function* to describe primary risk factors associated with the malaria incidences.
- Both spatial and attributed data were linked to analyze the risk factors associated with the malaria incidences.
- The API values for the year 2012 and 2013 were interpolated using IDW (Inverse Distance Weightage) method to map vulnerable zones in the study area.
- MIR-Red, NIR-Green and Green-Blue FCC (False Colour Composite) combinations were used to identify general land-use land-cover (LULC) pattern.

Uniform Data Generation Towards Mapping

In order to provide equal resolution of indicator to evaluate with epidemiological parameters, data from various layers was sectioned based on the percentage of area covered by the PHC, which is the unit for epidemiological data. For example, socio-economic parameters, such as population, child population, WFP and literacy, were generated at PHC level and a settlement map was produced using the following rationale. We first find the percentage settlement in any PHC and the percentage settlement of the district containing that PHC and then dividing former by latter and multiplying with WFP of that district, generate the WFP of PHC. Similarly, area based weighted values were calculated for all PHCs for the remaining three socio-economic indicators. A more detailed description of integrated mapping is described in the next section.

Single Point Data to Whole Geographical Area

- Thiessen polygons for respective PHCs were used to generate the geographic and socio-economic values.
- As the socio-economic data was represented for entire block boundary, hence area normalization method was used to find out socio-economic value for PHCs.
- The value for a PHC was calculated as the submission of various percentage shares of values covered under their respective Thiessen polygon.
- Whereas for the geographical values, the average value of pixels covered under their respective Thiessen polygon was considered.
- Finally, the normalised value for all parameters was interpolated for the entire study area using IDW method.

Integrated Mapping Methodology

Shape files of geographical features such as forest, water bodies, and settlements and climatic factors such as temperature, relative humidity and rainfall were generated and all six discrete elementary layers were prepared and were imported to ArcMap 10.1 environment. The entire study area, including all CHCs/PHCs, was geo-referenced through numerous GPS coordinates, adjusting the corresponding points in the software environment. Through ArcGIS 10 this set of information was used to develop maps for all the villages in the study area. The analysis was done using ArcMap GIS to describe primary risk factors associated with malaria endemicity. Later, the registered sub-centres with their GPS co-ordinates were imported into ArcGIS and spatial data was linked with their attributes. Similarly, various other layers were developed based on socio-economic parameters as well as geographical features as per the schematic flowchart (Figs. 9.1 and 9.2).

API value of year 2013 was interpolated using the IDW method to map vulnerable zones in the study area. FCC imagery was used to locate general land use in the study area. Vulnerable zones were overlaid on general land to analyze possible malaria causes. GIS-integrated mapping involves following steps:

1. GIS layers for 12 malaria factors (Fig. 9.1) were created individually based on natural breaks classes.
2. We had epidemiology data in PHC/CHC wise format, socio-economic data at block level and climatic data in gridded from. Therefore, to bring all different types of data at one platform:
    - *Thiessen polygons* for respective PHCs were used to generate the geographic data and socio-economic values.
    - As the socio-economic data was represented for entire block boundary, hence *area normalization method* was used to find out socio-economic values for PHCs.
    - The value for a PHC was calculated as the submission of various percentage shares of values covered under its respective Thiessen polygon. Whereas, for geographic values, the average value of pixels covered under its respective Thiessen polygon was considered.
3. These individual layers were integrated into three categories (Figs. 9.7 to 9.9) as per Table 9.2, using standard weights and mathematical equation:

   $$MHS = HS_{se} \times HS_{e} \times HS_{gf}$$

   Where, MHS = Malaria Hotspot, HS_{se} = Hotspot for socio-economic, HS_{e} = Hotspot for epidemiology, HS_{gf} = Hotspot for geographical features.
4. To obtain integrated malarial hotspot (Fig. 9.10), all 12 individual layers are combined using multiplicative function

(above equation) and weights and output was categorized using natural breaks. Multiplicative function is used to optimize the respective ranks (Table 9.2) of each malaria factor or GIS layers.

Malarial Hotspots Logics

Weights were used to produce three layers (L_{13}, L_{14} and L_{15}) initially which were later integrated to produce malaria hotspot (Layer L_{16}). The detailed process followed was:

1. PHC wise layers of all 12 factors (Fig. 9.2) $L_1, L_2 \ldots L_{12}$ was created.
2. All layers were integrated using Boolean operator 'Union' to get layer L_{13}.

   $$L_{13} = \bigcup_{i=1}^{2} (B_E) \in all\ L_i$$

   B_E stands for epidemiology for all layers from L_1–L_2
   Thus, layer $L_{13} = \{B_E: B_E \in \text{Layers } L_i;\ i = 1, 2\}$ (Fig. 9.7)
3. Similarly, for Socio-economic factors (B_S) L_{14}, for geographical/climatic factors (B_G) L_{15} and malaria hotspot was obtained by integrating layers L_{13}, L_{14} (Fig. 9.8) and L_{15} (Fig. 9.9) using Boolean operator 'Union' to get layer $L_{16} = \{B_{E,S,G}: B_{E,S,G} \in \text{each layers } L_k;\ k = 13, 14, 15\}$ (Fig. 9.10).

Generation of Weight Matrix

An evidence-based weighing method[22] was adopted which specifies the relationship of selected factors with malaria through weights. However, selected factors were decided based on scrutiny of a series of journals and research articles. The preferences were based on various research findings[14, 16, 19, 23-25] of related study regions and different regions as well. The weight system was derived from previously done researches in various regions. The information from the journals was integrated based on the relative weightage for a particular malaria factor and its frequency of repetition in research publications. A score out of 100 corresponding to these observations was assigned to each malaria factor to constitute the matrix for the weight factors.

Table 9.2: Integrated Factors for Malaria Hotspots Identification (Weight Matrix)

Factors	*Standard* weight (%)*	*Ranks*	*Degrees of Vulnerability#*
Socio-economics			
Population	8	1	Low
		2	Moderate
		3	High
		4	Very high
Child Population (0-6 years)	6	1	Low
		3	High
		4	Very high
Workforce Participation	3	4	Very high
		2	Moderate
		1	Low
Literacy	4	4	Very high
		2	Moderate
		1	Low
Epidemiology			
API	12	1	Low
		2	Moderate
		3	High
		4	Very high
Slides Collected and Examined	8	1	Low
		2	Moderate
		3	High
		4	Very high
Geographical Features			
Forest Cover	11	1	Non Forested - Low
		2	Plantation/Grassland - Moderate
		3	Wet Tarai Swamp - High
		4	Moist Deciduous - Very high
Settlements	5	1	Low
		2	Moderate
		3	High
		4	Very high
Temperature (°C)	8	3	22-25 - High
		2	26-27 - Moderate
		1	Above 27 - Low
Rainfall (mm)	13	1	60-74 - Moderate

(Contd.)

Table 9.2 (*Contd.*)

		2	75-85 - Very High
		3	85-106 - High
		4	Above 10 - Low
Water Bodies	12	4	Waterlogged - Very high
		3	Rivers/canals - High
		1	Other regions - Low
Relative Humidity (%)	10	1	< 60 - Low
		3	61-70 - High
		4	Above 70 - Very High

* Based on empirical observations guided by expert's opinion.
\# Natural breaks classification if value not mentioned (low to high downwards).

Malarial Hotspots Identification

Risk maps were prepared by overlaying twelve basic maps (Fig. 9.2). Overlay was done based on the weight system. The preferences were based on various research findings[14, 18, 24, 25] of related study regions and different regions as well. After collecting and evaluating expert response and integrating it with findings of a variety of researches, all the factors were divided into four categories, ranked 1-4. Factors ranked 1 were considered 'low', ranked 2 'moderate', ranked 3 'high', and ranked 4 'very high'.

Results

Land Use Pattern

The major use of land falls in open/current fallow (47 per cent) and agriculture land (39 per cent). Most of the land is either for cultivation or is under forest area. Considering available rainfall intensity, the region is good for rice cultivation. Rice fields and forests provide excellent breeding space for mosquitoes.[26] Land use pattern indicates the study region could be important malaria potent zone.

Epidemiology and rainfall vis-à-vis

For Maharajganj and Kushinagar seasonal variation of malaria incidence, slides collected and examined as well as monthly rainfall was plotted for years 2012 and 2013. It was observed during the rainy seasons (July-October) that malarial incidence was relatively high for both districts in 2012 as well as 2013 indicating possible strong correlation of rainfall with malaria. Seasonal variation of malaria during 2012 and 2013 was also similar in general (Fig. 9.4).

There was an increase in number of slides collected and examined in 2013 over 2012 and also during rainy seasons more slides were

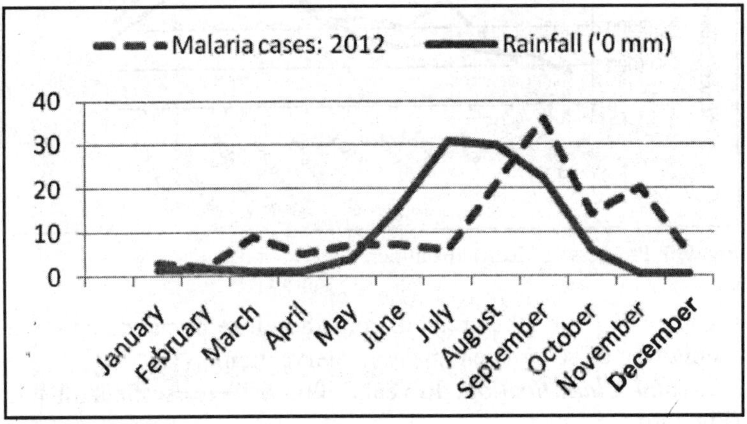

Fig. 9.4: Variation of Rainfall *vs.* Malaria.

collected and examined (Fig. 9.5) indicating medical facilities in terms of slides collected and examined had increased to reduce early detection of malaria incidence to reduce malarial deaths and is clear indicator of fine discharge of government medical facility and it also indicates the penetration of health facilities to the public. The districts of the study area could be declared 'sound' against the health facility available. It is important to note that the medical facility profile (Fig. 9.5) is indicative of governmental schemes reinforcing the expansion of the health infrastructure in the study area. Although API of the region falls below the national average, geographical characteristics, proximity to the Himalayan region and poor socio-economic conditions make the region sensitive to various vector borne diseases.

The study region has been epidemic for vector-borne diseases, such as Japanese Encephalitis, Dengue and Chikungunya. It is important to analyse the results to establish control measures against the deadly disease. It was found that the region in the vicinity of Partawal, Fazil Nagar, Motichak, Ramkola and Padrauna PHCs had

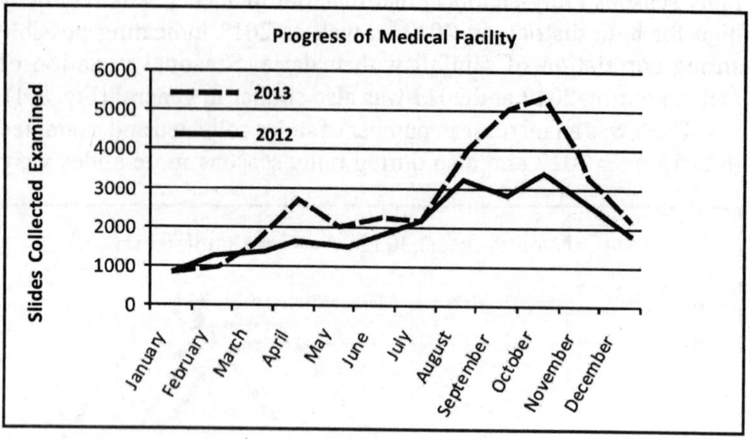

Fig. 9.5: Progress of Medical Facilities.

higher API over other regions and therefore demands strategic monitoring of government malaria intervention.

Land Classification: Reveals 5003 villages/settlement unit (Fig. 9.6).

GIS Maps for Epidemiology

Layers are produced for API 2013 and health facility indicator in terms of slides collected and examined. These two maps were overlaid to produce an integrated map for epidemiology (Fig. 9.7).

Mapping of Socio-economical and Demographic Features

Four socio-economic elementary layers on general population distribution, child population (0-6 years), WFP and literacy were produced. Elementary maps were overlaid in GIS environment to produce integrated map of socio-economic indicators (Fig. 9.8).

Geographical Indicator Maps

Six elementary layers covering major geographical malaria-related factors including vegetation, water bodies, rainfall, settlements, temperature, and relative humidity were developed to establish possible links between these indicators and malaria. The elementary

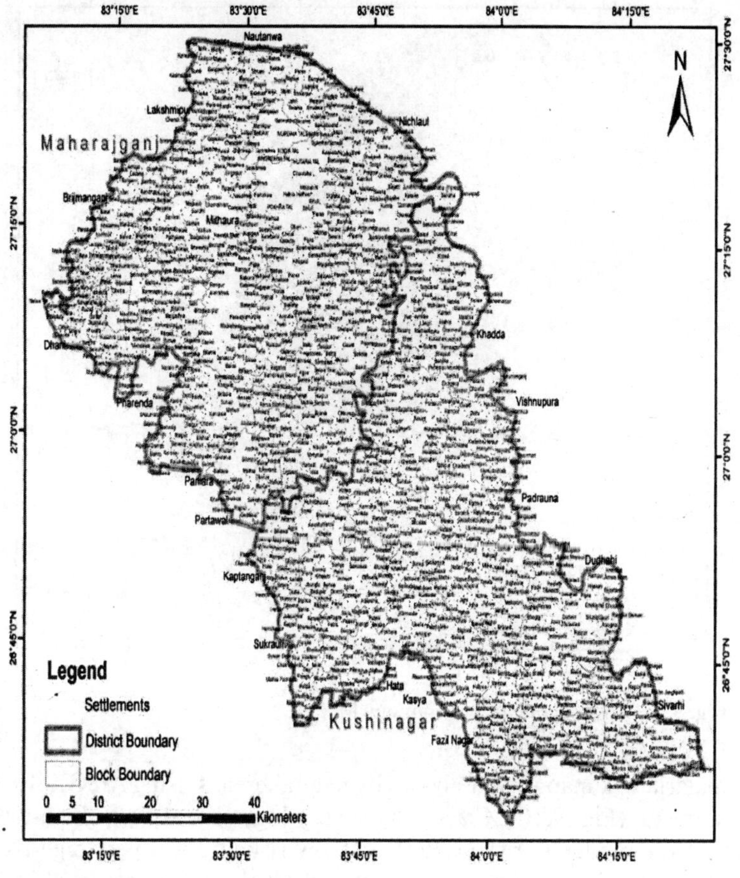

Fig. 9.6: Villages/Pockets Extracted from the Study Area.

maps were elementary units in developing GIS-integrated geographical indicator map (Fig. 9.9).

GIS Integrated Maps

To understand spatial distribution of malaria aspects, four layers of socio-economic factors, two layers of epidemiology factors and six layers of environment and geographic factors were rated, weighted and ranked (Table 9.2) on the basis of their importance on malaria incidence. Overlaying of these layers using calculated weights yielded

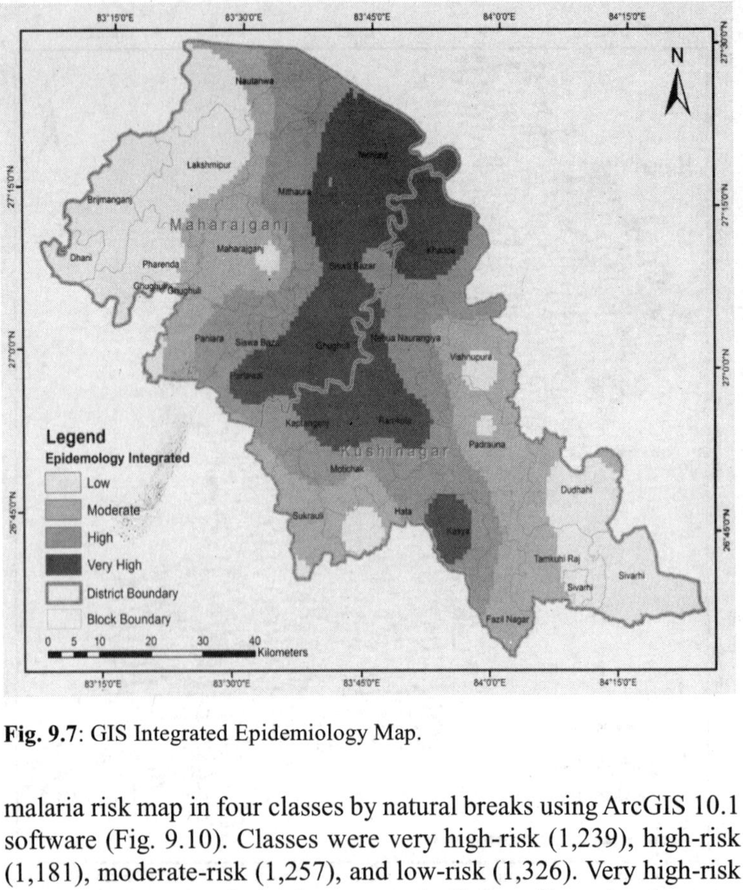

Fig. 9.7: GIS Integrated Epidemiology Map.

malaria risk map in four classes by natural breaks using ArcGIS 10.1 software (Fig. 9.10). Classes were very high-risk (1,239), high-risk (1,181), moderate-risk (1,257), and low-risk (1,326). Very high-risk class constitutes malarial hotspot and all the villages/pockets are mapped and also can be extracted (Fig. 9.12).

Epidemiology data for year 2012 was kept to verify the predictive model and results obtained in the study confer with the malaria observed in the villages of 'very high' or 'high' incidence. GIS mapping for year 2012 for same geographic region was done by Qayum *et al.,* 2013 and result was compared with the predictive model in the current study. Malaria incidence of year 2012 with 2013 was compared and also seasonal and monthly variation of malaria cases was plotted. In both districts malaria incidence is relatively high during months of July-September (rainy season). This establishes positive correlation of malaria cases with rainfall. In rainy seasons, the number

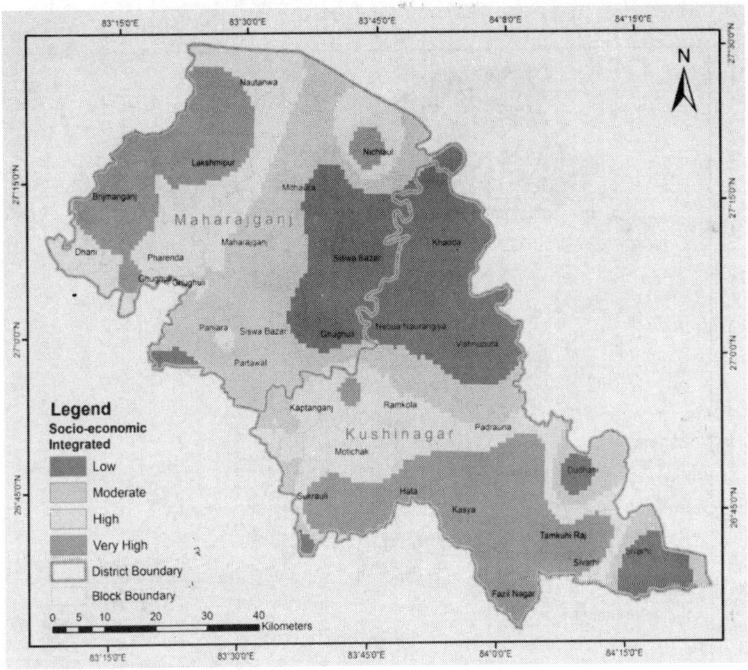

Fig. 9.8: GIS Integrated Socio-economic Map.

of breeding sites increases (because of waterlogging) leading to growth of malaria vectors. However, from 2012 to 2013 there was no significant increase in malaria eradication for the studied area. In general, it remained unchanged and the study area demands deeper investigation of the current malaria situation to bring change and satisfactory health achievements.

Malarial Hotspot Classes

Overlay of all 12 GIS elementary layers corresponding to epidemiology, socio-economics, and geographical/environmental/ climatic factors; revealed a total of 1,239 villages out of 5,003 villages studied were found to be malarial hotspots, while 1,326 villages/ pockets were found to be with least probability of malaria incidence and these are of least concern (Fig. 9.11). The entire villages/pockets/ settlement are overlaid to analyse vulnerability scenario (Fig. 9.12).

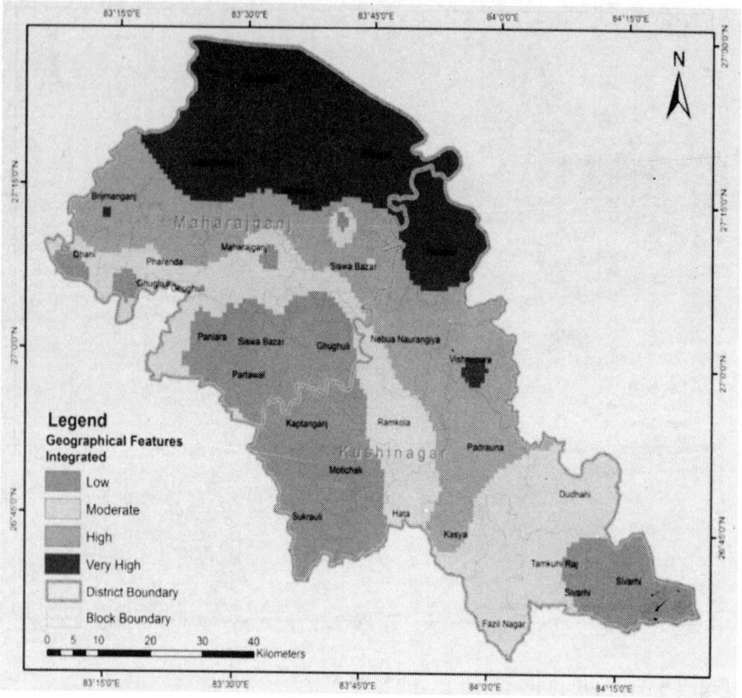

Fig. 9.9: GIS Integrated Geographical Features Map.

Weight Matrix

It was obtained based on the compilation of expert's opinion for a particular malarial factor derived from the findings of various research works done in similar geographical regions.

Correlation Matrix

It was drawn against various malarial factors to find interweaving nature, correlation indices, and to establish relationship between major malaria factors (Table 9.3). The correlation factors were computed by overlaying layers of malarial hotspot, epidemiology, geographics and socio-economics under ArcGIS. It was observed that epidemiology and geographic features were related to malaria incidence by 57 per cent, socio-economic factors were also largely

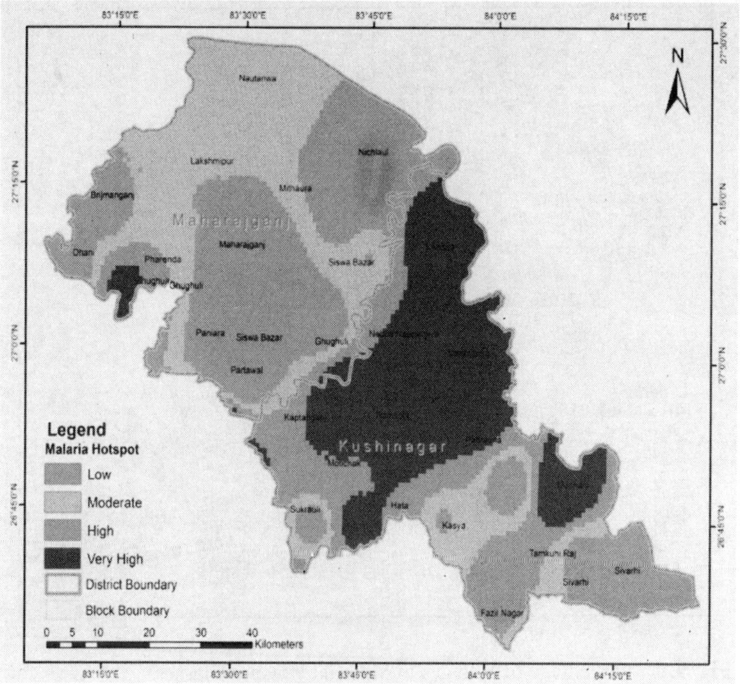

Fig. 9.10: GIS Integrated Malarial Hotspots Map

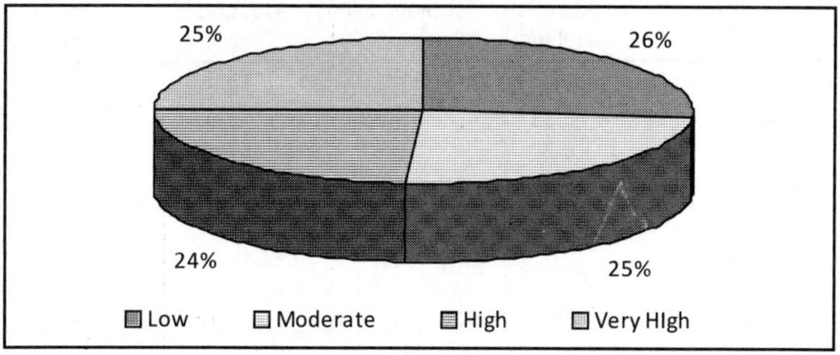

Fig. 9.11: Percentage of Villages in Malarial Hotspot Classes.

(53 per cent) related to geographic features, while socio-economic were not a major factor in determining malaria incidence in a given locality; the major factors remain epidemiology and geographic features.

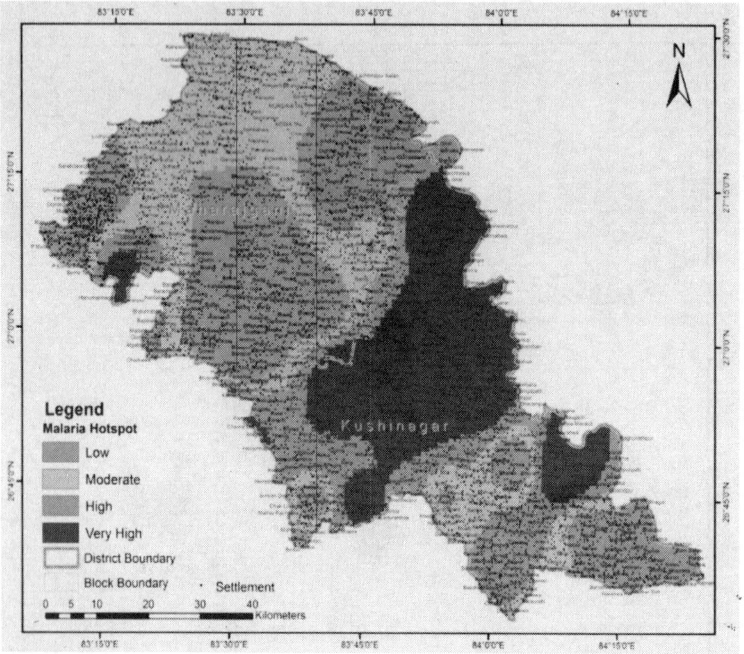

Fig. 9.12: Percentage of Villages in Malarial Hotspot Classes.

Table 9.3: Correlation Matrix

	Malarial Hotspot	Epidemiology	Geographics	Socio-Economy
Malarial Hotspot	1.00	0.31	0.38	0.10
Epidemiology	0.31	1.00	0.57	0.47
Geographics	0.38	0.57	1.00	0.53
Socio-Economy	0.10	0.47	0.53	1.00

Discussion

Malaria control action plans are dying out due to improper implementation, inadequate surveillance and lack of geo-referenced information to pinpoint the trouble spots for timely preventive actions.[8] The malaria situation has been found to dissuade social and economic progress in any state. The present work emphasizes the analysing of the malaria epidemic situation and attaches various dimensions of socio-economic situations, epidemiological circumstances and geographic conditions to develop an integrated map based on the application of GIS (Fig. 9.10). GIS has been widely accepted as a mapping device for anti-malarial plants to develop geo-referenced attributes of all such plants with anti-plasmodic actions.[9] Studies have already been done for geographic association with malaria prevalence and have established that a positive correlation for malaria exists with proximity to water bodies.[10] In Huang-Huai, China it was found that 74 per cent of malaria cases were located within 60 m of water bodies and the risk rate among the people living there was significantly higher than elsewhere.[11]

The socio-economic data, as well as quantitative and qualitative information on health facilities, have spatial basis and can be integrated.[27] GIS mapping has already been done for the study area[6] at PHC/CHC level but the aim here was to extend this up to the villages. Malaria can be said to be a disease affecting mainly poor and marginalized populations in remote rural areas, who are characterized by inadequate control measures and limited access to health infrastructure. Socio-economic and physico-chemical factors could also be important causes of malaria endemicity in the study region. The data in this work have been acquired from Landsat Thematic Mapper, from Census India 2011 and epidemiological data were collected from district malaria offices (DMO).

Water bodies play a pivotal role in malaria dynamics. Vicinity to water bodies is very important for malaria incidence. It varies inversely with distance from the water body. Based on the distance, factor weights are designed (Table 9.2). Most of the study area falls within cultivable lands. Rice is one of the major crops in the region requiring lots of water which makes a virtual water reservoir and high chance of malaria breeding sites. It was reported that mosquito breeding in rice fields is inversely proportional to the distance from village during a study in Madla District, Madhya Pradesh.[26] However, the precise role of rice fields in maintaining high malaria transmission could not be established but the rice fields contributed significant vector populations and thus high probability of malaria cases is expected.

Moderate rainfall can provide the conditions for breeding of *Anopheles* mosquito and enhances malaria hazard. The soil of Maharajganj and Kushinagar is clay and alluvial loam, which holds water and little additional rain leads to waterlogging. Thus, breeding sites are generated and this is the reason that this region has relatively high malaria incidence (Fig. 5.9). It was found that Siswa Bazar region has relatively low malaria incidence, the prime reason being heavy rainfall as it is the district with the highest annual rainfall in the whole state. The rainfall flushes out the larvae and excess rainfall possesses lower weight while the moderate (74-95 mm) rainfall that falls in southern Maharajganj and Kushinagar has high rank and these regions are malaria sensitive with respect to rainfall criteria.

This study could be useful in providing basic knowledge of malaria risk factors and to focus control measures on vulnerable populations alone, thus enabling optimal utilization of resources available, which is essential for developing countries with poor socio-economic indicators. Malarial mapping enables easy update of information and effortless accessibility of geo-referenced data to policy-makers to produce cost-effective measures for malaria control in endemic regions. The success of such control measures mainly depends on the precise identification and geographical reconnaissance of malarial hotspots. Malaria risks maps are a convenient tool for discussing targeted and cost effective control measures with government authorities. GIS enables the generation of revised maps as soon as new data are available.

Conclusion

This study could be useful in providing basic knowledge of malaria risk factors and to focus control measures on vulnerable populations alone, thus enabling optimal utilization of resources available, which is essential for developing countries with poor socio-economic indicators. Malarial mapping enables easy update of information and effortless accessibility of geo-referenced data to policy-makers to produce cost-effective measures for malaria control in endemic regions. The success of such control measures mainly depends on the precise identification and geographical reconnaissance of malarial hotspots. Malaria risks maps are a convenient tool for discussing targeted and cost-effective control measures with government authorities. GIS enables the generation of revised maps as soon as new data are available.

For the malaria hotspot identification, it was observed that the dimensions considered are primarily inter-weaving factors of malaria epidemic and closely affects malaria situations. The regions with waterlogging, high rainfall, and proximity to forest area supplemented with poor socio-economic condition are hotspot regions. The work at the microscopic level is presented through a series of maps, tables, figures and graphs to classify the entire area into 'very high', 'high', 'moderate' and 'low' category of malaria and to publish list of all such villages. 'Very high' categories of villages are termed as malarial hotspots which may be used to define government policy for the focused intervention towards malaria control measures.

Informatics tools such as GIS and remote sensing can be used in the field of vector-borne diseases including malaria. The malarial mappings enable easy update of information and effortless accessibility of geo-referenced data to policy-makers to produce cost-effective measures for malaria control in the endemic regions. Computerized spatial database and GIS mapping software provides powerful tools for the management and analysis of malaria control programme. Spatial distribution highlights the geographical location of anti-malarials and facilitates easy access of such anti-plasmodic plants. Mapping of plants would help researchers to source material suitable for the discoveries of lead molecules and novel anti-malarials.

Competing Interest: The authors declare that they have no competing interests.

Acknowledgements

We would like to acknowledge the huge support received from Dr. Andrew M. Lynn, Associate Professor at School of Computational and Integrative Sciences, Jawaharlal Nehru University, New Delhi, India for his critical evaluation of the work and for various technical supports.

Notes

1. World Health Organization, *World Malaria Report 2012*, Geneva, http://www.who.int/malaria/publications/world_malaria_report_2012/en/
2. Verma, A.K., Kumar M., Bussmann, R.W. (2007), Medicinal Plants in an Urban Environment: The Medicinal Flora of Banares Hindu University, Varanasi, Uttar Pradesh, *Journal of Ethnobiology and Ethnomedicine*, 3(35).
3. Mishra, S.B., Dwivedi, S., Shashi, A., Prajapati, K. (2008), Ethnomedicinal Uses of Some Plant Species by Ethnic and Rural Peoples of the Salem District of Tamilnadu with Special Reference to the Conservation of Vanishing Species, *Ethnobotanical Leaflets*, 12: 873-87.

4. Qayum, A., Arya, R., Kumar, P., Lynn, A.M. (2015), Socio-economic, Epidemiological and Geographic Features-based GIS-integrated Mapping to Identify Malarial Hotspot, *Malaria Journal*, 14:192, doi:10.1186/s12936-015-0685-4.
5. *Malaria Situation in India*, Delhi: National Vector Borne Disease Control Programme, Ministry of Health and Family Welfare, Government of India, Available from: http://nvbdcp.gov.in/malaria3.html
6. Qayum, A., Lynn A.M., Rakesh Arya, Jaiswal, S.K. (2013), GIS Integrated Epidemiological Indices for Risk Area Identification Towards Malaria Control Measures, *IJEAT*, *2(6)*:376-81.
7. National Vector Borne Disease Control Programme: *Guidelines for Diagnosis and Treatment of Malaria in India,* 2009.
8. Yadav, K., Nath, M.J., Talukdar, P.K., Saikia, P.K., Baruah, I, Singh, L. (2012), Malaria Risk Areas of Udalguri District of Assam, India: A GIS based study, *Int J Geogr Inf Sci.*, 26:123-31.
9. Qayum, A., Lynn, A., Arya, R. (2014), Traditional Knowledge System-based GIS Mapping of Antimalarial Plants: Spatial Distribution Analysis, *Journal of Geographic Information System*, 6:478-491. doi: 10.4236/jgis.2014.65041
10. Van der, H.W., Konradsen, F., Amerasinghe, P.H., Perera, D., Piyaratne, M.K., Amerasinghe, F.P. (2003), Towards a Risk Map of Malaria for Sri Lanka: The Importance of House Location Relative to Vector Breeding Sites, *Int. J. Epidemiol*, 32:280-285.
11. Zhou, S.S., Zhang, S.S., Wang, J.J., Zheng, X., Huang, F., Li, W.D., Xu, X., Zhang, H.W. (2012), Spatial Correlation between Malaria Cases and Water-bodies in Anopheles Sinensis Dominated Areas of Huang-Huai Plain, China, *Parasit Vector*, 5:106.
12. *Census of India* (2011), From Uttar Pradesh Administrative Atlas, Directorate of Census Operations, Uttar Pradesh.
13. Upadhyay, R.K. and Ahmad, S. (2012), Japanese Encephalitis Virus (JEV), it's Epidemiology, Disease and Vector Control with Special Reference to Immune Surveillance and Safety Measures: A Review, *Journal of Pharmacy Research*, 4(8): 2490-2499.
14. Adjuik, M., Bagayoko, M., Binka, F., Coetzee, M., Cox J., *et al.* (1998), *Towards an Atlas of Malaria Risk in Africa.*
15. Jepson, W.F., Moutia, A., Courtois, C. (1947), The Malaria Problem in Mauritius: The Bionomics of Mauritian Anophelines, *Bull. Entomol. Res.*, 38:177-208.
16. Pampana, E., (1969), *A Textbook of Malaria Eradication*, London: Oxford University Press.
17. Klinkenberg, E., Hoek, W.V.D., Felix, P. (2004), Amerasinghe : A Malaria Risk Analysis in an Irrigated Area in Sri Lanka, *Acta Tropica*, 89:215–225.
18. Musa, M.I., Shohaimi, S., Hashim, N.R., Krishnarajah, I. (2012), A Climate Distribution Model of Malaria Transmission in Sudan, *Geospatial Health*, 7(1): 27-36.

19. Salehi, M., Mohammad, K., Farahani, M.M., Zeraati, H. (2008), Spatial Modeling of Malaria Incidence Rates in Sistan and Baluchistan Province, Islamic Republic of Iran, *Saudi Med. J.*, 29(12):1791-96.
20. Srivastava, A., Nagpal, B.N., Saxena, R., Wadhwa, T.C., Mohan, S., Siroha, G.P., Prasad, J., Subbarao, S.K. (2004), Malaria Epidemicity of Mewat Region, District Gurgaon, Haryana, India: A GIS based study; *Curr Sci*, 86:1297-1303.
21. Berry J.K. (1995), *Beyond Mapping: Concepts, Algorithms and Issues in GIS. GIS World Books*, Fort Collins, USA.
22. Hana-Bojd, A.A., Vatandoosta, H. Oshaghia, M.A., Charrahyb, Z. *et al.* (2012), Spatial Analysis and Mapping of Malaria Risk in an Endemic Area, South of Iran: A GIS-based Decision-making for Planning of Control, Acta Tropica, 122:132-137.
23. Martens, W.J., Niessen, L.W., Rotmans, J., Jetten, T.H., McMichael, A.J. (1995), Potential Impact of Global Climate Change on Malaria Risk, *Environ Health Persp*, 103:458-464.
24. Haghdoost, A.A., Alexander, N., Cox, J. (2008), Modeling of Malaria Temporal Variations in Iran, *Trop. Med. Int. Health*, 13(12):1501-1508.
25. Cox, J., Craig, M., Le Sueur, D., Sharp, B. (2008), Mapping Malaria Risk in the Highlands of Africa, *MARA/HIMAL Tech Rep,* 114.
26. Singh, N., Singh, O.P., Soan, V. (1989), Mosquito Breeding in Rice Fields and its Role in Malaria Transmission in Mandla District, Madhya Pradesh, *Indian J Malariol*, 26(4):191-98.
27. Nath, M.J., Bora, A.K., Yadav, K., Talukdar, P.K., Dhiman, S., Baruah, I., Singh, L. (2013), Prioritizing Areas for Malaria Control using Geographical Information System in Sonitpur District, Assam, India, *Public Health.*
28. Park, K. (2013), *Textbook of Preventive and Social Medicine*, 22nd Ed., 234-35, 248.

10
Geographical Distribution of Cancer in India

Rais Akhtar

A Medico-geographical study of cancer distribution in any specific region is of vital importance in order to ascertain specific causes of the disease related to the geography of the area. For instance; the general relations, such as cigarette smoking and lung cancer and low socio-economic status, and inadequate genital hygiene and the incidence of cervix uteri, apply widely. On the other hand, the consumption of tapioca and thyroid cancer, and reverse smoking (burning end inside the mouth) and hard palate cancer are region-specific. Several studies have been carried out in different parts of the world, which highlight significant regional patterns and sometimes suggest factors that may be associated with the occurrence of different types of carcinomas. The geocan-cerology studies conducted by Tromp and Diehl[1], Chaklin[2], Howe[3], Pyle[4], Verhasselt[5] and Armstrong[6] are of importance and have paved the way for further regional studies.

However, very little work is being done in the field of geography of cancer in India, partly because of lack of interest in such studies and partly due to the limitations in the availability of systematic incidence data.

For the first time, a Cancer Registry was established in the Tata Memorial Hospital in Bombay, and incidence data were published for 1970-72 for 36 hospitals located in different geographic regions of the country.

Based on this data an attempt had been made to study the pattern

Reprinted from *International Journal of Environmental Studies,* 20, 291-298, 1983.

of cancer distribution on the basis of ranking.[7] The data were plotted in the Hospital Catchment Zones, which were identified on the basis of road/rail accessibility (Fig. 10.1). The study highlights the most important typical cancer regions which have been associated with the physical, biological, socio-economic and cultural factors. Thus, the larynx cancer in the north-eastern part of the country was associated with betel-nut cultivation on the oil-rich soils and its consumption; stomach cancer in the southern part of India with the consumption of hot food (over-fried food with considerable amount of chillies and other spices); the cancer of the hard-palate with reverse smoking (the burning end inside the mouth), locally known as *Chutta*

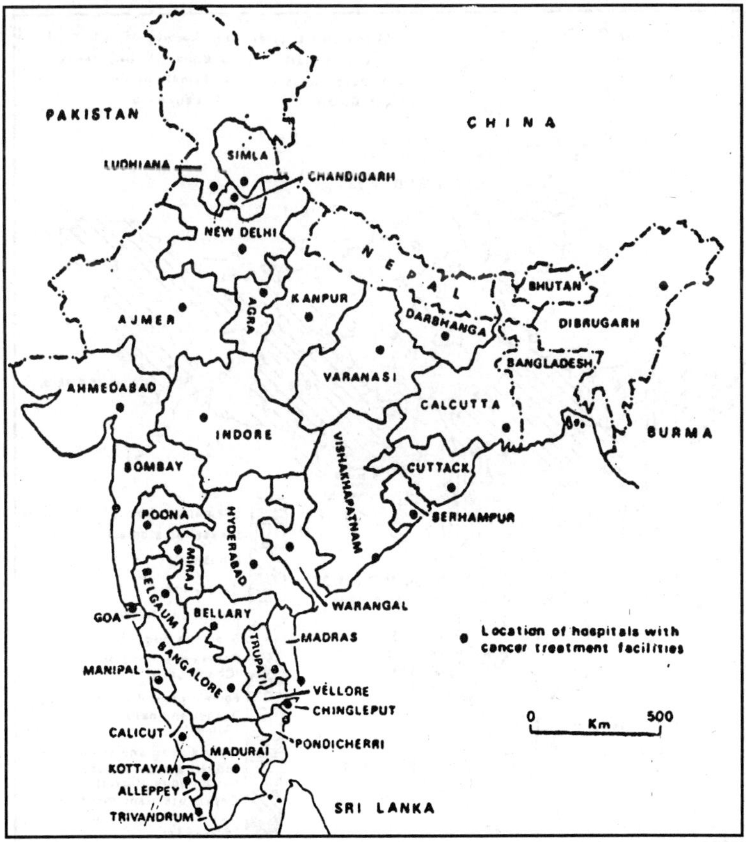

Fig. 10.1: Hospital Catchment Zones.

in the eastern coastal areas, and mouth cancer with tobacco consumption in the northern part of the country.[8]

In the present study, an attempt has been made to study the intensity of cancer occurrence in India, with special reference to stomach cancer, in order to pinpoint significant correlations.

Database

The maps (Figs. 10.2 and 10.3) are based on the morbidity data for various cancer sites published in the *Indian Journal of Cancer Supplement* (series I to IX) on the epidemiology of cancer in the

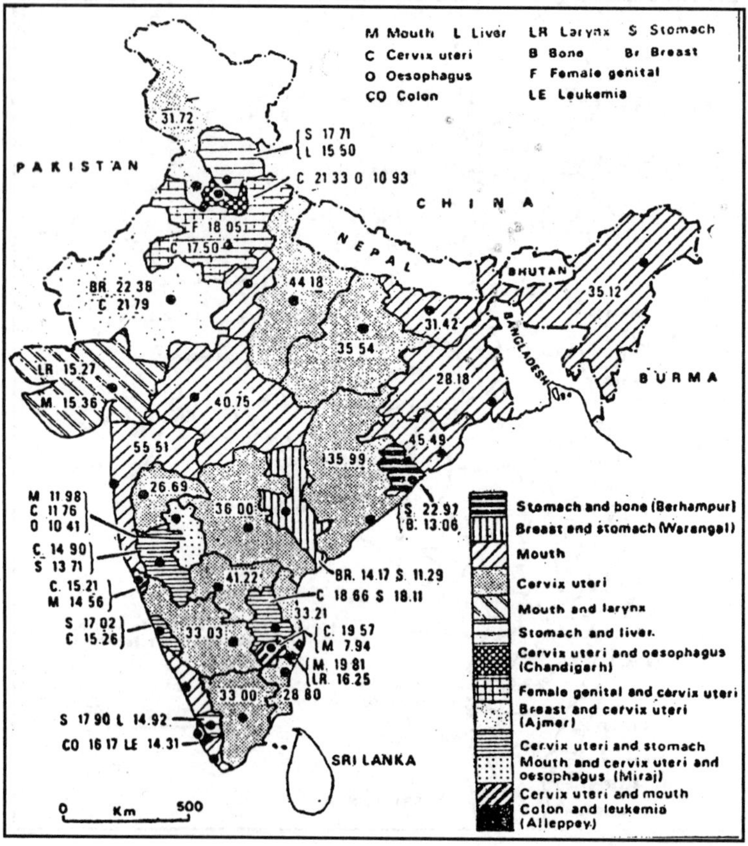

Fig. 10.2: Intensity of Cancer Occurrence in India (1970-72) (Percentage of Total Cancer Incidence in each Zone).

Indian subcontinent. The data pertain to the period 1970-72 and are presented for 36 hospitals where cancer cases were reported.

Methodology

The map (Fig. 10.2) shows the intensity of cancer occurrence in India. In each Hospital Catchment Zone[9] numbers of cases of all types of carcinomas were added and the percentage of each cancer type in the total was computed. A single cancer or a combination of different cancers with percentages of 25 or more were plotted in order to see the pattern of cancer intensity in each region. The map (Fig. 10.3)

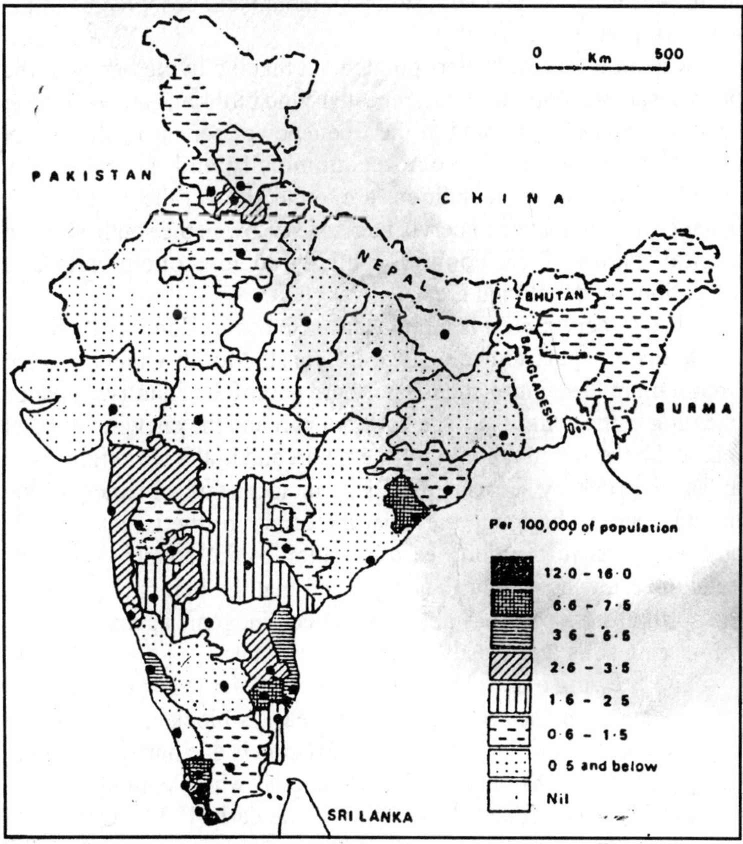

Fig. 10.3: Spatial Disribution of Stomach Cancer in India.

reveals the distribution of stomach cancer in the country, and is based on the incidence rate computed per 1,00,000 population in each zone.

Intensity of Cancer Occurrence

The map (Fig. 10.2) shows the patterns of the intensity of cancer occurrence in India, with marked regional variations. *Cervix uteri* is common both in the north as well as in the south, obviously because of the unhygienic living conditions mostly related to the poor economic status. *Cervix uteri* is also significant in combination with oesophagus and general genital cancer in the north-west, with breast in the western part, and with stomach, mouth and oesophagus in the southern part of the country.

A number of researchers pointed out that the living habits of the people, socio-economic status, repeated child births and an inadequate genital hygiene are related to the frequency of cancer of the cervix uteri.[10] Barring certain socio-economically and educationally developed areas, such conditions are found all-over the country. For instance, the incidence of cervix uteri is very low in the south-western coastal region of the country, a highly socio-economically and educationally developed area.

Next to cervix uteri is mouth cancer; it occurs dominantly in the north-eastern part and on the west coast. Mouth cancer is also important in the central and the northern part of the country. Tobacco chewing in the central and the northern part and the chewing of betel leaf and betel nut in the north-eastern part and in the western coastal areas are generally associated with the incidence of the cancer of the mouth. Sarma[11] has suggested that the cancer of the larynx and the adjacent parts in the north-eastern region of the country is due to betel nut chewing. He further suggested that the betel nut grown in the north-eastern part may absorb some carcinogenic agents from the oil-bearing soils and thus become more irritant.

The chewing of betel nut has also been regarded as the cause of mouth cancer in the western coastal areas. Niblock noted that the high frequency of mouth cancer in this region is due partly to the fact that people are in the habit of chewing "betel" which contains a large amount of caustic lime.[12] Much later in the early 1930s, Orr, while investigating the causes of mouth cancer on the western coast, noted that "the diet of the Travancore people is perhaps of all human diets the one in which the vitamin elements are most poorly represented."[13]

The diet consists entirely of rice and tapioca and is very deficient in protein and vitamin A. Orr quoted McCarrison who proved conclusively that the lack of vitamin A is responsible for the growth of epithelial growths and ulcers of the stomach.[14]

In view of this, Orr suggested that "a certain sum might be voted for the encouragement of vegetable gardening, dairying and poultry. Much of the land at present waste or devoted to tapioca might be diverted to this purpose."[15]

However, efforts were hardly made in that direction. Tapioca is still being cultivated widely. In the southern part of the western coast, particularly in the Quilon lowlands and Trivandrum, tapioca attains the first rank in the crop combinations. In fact, tapioca or cassava plays a dominant role in feeding low-income people and, in many tropical countries, it forms the basic ingredient of their diet.

Significantly, some research findings reveal that cassava contains linamarin, a cynanogenic glucoside, which, when acted upon by the enzyme linamarse contained in the plant, forms cyanide, which in humans is predominantly converted into thiocyanate, a known goitrogenic agent.[16] The author is of the opinion that the tapioca might contain some carcinogenic agents too. Thus, an investigation should be undertaken in order to ascertain the carcinogenic elements in the tapioca crop.

Mouth cancer is also widely common in the northern part of the country, although not as significant as *cervix uteri*. The practice of consuming Mainpuri tobacco has been proved in a number of research findings as the cause of oral cancer. In fact, the use of this type of tobacco dates as far back as 60 years, when it is said to have been started by a Raja of Mainpuri, spreading as a fashion among the people of this area.

Mainpuri tobacco is actually a mixture of tobacco with lime, finely cut betel nut and powdered clove or camphor. According to Wahi, tobacco carcinogens aided by possible carcinogens in the lime and the irritation of constant chewing could probably be playing an important aetiologic role in the production of oral cancer in northern India.[17]

Cancer of the oesophagus is predominant in the Chandigarh (Punjab) area of the north-western part of the country. This region is highly developed both agriculturally and industrially; the people in general are prosperous. One survey report says,

> though no direct link has been established between cancer and economic progress, some habits acquired with prosperity are said to lead to cancer. For example, excessive intake of alcohol causes cirrhosis of the liver, which in a considerable number of cases leads to cancer. The incidence of cancer of the oesophagus is also known to be higher among liquor addicts.[18]

This report further states that heavy drinking is quite widespread in Punjab. The consumption of liquor in the state has gone up many times following the prosperity brought about by the Green Revolution.

The incidence of breast cancer is highest in the Ajmer region of the western part and in the Warangal region in the south-eastern part of the country. Several researchers[19] have noted that Parsi and Sindhi women have a higher frequency of breast cancer. However, both in Ajmer and Warangal regions, the proportion of the Parsi community is negligible; again, the Sindhi community forms a small proportion in the Ajmer region. This highlights the fact that one should go beyond the idea that only Parsi and Sindhi women are the worst sufferers and investigate whether the environmental factors have any role to play in the incidence of breast cancer in Ajmer and Warangal regions, or do the communities in these areas have some similar customs and traditions to those of Parsi and Sindhi women?

Cancer of colon is concentrated in the south-western coast, namely the Kottayam and Alleppey area of Kerala. This area is industrially developed and most of the people are engaged in industrial activities, especially in mineral-based industries. The beach sands of southern Kerala are extremely rich in a number of relatively rare minerals such as ilmenite (the chief source of titanium), monazite (the source of thorium), cerium, uranium, zircon and garnet. They are believed to be the world's largest and wealthiest reserves of ilmenite and monazite. Rice and tapioca form staple food items in the diet of the rural population.

Burkitt noted that colon cancer is rare in communities which exist on a high residue diet and is common where a low residue diet has been adopted.[20] According to Stewart,

> a high rate of colonic cancer has not been reported from those countries in which the economic development is low

> and the people subsist predominantly on natural diets .... The rates for the cancer of the colon generally correlate with the degree of industrial development.[21]

An enquiry by the author regarding the diet intake in Kottayam and Alleppey area reveals that the people, particularly in urban areas, do take a low residue diet. Besides the area is the highly developed industrially and the rate of literacy is the highest in the country.[22] However, an investigation into the "self-specific environments" of the colon cancer patients and non-patients may reveal the factors which cause the cancer of the colon.[23] The significance of food crops grown on radioactive sands should also be studied.

Spatial Distribution of Stomach Cancer

Some outstanding medico-geographic oriented researches have been carried out which explain the incidence of stomach cancer in different regions. Among these, Voisin's study on the elements of soil and the occurrence of stomach cancer[24] and Armstrong's work on Diehl's milk and the incidence of stomach cancer in Iceland[25] are landmarks in this direction.

Besides, Tromp and Diehl, study on the stomach cancer in the Netherlands usefully highlights some geographical elements which cause its incidence.[26] Howe[27] and Chaklin[28] have also noted the regional variation in the distribution of stomach cancer. Various soil types were identified in relation to the level of incidence. Fig. 10.3 shows that, although cancer of the stomach has occurred all-over the country, its highest concentration is in the southern part, particularly along the south-west coast. The intensity is also high in the north-western part and the eastern coast.

An investigation into the possible causes related with the incidence of the stomach cancer in the north-western part and the south-western coastal areas leads to some interesting explanations which in fact need to be studied at a micro-level. As noted earlier, the people of Punjab in the north-western part of the country drink alcohol heavily. Such a habit causes the cancer of the oesophagus and possibly the same usages may also be suggested for the incidence of cancer of the stomach.[29] It should be added here that the author so far has not come across any study in which correlation between the alcohol consumption and the incidence of stomach cancer was obtained. High meat consumption may also be involved, perhaps in the high incidence of stomach cancer especially.

Cancer of the stomach is infrequent in the western and central parts of the country. According to Paymaster, the insignificant incidence of stomach cancer in Gujarat in western India is because of the strict vegetarian diet with fair amounts of milk and other dairy products.[30] While observing the food habits of Gujarat people, the author noticed that sugar or *gur* is mixed usually in the vegetables and pulses dishes—a typical style of food preparation not found anywhere in the country.

As it is evident from Fig. 10.3, the intensity of the occurrence of stomach cancer is highest in the southern part of the western coast. Several researchers working on the problem of stomach cancer highlighted that the habit of eating over-fried food with considerable amounts of chillies and other spices leads to the occurrence of stomach cancer. The author has found, while studying the dietary practices of the south Indians, that in general the consumption of over-fried food is common in all cultural groups. On the other hand, stomach cancer is widely reported only in the southern part of the western coast. Thus, a thorough investigation in the regional structure of the southern part of the western coastal area is required.

A general study of the regional structure of the south-western coastal area highlights some salient features typical to this area. For instance as mentioned earlier, the soils of the area contain abundant radioactive elements and tapioca or cassava is grown and is important in the diet. As has been noted, tapioca contains goitrogens, with the result that a large population especially in the rural areas suffer with enlargement of the thyroid gland, sometimes resulting in the carcinoma of the thyroid gland, noticed by Paymaster.[31] The author is of the opinion that tapioca might contain some carcinogenic substances, although no evidence in any tropical country has come to notice. The other suggestive correlation might be with the crops particularly tapioca, grown in the soils which contain radioactive elements which might develop cancerogens. The research investigations carried out by Voisin, Tromp and Armstrong reveal a positive relationship between the soil elements and the incidence of stomach cancer. According to Voisin, excessive soil moisture favours the development of cancer. He further elaborated that the variation in soil moisture affects the equilibrium of mineral elements in the soil water and the excessive soil moisture favours excess of potassium over magnesium and prevents the transformation of organic matter into humus. Thus, a further enquiry into the possible relationship of soil and cancer needs to be studied in the high rainfall areas of the south-western coast.

Tromp has carried out his studies on soil and stomach cancer in the Netherlands and obtained a positive correlation with certain types of soil characteristics and the incidence of cancer. Armstrong has clarified a soil-cancer relationship. According to him, soil is implicated with the cancer or other human disease by way of a complex food chain extending from plants and animals, through the cultural processes of food preparation, to the individual variability of human beings. Analysis of the element content of pasture grass and drinking water provide partial evidence of the amounts and preparations of elements transported from soil to man.[32] The radioactive elements in the soils, cultivation and consumption of tapioca, and the habit of eating hot food, fried in coconut oil might have a complex relationship that needs to be investigated in detail.

Conclusions and Suggestions

The study highlights the following points:

(1) There are regional variations in the distribution of cancer in India.
(2) Each region has a typical type of cancer, related to the region's characteristics; physical and cultural.
(3) Some cultural practices related with the occurrence of cancer, such as chewing of Mainpuri tobacco, and *Chutta*[33] smoking are deeply rooted and even the spread of education has not brought any change in the way of living of the people.
(4) Similarly, there are variations in the occurrence of the stomach cancer in India, the southern part having high intensity and certain areas in the north being free from it.
(5) The incidence of stomach cancer is high in the areas: (a) where the consumption of over-fried food, meat and locally prepared alcohol is very common, such as in Punjab; and (b) in areas where tapioca is a staple food and coconut oil is widely consumed, such as in Kerala. The areas largely subsisting on a vegetarian diet, with more fruits and milk

tend to have incidence rates that are either negligible or very low.

Thus, it may be concluded that the occurrence and distribution of cancer in India is function of certain deep rooted cultural practices, socio-economic standards and the diet intake. Physical environment also plays a role to the extent of altering the trace elements in the soil and water.

Obviously, cancer is a complex problem and to be studied at a micro-level. The study would be more comprehensive and the result would be more realistic if the "self-specific environment" of sample cases of patients and non-patients are studied in each intensity zone.

Acknowledgements

The author is very grateful to Professors Andrew Learmonth, Vola Verhasselt and R.W. Armstrong for their constructive suggestions.

Notes

1. Tromp, S.W. and Diehl, J.C. (1955), A Statistical Study of the Possible Relationship between Cancer of the Stomach and Soil, *Brit. J. Cancer,* 9, 349-357.
2. Chaklin, A.V. (1962), The Geographical Distribution of Cancer in the Soviet Union, *Soviet Geography,* 3, 59-68.
3. Howe, G.M. (1971), The Geography of Lung-bronchus Cancer and Stomach Cancer in the United Kingdom, *Scottish Geographical Magazine,* 87, 202-220.
4. Pyle, G.F. (1971), *Heart Disease, Cancer and Stroke in Chicago,* Chicago: University of Chicago, Department of Geography.
5. Verhasselt, Y. (1975), *Maps of Cancer Distribution,* Vrije Universiteit te Brussel Geografisch Instituut.
6. Armstrong, R.W. (1976), The Geography of Specific Environments of Patients and Non-patients in Cancer Studies, with a Malaysian example. *Economic Geography,* 52, 161-170.
7. Akhtar, R. (1978), Geography of Cancer in India, *Mèdicine Biologie Environment,* 6, 20-30.
8. *Ibid.*
9. In order to demarcate the catchment zone of each hospital (Fig. 10.1), the accessibility, in terms of road and rail communications was taken into consideration. Physical barriers, such as rivers and mountains which hamper people's movement were also given due consideration.

10. Wynder, E.L. (1955), Environmental factors in cervical cancer: an approach to its prevention, *Brit. Med. J.,* 1, 743-747; Gault, E.W. (1955), Geographic distribution of carcinoma of uterus and relative distribution of cervical and fundal carcinoma with special reference to South India; *Schweiz, Z. Path. Bakt.,* 18,732-749; Wahi, P.N., Mali, S. and Luthra, U.K. (1969), Factors Influencing Cancer of the Uterine Cervix in North India, *Cancer,* 23, 1221-1226; Luthra, U.K. (1976), Epidemiology of cervical cancer in India, in T. Hirayama (Ed.) *Cancer in Asia: Opportunity for Prevention, Detection and Treatment,* Tokyo: University Park Press, 161-166.
11. Sarma, S.N. (1958), A Study into the Incidence and Etiology of Cancer of Larynx and Adjacent Parts in Assam, *Indian J. Medical Research,* 46, 525-533.
12. Niblock, W.J. (1902), Cancer in India, *Indian Medical Gazette,* 161-163.
13. Orr, I.M. (1933), Oral Cancer in Betel-nut Chewers in Travancore, *Lancet,* 2, 575-580.
14. *Ibid.,* p. 577.
15. *Ibid.,* p. 579.
16. Ermans, A.M. *et al.* (1980) (Eds.), *Role of Cassava in the Etiology of Goitre and Cretinism,* International Development Research Centre, Ottawa, p. 5.
17. Wahi, P.N.; Lahiri, B. and Kehar, U. (1966), Epidemiology of Oral and Oropharyngeal Cancer: A Study of Regional Factors in Uttar Pradesh, *J. Indian Med. Assoc.*, 46, 175-181.
18. Cancer Incidence in Punjab (1979), *The Times of India,* 22nd February, New Delhi.
19. Jussawalla, D.J. (1970), Breast Cancer in India, in T. Hirayama (Ed.) *op. cit.,* pp. 265-273; Paymaster, J.C. and Gangadharan, P. Cancer in Parsi community in Bombay; *Intern. J. Cancer Res.,* 5, 426-431.
20. Burkitt, D.P. (1971), Colon Carcinogens: Their Metabolism and Mode of Action, *Cancer,* 28, 3.
21. Stewart, H.L. (1971), Geographic Pathology of Cancer of the Colon and Rectum, *Cancer,* 28, 25.
22. Traditional industries; such as coir, cashew, bricks and tiles, oil milling, handloom and timber continue to dominate the industrial sector in Kerala, employing nearly 83 per cent of the total workforce in the industrial sector. Other industries include rubber goods, cycle rim, shark liver oil, plywood, ceramics, soap and textiles and industries producing rayons, glass, fertilizers, cement, aluminium, and electrical goods.
23. Armstrong, R.W. (1976), The Geography of Specific Environments of Patients and Non-patients in Cancer Studies, with a Malaysian example. *Economic Geography,* 52, 161-170.
24. Voisin, A. (1959), *Soil, Grass and Cancer,* London.
25. Armstrong, R.W. (1967), Milk and Stomach Cancer in Iceland, *Acta Agriculturea Scandinavia,* 17, 30-32.
26. Tromp, S.W. and Diehl, J.C. (1955), A Statistical Study of the Possible Relationship between Cancer of the Stomach and Soil, *Brit. J. Cancer,* 9, 349-357.

27. Howe, G.M. (1971), The Geography of Lung-bronchus and Stomach Cancer in the United Kingdom, *Scottish Geographical Mag.*, 87, 202-220.
28. Chaklin, A.V. (1962), The Geographical Distribution of Cancer in the Soviet Union, *Soviet Geography,* 3, 59-70.
29. Cancer Incidence up in Punjab, *The Times of India, op. cit.*
30. Paymaster, J.C. (1964), Cancer and its distribution in India, *Cancer,* 17, 1031.
31. *Ibid.,* p. 1033.
32. Armstrong, R.W. (1964), Environmental Factors Involved in Studying the Relationship between Soil Elements and Disease, with an Iceland example, *Amer J., Public Health,* 54, 1536-1544.
33. *Kangri* Burn Cancer (in the Kashmir Valley in the Northern Part) and Hard Palate Cancer due to *Chutta* or Reverse Smoking in the Northern Part of the Eastern Coast have not Emerged as Significant in Fig. 10.2. Hence not dealt with.

11
Food Production Efficiency and Nutrition in India

Mohammad Shafi

This chapter is an attempt to make a comparative study of the food production efficiency and the availability of nutrition in terms of calories in India. Fig. 11.1 shows the per acre productivity of all food crops grown in the area in terms of Standard Nutrition Units. The procedure in the preparation of this map may be summarized as follows:

The district has been taken as the unit of study and the acre yields of each food crop grown in the district were converted into calories. These were added together and divided by the number of crops considered. The result thus obtained revealed the output of calories per acre. Considering the actual intake of 2,000 calories per person per day as the minimum requirements under Indian conditions (equivalent to a farm production of 8,00,000 calories, taking into account a loss of 10 per cent in the general range of extraction rates and known losses in food production) the author has converted the per acre calories into Standard Nutrition Units. It will be seen from Fig. 11.1 that the areas of food production efficiency have been grouped into five categories: very high (above 2.5 S.N.U. per acre), high (2-2.5), medium (1.5-2), low (0-1.5), very low (below 1).

The areas of very high food production efficiency lie in general in southern India, mostly in the states of Madras (now Tamil Nadu) and Andhra Pradesh while there are vast areas in India where the

Reprinted after having been edited from *The Geographer,* 14, 23-27, 1967.

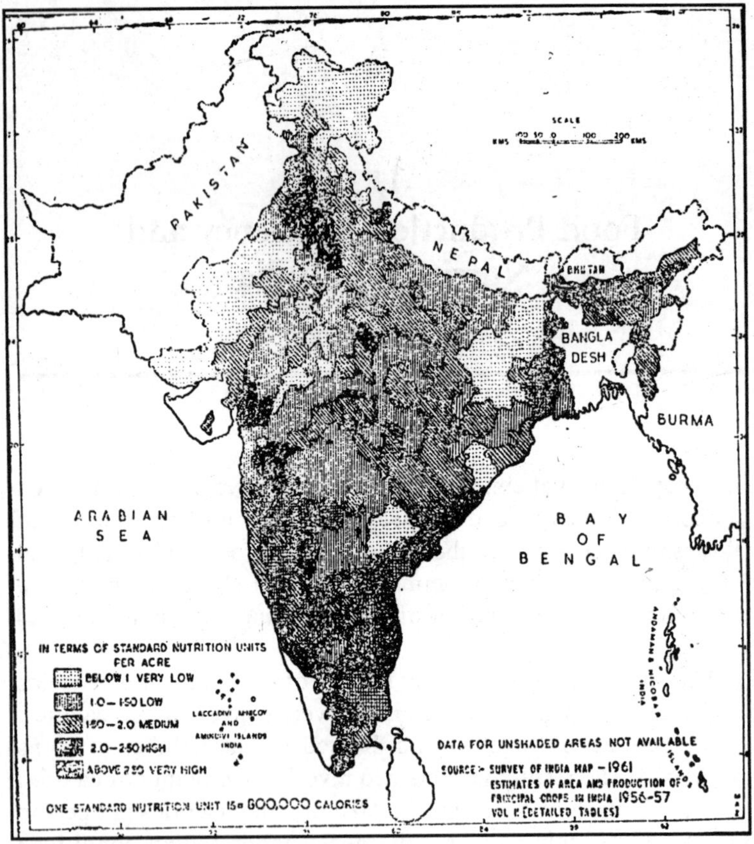

Fig. 11.1: India: Food Production Efficiency*

food production efficiency is low or very low. The northern parts of Punjab (now Punjab and Haryana) and a major portion of Uttar Pradesh show only medium production efficiency in spite of the fact that there is a zone of predominantly alluvial soil and a substantial area is under irrigation.

* Per Acre Productivity of all Food Crops in terms of Standard Nutrition Units.
The district has been taken as the unit of study. The district boundaries are based on the Survey of India Political Map, 1961.
Agricultural statistics used in this study have been taken from *Estimates of Area and Production of Principal Crops in India—1956-57,* Vol. I.
Data for unshaded areas were not available.

The differences in the good production efficiency over the different parts of the country are partly due to the differences of climate and soil and partly due to the differences in the progress of agricultural development programmes between different states. The varying use of inputs like fertilizers, improved seeds, irrigation water, and insecticides shows a close correlation to the productivity per acre, as is shown in Table 11.1.

Table 11.1: Variation in Inputs

States	*Co-operative loans advanced (1959-60)*		*Use of chemical fertilizers (1959)*			
	Total ₹ in lakhs	*Per acre cropped area (in Rs.)*	*Total Tons*	*Per acre of agri-cultural land*	*Gross irrigated area as (000 acres)*	*Gross irrigated area as percentage of gross area sown*
Andhra Pradesh	1750	5.86	36,911	2.64	8,640	28.0
Madras (T. Nadu)	1737	10.36	40,232	5.38	7,312	42.8
Mysore (Karnataka)	1203	4.62	11,847	1.03	2,141	8.2
Maharashtra and Gujarat	5063	15.43	42,664	1.36	4,286	6.1
Uttar Pradesh	2922	5.43	44,170	1.87	13,238	24.6
Punjab	1129	4.60	7,124	0.67	9,514	38.8
Rajasthan	539	1.59	3,158	0.21	4,067	12.0
Madhya Pradesh	1301	2.97	9,913	0.51	2,096	4.8
Assam	67	1.11	1,644	0.62	1,533	26.5
West Bengal	227	1.51	12,283	1.83	3,379	22.4
Bihar	129	0.47	15,129	1.36	5,090	18.6
Orissa	235	1.57	5,172	0.77	2,820	18.0

It will be seen from Table 11.1 that the amount of co-operative loans per acre of cropped area, use of chemical fertilizers per acre of agricultural land and the percentage of the irrigated area to the gross cultivated area are substantially high in the States of Madras, Andhra Pradesh, Maharashtra and Gujarat and these factors correspond with the high production efficiency of these States, while the low and very low production efficiency of Orissa, Madhya Pradesh and Rajasthan corresponds to the low amount of fertilizers and co-operative loans available to these States.

Agricultural policy should be formulated in such a manner as the medium, low and very low efficiency areas are at least raised to the level of high efficiency areas, if not to the level of very high efficiency areas, and this will substantially raise the agricultural production in the country.

The writer has further attempted to calculate the total existing production of Standard Nutrition Units (S.N.U.) and the additional production of S.N.U. if the food production efficiency of the lands of the three categories are brought to the level of the lands of the high production efficiency.

Excluding the areas for which data were not available, the existing production of 375 million S.N.U. falls far short of the requirement if the total population of India is taken at 480 millions in 1966. The per head S.N.U. amounts to 0.78 whereas the average requirements should not be less than 1 S.N.U. However, if the existing and the additional S.N.U. are taken into account, the total would amount to 608 million S.N.U. The year 1968, when the population would be 500 millions, is fixed as the target to raise the additional S.N.U. Each individual would not only be provided with one S.N.U. but there would be a balance of 100 million S.N.U. and would make India self-sufficient for a decade to come.

The pattern of production efficiency, particularly in the range of medium to very low, broadly corresponds with the pattern of caloric intake of the population. Fig. 11.2 is an attempt to show the Standard Nutrition Unit per person per annum. The district has been taken as the unit of study. The total production of all food crops has been converted into calories and divided by the number of people in that district. The result thus obtained was further divided by 8,00,000 calories to obtain Standard Nutrition Units per person.

An examination of Fig. 11.2 shows that there are eight districts where the S.N.U. is over 2.5 and these districts fall in the States of Andhra Pradesh (Kurnool), Mysore (now Karnataka), (Bellary and Bijapur), Madhya Pradesh (Hoshangabad), and Punjab (now Punjab and Haryana) (Bhatinda, Hissar, Rohtak, Narnaul and Mahendargarh).

There are nine districts where the S.N.U. is between 2 and 2.5. These lie in the States of Andhra Pradesh (West Godavari); Maharashtra (Osmanabad, Sholapur); Madhya Pradesh (Chhindwara, Sagar, Damoh); Gujarat (Palanpur); Rajasthan (Sri Ganganagar). There are 22 districts in the category of 1.5 to 2 S.N.U. These fall in the States of Andhra Pradesh (Nellore); Mysore (now Karnataka)

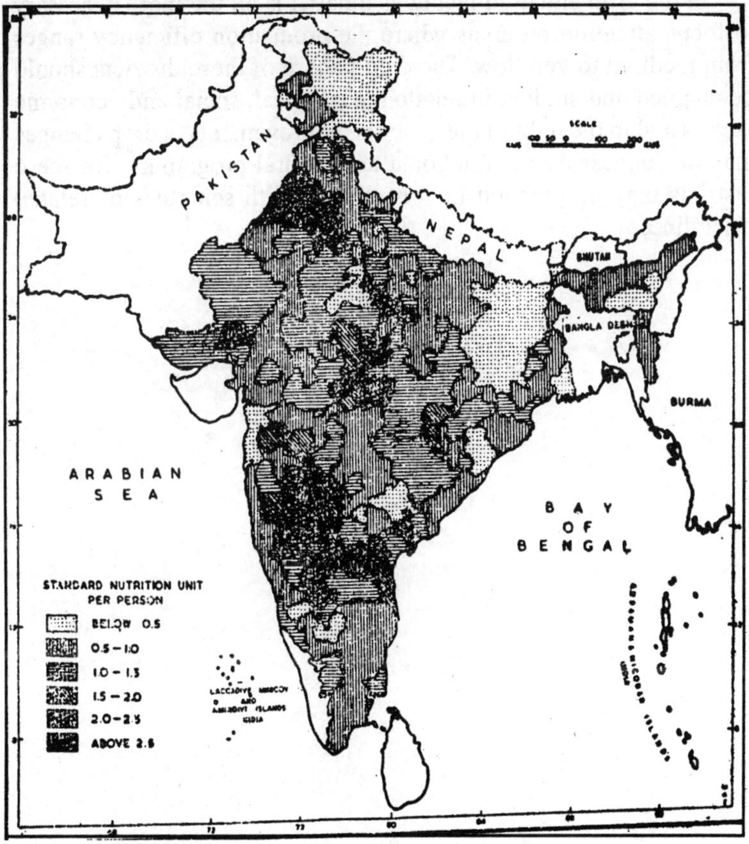

Fig. 15.2: Standard Nutrition Units Per Person Per Annum.

(Bidar, Gulbarga, Raichur, Belgaum and Chitaldrug); Maharashtra (Nasik, Aurangabad, Satara, Sangli); Madhya Pradesh (Raipur, Guna, Vidisha, Raisen and Bhind); Uttar Pradesh (Banda and Jalaun); Punjab (now Punjab and Haryana) (Gurgaon, Karnal, Sangrur, Ferozepur).

Thus, there are 39 districts where the S.N.U. is above 1.5 and if we add to these 74 districts which have S.N.U. between 1 and 1.5, it will be seen that 113 districts or about one-third of the total districts of India are above the critical level while two-thirds fall below that level. Those districts where the level of nutrition of the people is critical are the district where the food production efficiency ranges from medium to very low.

In the grim situation facing us today it is all the more necessary to focus attention on areas where the production efficiency ranges from medium to very low. The crop pattern of these districts should be mapped and studied in relation to physical, social and economic factors and in the light of the analysis, improvements in crop changes may be suggested and a national agricultural programme for these districts may be planned in consultation with scientists of related disciplines.

12

Food Insecurity in Rural Areas of Bandipore District, Jammu & Kashmir

Rais Akhtar

"Mountain water, forests, flora, and fauna constitute a rich global resource.
Yet in many places, the people living in mountain environments are exposed to harsh climatic conditions and soil and terrain constraints that make sustainable agricultural production difficult. In many locations, their relative isolation also limits non-agricultural options."

—**Barbara Huddleston** *et al.* (2003)
(Towards a GIS based analysis of mountain environments and population, FAO, Rome)

Introduction

The objectives of the chapter are to examine the environmental framework of food production and its availability in 100 households in four randomly selected villages in Bandipore district. The data obtained through a structured questionnaire survey. The aim of the analysis is to study various drivers of food insecurity in the region, and identify coping strategies when faced with shocks. This survey was based on a stratified random sampling and analysis of data shows that rural food needs are mainly met with food imported from outside the mountain region. Nearly 44 per cent of potatoes are purchsed from the nearby town as this rural area supply only 23 per cent of their needs. Regarding the supply of tomatoes, nearly 32 per cent come from outside the mountain region. About 50 per cent chickens consumed are obtained from the town. However, milk supply is satisfactory in the rural areas. The analysis shows that about 58 per cent households draw down on savings when faced with shocks, with only 21 per cent borrow money from other sources. Important key drivers in food insecurity in the rural areas include shortage of food and insufficient food production comprise 44 per cent. Sixty per cent respondents are of the opinion that temperature has risen in the area in the last one decade. However, in view of the importance of non-agricultural activities, people are financially well off and this is evident from the diet intake and the level of nutrition (k.cal.) Adaptation to increased risk of floods and droughts are among new climatic realities and the rural people are unable to cope with their traditional coping strategies. Government have to find ways to develop infrastructure network particularly all weather roads, marketing and health care facilities to support improved livelihood strategies.

Introduction: Geo-Ecology of the Region

Bandipore district of Jammu & Kashmir state falls in the Western Himalaya that constitute 25 per cent of the total population of the Himalaya (Fig. 12.1). It is located on the banks of the Lake Wular which is said to be the largest fresh water lake in the whole Asia. This lake is the home to many migratory birds. Nearly 50 per cent of cultivated land producing paddy, maize and fodder is irrigated.

The average rainfall recorded in the region is 589 mm and the number of rainy days is 82. The topography of region includes plains, karewas, hill and wetlands and water bodies. The kind of topography in general makes the areas prone to flooding and drought (Raina, 2002). Among the various tahsils of Bandipur district, Bandipore tahsil has the least number of villages as much of the area is under forest or water bodies. In most villages the water is lifted by pumps and distributed through irrigation canals. The predominant clay soils become very loose when wet, and hard when dry. Women and the young ones are engaged in the production of handicrafts like carpet making, embroidery and shawl weaving. The people mostly belong to low income group (GoI, 2001).

The situation is exacerbated by low productivity, unemployment and underemployment. The region lacks basic services including

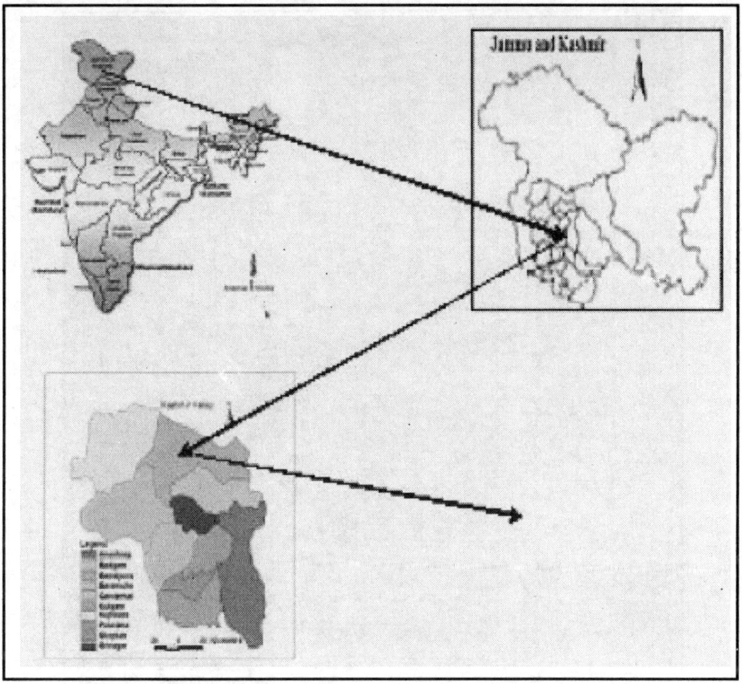

Fig. 12.1: Location Map of the Study Area.

Source: Delineated from SOI Toposheets in GIS Environment.

sanitation (Plate 1) and safe drinking water. Average literacy rate is 51 per cent that is lower than the national average (59.5%). Most people in the region suffer from waterborne diseases and malnutrition.

Methodology

The study is based on survey of four villages of Bandipore Tahsil. Twentyfive households were selected from each village using stratified random sampling. The questionnaire administered was the same as used for similar surveys in other mountainous areas. The questions pertained to purchase of food items by location, response of people when faced with negative shocks, particularly the rising prices of food items, and major key drivers of food insecurity in the study area. The study is basically based on primary data obtained through the questionnaire.

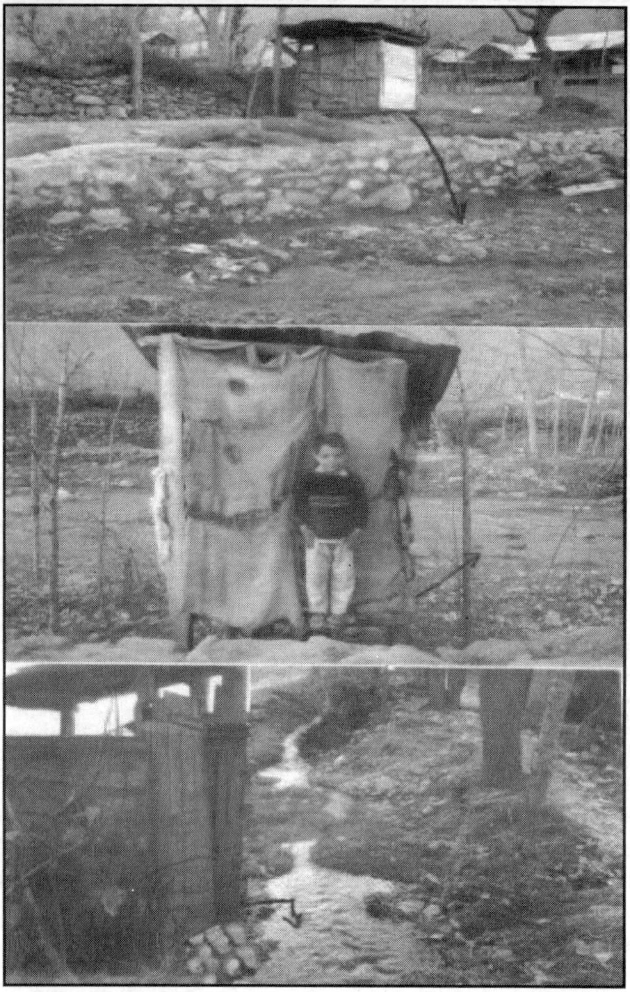

Plate 1: State of Sanitation in Bandipore.

Purchase of Food Items by Location

Fig. 12.2 gives the distance from which people purchased rice. Rice is a staple food and constitutes major part of people diet. The region supplies only about half (52%) of its requirements. Twenty two per cent is obtained from other village, 16 per cent from the town, and 10 per cent from outside the mountain.

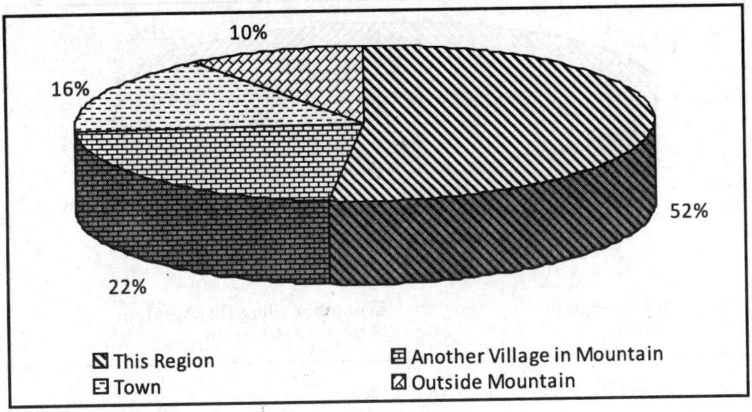

Fig. 12.2: Supply of Rice by Location.

Potato also constitutes a major component of the diet of the people. But only 44 per cent of the demand is met locally and the rest comes from other villages, Bandipore town or from outside the mountain (Fig. 12.3).

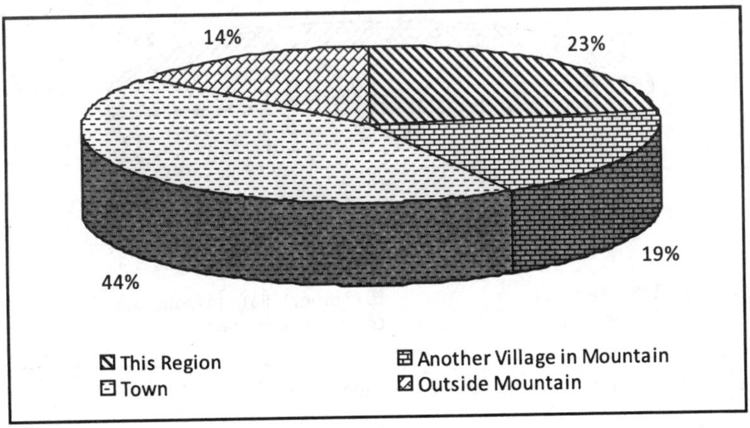

Fig. 12.3 : Supply of Potatoes by Location.

Onion is utilized in the preparation of different food items. About 32 per cent of the requirements is met purchased from outside the mountain; 26 per cent from the region, and another 26 per cent from neighbouring village (Fig. 12.4).

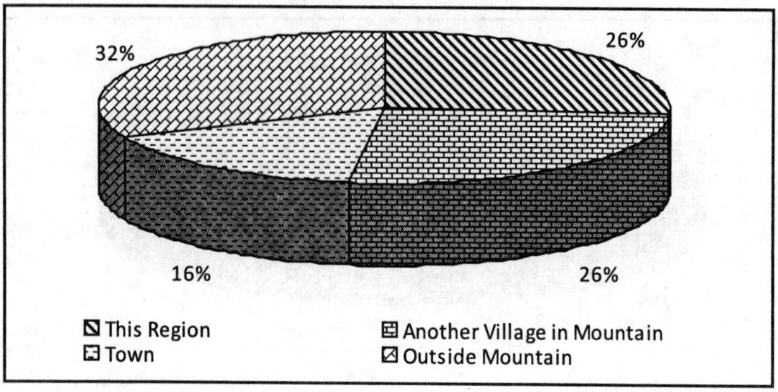

Fig. 12.4: Supply of Onions by Location.

The region is not self-sufficient even in vegetables like tomatoes. About 32 per cent of the need is met from outside mountain and 20 per cent and 19 per cent from another village and town respectively. The region produces only 29 per cent of the requirements of the study area (Fig. 12.5).

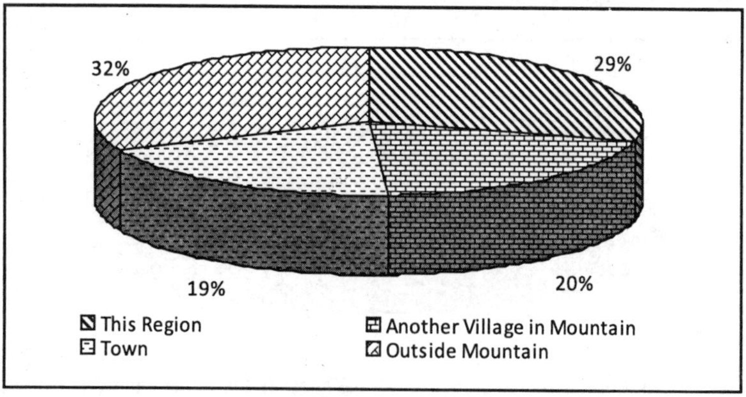

Fig. 12.5: Supply of Tomatoes by Location.

For poultry people are heavily dependent on Bandipore. The region produces only 19 per cent of its requirements and about 21 per cent of it is obtained from other village (Fig. 12.6).

The region is, however, well off in milk. It produces 83 per cent of its requirements. The rest comes from a neighbouring village (13%); from the town (3%) and outside mountain (1%) (Fig. 12.7).

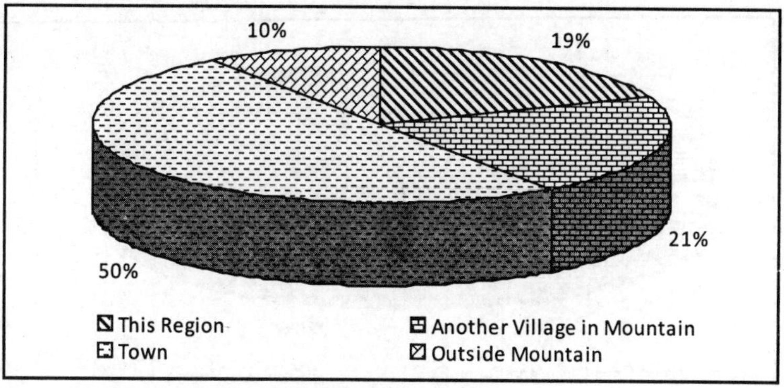

Fig. 12.6: Supply of Chicken by Location.

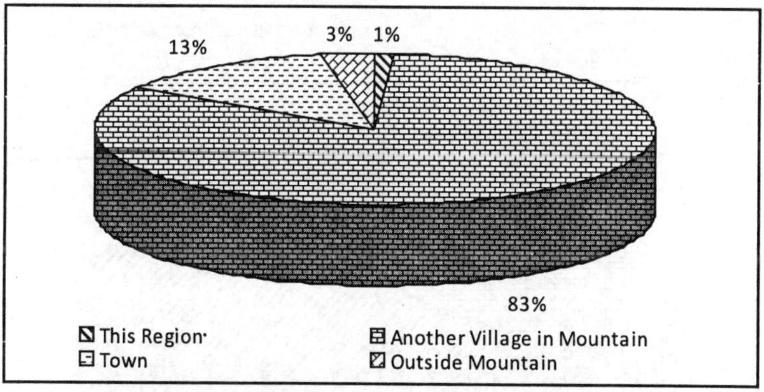

Fig. 12.7: Supply of Milk by Location.

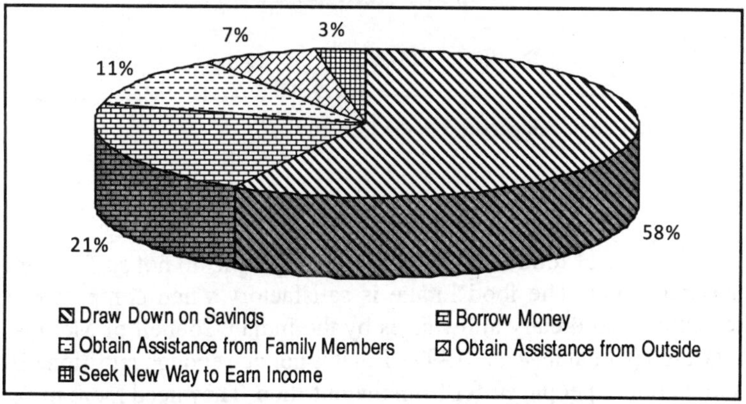

Fig. 12.8: Response of the People when Faced with Negative Shocks.

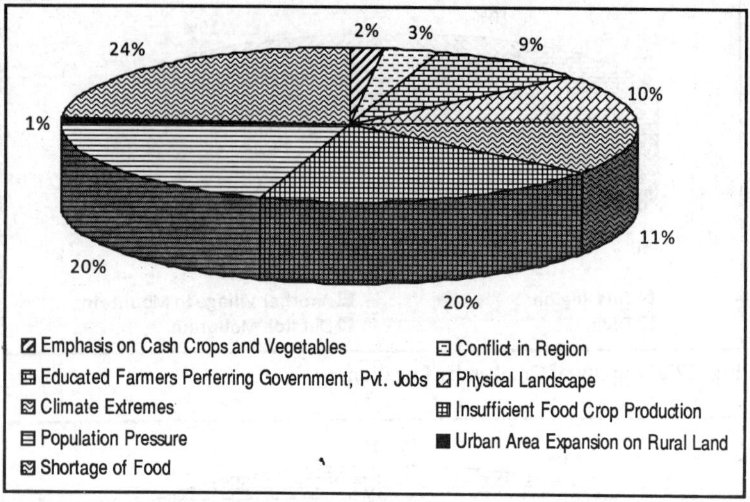

Fig. 12.9: Key Drivers in Food Insecurity.

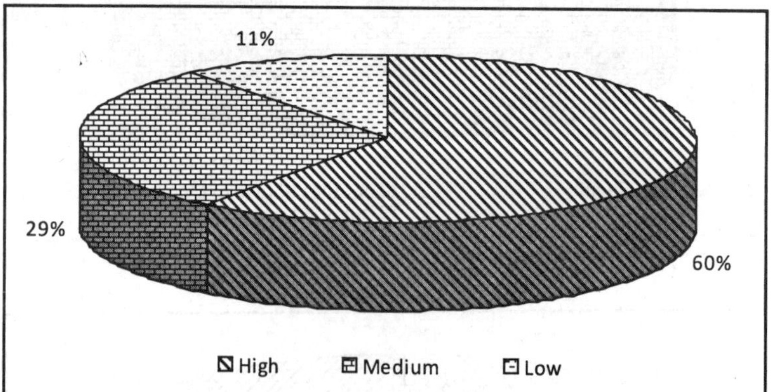

Fig. 12.10: Rise in Temperature in the Last 20 Years.

Diet and Nutrition Intake

The shortage of food notwithstanding, the people do not suffer from undernutrition. The food intake is satisfactory when compared to recommended dietary allowances by the Indian Council of Medical Research (Gopalan, *et al.,* 1999). But it is not rich enough nutritionally and therefore people suffer from malnutrition. They need more milk, meat, fruits and vegetables.

The diet intake of Chattibandy village is shown in Tables 12.1 and 12.2 to demonstrate the status of the nutrition in the villages.

Table 12.1: Food Intake in the Village (per head) in Chattibandy Village

	Chapattis	*Egg. No.*	*Butter gm*	*Rice gm*	*Vegetables gm*	*Meat gm*	*Curd gm*	*Fruits gm*	*Sugar gm*	*Oil Fat gm*
Average of the Day	3.07	1.00	58.33	216.90	206.70	100.00	110.10	30.00	40.00	40.00
Average of the Week	21.48	7.00	350.58	1518.30	1446.90	700.00	770.70	210.0	280.00	280.00

Note: One chapatti is made of 70 grams of wheat/maize flour; Eggs are in number Tea-number of cups, other items in grams.

Source: Based on fieldwork in the village.

Table 12.2: Nutrition Intake (k. cal.) Per head in Chanttibandy Village

	Chapattis	*Eggs*	*Butter*	*Rice*	*Vegeta-bles*	*Meat*	*Curd*	*Fruits*	*Sugar*	*Oil Fat*	*Total*
Average of the Day	716.00	86.00	380.00	851.00	26.00	194.00	66.00	20.00	168.00	360.00	2867

Note: Recommended Dietary Allowances (K. cal.) for a Person with Moderate Work is – 2545.

Based on *Nutritive Value of Indian Foods*, by C.Gopalan *et al.*, ICMR, National Institute of Nutrition, Hyderabad, 1999.

Conclusions and Suggestions

The study reveals that agriculture does not produce enough food for the population of the villages studied. As a result of this, there is shortage of food and resulting malnutrition. The analysis shows that most of the food items are purchased from outside the villages under study. Nearly 50 per cent poultry comes from a distance of 300-500 km from across the mountains.

Nearly 58 per cent people draw money from savings when faced with negative shocks, and 21 per cent borrow money (Fig. 12.8). Major drivers related to food insecurity in the region are shortage of food (44%), population pressure (20%), extreme weather events (11%) and physical landscape (10%) (Fig. 12.9). However, the diet survey carried out in one of the four villages does show that at least in terms of k.calories majority of the population is better off, though they suffer from diseases as a result of malnutrition.

The agicultural situation as it prevails in the region under study can be improved and food security achieved through regular supply of food from outside. In a situation where land is not able to support the people, there is a need to promote non-agricultural activities in the rural areas of the mountains to enable people to increase their capacity to purchase food from the market.

In order to make agriculture sustainable rainwater harvesting and revival of traditional and new water storage system are crucial especially when the weather conditions are adverse. There is a need to restrict conversion of rice producing land into orchards.

In order to make farmers self-sufficient in food production and thus improve food security and livelihood, Jammu & Kashmir Government encourages farmers to use high yielding variety of seeds, provides lift irrigation pumps and foot spray pumps on 50 per cent subsidy basis. The farmers are being encouraged to grow saffron and mushroom particularly in tribal belts. Agricultural land is covered under land development programme, i.e. land leveling and bench terracing, animal husbandry, fisheries, and horticulture are being encouraged by the State Government (J&K, 2001). Besides, there is need to promote non-agricultural activities in agriculturally low productive areas with objective to enhance food purchasing capacity of the people. These include poultry and fish farming, sericulture and bee keeping apart from promoting handicrafts.

Acknowledgements

I am grateful to the field investigator Dr. Ravi Kumar Bhat and his team from Bandipore for conducting the sample survey in the four selected villages of Bandipore tahsil. I am thankful to him for conducting diet survey in one of the villages in June-July 2010, despite political disturbances in the region. I am also thankful to the respondents for their understanding and logical response.

I am also indeted to Profs. Gregory Greenwood and Markus Ginger for his valuable comments.

References

Gopalan, C., *et al.*, (1999), *Nutritive Value of Indian Foods*, Hyderabad: Indian Council of Medical Research.

Government of India (2001), *District Census Handbook Baramulla*, Jammu & Kashmir, New Delhi: Registrar General's Office.

J&K (2001), *Jammu and Kashmir Development Report,* Chapter 3, Srinagar, J&K: Socio-Economic and Administrative Development.

Raina, A.N. (2002), *Geography of Jammu and Kashmir State*, Jammu: Radha Krishan Anand & Co.

13

The Geographic Distribution and Trends in Cholera Incidence in Tamil Nadu

B. Hyma and *A. Ramesh*

This study reviews epidemiology and the problem of endemicity of cholera in the State of Tamil Nadu, India, during the period 1961-1974, for the purpose of effecting better prevention and control methods and the eventual eradication of the disease.

One objective of this study is to identify those geographic areas in the State of Tamil Nadu, India, in which significant levels of cholera were found during the period 1961-1974. Concentrating mainly on aspects of medical geography, this research paper describes the extent of areal and seasonal variations in incidence and mortality; information necessary for predicting cholera patterns in future control and prevention planning. A study of the geographic distribution and incidence trends of cholera is necessary in tracing areal as well as seasonal patterns; vital information for planning the health care programme of a State. The problem of endemicity of cholera, with particular reference to the study area, is presented.

Another objective of this research is to determine the extent to which there has been reappearance or re-establishment of cholera in areas from which it had apparently disappeared or declined some years ago. A study of disease patterns in the period 1955-1964 by the World Health Organization showed that the recrudescence of certain diseases regarded as either quiescent or under control is a troublesome event, but even more troublesome is the extension of the

Reprinted after having been edited, from *The Indian Geographical Journal,* **51**, 1-32, 1976.

communicable diseases such as cholera El Tor, infectious hepatitis and hemorrhagic fever within or beyond the territories in which they usually occur. The El Tor biotype invaded India, in 1963-64 from its endemic foci in Sulawesi through south-east Asia. The study noted the similarity between the menacing extension of cholera El Tor from the Philippines to Iran and Asiatic cholera in its classic period.[1] Although mortality from cholera has declined considerably throughout this region in recent years, incidence rates have risen. Characteristics of cholera differ from area to area, adding to the complexity of finding effective prevention and control methods.

Sources of data and information

For the State of Tamil Nadu, the subject of this study, health data are not readily available according to both Madras Census Report[2] and the authors' recent experience. The data are obtained from public health records with great difficulty. The morbidity and mortality of cholera in the major administrative districts of the State of Tamil Nadu were studied for the period between 1956-1974 utilizing monthly statistics. Sources available for compilation of mortality and morbidity statistics are: (1) public health records, containing notification of diseases in different administrative divisions; (2) the Census of Madras; and (3) hospital in-patient records. Hospital and clinic sickness and deaths records are not always accessible, nor are they considered consistent or complete.[3] Therefore, this study uses, as its main source, the annual statistics published by the Public Health Department of the Government of Tamil Nadu; specifically, these statistics are to be found in an annual publication entitled "Report on Health Conditions in the Madras State" available from 1955 to 1970. It contains selected health data for districts, and municipalities with populations of 30,000 and above.

No published data are available for the smaller administrative units such as panchayat unions, taluks or villages. However, the data from taluks are maintained in raw data sheets at the Statistical Division of the Directorate of Public Health. No attempt has been made so far to have these particulars compiled and consolidated in a tabular form.

The Public Health reports containing statistics, for deaths due to cholera, smallpox, plague, fevers (including malaria), dysentery, diarrhoea and respiratory diseases, are given by months for each year for each district unit, from 1950 to 1970. Morbidity data for cholera are available only from 1961 to the present; previous reports were found to be missing.

The Census of Madras (Demography and Vital Statistics), published in 1965[4] is the only other valuable publication containing comprehensive information on health and vital statistics of the State of Tamil Nadu and selected aspects of the Public Health system in the State. Intensive fieldwork was necessary in order to compile data for this study from public health returns available from 1961 to 1974.

Trends in Death Rate from Cholera in Tamil Nadu, 1921-1976

Figure 13.1 presents the death rate patterns in the State during the period 1921-1976. Although fluctuations are apparent (Table 13.1), cholera mortality was high prior to 1950. The overall death rate decreased gradually from 1924 to 1933. Two significant peaks, observed in 1935 and in 1943 were followed by a smaller peak in 1950. The epidemic in 1953 claimed 71,156 lives, the highest number of deaths during a single epidemic.

Studies of periodicity of cholera outbreak suggest a six-year cycle in its occurrence in epidemic form.[5] Although the number of deaths registered from cholera has decreased since 1950, the trend has not been continuous. It is clear that improved health facilities and preventive measures (mainly inoculations) following the planning period have reduced the mortality rate. Although two small peaks were noticed during 1957-58 and 1963-64, they were much lower than those of 1943 and 1950. The epidemic status has declined progressively since 1965. The data clearly indicate effective control over the mortality of this disease.

The overall (1921-1976) frequency of disease occurrence shows a definite pattern (Table 13.1).

As the rate of mortality increases, the number of years in which each frequency occurs decreases, indicating that high mortality rate is found only in few selected (epidemic) years. The very high frequency of 11 years of the 54-year total in the category greater than 100 is mainly due to the high mortality during the epidemic years before 1950.

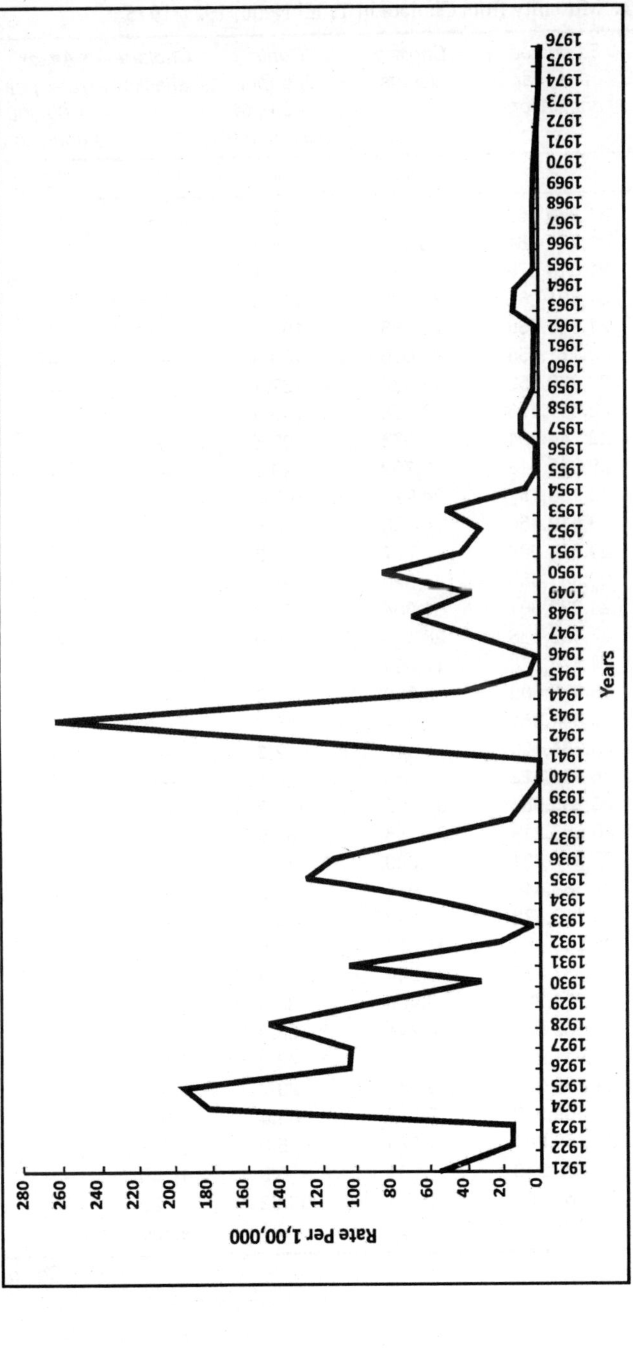

Fig. 13.1: Death Rates from Cholera, Tamil Nadu, 1921-76.

Source: Tamil Nadu Public Health Records, Statistical Division, Directorate of Health Services and Family Planning, Government of Tamil Nadu.

Table 13.1: Mortality from Cholera in Tamil Nadu, 1921-1975

Year	*Estimated mid-year population*	*Cholera deaths*	*Death rate (per 1,00,000) population)*	*Cholera attacks*	*Attack rate (per 1,00,000 population)*
1	*2*	*3*	*4*	*5*	*6*
1921	21,260,853.	12,170	57.2	—	—
1922	21,438,964	3,507	16.4	—	—
1923	21,619,078	3,265	15.1	—	—
1924	21,801,266	39,678	182.0	—	—
1925	21,985,556	43,138	196.3	—	—
1926	22,171,954	23,036	103.9	—	—
1927	22,360,552	22,836	132.1	—	—
1928	22,551,476	33,435	148.3	—	—
1929	22,744,704	23,532	103.5	—	—
1930	22,940,013	6,792	29.6	—	—
1931	23,158,151	24,974	107.8	—	—
1932	23,419,450	4,788	20.4	—	—
1933	23,684,028	777	3.3	—	—
1934	23,951,960	11,520	48.1	—	—
1935	24,223,301	31,304	129.2	—	—
1936	24,498,136	28,430	116.0	—	—
1937	24,776,528	17,554	70.9	—	—
1938	25,058,605	3,990	7.2	—	—
1939	25,644,381	1,837	15.9	—	—
1940	25,634,100	112	7.2	—	—
1941	26,956,322	120	0.4	—	—
1942	26,295,986	30,703	116.8	—	—
1943	26,653,219	71,156	267.0	—	—
1944	27,017,281	10,029	37.1	—	—
1945	27,388,440	914	3.3	—	—
1946	28,153,470	172	0.6	—	—
1947	28,548,064	11,217	39.8	—	—
1948	29,837,377	20,254	70.9	—	—
1949	30,231,324	9,409	32.0	—	—
1950	30,569,545	26,341	88.3	—	—
1951	30,911,994	12,692	42.0	33,613	—
1952	31,258,801	9,081	29.7	29,933	—
1953	31,609,949	16,517	53.4	43,948	—
1954	31,258,801	1,575	5.0	3,917	—
1955	31,609,949	291	0.9	1,140	—
1956	31,965,591	6	0.002	29	—
1957	32,325,837	2,930	9.1	9,150	—

(Contd.)

Table 13.1 (*Contd.*)

1	*2*	*3*	*4*	*5*	*6*
1958	32,690,825	2,312	7.1	6,508	—
1959	33,060,567	206	0.6	460	—
1960	33,435,162	20	0.06	26	—
1961	33,769,000	29	0.085	59	0.17
1962	34,162,000	69	0.201	827	2.14
1963	34,519,000	4,704	13.63	11 ,412	33.06
1964	34,876,000	3,935	11.28	10,378	29.75
1965	35,233,000	838	2.38	2,916	8.27
1966	35,590,000	681	1.91	2,693	7.56
1967	35,947,000	647	1.79	3,552	9.88
1968	36,304,000	568	1.56	5,980	16.47
1969	36,661,000	632	1.72	5,471	14.92
1970	37,018,000	248	0.67	1,280	3.45
1971	41,448,000	156	0.38	2,385	5.75
1972	42,193,000	197	0.47	3,281	7.77
1973	42,938,000	226	0.52	3,028	7.05
1974	43,683,000	109	0.24	3,586	8.2
1975	44,428,000	37 (up to May)	—	1,418 (up to May)	—

Sources: 1. India, *Census of India* 1961, Vol. IX, Madras: Demography Statistics (Report), Part I-B (i) (Madras: Government of Madras Press, 1965), pp. 131-132.

2. Unpublished records from Statistical Division, Directorate of Public Health and Family Planning Services, Government of Tamil Nadu.

— Data not available.

Deaths/100,000 population	Number of Years of Occurrence
Less than 20-	30
20-40	6
40-60	4
60-80	2
80-100	1
Greater than 100	11

Trends in Mortality Rate by Districts, 1956-1974

Cholera death rate figures for the districts of Tamil Nadu indicate a gradual decrease since 1957 (Fig. 13.2). Fifty per cent of the districts indicate a high peak during 1957-58; Madras (Now Chennai) (23.58), Tiruchirapalli (15.86), Thanjavur (29.34), Tirunelveli (15.21) while in the other districts the rate falls below 5.0.

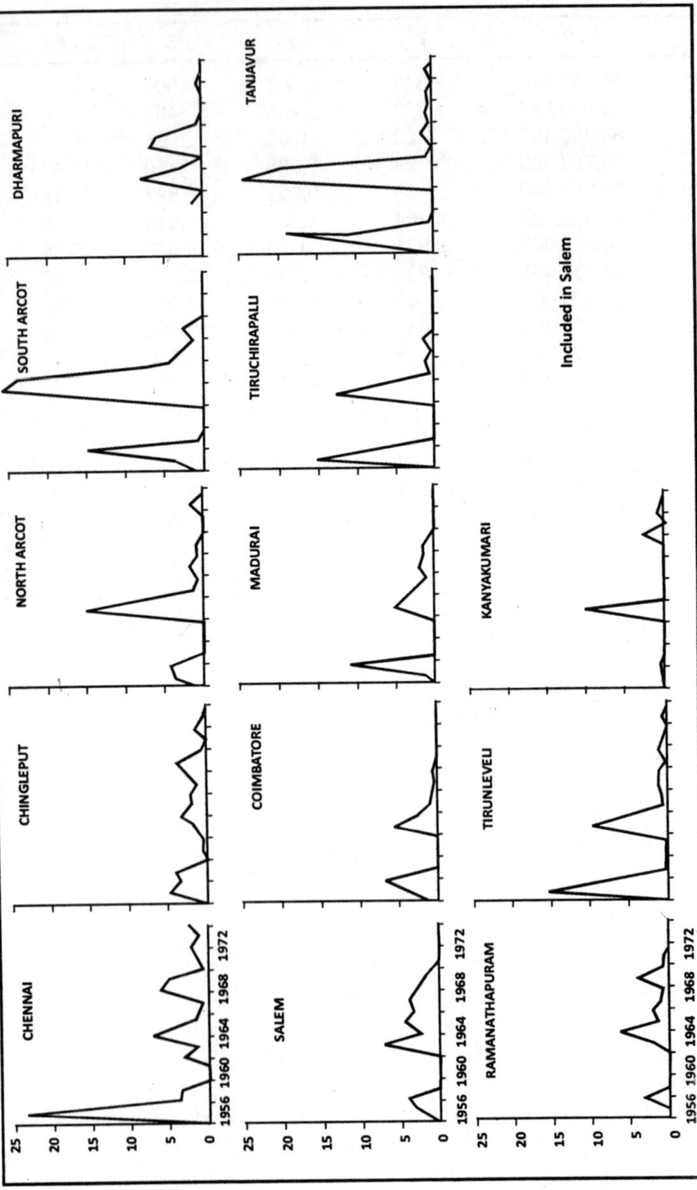

Fig. 13.2: Mortality Rate from Cholera by District, Tamil Nadu, 1956-74.

The Annual Health Report of the Public Health Department (1958) states the sharp increase in mortality during 1957 was much less than the average mortality for the entire period of 1951-57. Cholera was responsible for only 0.3 per cent of all deaths in 1957.

In the whole state a seasonal pattern in incidence was seen, tending to peak in the latter half of the year. The entire state was free from cholera during the first quarter of 1957. In August, 1957, a serious epidemic broke out in Tirunelveli and Madras (Now Chennai), it gradually declined towards the end of the year. An epidemic in Thanjavur and other deltaic districts during November and December, continued into the first quarter of 1958. The infection was reported to have been carried from district to district by the movement of agricultural labourers, and through irrigation canals.

A general decrease in death rates occurred during 1959-62 in almost all the districts, and in 1960-61, the State was practically free from cholera. According to the Public Health Report that year, out of the recorded 20 deaths, 6 occurred in two municipal towns and 14 in rural areas. Large-scale inoculation campaigns conducted during 1956-62 were responsible for this significant decline in incidence. In 1962, deaths were reported in five districts (Thanjavur, North Arcot, South Arcot, Chingleput and Madras) except for Madras (3.05) the rate was insignificant in the eight other districts.

In the latter part of 1963 and the early part of 1964, increases in death rates were noted in all districts. The Annual Health Report[6] states that during the third week in January this epidemic peaked, involving a large number of villages situated on river banks, mainly in the districts of South Arcot, Thanjavur, Tiruchirapalli and North Arcot. By the end of February, 1954, the incidence was almost under control; from March to October only sporadic cases were reported. Heavy rains in the month of November resulted in another increase in infection, raising the death rate once again, in South Arcot (60.32), Madras (7.30), Ramanathapuram (6.31) and Chingleput (5.84). The district of South Arcot showed a very high death rate (60.32) in 1964 and, in fact, during the entire period of 1956-74, Thanjavur followed during 1963 and 1964 with peak of 39.76 and 19.77. During 1964-65, the districts of Nilgiris and Kanyakumari were free from cholera incidence.

After 1965, the death rate in all districts declined with some slight variations observed during 1966-68. For instance during 1967, South Arcot was conspicuous with 4.5, Salem with 4.2 and Dharmapuri with 6.69. According to the Annual Health Report, cholera incidence continued to be prevalent during the beginning of 1967, but a decline was noticed after April, followed by an upward trend in November and December. Higher incidence in the following January and February was attributable to heavy rains and the beginning of harvest season which attracted a large number of migrant labourers. During 1968, cholera was prevalent in epidemic form only in the districts of Madras, Madurai and Chingleput; the districts of Kanyakumari and Nilgiris were free from infection. Madras City reported the largest number of deaths (114) in 1968; in 1969, high death rates were reported from Ramanathapuram (4.02) and Madras (4.91). The epidemic in the Ramanathapuram district which claimed 110 lives was reported to have been caused by dry, acute drought conditions and scarcity of food.

For the year 1970, cholera deaths were reported in all districts except Nilgiris. In order of severity of deaths, the affected areas were: Kanyakumari (31 deaths); Thanjavur (30); North Arcot (27); Madurai (6); and Salem (26). Rates were found to be lower (below unit level) than in previous years. In 1971, cholera was prevalent in Thanjavur, Ramanathapuram, Madras and Tirunelveli, however, rates were below one unit. In 1972, cholera was reported in all districts except Ramanathapuram and Nilgiris. In 1974, out of a total of 109 deaths reported in Tamil Nadu (Table 13.3a), the highest was found in Madras (71) followed by Salem (9), North Arcot (8), Tiruchirapalli (7), and South Arcot (5). By May of 1975, districts reporting deaths were Madras (13), Tiruchirapalli (11), Madurai (4), Ramanathapuram (4), North Arcot (3), Coimbatore (2), with a total of 37 deaths for all of Tamil Nadu (Table 13.3b). Death rates in all districts declined below unit after 1970.

Average Annual Death Rate by Districts

It is interesting to examine the earliest possible picture of cholera in Tamil Nadu. Table 13.2 indicates the high death rate to be in the Thanjavur district, followed by Tirunelveli and South Arcot.

High death rates correlate to the important river basins, especially in the lower reaches, such as the Tambaraparani basin in Tirunelveli district, the Palar River tract in the Chingleput district and the Ponnaiyar River basin in the South Arcot district. These were not free from cholera during this entire period.

Table 13.2: Mean Death Rate from Cholera, 1896-1960

District		*1956-60*	
	1896-1926	*Average Annual death*	*Rate (per 1,00,000 persons)*
Madras	91	108	6.59
Chingleput	101	49	2.30
North Arcot	115	51	1.66
South Arcot	118	115	3.87
Salem	132	59	1.60
Coimbatore	139	83	2.41
Nilgiris	—	—	—
Madurai	126	84	2.69
Tiruchirapalli	144	138	4.42
Thanjavur	257	268	8.44
Ramanathapuram	126	18	0.77
Tirunelveli	190	119	4.46
Kanyakumari	—	2	0.21
State	—	**1,094**	**3.35**

Source: India, *Census of India 1961*, Vol. IX, Madras: Demography and Vital Statistics (Report), p. 170.

1956-60

Figure 13.3 shows a different spatial pattern from that of 1896-1926; concentrations were found in several different zones, the endemic tracts of Thanjavur and Madras, in the adjoining two districts of South Arcot and Chingleput, and further South in the Tiruchirapalli and Tirunelveli districts. During this period the death rate was only one-twentieth of the rate that prevailed half a century before. This reduction, as reported in Public Health Records, was mainly due to a concerted effort to improve water quality and sanitation, to expand the preventive health staff for communicable diseases, and effect other preventive measures such as inoculation campaigns during this period.

1961-65

Exceptionally high death rates were found in South Arcot (22.05), Thanjavur (12.21), North Arcot (5.08) and Tiruchirapalli (4.37). Other interior districts and southern regions showed a lower rate (Fig. 13.3).

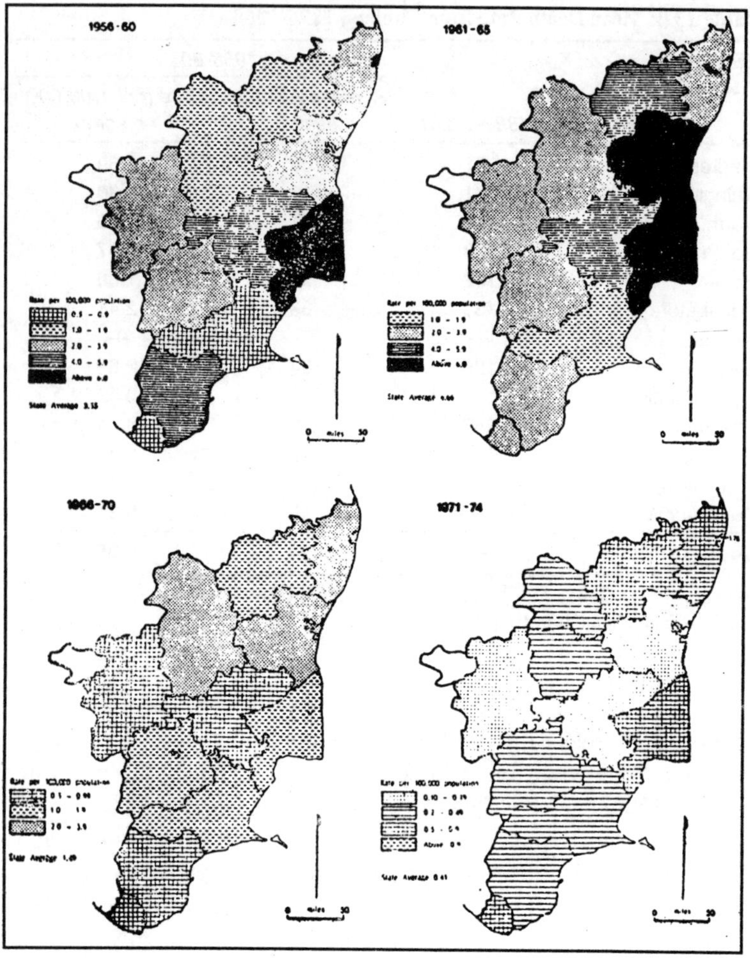

Fig. 13.3: Average Annual Cholera Death Rate by District, Tamil Nadu, 1956-74.

1966-70

A comparatively lower rate was found during this period than during previous periods, differing also in spatial pattern, from previous years (1961-65), in that the concentration seems to have moved northward covering both the interior districts; Salem and Dharmapuri and the coastal districts of South Arcot and Chingleput (Fig. 13.3).

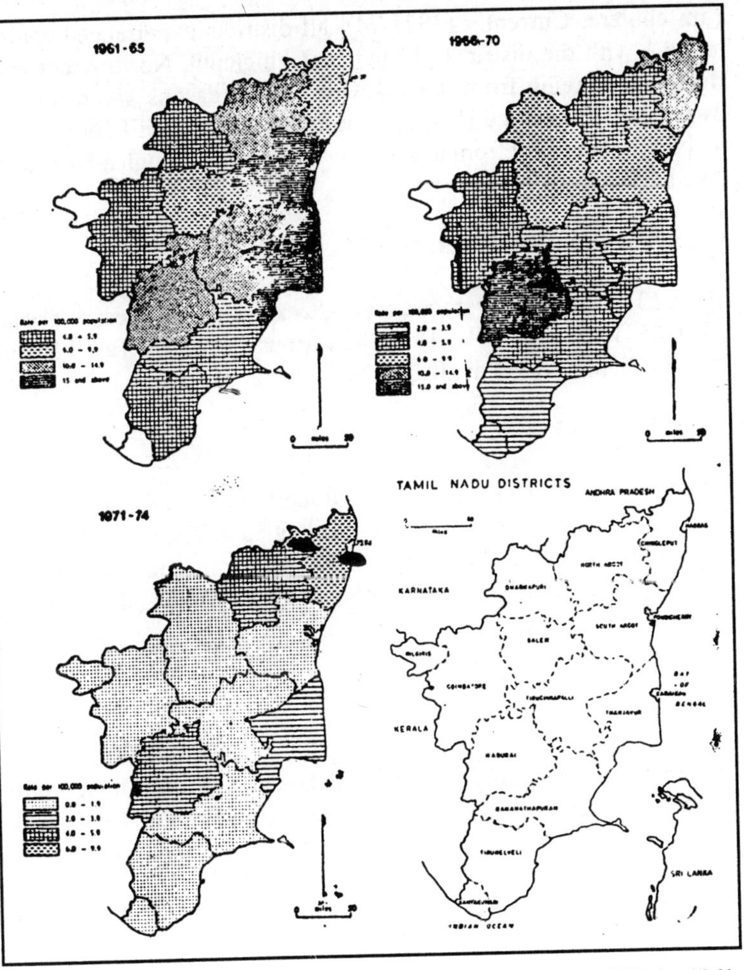

Fig. 13.4: Average Annual Cholera Attack Rate by District, Tamil Nadu, 1961-74.

1971-74

Madras City with a rate of more than 1.5 appears to be the centre of a highly concentrated zone. All other districts show a figure less than 1 [North Arcot (0.68), Thanjavur (0.59), Chingleput (0.56), and Kanyakumari (0.51)].

Overall patterns indicate that from 1896 to 1965 Madras and Thanjavur had comparatively high annual death rates (above 5.0) from cholera. Currently (1971-74), all districts experienced a rate below 1 with the districts of Madras, Chingleput, North Arcot and Thanjavur ranging from 0.5-1.0. One of the reasons given for the lower death rates since 1964 is the introduction of the El Tor biotype of cholera; mortality from this variety is low even though attack rates have been relatively higher.

Average Annual Attack Rate by Districts, 1961-1974

Figure 13.4 compares average annual attack rates at five-year intervals (1961-65, 1966-70, 1971-74) for the various districts of Tamil Nadu. Data for districts were available only from 1961.

1961-65

The nucleus of attacks was centred around the coastal zones of the districts of Madras, South Arcot and Chingleput. The rate decreased further westward and southward in the State. Again, some correlation is apparent between the lower reaches of river basins and the higher incidence of cholera.

1966-70

The rates were much lower during this period than during the previous period 1961-65. The inland areas of Madurai, Salem and Dharmapuri reported the higher rates, although Madras and adjoining Chingleput also continued to report high rates.

1971-74

Average annual attack rates for the period of 1971-74, have declined significantly compared with previous periods. Madras City and Salem reported high figures, 2,860 cases and 168 cases respectively, of a total 3,586 cases for the State for the year 1974; Up to May 1975, Madras (893 cases) and Madurai (252) rank highest out of a total of 1,418 cases reported for the entire State of Tamil Nadu. The average annual rate for this period was highest in Madras (73.94), followed by Chingleput (9.64), Madurai (5.76), North Arcot (4.99), Thanjavur (2.41) and Salem (2.18). The concentration seems to be in the northern part of the State; the south and the interior, except for Madurai, were less susceptible to attack.

The Madras district is in the forefront with a very high annual attack rate (more than 30). Districts like Madurai and South Arcot fluctuate between 5 and 30, indicating that these districts were only moderately susceptible. During the period 1961-65, only about 15 per cent of the total districts (14) were found in the group below 5, the remainder were above this rate. These percentage figures have increased gradually, that is from 1966-70, 46 per cent of the districts were below 5, and from 1971-74, 50 per cent were below 5, indicating that more and more districts have become free from high rates of cholera attack.

The largest number of cholera cases through May, 1975 were reported from Madras City (893), Madurai (252), Tiruchirapalli (93), Dharmapuri (41), South Arcot (61), Ramanathapuram (10), of the total 1,418 attacks reported for the State (Table 13.3b). This may be partially due to acute drought conditions prevailing in some districts, the failure of monsoons, and the scarcity of water in recent months.

Number of Registered Deaths Due to Cholera by Districts, 1901-1974

Up to 1950, Thanjavur and South Arcot districts had the highest number of registered deaths computed at five year intervals (Table 13.4a). Until 1930, Thanjavur held the highest rank (from 1919 to 20) then during the period 1951-55, Kanyakumari took over the top rank. For the period 1971-74, Madras City has ranked first, followed by North Arcot. Strangely, endemic South Arcot is nowhere in the picture. Similarly, districts like Tirunelveli and Tiruchirapalli, which were holding second and third rank during 1956-60, do not enter the ranking column at all during 1971-74. Madurai appears to be the only interior district in the ranking column. Another striking feature in 1971-74 is that the first five districts show very low figures with regard to registered deaths as compared to earlier periods.

Total Number of Notified Cases of Cholera by Districts, 1961-1974

Table 13.4b presents the districts at five-year intervals ranked according to the notified attacks of cholera since 1961. A somewhat different picture emerges when compared with Table 13.4a. In the epidemic year, 1963, the districts of Thanjavur, South Arcot, North

Arcot, Madras and Madurai reported a higher number of cases. Between 1967 and 1971, Madras and Madurai continued to register large numbers of cases and occupied the first and second ranks, Endemic South Arcot, having disappeared from the scene after 1966, later appeared in the fifth column in 1973. The decline in incidence in this district may have been due to the preventive measures that were introduced, while the later increase may have been due to the re-appearance of the epidemic cycle after seven years. Thanjavur continued to be endemic; it has occupied the third position more or less since 1967. Since 1974 and early 1975, the interior districts of Salem, North Arcot, Tiruchirapalli and Coimbatore have been reporting cases of cholera (Tables 13.3a and 13.3b) for which explanations are not available at the present time.

Notified Cases and Registered Deaths Due to Cholera by Districts, 1951-1974

During the last 23 years, there have been an average of 7,900 cases per annum of cholera of which deaths numbered 2.798 (Table 13.5a). The average fatality rate was 35 per cent of the notified cases. Fluctuations have occurred in the number of attacks as well as deaths, and in the decennium under consideration, the maximum was recorded in 1953 (Table 13.5a). There was a gradual decrease in the percentage figures from 1953 to the present, but a significant increase during the epidemic years 1958 to 1967. During the last three years, there have been fewer deaths (less than 7.5%) than attacks.

In general, in almost all of the districts of Tamil Nadu (Table 13.5b), the ratio of deaths to attacks has been declining from 1961-65 to 1971-74. However, Tiruchirapalli, Tirunelveli, Kanyakumari, and Thanjavur districts do show consistently higher percentage figures than the other districts. The reason is not known. Deaths are reported more accurately, however, than attacks.

1961-65

Madras City registered a low fatality rate (Table 13.5b), while endemic South Arcot, Tiruchirapalli, Dharmapuri and Tirunelveli registered a very high figure, due perhaps to the backwardness of medical facilities for cholera control. More than 70 per cent of the districts (10) of Tamil Nadu registered above the State average of 37.8 per cent during this period.

Table 13.3(a): Monthly incidence of cholera by district, Tamil Nadu, 1974

A=Notified Attacks • D=Registered Deaths

Districts	Jan.		Feb.		Mar.		Apr.		May		June		July		Aug.		Sept.		Oct.		Nov.		Dec.		Total	
	A	D	A	D	A	D	A	D	A	D	A	D	A	D	A	D	A	D	A	D	A	D	A	D	A	D
1. Madras City	330	6	203	3	253	7	383	11	352	12	203	3	241	2	469	17	155	2	110	3	113	3	48	2	2,860	71
2. Chingleput	—		2	0	1	0	1	0	2	0	3	0	2	0	2	0	1	0	—		—		—		14	0
3. North Arcot	—		1	1	8	0	18	2	8	2	11	0	25	1	13	0	35	0	8	0	4	1	3	1	134	8
4. Scuth Arcot	15	4	6	0	3	0	—		—		—		1	0	3	0	2	0	7	1	12	0	—		49	5
5. Dharmapuri	—		—		—		3	1	1	0	—		4	0	4	0	1	0	—		—		—		13	1
6. Salem	8	2	18	0	33	1	23	3	—		18	0	12	0	26	0	3	1	11	1	9	0	7	1	168	9
7. Coimbatore	11	2	17	0	5	0	8	0	3	0	1	0	6	0	9	0	28	1	4	0	12	0	3	0	107	3
8. Nilgiris	—		—		—		—		—		—		—		—		—		—		6	0	1	0	7	0
9. Madurai	3	0	4	0	5	0	—		15	0	—		3	0	—		5	0	2	0	8	0	1	0	46	0
10. Tiruchirapalli	14	0	18	0	—		8	3	4	2	2	0	—		—		13	1	4	0	4	1	53	0	120	7
11. Thanjavur	4	1	10	0	—		—		—		—		—		1	0	—		—		—		—		15	1
12. Ramanathapuram	—		5	0	—		—		6	0	1	0	—		—		1	0	3	1	20	0	6	0	42	1
13. Tirunelveli	—		—		5.0		—		—		—		—		—		—		—		1	0	2	2	8	2
14. Kanyakumari	—		—		—		—		—		—		—		—		1	1	2	0	—		—		3	1
Total	**385**	**15**	**284**	**4**	**313**	**8**	**444**	**20**	**391**	**16**	**239**	**3**	**294**	**3**	**527**	**17**	**245**	**6**	**151**	**6**	**189**	**5**	**124**	**6**	**3,586**	**109**

Source: Unpublished Data, Statistical Division (Epidemiology Section), Directorate of Public Health Services and Family Planning, Government of Tamil Nadu.

Table 13.3(b): Monthly Incidence of Cholera by District, Tamil Nadu, 1975

A=Notified Attacks • D=Registered Deaths

District	January		February		March		April		May		Total	
	A	*D*	*A*	*D*	*A*	*D*	*A*	*D*	*A*	*D*	*A*	*D*
1. Madras City	104	1	233	5	300	3	169	4	97	0	893	13
2. Chingleput	—		—		—		—		3	0	3	0
3. North Arcot	1	0	—		7	3	1	0	4	0	13	3
4. South Arcot	3	0	—		32	0	6	0	—		41	0
5. Dharmapuri	—		1	0	—		—		—		1	0
6. Salem	8	0	10	0	3	0	21	0	5	0	47	0
7. Coimbatore	3	1	6	0	1	1	—		—		10	2
8. Nilgiris	—		—		—		—		—		—	
9. Madurai	4	0	42	1	76	2	72	0	58	1	252	4
10. Tiruchirapalli	22	0	23	1	34	10	14	0	—		93	11
11. Thanjavur	21	0	5	0	—		—		—		26	0
12. Ramanathapuram	7	2	2	0	—		11	1	4	1	24	4
13. Tirunelveli	12	0	3	0	—		—		—		15	0
14. Kanyakumari	—		—		—		—		—		—	
Total	**185**	**4**	**315**	**7**	**453**	**19**	**294**	**5**	**171**	**2**	**1,418**	**37**

Source: Statistical Division, Directorate of Public Health Services and Family Planning, Government of Tamil Nadu.

Table 13.4(a): Total Dumber of Registered Deaths Due to Cholera by District, Tamil Nadu, 1911-1974 (Ranking the District According to Total Cholera Deaths Reported)

Year	*(Rank)*				
	1	*2*	*3*	*4*	*5*
1911-1915	Thanjavur (33,482)	South Arcot (19,854)	Madurai (13,868)	Tiruchirapalli (13,464)	North Arcot (13,409)
1916-1920	South Arcot (17,353)	Salem (17,292)	Madurai (17,284)	Tirunelveli (16,148)	Thanjavur (15,918)
1921-1925	Thanjavur (17,094)	Madurai (14,599)	South Arcot (12,127)	Tirunelveli (11,697)	Coimbatore (11,776)
1926-1930	Thanjavur (28,000)	South Arcot (14,720)	Tirunelveli (12,358)	Tiruchirapalli (10,531)	Madurai (7,335)
1931-1935	South Arcot (18,539)	Thanjavur (8,949)	North Arcot (8,710)	Madurai (6,400)	Tiruchirapalli (5,686)
1936-1940	Thanjavur (10,024)	South Arcot (6,589)	Coimbatore (5,930)	Madurai (5,816)	Tirunelveli (5,011)
1941-1945	South Arcot (17,725)	North Arcot (15,631)	Thanjavur (14,926)	Tirunelveli (13,245)	Coimbatore (11,505)
1946-1950	Thanjavur (12,445)	Madurai (9,359)	South Arcot (9,065)	Tiruchirapalli (6,571)	Tirunelveli (6,057)
1951-1955	Kanyakumari (5,983)	Thanjavur (5,004)	South Arcot (4,760)	Tiruchirapalli (4,714)	Madurai (4,058)

(Contd.)

Table 13.4(a) (*Contd.*)

Year	*(Rank)*				
	1	*2*	*3*	*4*	*5*
1956-1960	Thanjavur (131)	Tiruchirapalli (692)	Tirunelveli (597)	South Arcot (576)	Madras (541)
1961-1965	South Arcot (3,452)	Thanjavur (2,023)	North Arcot (818)	Tiruchirapalli (713)	Madurai (441)
1966-1970	South Arcot (410)	Salem (340)	Madurai (300)	Madras (246)	Chingleput (245)
1971-1974	Madras (183)	North Arcot (107)	Thanjavur (93)	Chingleput (68)	Madurai (34)

Source: Compiled from: *Census of India, 1961*, Vol. XI, Madras: Demography and Vital Statistics (Report), pp. 91-101. Unpublished Public Health Records, Statistical Division, Directorate of Public Health Services and Family Planning, Government of Tamil Nadu.

Table 13.4(b): Total Number of Notified Cases of Cholera by District, Tamil Nadu, 1961-1974

Year	*(Rank)*				
	1	*2*	*3*	*4*	*5*
1961-1965	South Arcot (6,991)	Thanjavur (4,426)	Madras (3,678)	North Arcot (2,126)	Madurai (1,997)
1966-1970	Madras (7,571)	Madurai (2,646)	Chingleput (1,493)	Salem (1,303)	South Arcot (1,071)
1971-1974	Madras (7,632)	Chingleput (1,160)	Madurai (926)	North Arcot (778)	Thanjavur (379)

Source: Unpublished Public Health Records, Statistical Division, Directorate of Public Health Services and Family Planning, Government of Tamil Nadu.

Table 13.5(a): Notified Cases and Deaths due to Cholera in Tamil Nadu, 1951-1974

Year	Notified Cases	Deaths	Percentage (Deaths per 100 Cases)
1951	33,613	12,552	37.3
1952	29,993	9,081	30.3
1953	43,948	22,445	51.1
1954	3,917	1,592	40.6
1955	1,140	291	25.5
1956	29	6	20.7
1957	9,150	2,930	32.0
1958	6,508	2,312	35.5
1959	460	206	44.8
1960	26	20	76.9
1961	59	29	49.1
1962	827	69	8.3
1963	11,412	4,704	41.2
1964	10,378	3,935	37.9
1965	2,916	838	28.7
1966	2,693	681	25.2
1967	3,552	647	18.2
1968	5,980	568	9.4
1969	5,471	632	11.5
1970	1,280	248	19.3
1971	2,385	156	6.5
1972	3,281	197	6.0
1973	3,028	226	7.4
1974	3,586	109	3.03

Source: Public Health Records, Statistical Division, Directorate of Public Health Services and Family Planning, Government of Tamil Nadu.

1966-70

Although the fatality rate declined during this period, South Arcot still occupied the top position (38.2) followed by two new entrants, Dharmapuri and Ramanathapuram (Table 13.5b). The State average was low compared to previous years, yet more than 70 per cent of the districts were found to be above this figure. The number of cases reported in Madras during this period was double that of 1961-65 (perhaps due to improved registration systems) but the percentage of deaths relative to attacks is very low (3.2), obviously indicating better health care facilities in the corporate city. Some districts like

Table 13.5(b): Notified Cases and Deaths due to Cholera by District, Tamil Nadu, 1961-1974

Districts	*1961-1965*			*1966-1970*			*1971-1974*		
	Total Cases	*Total Deaths*	*Deaths per 100 Cases*	*Total Cases*	*Total Deaths*	*Deaths per 100 Cases*	*Total Cases*	*Total Deaths*	*Deaths per 100 Cases*
1. Madras	3,678	245	6.6	7,571	246	3.2	7,632	183	2.39
2. Chingleput	832	249	29.9	1,493	245	16.4	1,160	68	5.86
3. North Arcot	2,126	818	38.4	738	215	29.1	778	107	13.75
4. South Arcot	6,991	3,452	49.3	1,071	410	38.2	195	18	9.23
5. Dharmapuri	392	175	44.6	524	194	37.0	116	21	18.10
6. Salem	863	363	42.0	1,303	340	26.0	273	31	11.35
7. Coimbatore	868	370	42.6	848	119	14.0	217	20	9.21
8. Nilgiris	—	—	—	—	—	—	7	—	—
9. Madurai	1,999	441	22.0	2,646	300	11.3	920	34	3.67
10. Tiruchirapalli	1,782	713	40.0	800	152	19.0	211	28	13.27
11. Thanjavur	4,423	2,023	45.7	769	175	22.7	379	93	24.53
12. Ramanathapuram	606	240	39.6	719	239	33.2	159	31	19.49
13. Tirunelveli	755	376	49.8	369	103	28.1	146	28	19.17
14. Kanyakumari	269	108	40.1	125	37	29.6	81	26	32.09
State Total	**25,585**	**9,573**	**37.8**	**18,976**	**2,776**	**14.6**	**12,284**	**688**	**5.60**

Source: Public Health Records, Statistics Division, Directorate of Public Health Services and Family Planning, Government of Tamil Nadu.

Table 13.5(c): Case Fatality Rate by District, Tamil Nadu, 1961-1974

(Deaths per 100 Cases)

Year	*(Rank)*				
	1	*2*	*3*	*4*	*5*
1961-1965	Tirunelveli (50)	South Arcot (49.3)	Thanjavur (45.7)	Dharmapuri (44)	Salem (42)
1966-1970	South Arcot (38.2)	Dharmapuri (37)	Ramanathapuram (33.1)	North Arcot (29.6)	Kanyakumari (29.6)
1971-1974	Kanyakumari (32.1)	Thanjavur (24.5)	Ramanathapuram (19.5)	Tirunelveli (19.2)	Dharmapuri (18.1)

Source: Compiled by Authors from Table 11.5(b).

Kanyakumari, Tirunelveli, Thanjavur, Tiruchirapalli, Madurai, North Arcot and South Arcot indicated a remarkable decline in total cases but maintained fatality rates well above the State average.

1971-74

Although the average figure for the State is low in this period, there are ten districts well above the State average (Table 13.5b). It is significant to note that Kanyakumari occupies the first place (Table 13.5c), when, in the past, this district has consistently registered the lowest number of cases. The concentration appears to centre around the endemic tracts of Thanjavur and Ramanathapuram districts. The Madras, Chingleput and Madurai districts have low fatality rates despite a larger number of cases reported in the State (Table 13.5b) during this period.

Seasonal Incidence of Deaths and Attacks due to Cholera by Districts, 1956-1974

Cholera is a disease that is strongly influenced by geographic and climatic factors. Several studies have shown that rainfall, humidity and temperature are closely connected to the prevalence of cholera.[7] Certain seasonal conditions are more favourable for the development and transmission of cholera than others. Rainfall is found to have the closest connection to incidence for example, in many areas cholera grows to epidemic proportions during or immediately following the rainy season. Earlier studies indicate that districts of Tamil Nadu can be mapped into areas of cholera prevalence in certain seasons of the year, that cholera follows monsoons with great regularity.[8]

Four climatic seasons are recognized in the State: (1) the hot, dry period from mid-February to the end of May; (2) the period of the advancing monsoon, with a hot, humid season, June to August (the period of south-west monsoon rains fall in the second half of June); (3) post-monsoon, the cool, dry period from mid-December to mid-February. The central districts of Tamil Nadu, consisting of Salem, Tiruchirapalli, Coimbatore, Madurai, and Ramanathapuram, receive rainfall from both monsoons, however, the main rainfall season results from the retreating north-east monsoon. The northern coastal districts of Thanjavur, South Arcot, Chingleput, Madras and North Arcot, receive their annual rainfall from the north-east monsoon. The south-west monsoon prevails mainly in Kanyakumari, Tirunelveli and Nilgiris districts.

The major peak of cholera incidence occurs in Tamil Nadu, with the arrival of the north-east monsoon during November and December (Figs. 13.5 and 13.6). January and February considered the post-monsoon cool, dry season provide favourable conditions for the persistence of incidence in the, State following the monsoon rains. During 1971-74, the total attacks due to cholera, though less in intensity were somewhat evenly distributed over all months, there were two small peaks, one during the 4-month period from October to January and the other in the summer months of June and July (Fig. 13.6).

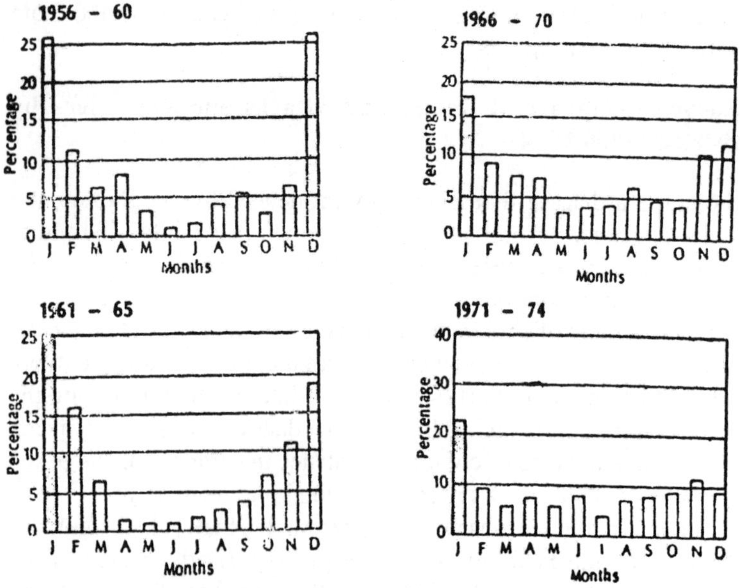

Fig. 13.6: Seasonal Incidence of Death Due to Cholera,, Tamil Nadu, 1956-74 (monthly percentage of deaths).

The major occurrence of cholera tend to follow the chief monsoons, however, when severe dry conditions exist, cholera epidemics are also liable to occur due to the use of contaminated water, safe supplies having dried up. Cholera decreases as the water supply improves with the rains.

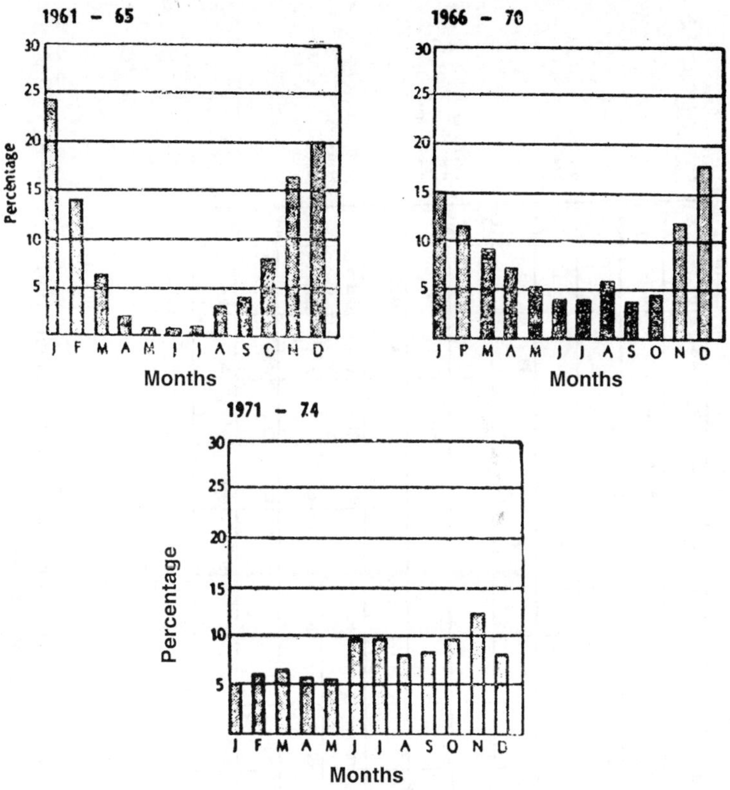

Fig. 13.6: Seasonal Incidence of Attacks due to Cholera, Tamil Nadu, 1961-74 (monthly percentage of attacks).

Monthly death and attack rates exceeding 10 per cent are given in Figs. 13.7 and 13.8 for every district of Tamil Nadu at the five-year intervals of 1961-65, 1966-70 and 1971-74. The chart indicates two clusters during the post-monsoon (cool) period, *viz.* December through February in the case of deaths (Fig. 13.7) and November through February in the case of attacks (Fig. 13.8). Almost all districts of Tamil Nadu fall into this group, indicating that cholera incidence is more pronounced during the cool, dry season. For a few districts like Tirunelveli and Kanyakumari, the incidence is found to be noticeable during the retreating monsoon period (October-December).

The season next in importance with regard to cholera incidence and deaths is the hot, dry season (March to April) when

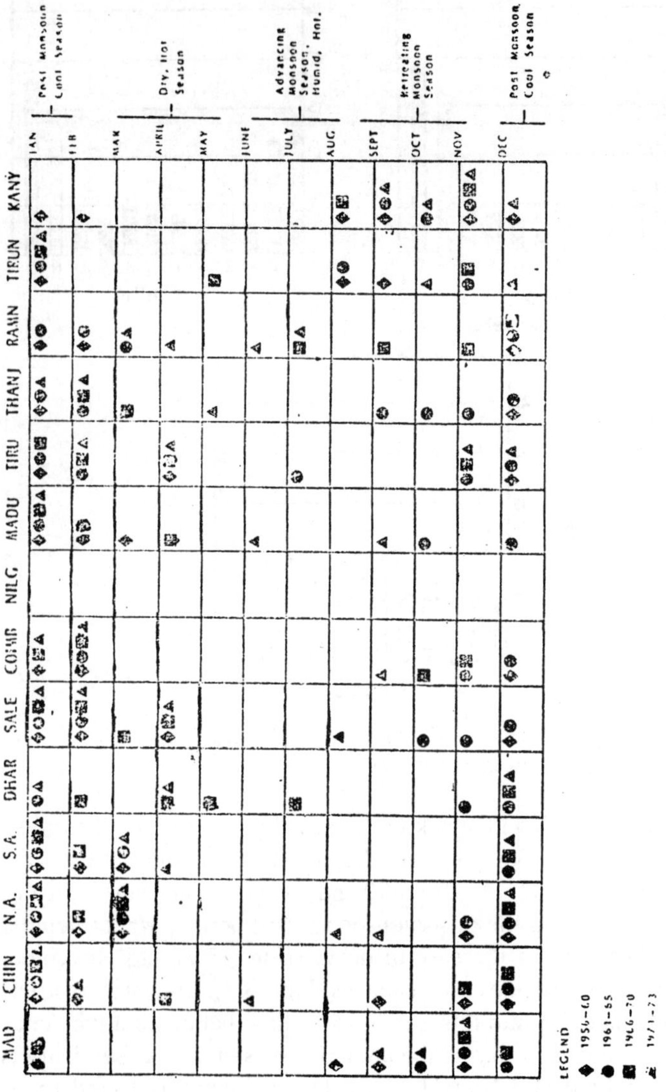

Fig. 13.7: Seasonal Incidence of Deaths due to Cholera by district, Tamil Nadu, 1956-60, 1961-65, 1966-70, 1971-74 (monthly percentage of deaths 10 per cent and over).

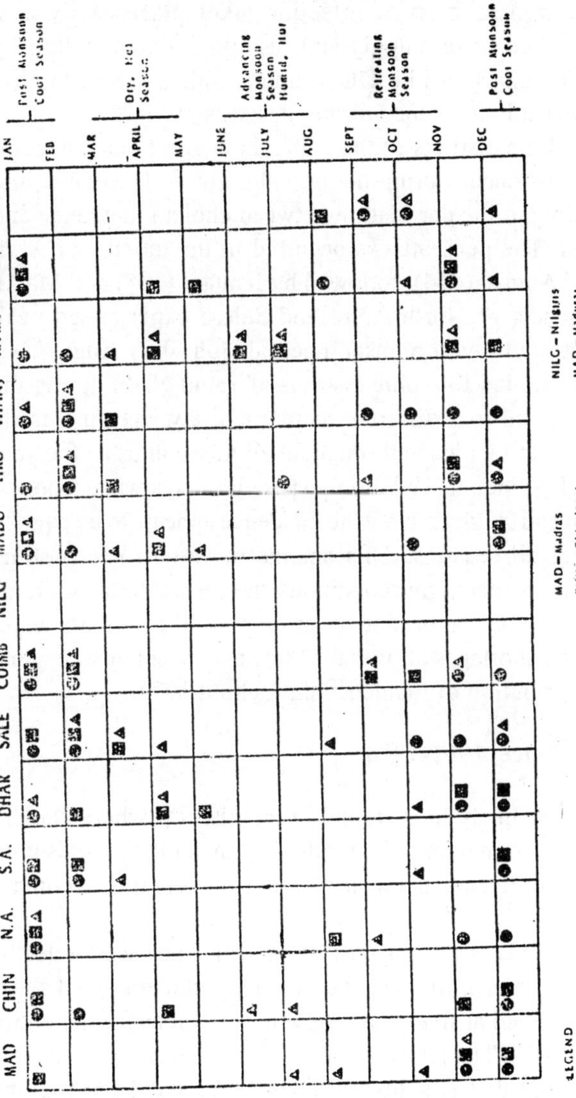

Fig. 13.8: Seasonal Incidence of Attacks due to Cholera by district, Tamil Nadu, 1961-65, 1966-70, 1971-74 (monthly percentage of deaths 10 per cent and over).

water supplies are at their lowest and large numbers of fairs and festivals occur in the State. Huge populations are attracted to the centres, where transmission of infection takes place easily as a result of the limited water supply and resulting contamination by carriers. Interior districts like Dharmapuri, Salem, and Madurai experience noticeable incidence during this season.

In almost all the districts of the State, the highest percentage of deaths and attacks occur during the period between December and February, pointing to the correlation between cholera incidence and the cool season. The peak attacks occurred in the months of April (527 cases) and August (444), followed by January (385) and March (313). The districts of North Arcot and Salem experienced peak incidence in the south-west monsoon period (June-July-August).

The data compiled for some districts of Tamil Nadu during the years 1971-74, point to a different picture entirely, that of a fairly even distribution in incidence throughout all the months of the year (Table 13.3b). Previous to 1973, only sporadic cases were reported between March and October. Now the incidence appears to be equally distributed over all seasons. This change in pattern needs some explanation. Adverse economic conditions, the general failure of rains in the 1973-74 period, evaporating water supplies, the resultant water scarcity and food shortages allover the State may account somewhat for the even distribùtion of incidence throughout 1974.

Level of Persistence, 1961-1974

Endemic areas are likely to be found in the districts where cholera incidence persists from month to month. The longer the periods with no cholera cases or deaths in a district, the less likely it is to contain endemic foci.

There are periods of varying duration in which no cases or deaths were recorded. For each district, total monthly cholera attacks and deaths were compiled at five-year intervals, as well as for the entire period of 1961-1974. The total number of months in which no deaths or cases were recorded is shown (Tables 13.6a and 13.6b) as the percentage of total months (60) for the five-year period considered. This classification affords another method of determining the relative significance of different districts with regard to their endemicity.

Table 13.6(a): Cholera Persistence Level by District, Tamil Nadu, 1961-1974

Percentage of months free from cholera deaths	*1961-1965 (Total number of months=60)*	*1966-1970 (Total number of months=60)*	*1971-1974 (Total number of months=48)*	*1961-1974 (Total number of months=168)*
1	*2*	*3*	*4*	*5*
91-100	Nilgiris (100.0) Kanyakumari	Nilgiris Kanyakumari	Nilgiris	Nilgiris Kanyakumari
81-90	Dharmapuri Coimbatore Salem Tirunelveli	—	Kanyakumari South Arcot Coimbatore Ramanathapuram Chingleput Tirunelveli	—
71-80	Madurai Tiruchirapalli Ramanathapuram Madras Thanjavur	Coimbatore	Tiruchirapalli Thanjavur Dharmapuri Madurai	Coimbatore Tirunelveli Dharmapuri
51-70	Chingleput	—	Salem	Thanjavur Ramanathapuram Tiruchirapalli South Arcot Chingleput

(Contd.)

Table 13.6(a): (*Contd.*)

1	*2*	*3*	*4*	*5*
51-60	—	Tirunelveli	North Arcot	Salem
		Thanjavur		Madurai
		Dharmapuri		
		South Arcot		
41-50	North Arcot	North Arcot	—	North Arcot
		Tiruchirapalli		Madras
		Ramanathapuram		
		Chingleput		
31-40	—	Madras	—	—
21-30	—	Salem	Madras	—
11-20	—	—	—	—
0-10	—	Madurai	—	—

Note: Compiled by the Authors from Unpublished Public Health Records.

Table 13.6(b): Cholera Persistence Level by District, Tamil Nadu, 1961-1974

Percentage of months free from cholera attacks	*1961-1965 (Total number of months=60)*	*1966-1970 (Total number of months=60)*	*1971-1974 (Total number of months=48)*	*1961-1974 (Total number of months=168)*
1	*2*	*3*	*4*	*5*
91-100	Nilgiris (100) Kanyakumari	Nilgiris	Nilgiris	Nilgiris
81-90	Dharmapuri Salem Coimbatore Tirunelveli	Kanyakumari	Kanyakurnari	Kanyakumari
71-80	Madurai Thanjavur Tiruchirapalli Ramanathapuram		Ramanathapuram South Arcot	
61-70	Madras South Arcot North Arcot		Tirunelveli Thanjavur Tiruchirapalli	Tirunelveli Thanjavur Ramanathapuram Climbatore

(Contd.)

Table 13.6(b): *(Contd.)*

1	*2*	*3*	*4*	*5*
51-60	Chingleput —	Coimbatore	Dharmapuri Chingleput	Dharmapuri South Areot Tiruchirapalli
41-50		Madras Thanjavur South Arcot Dharmapuri Tirunelveli North Arcot Ramanathapuram	Salem Coimbatore	North Arcot Salem Chingleput
31-40	—	Chingleput Tiruchirapalli	North Arcot	—
21-30	—	—	—	Madurai Madras
11-20	—	Salem	Madurai	—
0-10	—	Madurai	Madras	—

Note: Compiled by the Authors from Unpublished Public Health Records.

1956-60

Madurai, Ramanathapuram, Salem and North Arcot had the highest percentage (above 80) of months free from cholera deaths. Persistence is of a noticeable level in Coimbatore (69.4), South Arcot (69.4) and Thanjavur (69.4).

1961-65

The persistence level was found to be significant in North Arcot (46.6), followed by South Arcot (61.6) and Chingleput (68.3). Districts with months free from attacks closely follow this pattern, but with slightly higher figures, except for Chingleput (58.3) and North Arcot (63.3) (Table 13.6a). The interior districts exhibited a greater freedom from attacks than the northern coastal districts. The Nilgiris and Kanyakumari continued to enjoy a higher percentage of freedom from cholera incidence than all the other districts for the entire period studied. North Arcot exhibited a high frequency of incidence during this period.

1966-70

During this period, the persistence level is significant in terms of both attacks and deaths in all the districts of Tamil Nadu. Madurai exhibited the lowest number of free months, 8.3 per cent for deaths, 1.6 per cent for attacks, followed by Salem, Madras, Tiruchirapalli, Chingleput, North Arcot and Ramanathapuram which showed high persistence levels in the 40-50 per cent range (Tables 13.6a and 13.6b). This period appears to have the lowest percentage of cholera-free months recorded in any district in any period considered. The Madras district, which experienced a high percentage of cholera-free months during the earlier periods, has come down remarkably (36.6% death-free months) in 1966-70, again reporting frequent incidence of cases and deaths.

1971-74

A change in overall pattern is noticed with regard to the distribution of percentage figures. Death-free months were fairly high for most of the districts except Madras (22.9), North Arcot (56.2), and Salem

(68.7). However, in the case of attack-free months, all districts fluctuated, with a higher frequency of attacks occurring in Madras (only 10.4% attack-free months), Madurai (2.0), North Arcot (35.4), Salem (45.8), Coimbatore (45.8), Dharmapuri (52.0) and Chingleput (50.0). Ramanathapuram and endemic South Arcot, however, enjoyed a higher proportion of freedom from cholera incidence.

1961-74

The overall pattern of death-free months observed for the entire eleven-year period (1961-74) indicate that Madras ranked high in its level of persistence (46.4 per cent), followed along with North Arcot, the same followed by Madurai (51.2), Salem (57.7), Chingleput (51.9), and South Arcot (64.9). The northern coastal districts and one interior district (Salem) appeared to contain endemic foci during this period.

In terms of attack-free months, high persistence levels were again found in Madras, Madurai, Chingleput, Salem, North Arcot, Tiruchirapalli, South Arcot and Dharmapuri (Table 13.6b).

Degree of Endemicity of Cholera by Districts, 1956-1974

The degree of endemicity of individual districts was determined by examining the average cholera death rate for the five-year period and recording the three lowest monthly incidence rates for each year. This rate gives the minimum level at which the incidence of disease occurs in each district. The lower the level attained by the disease, the lower the degree of endemicity.[9] The term "endemicity" must be used with caution; here it is used in a relative sense. The terms "highly endemic", "moderate" and "low endemicity" are used only relatively to each other. The relative values for each district for each selected interval are shown in Figures 13.9 and 13.10. Although this analysis does not demarcate endemic areas in an absolute sense, broad patterns at district levels are illuminated. The index is calculated as follows: the three lowest monthly death rates and attack rates per 1,00,000 were taken for each year of the five-year period and were added (a total of 15 figures) and, divided by 15 to give the average minimum monthly incidence rate (Tables 13.7a and 13.7b).

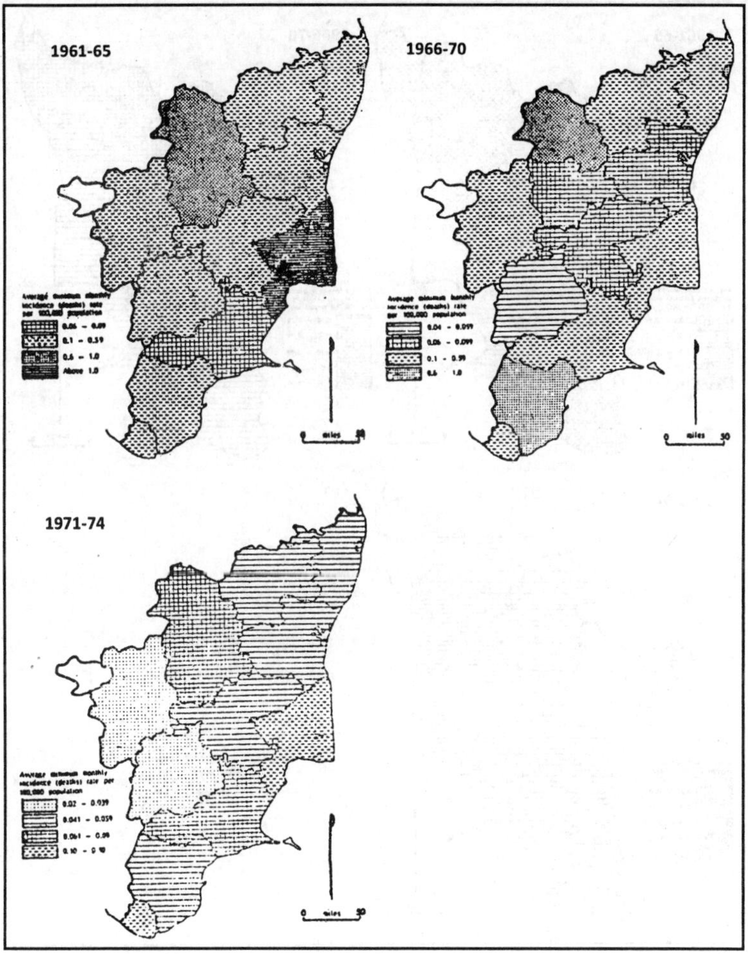

Fig. 13.9: Degree of Endemicity of Cholera by District, Tamil Nadu, 1961-74.

1951-65

Relatively high endemic districts were Thanjavur, Dharmapuri, Madras and Salem. Moderate endemic areas were found in Coimbatore, South Arcot, Madurai, Tirunelveli, Tiruchirapalli, Chingleput and Kanyakumari. More districts fell into the moderate endemicity category (Fig. 13.9). Ramanathapuram ranked low preceded by endemic North Arcot (Table 13.7a).

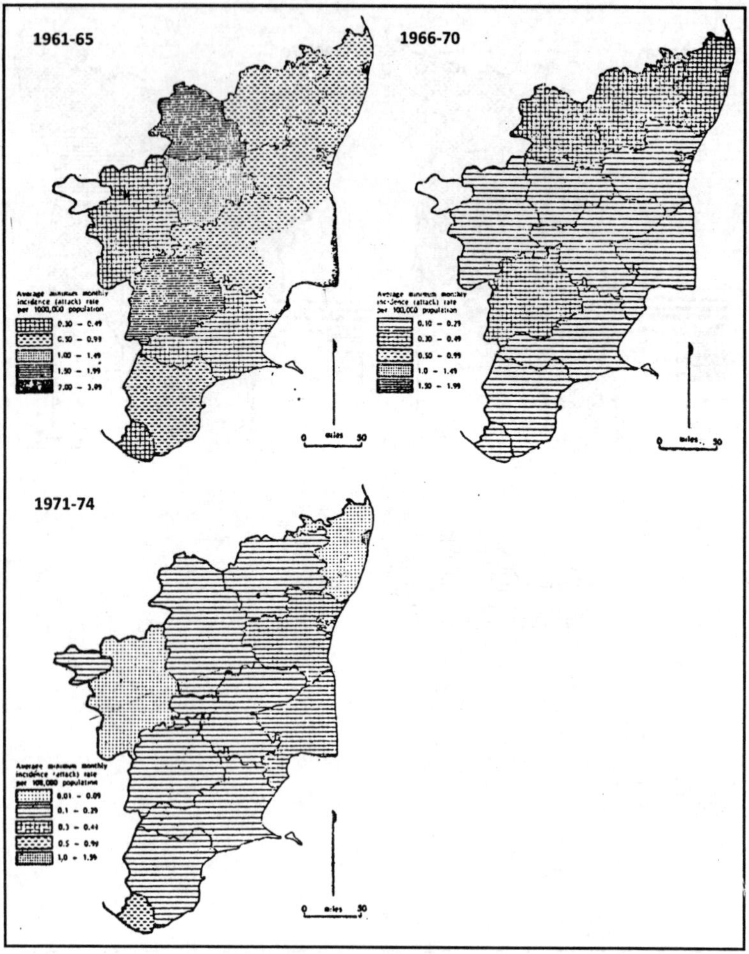

Fig. 13.10: Degree of Endemicity of Cholera by District, Tamil Nadu, 1961-74.

1966-70

The intensity of endemicity has decreased, as shown by the fact that no district's averge monthly death rate exceeds 1:1,00,000. In the overall pattern, Dharmapuri continued to have a high value along with Madras and Tirunelveli. Madurai exhibited a low index, followed by Tiruchirapalli and South Arcot, while the rest of the districts

Table 13.7 (a): Endemicity of Cholera by District, Tamil Nadu: Endemicity Index (Average minimum monthly incidence (cases) rate per 1,00,000 population)

District	*1961-1965*	*1966-1970*	*1971-1974*	*1961-1974*
Madras	3.78	1.53	1.32	2.21
Chingleput	0.69	0.32	0.04	0.35
North Arcot	0.51	0.31	0.17	0.33
South Arcot	0.88	0.17	0.34	0.46
Dharmapuri	1.86	0.30	0.14	0.77
Salem	1.03	0.16	0.19	0.46
Coimbatore	0.36	0.20	0.04	0.20
Madurai	1.52	0.46	0.11	0.69
Tiruchirapalli	0.89	0.14	0.21	0.36
Thanjavur	3.68	0.30	0.35	1.44
Ramanathapuram	0.34	0.21	0.20	0.25
Tirunelveli	0.56	0.12	0.26	0.31
Kanyakumari	0.44	0.12	0.54	0.36
Nilgiris	—	—	0.11	—

Note: Compiled by Authors.

Table 13.7 (b): Endemicity Index (Average minimum monthly death rate per 1,00,000 population)

District	*1956-1960*	*1961-1965*	*1966-1970*	*1971-1974*	*1956-1974*
Madras	0.29	0.82	0.78	0.08	0.49
Chingleput	0.26	0.26	0.11	0.05	0.17
North Arcot	0.32	0.19	0.13	0.05	0.17
South Arcot	0.28	0.35	0.10	0.04	0.19
Dharmapuri	—	0.83	0.10	0.08	0.36
Salem	0.27	0.52	0.81	0.07	0.41
Coimbatore	0.31	0.49	0.11	0.04	0.23
Madurai	0.50	0.34	0.04	0.03	0.22
Tiruchirapalli	0.05	0.30	0.06	0.05	0.11
Thanjavur	0.05	1.71	1.3	0.14	0.80
Ramanathapuram	0.19	0.08	0.12	0.61	0.25
Tirunelveli	0.60	0.33	0.67	0.07	0.41
Kanyakumari	0.04	0.24	0.22	0.17	0.16
Nilgiris	—	—	—	—	—

Note: Compiled by Authors.

occupied relatively moderate categories. Zones of high values were scattered throughout different parts of the State, with the least endemic zone located in the central part. As compared with previous periods, the higher figures have shifted from Thanjavur to Dharmapuri and Tirunelveli, both of which occupy the upper part of the river basins, Kaveri and Tambaraparani respectively (Fig. 13.9).

1971-74

The index values have come down significantly, obviously indicating the decreased intensity of the disease. Kanyakumari appeared to be the endemic area followed by Thanjavur. The present high index represents the lowest index value of the earlier periods; the lowest index ranging from 0.02 to 0.05, was not seen during the earlier periods (Fig. 13.9). Madurai represents the lowest figure followed by South Arcot, Chingleput and North Arcot. Spatial shifts in endemic zones show Thanjavur once again in the endemic zone as noticed in 1961-65. However, the value of the index is definitely low, that is, less than 1.0.

1961-74

The average minimum monthly death rate for the entire period identifies 3 high endemic districts; Thanjavur, Dharmapuri and Madras. These values are extremely low (less than one), notwithstanding the fluctuations observed over the five-year period. Moderate incidence persisted in the interior districts of Salem, Dharmapuri and Coimbatore, apart from Thanjavur and Madras. Low endemicity was observed in the northern coastal districts, the central parts of Madurai and Tiruchirapalli districts and the southern districts of Tirunelveli and Ramanathapuram.

1961-65 Endemicity Index-based on Cholera Attacks

Regarding cholera attacks, all the districts of the State, with the exception of Nilgiris, were affected. Madras and Thanjavur ranked high in this time period, whereas Salem, Madurai and Dharmapuri were moderately affected. Both the upper and lower part of the Kaveri Valley were significant zones of attacks (Fig. 13.10).

1966-70

The lower values of the endemicity index during this period clearly show a lesser intensity of attack all over Tamil Nadu. The highest is found in Madras followed by Madurai. Significant zones were found in the north in the districts of Madras, Chingleput, North Arcot and Dharmapuri.

1971-74

Endemicity values were extremely low (less than one) during this period, as compared to previous periods; a large number of districts (6) in the relatively moderate endemicity group (0.30-0.49) indicate that attacks were more prevalent than deaths in Tamil Nadu. Noticeable attacks were concentrated in South Arcot, Thanjavur, and Kanyakumari districts. Madras continued to occupy the most prominent position. The interior districts, except Coimbatore, appeared to have experienced some cholera incidence. Patterns appear to be diffused, and no easy explanations have been available for the somewhat alternating zones of attacks occurring in the State during 1971-74.

1961-74

The overall pattern with regard to endemicity (attack rates) for a period of 14 years shows Madras and Thanjavur as the high concentration zone, followed by Dharmapuri and Madurai (Fig. 13.10).

Total Number of Registered Deaths due to Cholera by Taluk, 1961-1973

1961-65

The highest number of deaths were reported from taluks of Chidambaram (955) and Tirukoilur (893) in the South Arcot district, followed by two other taluks, Vriddhachalam (410) and Villupuram (373), in the same district (Fig. 13.11). A significant number of deaths (200-300) were reported from five taluks in the endemic Thanjavur district (100-200) from isolated pockets in Madras, three taluks in North Arcot, Salem, Erode, Tiruchi, Madurai, Ambasamudram, etc. Except for fifteen taluks, all taluks reported cholera during this five-year period.

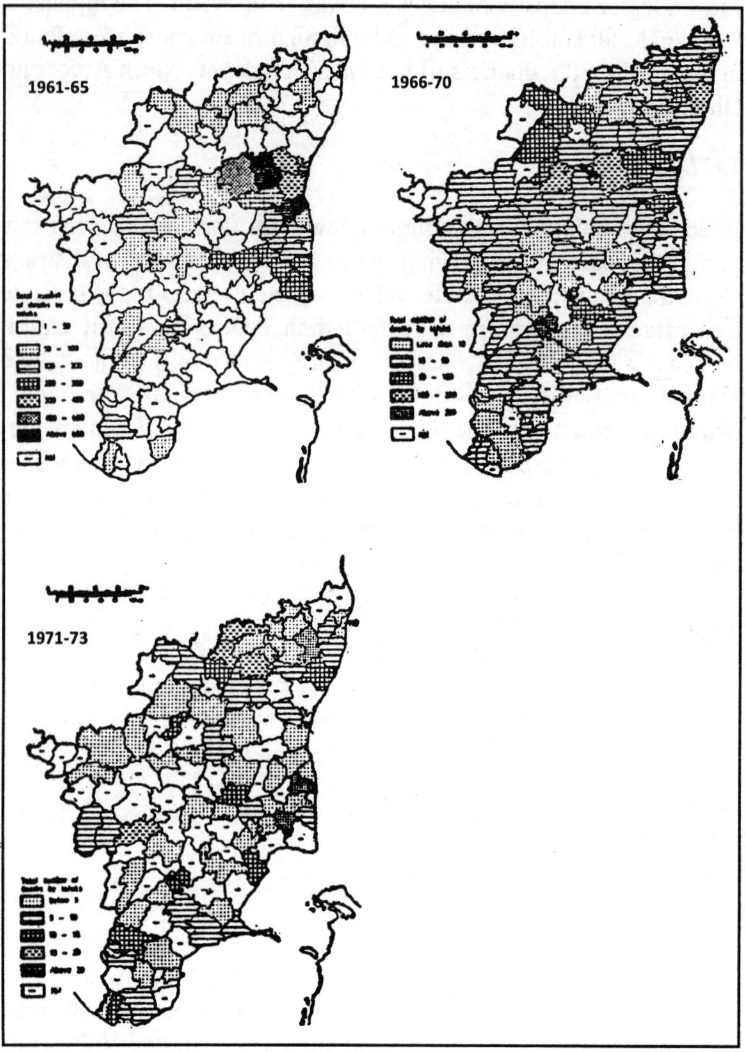

Fig. 13.11: Registered Deaths from Cholera by Taluk, Tamil Nadu,1961-73.

1966-70

Deaths were significantly lower than during previous periods. The highest rate was reported in Madras (246), followed by Madurai (202), Salem (136) and Kallakurichi (106) in South Arcot reported more than 100 deaths. Endemic tracts were found mainly in the South Arcot and Dharmapuri districts. Most of the taluks were concentrated in the range of 1-30, while only 15 taluks reported no deaths. A diffused pattern is apparent during this period.

1971-73

Total registered deaths were even lower than in the period 1966-70. A larger number of taluks (41) did not report deaths during this period than during 1966-70. Highest reports for this period were concentrated in Madras (112) and Kanncheepuram (39) in the Chingleput district, followed by two taluks, Mayuram (37) and Mannargudi (20), in the Thanjavur district. Four North Arcot taluks, Gudiyatham, Polur, Vaniambadi, and Tirupathur reported deaths in the range 15-20 (Fig. 13.11).

Notified Cases of Attacks by Taluk, 1961-1973

Twelve taluks did not report cases; all others reported cases of cholera. The largest number of cases was reported from Madras (3,678) and Madurai (1,183), while endemic taluks in the South Arcot and Thanjavur districts reported the next highest, ranging between 600-1,000 in the South Arcot and 200-600 in Thanjavur (Fig. 13.12). North Arcot emerges a second smaller foci, in the range of 200-400. Scattered cases were reported (range 100-200) mainly from the taluks in Coimbatore, Salem, Dharmapuri and Madurai.

1966-70

All the taluks except fifteen reported cases of cholera during this period. Madras (7,571) and Madurai (2,135) continued to report the largest number of cases. A diffused pattern again appeared. Taluks reporting cases in the range of 200-400 were in South Arcot, Salem and Dharmapuri, while smaller numbers of attacks (100-200) were reported from various taluks in all the districts (Fig. 13.12).

1971-73

Madras (4,772) and Madurai (724) continued to occupy the most prominent positions. A large number of taluks in the North Arcot and

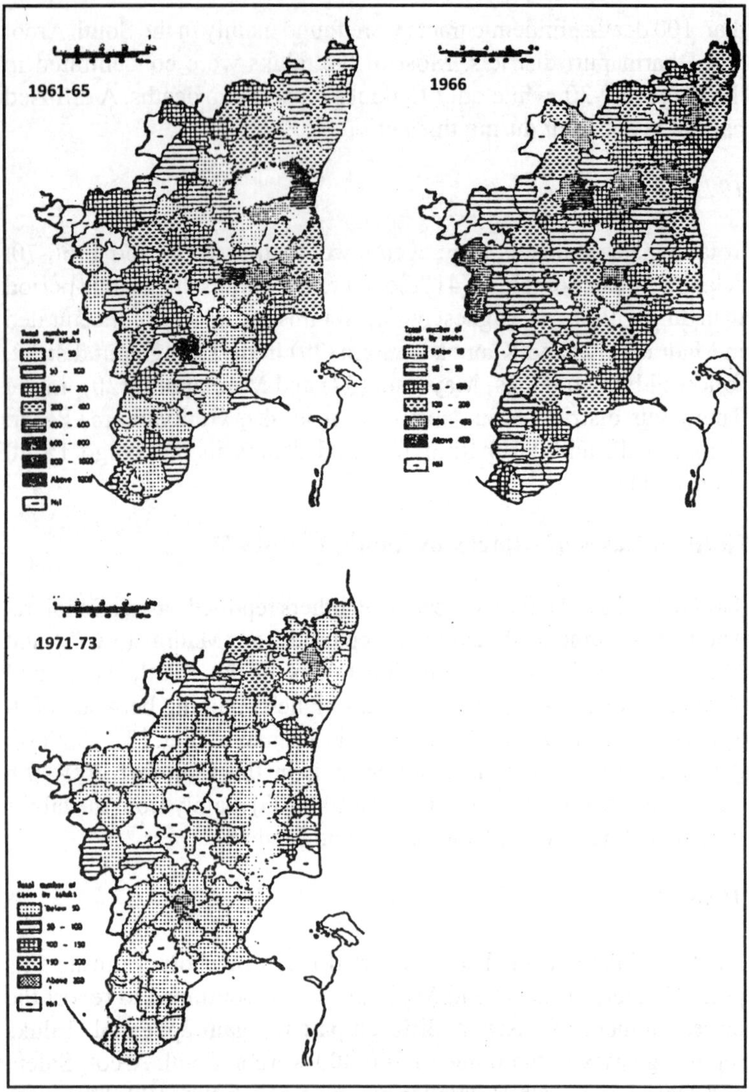

Fig. 13.12: Notified Cases of Cholera by Taluk, Tamil Nadu, 1961-73.

Thanjavur districts exhibited endemicity during this period. A large number of taluks (25) scattered throughout the State did not report cases of cholera (Fig. 13.12).

The Overall Pattern of Changes in the Incidence of Cholera from 1961 to 1974

In order to assess the endemic significance of the areas studied, several measures were used in this article to study the distribution pattern of cholera deaths and attacks in different districts of Tamil Nadu. The following categories of figures were examined at five-year intervals for each district of Tamil Nadu: (1) average annual death rates and attack rates; (2) total number of registered deaths and cases due to cholera; (3) persistence level as measured by free periods (monthly percentages) from cholera attacks and deaths; and (4) endemicity index, showing average minimum monthly incidence rates. The districts were ranked according to high, moderate and low figures to study the persistence level.

During the period 1961-65, the Thanjavur and South Arcot districts emerged as major endemic foci (Table 13.7). Minor foci were identified in North Arcot, Madras and Tiruchirapalli.

However, a shift took place during 1966-70. Even though Madras and Madurai continued to report cholera cases, higher numbers of deaths were reported from the interior districts of Dharmapuri and Salem. The northern coastal and adjoining districts of Chingleput and North Arcot began to appear as endemic foci. The persistence level was no longer noticed in the endemic Thanjavur district, but in Salem, it seemed to continue at a low level. During 1966-70, a fairly large number of districts in Tamil Nadu experienced cholera incidence as compared to the previous years, 1961-65. The pattern was somewhat diffused rather than being concentrated in a few small foci.

During 1971-74, the northern coastal districts (North Arcot, Chingleput, and Madras) of Tamil Nadu appeared to be the major zones of incidence. Madurai and Thanjavur also continued to remain in the picture. An epidemic in Kanyakumari brought it to the forefront in 1973, whereas in previous years Kanyakumari was less noticeable. The interior district of Salem and Dharmapuri also began to exhibit relatively high persistence levels during this period.

Conclusion

This chapter presents the level of endemicity of each district due to cholera infection during different periods. For the entire period covered cholera incidence persisted at relatively moderate levels in

Table 13.8 : Districts in Order of Importance as Regards Endemicity of Cholera, Tamil Nadu, 1961-1974 (Districts in first four high ranks are shown)

Endemicity Level	*1961-1965*		*1966-1970*		*1971-1974*	
	Rank 1&2	*Rank 3&4*	*Rank 1&2*	*Rank 3&4*	*Rank 1&2*	*Rank 3&4*
1	*2*	*3*	*4*	*5*	*6*	*7*
1. Average annual death rate	South Arcot Thanjavur	North Arcot Tiruchirapalli	Dharmapuri Salem	Madras Chingleput	Madras North Arcot	Thanjavur Chingleput
2. Average annual attack rate	South Arcot Madras	Thanjavur North Arcot	Madras Madurai	Chingleput Salem	Madras Chingleput	Madurai North Arcot
3. Total number of registered rate due to cholera	South Arcot Thanjavur	North Arcot Tiruchirapalli	South Arcot Salem	Madurai Madras	Madras North Arcot	Thanjavur Chingleput
4. Total unmber of notified cases of cholera	South Arcot Thanjavur	Madras North Arcot	Madras Madurai	Chingleput Salem	Madras Chingleput	Madurai North Arcot
5. Persistence level (percentage of months free from cholera deaths)	North Arcot South Arcot	Tiruchirapalli Ramanathapuram	Madurai Salem	Chingleput Ramanathapuram	Madras Madurai	Salem Coimbatore
6. Persistence level (percentage of months free from cholera deaths)	Chingleput South Arcot	North Arcot Madras	Madras Madurai	Tiruchirapalli Chingleput	Madras Madurai	Salem Chingleput

(Contd.)

Table 13.8 (*Contd.*)

1	*2*	*3*	*4*	*5*	*6*	*7*
7. Average minimum monthly incidence rate (deaths)	Thanjavur Madras	Dharmapuri Salem	Dharamapuri Madras	Tirunelveli Kanyakumari	Kanyakumari Thanjavur	Madras Dharmapuri
8. Average minimum monthly incidence rate (attacks)	Madras Thanjavur	Dharrnapuri Madurai	Madras Madurai	Chingleput North Arcot	Madras Kanyakumari	South Arcot Thanjavur

Note : Compiled by authors.

the northern coastal districts of Madras, Chingleput, North Arcot, South Arcot and Thanjavur, and in the interior districts of Salem, Dharmapuri, Coimbatore, Tiruchirapalli and Madurai. In the remaining southern districts of Ramanathapuram, Tirunelveli and Kanyakumari (except in 1973) only sporadic cases were reported.

There are difficulties in attempting to draw inferences regarding the comparative cholera incidence patterns of different districts. For instance, the registration efficiency in the districts may not be uniform throughout the periods considered. However, some generalisations are made concerning persistence and endemicity in different areas by examining the trends in mortality and case occurrence for fourteen years. The distribution of disease, its changing pattern of incidence, if any, and the degree of intensity clearly show the amount of control that has been achieved. The declining trend in cholera occurrence, indicates the extent of control over incidence and spread, in Tamil Nadu, particularly since 1960.

The Problem of Cholera in Endemic Areas of Tamil Nadu : An Overview

In characterizing the disease in the previous section, a general pattern of distribution was clearly identified. The distribution maps were found to present no definite pattern or consistency which made it difficult to formulate relationships explainable in strictly geographic terms. Because of the limited information available on the epidemiology of the disease in different areas of the State, existing patterns observed from maps could not be explained. Collection of information was difficult. Printed documents or research studies relating to the epidemiological significance of the disease to the natural and cultural environment in the study area were scarce. Hence, it was not possible without intensive field surveys to find direct relationship between the environment and the incidence and spatial distribution of the disease. However, after personal discussion with health officials, epidemiologists for the State, and epidemiologic statisticians in the Department of Public Health, and information obtained from the recent Perspective Plans for health and rural development programmes in the state, the following observations were made on the status of cholera incidence in Tamil Nadu.

Because cholera is primarily water-borne in Tamil Nadu, it appeared traditionally in those areas encompassing the confluence of rivers and streams, in wet areas such as paddy fields, etc., and in river valley deltas and coastal tracts.

The Kaveri River Delta was found to be the main endemic area in the State, followed by other river valleys like Vaigai in the Madurai district, Tambaraparani in the Tirunelveli district, Palar in North Arcot and Chingleput districts, and Pennar in South Arcot. Thanjavur, South Arcot, North Arcot and Tiruchirapalli are considered the main endemic districts in the State; other districts such as Madurai, Dharmapuri are endemic to a lesser degree. Recently, Madras city and Madurai city have been reporting year-round cases of cholera, thereby indicating an increase in urban incidence, increasing with the rates of urbanization. Also, their status as corporate cities have provided them with better registration and notification systems than other areas.

Before an advanced transportation network was introduced by British India, incidence followed the river systems in its pattern of spread. Infection often spread downstream along the rivers, such as in the Kaveri River basin pattern, which spread downstream from Mysore now Karnataka State through the Dharmapuri and Salem districts to Tiruchirapalli, and to the deltaic regions of the Thanjavur district. This pattern appeared to change with the development of rail road systems, although some part of this systems follow riverine routes. Now the infection can be easily transmitted from Madras city to Coimbatore, for example. Thus, a 'leap frog' effect is seen outside these endemic foci, illustrating that there is no definite route now which can be traced easily.

This pattern is further complicated by agricultural and labour migrations, both internal and external, in the State. Lack of information or study on migratory routes adds to the difficulty of explaining incidence patterns. For example, certain taluks which are considered the most important groundnut-growing areas in the State attract a large number of migrants from the southern districts during groundnut season. Incidence of cholera seems to increase during the groundnut season in these areas which include taluks like Coimbatore and Pollachi (in the Coimbatore district) and others in the districts of North Arcot, South Arcot, Tiruchirapalli and Thanjavur. This was explained by Swaroop in his study in the Thanjavur deltaic region,[10] Detailed studies are needed to prove this relationship; at present there is no clear-cut evidence to form conclusions around migration and incidence of cholera.

However, the environmental and cultural conditions on the East Coast of Madras (comprising the districts of Chingleput, North Arcot, South Arcot, and Thanjavur) provide endemic foci for cholera occurrences here. This region enjoys ample rainfall during the retreating monsoon season (October-January), the highest proportion of net sown area under irrigation in the State and an extensive canal and tank irrigation system, as well as high density of rural population, and high death rates. Other cultural factors involved in the existence of endemic foci here are low standards of environmental hygiene and sanitation and marked population mobility, facilitated by agricultural activities and by many annual and seasonal fairs and festivals.

The importance of the study of the distribution of communicable diseases like cholera cannot be over-emphasized. It helps in determining the nature of health services and preventive medicine required and where they are needed. Diseases may change subtly and unnoticeably in distribution and occurrence, due to such factors as environment, population movement and carriers; this calls for a well-established surveillance network for early detection and the control of spread.

This research found that medical geography work and literature in the study area in recent times are almost nil. Hardly any research had been undertaken by geographers or epidemiologists to examine geographic distribution and changing patterns of communicable diseases in the study area. Vast potential exists in terms of further level of medical geographic research to promote health care systems in development planning. There is a definite need for filling the gap at macro and as well as at micro level in the geography of the study of diseases.

Acknowledgements

This article is extracted from a research report entitled "Cholera Incidence in the State of Tamil Nadu: A Case Study in Medical Geography", submitted to the International Development Research Center, in Ottawa, Canada, with whose research grant to one of the authors, B. Hyma, this research project was made possible at the University of Madras.

Appreciation and gratitude are acknowledged to Dr. C.A.K. Shanmugam, Additional Director, Directorate of Health Services and Family Planning, Government of Tamil Nadu, for his interest, cooperation and effort in providing us with the required data and information for this research project.

Notes

1. W.H.O., *Third Report on the World Health Situation, 1961-64*, No. 155, Geneva, 1967.
2. Government of India, *Census of India, 1961*, IX, *Madras: Demography and Vital Statistics* (*Report*), p. 240, Part I-B (i), Madras: Government of Madras Press, 1965.
3. *Ibid.*
4. *Ibid.*
5. Swaroop, S. and Pollitzer, R. (1928), World Distribution of Cholera Endemicity, *Epidemiological and Vital Statistical Report, World Health Organization* 5, 569-589, 1952, Russell, A.J. and Sundararajan, F.R., The Epidemiology of Cholera in India, *Indian Medical Research Memoir,* 12.
6. Government of India, *op. cit.*
7. Park, C.L. (1942), The Relation between Geographical Distribution and Climatic Factors and Spread of Plague, Cholera and Smallpox, *Proceedings of the Sixth Pacific Science Congress, Berkeley,* Los Angeles: University of California Press, 5, 506; Russell, A.J. and Sundararajan, F.R. *op. cit.*
8. Russell, A.J. and Sundararajan, F.R., *Ibid.* Hesterlow, A.M.V. (1929), The Geographical Distribution of Disease, *The Journal of the Madras Geographical Association,* 4, 81-97.
9. Swaroop, S. (1951), Endemicity of Cholera in India, *Indian Journal of Medical Research,* 39, 141-157.
10. Swaroop, S. (1951), Epidemiology of Cholera in Madras Presidency, *Indian Journal of Medical Research,* 39, 185-196.

14

Goitre Zonation in the Kumaon Region*

Rais Akhtar

The purpose of this study is to identify geochemical aspects of the environment and agricultural lifestyles as factors contributing to the endemicity of goitre in the Kumaon region of India. Regional variations in the incidence of goitre can be identified, and there are hypothesized associations with bedrock material, soil types, and mineral content of local waters. A general geochemical approach in understanding environmental aspects of disease is explained in a publication edited by Cannon and Hopps in 1971.[1] More specifically, Schiel and Wepfer have examined goitre incidence in the United States[2] and Ishankulov *et al.* have studied natural cause and effect relationships of endemic goitre in the Kazakhstan region of the Soviet Union.[3] Interestingly, the areas with highest goitre incidence in the United States and that part of the Soviet Union mentioned, experienced forms of Pleistocene glaciation not all that different from the Kumaon region of India. In general, movements of the glacial ice may in fact have removed important chemical ingredients from the bedrock and hence soils necessary to human systems, including iodine. Iodine

* The present study is confined to the Naini Tal and Almora districts and Champawat tahsil of Pithoragarh district of Uttar Pradesh, lying between 28° 43' 55" and 30° 20' 12" North latitudes and 78° 44' 30" and 80° 18' 45" East longitudes. The northern part of the region consists of mountain ranges, sometimes rising to an elevation of 25,689 ft (7706.7 m) above sea level, and from this mountainous terrain one passes with rapid transitions through the curious phenomena of the Bhabar and Tarai areas to the ordinary alluvial plain.

Reprinted from *Social Science and Medicine,* 12 D, 152-163, 1978.

deficiency has long been known as a major cause of goitre. Also, such localized aspects as consumption of canal and stream water as well as the consumption of food grown in local agricultural areas can help explain to some extent the endemicity of goitre in Kumaon.

For purposes of the present study, the prevalence of goitre in different parts of Kumaon was determined on the basis of a stratified purposive sampling technique, utilizing representative villages. Twenty villages were selected on the basis of differential elevation and cropping zones (Fig. 14.1). Data were collected from each of these villages pertaining to the prevalence of goitre, mineral content

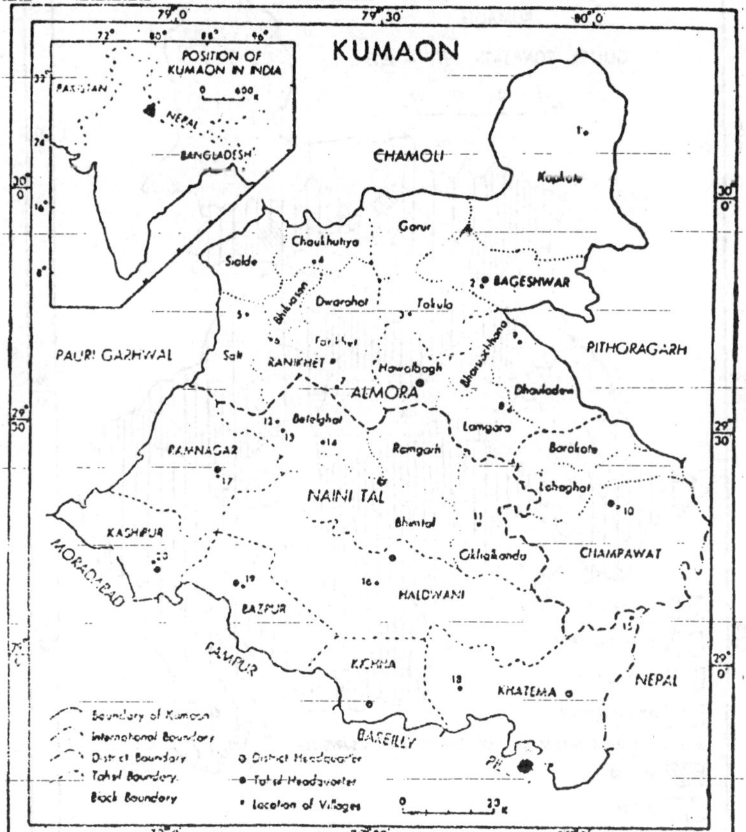

Fig. 14.1: The Kumaon Region with Settlements Listed within Tables 14.1 and 14.2.

of drinking water, general lifestyles, economic patterns, and diet. Fig. 14.2 is the resultant endemicity map prepared on the basis of information collected from 1970 to 1975. In addition to obtaining information from local inhabitants pertaining to their perception of goitre prevalence, data were obtained from various hospitals and dispensaries functioning within the region. Additional assistance was obtained from medical personnel in the development of the pattern shown in Fig. 14.2.

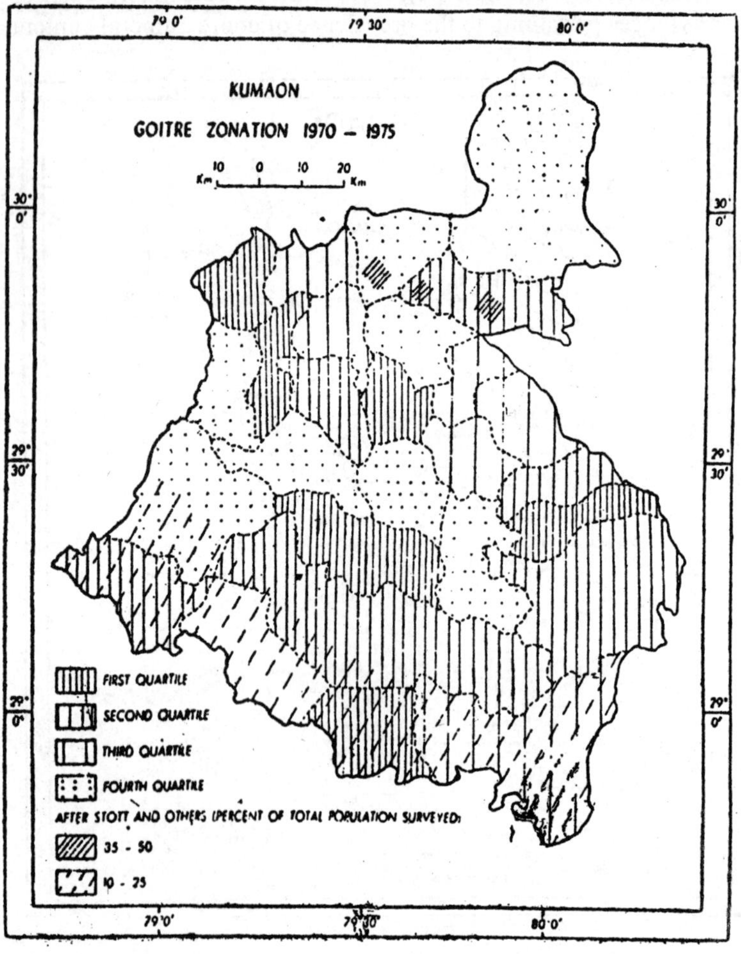

Fig. 14.2: Goitre Zonation in Kumaon, 1970-75.

Historical Assessments

Endemic goitre has been recognized in the Kumaon region for centuries. Local inhabitants, on the basis of their own experiences, postulated different causes for this disease over time. Early investigators observed goitre while touring the Kumaon area, usually in conjunction with general Himalayan studies. Most historical accounts agree that goitre was indeed common in the Kumaon hill country, with the malady occurring amongst all classes. Early accounts showed also that goitre was common for inhabitants of valleys as well as people living on mountain slopes, and also seemed to prevail in populations basically consuming river water as well as those who relied heavily on springs for water supplies.

In his work on the cause of goitre, McClelland dwelt at length on the question of causation.[4] He believed that by comparing the statistics about goitre that he collected in a large number of Kumaon villages with different altitudes and climates he might be able to establish a particular zone of the geologic strata contributing heavily to goitre. He was particularly interested in limestone materials. In addition, McClelland found an absence of goitre among inhabitants of villages in areas with formations of granite, gneiss and mica. In villages built over clay slate materials only one in 176 of the inhabitants were affected by goitre. In villages built over certain kinds of transition slate materials only one in 249 appeared to be affected. Conversely, in areas of settlement in regions of calcareous bedrock, as many as one in three suffered from the disease.

A study by Gordon published in 1884 lends some interesting insights into the particular problem. In a survey carried out in the north-western part of Kumaon, Gordon stated, "We met one or two men suffering from goitre—most hideous deformity—the penalty of drinking ice water. Undoubtedly in the exceeding heat of the low-lying valleys it must be a sore temptation both in the bath and in the drinking of water of the cool streams, even though they do come direct from the glacier and are fraught with such danger."[5] Atkinson noticed that goitre appeared to be confined to certain localities within the area and that perhaps no single general rule could be established pertaining to this localisation.[6] According to Atkinson, the presence of goitre may have been due to a combination of debilitating influences: for example, humidity, infected valley air, marshy soil, lifestyles of the local inhabitants, abrupt changes in temperature, and water from calcareous sources. In the process of preparing settlement reports on Kumaon, Batten observed that goitre prevailed to a large extent in Chogurkha especially in the settlements of Rungoor and Daroon.[7] Chogurkha is bounded on the north and east by the Sarju River which separates the area from Ganges as far as the junction of the Panar River in the western part of the Kumaon Himalayas.

Thus, even these early accounts associated glaciation somehow with the incidence of goitre. Not only were minerals often removed from soils and underlying bedrock, but intense flooding also was associated with melting of glaciers, leading to leaching or excessive washing away of the soil.[8] The resultant soil deficiency in many minerals and chemical elements, including iodine, was thus established very early. Mature iodine-rich soils had apparently been swept away and replaced by new soil types of crystalline origin with about one tenth the average iodine content. There is, therefore, the definite possibility that many parts of the world suffering from endemic goitre can be associated with the length of the post-glacial period of iodine replenishment. These factors might also help explain the prevalence of much lower goitre in tropical parts of the world. In addition to iodine loss through natural causes, centuries of repeated kinds of cropping patterns in Kumaon have contributed to the loss of what little iodine there is, removing perhaps as much 2-3 g per acre during a single harvest season, depending on the nature of the crop.

Etiology of Himalayan Goitre

While it is generally understood that the immediate cause of simple goitre is the failure of the thyroid gland to obtain a sufficient supply of iodine to maintain its normal structure and function, such factors as simple environmental deficiency of iodine are not so clearly understood. The geographic distribution of endemic goitre is not always so uniform as it might appear on a small-scale map. In Kumaon, for example, endemic goitre in the plains appears to be widely distributed. Conversely, in the more hilly regions, goitre is found scattered in different and often non-adjacent villages. Stott and others[9] hypothesized that goitre was found in endemic villages situated in hot, moist river valleys where maize was often freely cultivated. However, field investigations carried on during this study in relation to cropping patterns found no such clear-cut association between goitre prevalence and the cultivation of maize. In the Kumaon

Himalayas, maize is widely grown and locally consumed, particularly in the Okhalkanda area in the south-central part of the Kumaon region. Reference to Figures 14.1 and 14.2 indicates that the Okhalkanda area ranked fourth in the prevalence of goitre. However, villages over 7000 ft above sea level in the cooler climates appeared to be relatively free of goitre. Goitre was also found to be prevalent in the foothill areas of Naini Tal district where soils are fragile and porous, consisting of a thin covering of alluvium over harder materials. Water for human consumption is derived either from springs or open artificial channels bringing water from higher levels, often from some distance.

When Stott and his colleagues made the first truly systematic attempt to measure the prevalence of goitre in the Kumaon region in 1930 they conducted a survey in the Almora district and found a 40 per cent prevalence rate. Clearly a case for endemic goitre. Stott and his team also demarcated four areas where the prevalence rate ranged from 10 to 50 per cent. These patterns are also contained within Figure 14.2. In the early 1960s, the Goitre Control Division of the government of Uttar Pradesh resurveyed the mountainous area of Naini Tal and found a prevalence rate of 29.61 per cent. In the Bhabar and Tarai areas, results of a resurvey indicated a goitre rate of about 10 per cent. On the basis of the earlier and more recent studies of Kumaon, the following relationships can be put forth.

Geology, Mineralogy and Soil

While it can be established that limestone and lime-bearing rock materials are most closely associated with endemic goitre, the disease is not restricted to calcareous areas. Still, the explanation of the frequent association of goitre with limestone materials is considered important by some because the limestone rocks are among the most porous as well as most widely distributed within the area. In addition, limestone areas are also among the most freely cultivated and inhabited. Water derived from such rocks does contain excessive quantities of lime; the ingestion of which while not perhaps directly a cause of goitre throws an additional burden on the functional resources of the thyroid gland. According to Rundle, "the presence in the soil of decaying vegetable or animal matter may convert any soil, no matter what its geologic origin, into a suitable habitat for a *contagium vivium* of the disease. A manure heap or cess pit, for example, will be far more effective in this direction than the remains of extinct flora or fauna. A wooden tank or a wooden cage in which fish or animals are confined, and which becomes saturated with their own alive discharges, and with the decaying remnants of their food, a human habitation similarly soiled, all provide the conditions essential for the life of the living existence outside the body of the goitrous subject."[10] While such associations are almost endless in this kind of analysis, it is a fact that most of the soils in the Kumaon region belong to the limestone-bearing Siwalik Hills. However, the information collected and analyzed here also indicates that the prevalence of goitre can be associated with quartzite and granite formations.[11]

The incidence of goitre in relation to local sites, elevation and bedrock material is contained within Tables 14.1 and 14.2. The highest intensity of goitre occurred in the Hawalbagh block in the central, Bhikasen and Syalde in the north-western part of Kumaon. In addition, other areas of higher intensity included Lohaghat in the west, Bhimtal in the south-central, and Rudrapur in the southern part of Kumaon. It is only in Bhimtal that limestone bedrock materials are found; the other areas contain either granite or quartzite bedrock materials. Areas which were ranked second in terms of goitre intensity also had quartzite bedrock materials. Examples include Bageshwar in the north-east, Tarikhet in the central portion and Champawat in the eastern part of the region. On the basis of the village surveys, the prevalence of goitre in the latter areas ranged from 13 to 19 per cent.

Goitre in Relation to Surface and Sub-surface Hydrology

A common belief prevails among many villagers of the Kumaon area that the cause of goitre lies in the water, and this belief is in fact supported by a large mass of evidence collected by many researchers, medical and others, investigating goitre in the identified endemic areas. For example, there are portions of villages more markedly "goitrous" than others. In some of these villages, local inhabitants directly attributed the condition to water. Some water supplies indeed were known as "goitrous springs" by villagers who preferred to use river water for consumption in order to prevent the disease. In a detailed study of Ghorakhal village in the Betalghat area, it was noticed that goitre prevailed among people utililsing water flowing through rivulets orginating from limestone rocks. In that area river water is much more difficult to obtain and it is often necessary to carry it about 1000 m to the village. This results in a condition wherein

Table 14.1: Incidence of Goitre in the Kumaon Region (1970-75)

Survey No.	*Blocks*	*Prevalence rate per cent to the total cases in the region*
1.	Kapkote	0.02
2.	Bageshwar	4.3
3.	Garur	0.1
4.	Takula	1.2
5.	Bhaisiachhana	2.9
6.	Dhaula Devi	1.6
7.	Hawalbagh	14.4
8.	Lamgara	2.4
9.	Barakote	4.1
10.	Lohaghat	7.5
11.	Champawat	5.3
12.	Tarikhet	4.6
13.	Dwarahat	2.2
14.	Chaukhutia	2.3
15.	Bhikiasen	9.4
16.	Salt	1.1
17.	Syalde	8.9
18.	Ramgarh	0.3
19.	Bhimtal	8.1
20.	Okhalkanda	0.4
21.	Betalghat	1.3
22.	Haldwani	3.3
23.	Ramnagar	0.3
24.	Kashipur	4.0
25.	Bazpur	0.6
26.	Rudrapur	6.6
27.	Khatema	3.0

Based on Data Collected from Different Health Centres in the Kumaon Region.

many will take their chances with the local water source, resulting in about 60 per cent—most of them women—found suffering from advanced goitre. In addition, those who did not suffer from goitre for the most part made the extra trip to obtain water from farther away and at a lower elevation.

Many villagers in parts of Kumaon recognise that it is "chuna" water containing excessive amounts of lime that may be contributing to goitre. Characteristics of so-called goitrous water recognised by these villagers include the following: hardness; heavy consistency; astringent taste; lime smell; containing a consistently warm

Table 14.2: Incidence of Goitre in the Kumaon Region (1975)

Survey No.	*Village*	*Location*	*Height above sea level (ft.)*	*Bedrocks*	*River water* polluted/unpolluted*	*Incidence rate (%)*
1.	Khaljhuni	Upland	9790	gneisses	—	0
2.	Bamsera	Sarju Valley	3000	quartzite	polluted	16
3.	Palyurah	Kosi Valley	3000	quartzite	polluted	13
4.	Akheti	Ramaganga Valley	3000	limestone	unpolluted	3
5.	Jalikhan	Upland	6000	quartzite	poor and monotonous diet	1
6.	Sen Sera	Ramganga Valley	3000	quartzite	polluted	19
7.	Jaitha	Upland	6000	quartzite	—	5
8.	Kotila	Upland	6000	quartzite	poor and monotonous diet	7
9.	Padhya	Upland	5900	quartzite	—	11
10.	Mazgaon	Upland	5700	granite	—	0
11.	Bagaur	Upland	6200	limestone	poor and monotonous diet	7
12.	Bishguli	Kosi Valley	2800	limestone	unpolluted	5
13.	Ropa	Kosi Valley	3500	limestone	unpolluted	3
14.	Ghorakhal+	Upland	7500	limestone	poor and monotonous diet	60
15.	Ucholi	Bhabar	—	—	—	3
16.	Malli Bamori	Bhabar	—	—	—	4
17.	Chorpani	Tarai	—	—	—	2
18.	Chaumehla	Tarai	—	—	—	5
19.	Thotupura	Tarai	—	—	—	4
20.	Raipur Khurd	Plain	—	—	—	4

* Based on chemical examination done at the nearest health centre's lab.

\+ Ghorakhal is an exceptional village where a high endemicity was found. The writer came across no other area in the region with such a high rate of endemicity.

Note: Author's Study.

temperature during all seasons; chalky depositions resulting from boiling in containers; and "milky" deposits left in utensils. As already mentioned, a higher goitre incidence was noted by Stott and his colleagues in the early 1930s in many of these areas. In general, the Himalayan rivers and streams carry dissolved calcium suspended in their waters from the mountainous limestone. As the calcium becomes more diffused, it is eventually carried with alluvium. Given sufficient dispersal away from sources, the calcium is eventually sedimented and areas farther downstream in general have a lower incidence of goitre.

Another hypothesis much more difficult to substantiate because of the prevalence of water pollution in India is that made by McCarrison, who suggested that water pollution may also influence thyroid enlargement.[12] In an investigation of a village in Bhikiasen, the author found a 19 per cent goitre rate. The author also noted another area closeby with a lower pollution level and found less goitre. Such a contention is much more difficult to prove and in fact may be simply related to the carrying of excessive fluorides, elements that do not totally break down when passing through human and animal systems, into waters downstream.

Goitre and the Farming Culture

There is some reason to believe that such factor as agricultural practices, general lifestyles and the possibility of trace elements in food may also result in goitre endemicity to some degree. Some caution should be taken with the dietary approach because it is difficult to relate illness to trace elements without detailed long-term scientific studies. Nonetheless, some associations are believed to exist in Kumaon. To begin with, in areas where cultivated land is used intensively, including for double cropping, there is a clear lack of iodine content in the soils. One such area which is intensively used is the cultivated portion of the Ramganga Valley near Bhikiasen. As already mentioned, goitre is endemic in that area and this may be a result of both iodine deficiency in the soils as well as conditions of water consumed in the area. The Dhauladevi area of the eastern Kumaon Himalayas offers contrasting results. In that area goitre is not widely reported. In addition, the soils are not intensively cultivated, primarily because slopes are very steep.

In terms of dietary intake, some interesting associations have been made. For example, the cultivation of Pinallo, a root crop, has been generally related with the prevalence of goitre. Pinallo utilises large amounts of soil iodine in actual growth, so a curious situation results wherein a root crop utilising iodine for growth is depleting the soil of the mineral but apparently not in sufficient quantities to supply human systems with iodine. Where the land is not suitable for growing other crops, villagers are often compelled to cultivate Pinallo. In many Pinallo growing areas, particularly in western Kumaon, the prevalence rate of endemic goitre ranges from 3 to 5 per cent. This particular association is one area that definitely requires further detailed research.

Researchers have long attempted to associate endemic goitre in the Himalayan tract with poverty level, general living conditions and insufficient and imperfect diets. Some of the early researchers including Macnamara and McCarrison, in discussing the genesis of goitre, attached much importance to unbalanced diets.[13] In a study of "the geographic pathology of thyroid disease", Greer and Astwood listed peaches, pears, strawberries, spinach and carrots as having a moderate effect in terms of producing goiter.[14] Also, 19 other plants including cabbage, green pepper and beets were put forth as having some questionable effect. Apart from specific items which might be causing goitre, poor or monotonous diet is very common in almost all of the upland villages of Kumaon. In these upland areas dietary staples include madua and barley in the form of bread, and bhat and gohat pulses. A balanced diet of vegetables, citrus fruit, meat and milk are not within reach of perhaps up to 95 per cent of the population of many of the villages in the north-eastern and southern Kumaon Himalayas. Environmental conditions and general poverty restrict acquisition of many of these items. There is also little seasonal dietary change except on important festivals when wheat flour is used to prepare a special dish. Surveys show the incidence of goitre in these areas is from 7 to 11 per cent. Contrasting evidence related to diet was found in the Ropa and Bishguli villages in the southern part of the Kumaon Himalayas where diets and living conditions are similar but the goitre prevalence rate is from 3 to 5 per cent. These examples help explain why additional research into the possibility of dietary intake and goitre prevalence needs to be accomplished.

National Policy Aspects of Goitre Control

In 1964, the Government of India started a goitre control programme primarily consisting of promoting the use of iodized salt in goitrous areas. In fact, efforts are being made for increased use of iodine by inhabitants along the entire northern part of the country draining from the Himalayas. The programme has not been entirely successful.[15] For example, in 1969, non-iodized salt was still freely flowing in the market in Bijnor district of Uttar Pradesh and a resurvey of the population indicated that no significant impact had been made in terms of goitre control. Similar results were found in other provinces of the goitre control target area. Another problem resulted when it was found that the amount of iodine in the so-called "iodized salt" produced by manufacturing sources was below the prescribed standard indicated by the World Health Organization as necessary to control goitre. Part of the problem also appears to be due to apathy at certain state government levels. For example, until recently in West Bengal, iodized salt was being supplied to some districts; but the state government had not banned the entry of non-iodized salt into the area. Given such lack of control, no highly successful control measures can be taken. Quite recently health officials have found it necessary to actually ban the entry of non-iodized salt into endemic goitre areas. Even these measures have not been totally successful. In January 1976, the Jammu and Kashmir government actually lifted the ban on the entry of non-iodized salt. Persuasion from the national government resulted in imposing the ban on the entry of non-iodized salt once again. In Assam, similar kinds of apathy reached a peak. The Assam government has had survey teams allegedly carrying out goitre surveys since 1958, but to date no survey has been completely accomplished. National policy now calls for resurveys of endemic goitre areas in 1978, including Manipur, West Bengal, Tripura, Assam, Meghalaya, and the hilly areas of Uttar Pradesh. As a matter of national policy, these surveys should pay particular attention to environmental factors in association with goitre endemicity.

The findings of this chapter highlight certain environmental factors associated with goitre prevalence in Kumaon, and it is assumed that similar associations can be found in other government target areas. However, it should be understood that no single factor appears to be responsible for causes of goitre in different regions. Clearly, the main cause is iodine deficiency, but elements governing the supply of iodine in the diet are many and complicated when viewing regional systems. In addition to increasing supplies of iodized salt, some improvement might be made by diversifying diets, and ultimately cropping patterns, in particular sub areas. In many Himalayan areas, geographical conditions are such that a variety of crops, including important vegetables, may be grown, but centuries of particular agricultural practices giving emphasis to certain kinds of foodgrains are instilled in local populations. If State Governments cannot follow through with effective resurveys and comprehensive goitre control programmes, it must be a matter of national policy if this disease is to be brought under control in India.

Acknowledgements

I am grateful to Professor Andrew T.A. Learmonth of the The Open University, U.K. for supervising the work. Thanks are also due to Professor D. Banerjee, Professor Moonis Raza and Dr. I. Qadeer for their important suggestions.

Notes

1. Cannon, H.L. and Hopps, H.C. (Eds.) (1971), *Environmental Geochemistry in Health and Disease,* Colorado: The Geological Society of America, Boulder.
2. Schiel, J.B. and Wepfer, A.J. (1976), Distributional Aspects of Endemic Goitre in the United States, *Econ. Geog.,* 52, 116.
3. Ishankulov, M. Sh., Aydarkhanov, B.A. and Zeltser, M. Ye. (1975), Natural Cause-and-effect Relationships and the Prediction of Endemic Goitre, *Soviet Geog.*, 16, 169.
4. McClelland, J. *Geology of Kumaon* (1834), Quoted from Macnamara F.N. *Climate and Medical Topography in their Relation to the Disease Distribution of the Himalayan and Sub-Himalayan Districts of British India; with Reasons for Assigning a Malarious Origin to Goitre and some other Diseases,* p. 317. London, 1880. See also *Asiat. Re* XVI, 1928.
5. Gordon, C.F. (1884), *In the Himalayas and on the Indian Plains,* p. 348, London.
6. Atkinson, E.T. (1886), *Himalayan Districts of the North-Western Provinces of India,* Vol. III, p. 533, Allahabad.
7. Batten, J.H. (1863), *Report on the Settlement of the District of Kumaon,* p. 615, Banaras.
8. The first major Himalayan glaciation began during the culminating phase, and the overthrusting of the Siwaliks was followed by fluvioglacial

deposition which generally produced boulders much larger than those of the Siwalik conglomerates, Quoted from Gansser, A. (1964), *Geology of the Himalayas,* p. 245, London.

9. Stott, H., *et al.* (1931), The Distribution and Causes of Endemic Goitre in the United Provinces, *Ind. J. Med. Res.,* 18, 1069.
10. Rundle, F.F. (1951), *Joll's Diseases of the Thyroid Gland,* p. 84, London,
11. Gansser, A., *op. cit.,* p. 245.
12. McCarrison, R., *et al.* (1927), The Relation of Endemic Goitre to the Iodine Content of Soil and Drinking Water, *Ind. J. Med. Res.,* 15, 207.
13. *Ibid.*
14. Greer and Astwood also listed peaches, pears, strawberries, spinach and carrots as having a moderate goitrogenic effect, as well as 19 other plants including cabbage, green peppers and beets, as having a questionable effect and 31 others, among which were mustard, corn, black beans and onions. Quoted from Scrimshaw, N.S., The Geographic Pathology of Thyroid Disease, In : *The Thyroid* (Edited by Hazard, B.J. and Smith, D.E.), p. 112. Baltimore, 1964).
15. Goitre Control Programme a Failure, *Indian Express,* 25 September, 1969.

15
Geomedical Study of Iodine and Thyroid in North Kashmir Himalayas—India

G.M. Rather and *T.A. Kanth*

Introduction

Trace elements are the elements present in the earth's crust in concentrations less than 0.1 per cent (<1000 mg kg^{-1}) or those elements that are ordinarily present in plant or animal including human beings tissues in concentrations less than 0.01 per cent (<100 mg kg^{-1}) of the organism's dry weight.[1]

Trace elements in the soil are derived from Atmosphere, Hydrosphere, and Lithosphere. Model shows the pathways whereby the trace elements may find their way to human body and thus influencing the quality of health (Fig. 15.1).

The concentration of trace elements in soil, water or food items is mainly determined by the geological conditions of the area[2] and regional differences in essential minerals in the soil, water or air and hence human diet occur both in developed and developing countries, but their effects are usually more evident in the latter, largely because of imbalance and mismanaged nutrition and reliance on local food products.[3]

Each trace element has a standard requirement adequate for human health recommended by W.H.O.[4] All essential trace elements either in imbalance states[5] or in deficiency states[6] are known to create serious health problems particularly in the areas where these are regionally deficit.[7, 8] Diseases due to trace element deficiencies as well as excess are known for iodine, copper, zinc, selenium,

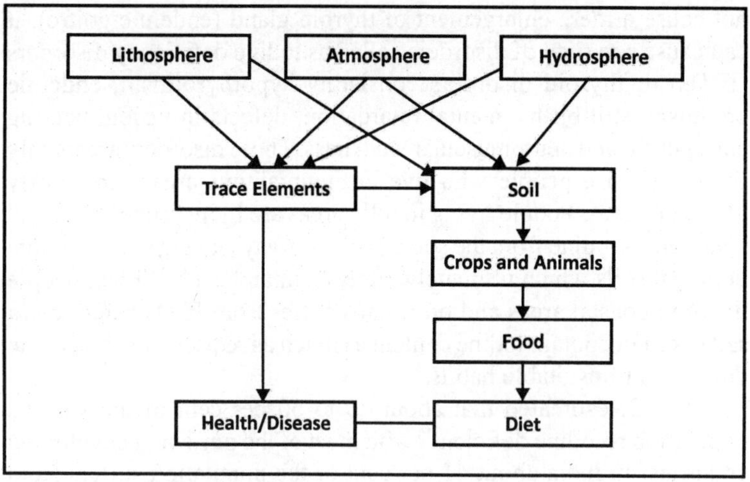

Fig. 15.1 : Schematic Drawing Showing Path by which the Trace Elements May Find their Way to Humans and Other Animals thus Influencing the Quality of IIealth.

Source: Compiled by Authors.

molybdenum, manganese, iron, calcium, arsenic and cadmium.[9] Endemicity of many chronic or mild disorders such as goitre, dental fluorosis[10] cancers[11], skin disorders etc. is quite prevalent across India because of the variable concentrations of certain trace elements such as arsenic, fluoride, iodine, cerium etc.[12]

Iodine is an essential element that is critical for the normal growth and development, and well-being of all humans. The human body does not make iodine and is dependent on dietary sources; making it an essential part of our diet. The healthy adult human body contains 15-20 mgs of iodine, of which about 70-80 per cent is in the thyroid gland. The normal intake and requirement of iodine is 100-150 $\mu g\ d^{-1}$.

The distribution of iodine is uneven in the biosphere. Both natural process such as leaching[13], volcanism[14] and human activities are responsible for redistribution of trace elements in the soils and water and organic environments (plants, animals and humans) through a network of pathways called as biogeochemical cycles.[15]

Iodine deficiency is associated with reduced thyroid hormone synthesis, leading to increased thyroid stimulating hormone levels, which stimulates thyroid over growth and goiter.[16] Its deficiency does not cause a mere enlargement of thyroid gland (endemic goitre), it can cause a variety of disorders called as iodine deficiency disorders (IDDs) or thyroid disorders consisting hypothyroidism, endemic cretinism, still-births, mental retardation, defects in vision, hearing and speech, and neuromuscular weakness. These disorders are mainly found in those people who live in mountainous areas, previously glaciated areas. People living in hilly areas are more prone to thyroid disorders as iodine from the soil is washed away leaving behind iodine deficient soils which ultimately effects human health.[17] Even people living in coastal areas and on islands suffer from IDDs because sea salt does not contain iodine content as much as required by the people due to their unsuitable habits.[18]

W.H.O. estimated that about 20 to 60 per cent of the world's population is iodine deficient[19] with most of the burden in developing countries. In India about 41 per cent of the population suffers from iodine deficiency and in the state of Jammu and Kashmir nearly 33 per cent of the population suffers from iodine deficiency.[20] According to a recent research conducted in 2013 on school children of Kulgam district, it was found that 18.9 per cent suffer from Total Goiter Rate (TGR); 21.2 per cent boys and 16.7 per cent girls.[21] Present study was an attempt to find out the concentration of Iodine in soils, drinking water and staple foods and incidence of thyroid in North Kashmir Himalayas.

Study Area

North Kashmir Himalayas is a part of Great Kashmir Himalayas and lies between 34°16'15.09" – 34° 12'41.35" North latitude and 74°48'00.00" – 75°05'09.58" East longitude. The mountain range has an average altitude of 2324 meters and stretches over an area of 5110.60 sq. kms. It is at a point near Zojila that Great Kashmir Himalayas takes a blend towards the south-west and is described as the North Kashmir range (Fig. 15.2). North Kashmir Range acts as a water divide between Jhelum in Kashmir Valley and Kishanganga of Gurez Valley. Paleozoic sedimentary rocks, Triassic limestone, Karewa and Alluvium are the predominant geological formations of the area with limestone, shale, sandstone and unconsolidated sediments as the dominant lithology. The soils of the concerned area vary in origin from alluvial to lacustrine and glacial[22] (Fig. 15.3 and Table 15.1).

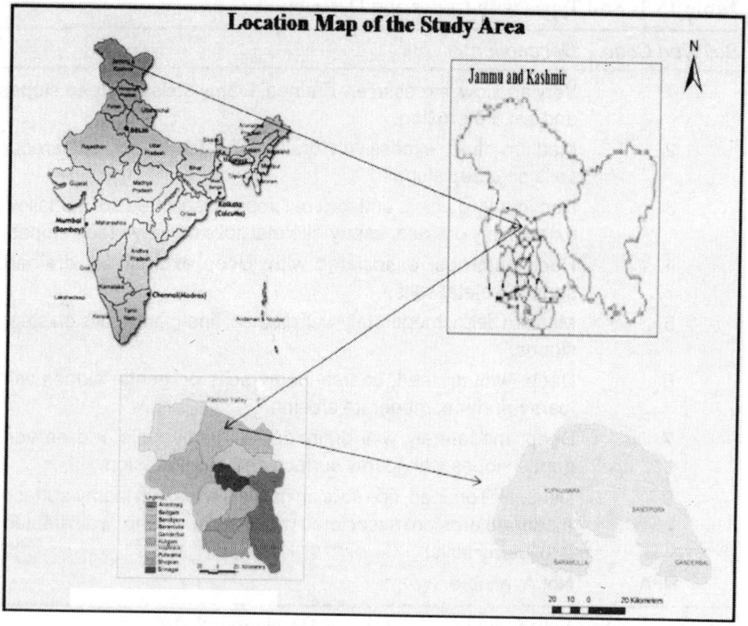

Fig. 15.2: Location Map (Generated from SOI Toposheets, 1971).

Source: SOI Toposheets.

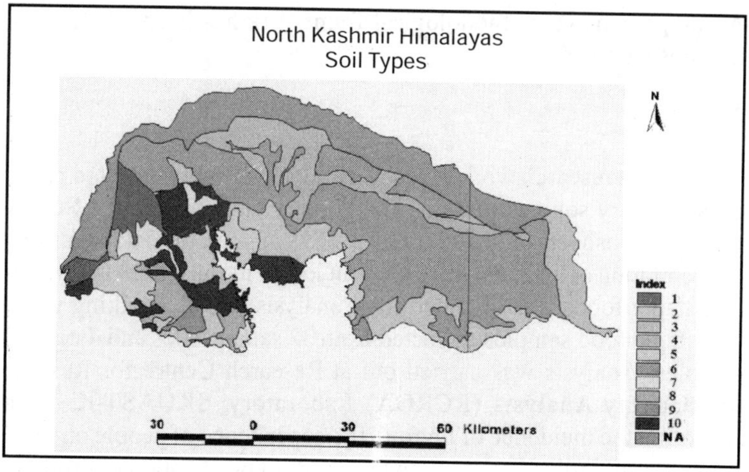

Fig. 15.3: Soil Map of the Study Area (Generated from Soil Map of J. and K., ICAR, Nagpur-2010).

Source: Modified from ICAR, Nagpur.

Table 15.1: Soil Types with Codes and Description

Soil type Code	*Description*
1	Very shallow, excessively drained, loamy soils on steep slopes and severe erosion.
2	Medium deep, excessively drained, coarse-loamy, calcareous soils on steep slopes.
3	Dominantly glaciers and rock outcrops; associated with: Shallow, extensively drained, sandy-skeletal soils on very steep slopes.
4	Rock outcrops; associated with: Deep extensively drained, sandy-skeletal soils.
5	Medium deep, moderately well drained, fine-loamy soils on steep slopes.
6	Deep, well drained, coarse-loamy soils on gentle slopes with loamy-surface, moderate erosion.
7	Deep, moderately well drained, fine loamy soils and on very gentle slopes with loamy surface and slight erosion.
9	Deep, well drained, fine soils on gentle slopes with loamy-surface, moderate erosion; associated with: Medium deep, well drained, fine loamy soils.
N. A.	Not Available.

Source: Modified from Soil Map of J. & K., ICAR, Nagpur-2010.

Data Base and Methodology

A comprehensive methodological framework has been adopted for the present research.

Data Base

The present research work is based mainly on primary data and partly on secondary sources of data. The primary data include the Survey of India toposheets on 1:50,000 scale of 1971 year, the data regarding concentration of essential trace element iodine in soils, drinking waters and staple foods was obtained from analysis of soil, drinking water and staple food samples collected from 32 sample sites and 4 control samples. Analysis was carried out at Research Centre for Residue and Quality Analysis (RCRQA) Laboratory, SKUAST-K. Data regarding the incidence of thyroid, the dependence of people on local foods, use of iodized salt, use and methods of purification of drinking water was obtained by conducting household survey through a well structured Schedule/Questionnaire.

Methods Used

The methodology has been divided into many steps based on the materials and techniques used. An outline of the various methodological steps is provided in the Fig. 15.4 and described under the following headings.

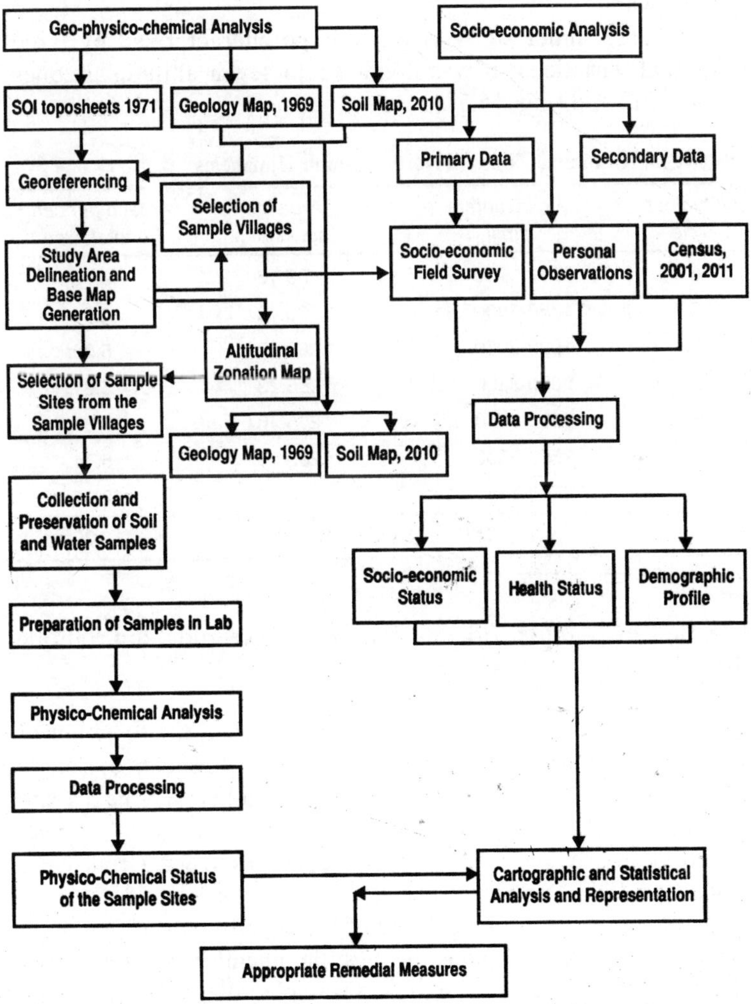

Fig. 15.4: Flow Chart of Methodology.

Delineation of Study Area Altitudinal Zone Mapping and Thematic Mapping

The study area was delineated from thirteen SOI toposheets of 1:50, 000 scale of 1971 with numbers as (43 series, j/2, j/3, j/6, j/7, j/10, j/11, j/14, j/15, N/3, N/4, N/7, N/8 and O/1. The toposheets were processed under GIS environment with the help of Arc View 3.2a software.

The area under study is fairly large characterized by large altitudinal variations; it was divided into seven altitudinal zones (Table 15.2) and (Fig. 15.5).

Table 15.2: Altitudinal Zones in North Kashmir Himalayas

Altitudinal Zone	*Alt. in meters amsl*	*Area in sq. kms.*	*Area in per cent to total Area*
A	1600-1750	499.18	9.76
B	1750-1900	308.43	6.04
C	1900-2050	269.87	5.28
D	2050-2200	286.23	5.61
E	2200-2350	275.50	5.39
F	2350-2500	293.19	5.74
G	2500 and Above	3178.20	62.18
	Total	**5110.60**	**100**

Source: SOI Topo-sheets.

Selection of Sample Villages, Sample Households and Sample Sites

Stratified Random Sampling technique was used for selection of around 15 per cent of sample villages (32) and 20 per cent of sample households (4000) in proportion to total number of villages and households from each altitudinal zone.

From each sample village soil sample site was selected from major agricultural field, Drinking water sample site was selected as the most common source of drinking water of the sample village (tap/river/tube well) and staple food as the most dominant crop (Table 15.3). Geo-coordinates and altitude of each sample village was measured with the help of GPS during field survey (Table 15.4).

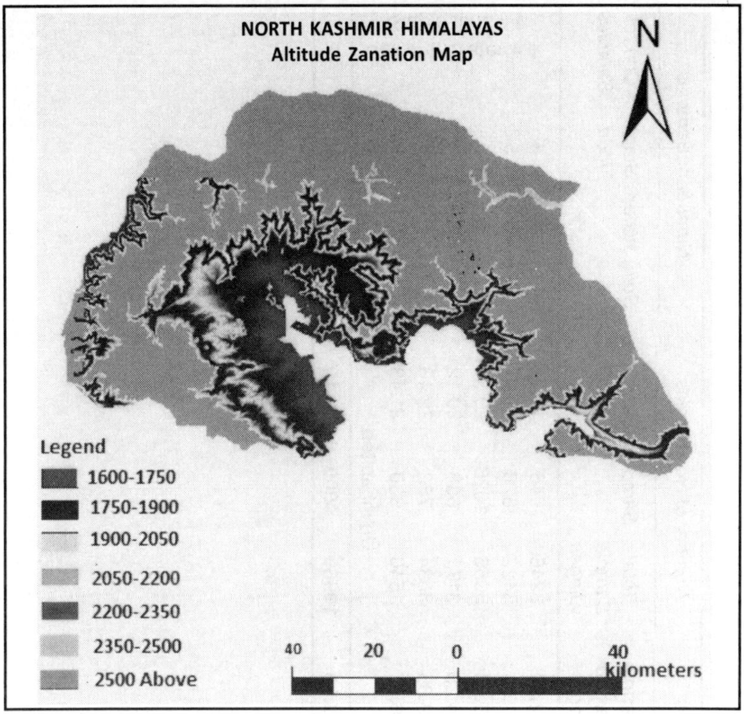

Fig. 15.5: Altitudinal Zonation Map.

Source: SOI Toposheet.

Sample Collection and Sample Codification

An intensive and multifaceted field-work was undertaken to collect the soil water and staple food. One soil, one water and one staple food samples were collected from each sample village making a total of thirty two (32) of each soil, water and staple food. One soil, one water and one staple food samples were collected from 4 control sites of Bandipora, Ganderbal, Kupwara and Baramulla having high agricultural productivity, good crop health and good human health status to make standard for comparative analysis. Soil samples were collected in clean unused polythene bags and were labeled properly. Soil samples were taken only from surface soil (depth of 0-30 cm) for the reason that these soils are under the cultivation of paddy, vegetables and maize and this is the major zone of root development

Table 15.3: Sample Frame

Altitude Zone	Altitude (meters)	Area (sq. kms.)	Revenue Villages			Number of Households			Number of Samples			
			Total	Sample	Sample (percentage)	Total Sample villages	Sample	Sample (percentage)	Soil	Water	Staple food	Control Samples
A	1600-1750	499.18	32	4	12.50	3246	546	16.82	4	4	4	Soil = 4, Water = 4, Staple food =4
B	1750- 1900	308.43	43	5	11.63	3422	678	19.81	5	5	5	
C	1900- 2050	269.87	51	8	15.68	5056	1026	20.30	8	8	8	
D	2050- 2200	286.23	42	6	14.28	3171	638	20.12	6	6	6	
E	2200- 2350	275.50	31	6	19.35	3534	782	22.13	6	6	6	
F	2350- 2500	293.19	18	3	16.67	1540	330	21.43	3	3	3	
G	2500-6000	3178.20					Un inhabited					
Total		**5110.6**	**217**	**32**	**15.00**	**19969**	**4000**	**20.10**	**32**	**32**	**32**	**12**

Table 15.4: Sample Villages with Geo-coordinates and Sample Site Codes

Sl. No.	*Sample Village*	*Latitude Longitude*	*Average Altitude (meter)*	*Soil Sample site code*	*Water Sample site code*	*Staple cereal Sample site code*
1	*2*	*3*	*4*	*5*	*6*	*7*
1.	Gund	34°17'44" N 74°48'30" E	1847	GSSI	GWS1	GFS1
2.	Chont Wali war	34°47'14" N 74°54'28" E	2370	GSS2	GWS2	GFS2
3.	Chhatragul peth	34°14'28" N 74° 58'05" E	1730	GSS3	GWS3	GFS3
4.	Khanan	34°18'47" N 74°51'59" E	2030	GSS4	GWS4	GFS4
5.	Wangat	34°19'33" N 75°06'50" E	2345	GSS5	GWS5	GFS5
6.	Waniarm	34°04'16" N 74°38'45" E	2295	GSS6	GWS6	GFS6
7.	Ajas	34°24'23" N 74°44'05" E	1690	BSS1	BWS1	BFS1
8.	Aragam	34°22'31" N 74°40'58" E	1765	BSS2	BWS2	BFS2
9.	Chithi Bandi	34°22'46" N 74°41'13" E	2190	BSS3	BWS3	BFS3
10.	Sumlar	34°24'39" N 74°43'41" E	1935	BSS4	BWS4	BFS4
11.	Arin Dardpora	34°25'43" N 74°42'16" E	2050	BSS5	BWS5	BFS5
12.	Kitsan	34°27'18" N 74°34'38" E	2355	BSS6	BWS6	BFS6
13.	Qoyal Muqam	34°26'58" N 74°34'36" E	2250	BSS7	BWS7	BFS7
14.	Malangam	34°26'12" N 74°33'26" E	2150	BSS8	BWS8	BFS8
15.	Aloosa	34°26'57" N 74°34'36" E	1835	BSS9	BWS9	BFS9
16.	Kandi	34°39'55" N 74°45'30" E	2250	KSS1	KWS1	KFS1
17.	Shirihama	34°21'45" N 74° 20'52" E	1745	KSS2	KWS2	KFS2
18.	Laeche	34°19'45" N 74°12'20" E	2045	KSS3	KWS3	KFS3
19.	Kualmabad	34°42'15" N 74°45'40" E	1815	KSS4	KWS4	KFS4

(Contd.)

Table 15.4 (*Contd.*)

1	2	3	4	5	6	7
20.	Waderbala	34°18'24" N 74°10'20" E	2010	KSS5	KWS5	KFS5
21.	Haril	34°30'25" N 74°12'42" E	1990	KSS6	KWS6	KFS6
22.	Shalthur	34°19'14" N 74°12'08" E	1835	KSS7	KWS7	KFS7
23.	Zachaldara	34°18'26" N 74°11'06" E	2360	KSS8	KWS8	KFS8
24.	Manebal	34°30'15" N 74°30'15" E	2055	KSS9	KWS9	KFS9
25.	Rishwar	34°40'55" N 74°48'45" E	2310	KSS10	KWS10	KFS10
26.	Nowgam	34°30'50" N 74°30'35" E	1935	KSS11	KWS11	KFS11
27.	Inderdaji	34°20'12" N 74°08'54" E	1950	KSS12	KWS12	KFS12
28.	Pothwari	34°28'19" N 74°14'25" E	1980	KSS13	KWS13	KFS12
29.	Potus	34°45'20" N 74°12'28" E	2146	BLSS1	BLWS1	BFS1
30.	Wahalutar	34°46'22" N 74°14'32" E	2253	BLSS2	BLWS2	BLFS2
31.	Wanpur	34°28'12" N 74°16'30" E	2036	BLSS3	BLWS3	BLFS3
32.	Naidhu	34°25'23" N 74°16'55" E	1684	BLSS4	BLWS4	BLFS4

Source: Based on GPS Readings during Sample Survey, 2013.

of crops.[23] Water samples were collected in clean unused plastic bottles from the selected sample sites. Staple food samples were taken as the most dominant crop locally cultivated from the soil. All the samples were properly packed, coded properly and reached to the lab within 24 hours for trace element-iodine, copper and zinc analysis.

Proper codification scheme was followed for identification of the samples.

Codes were used as:

1st alphabet for Macro region

2nd alphabet for Geo-chemical component
(S= Soil, W= Water, F= Staple Food)

3rd alphabet as simply S for sample in all components

4th alphabet as a numerical number of the village (1, 2, 3, 4 etc.)

In case of control samples alphabet C for control is added.

Lab Work

The soil, water and staple food samples were analyzed for concentration of trace element iodine at Research Centre for Residue and Quality Analysis (RCRQA) Laboratory, SKUAST-K, under Atomic Absorption Spectrophotometer (AAS-4141, Electronic Corporation Limited, India). A total concentration of I was determined after 4-acid digestion (HF, $HClO_4$, HNO_3 and HCl) by AAS.

Sample Household Survey

The socio-economic field survey of 4000 households was carried out through the structured schedules to study different socio-economic aspects like literacy, levels of education, occupation, dependence of people on local food items, use of iodized salt and the methods of purification of drinking water. The data regarding the prevalence of trace element related disease thyroid was obtained from household after proper verification from the prescriptions given by the registered practitioners.

Data Analysis and Map Work

Data obtained from the analysis of soil, water and staple food analysis from the RCRQA Laboratory, SKUAST-K and data obtained after tabulation of data from Questionnaire/Schedule was statistically analyzed. Composite score method was employed for identification of different categories of risk. Map work has been carried out under GIS environment.

Results and Discussions

Concentration of Iodine in Soils of Sample Villages

The soils of the study area have average concentration of iodine as 1.570mg/kg with a considerable negative mean deviation of -0.030 mg/kg from control samples. The concentration decreases from an average concentration of 1.617 mg/kg in altitudinal zone A to an average concentration of 1.524 mg/kg in altitudinal zone F. Average concentration of iodine shows positive deviations of + 0.017 mg/kg from control sample in altitude zone A and decreases with altitude to

Table 15.5: Concentration of Iodine in Soils

Altitudinal Zone	*Sample villages*	*Soil Sample Site*	*Concentration of Iodine with deviation from Control sample (mg/kg)*	*EC (ms)*	*pH*	*Org. Matter*
A (1600- 1750)	Chatragul, Ajas, Shirhama, Naidhu	GSS3, BSS1, KSS2, BLSS4	1.617 (+0.017)	1.567	7.47	1.42
B (1750-1900)	Gund, Aragam, Aloosa, Shiltra, Kalamabad	GSS1, BSS2, BSS9, KSS7, KSS4	1.562 (–0.038)	2.79	6.78	1.29
C (1900-2050)	Khanan, Arin, Sumlar, Haril, Mawar, Inderdeji, Potwari, Wanpur	BSS4, BSS5, BSS4, KSS6, KSS11, KSS12, KSS13, BLS3	1.588 (–0.012)	2.63	6.93	1.39
D (2050-2200)	Chitibani, Malangam, Waderbala, Monabal, Laeche, Potus	BSS3, BSS8, KSS5, KSS9, KSS3, BLSS1	1.546 (–0.054)	1.69	7.03	1.47
E (2200-2350)	Wangat, Waniarm, Mukam, Rishwari, Kandi, Walthur	GSS5, GSS6, BSS7, KSS10, KSS1, BLSS2	1.518 (–0.082)	1.71	5.64	1.38
F (2350-2500)	Chontiwaliwar, Kitsan, Zachaldara	GSS2, BSS6, KSS8	1.524 (–0.076)	1.73	7.00	1.35
G (2500 and Above)	—	Uninhabited				
Average	**32**	**32**	**1.559 (–0.030)**	**2.19**	**6.80**	**1.38**

Note: Figures in parenthesis represent deviation from Mean of Control Samples.

Concentration of I in Control Soil Samples

Control Soil Sample	*Con. of I (mg/kg))*	*Ecms*	*pH*	*OC*
GCSS	1.55	1.10	6.86	1.73
BCSS	1.68	0.80	7.62	0.90
KCSS	1.68	1.11	7.57	1.13
BLCSS	1.49	8.08	7.34	1.05
Mean	**1.60**	**2.77**	**7.34**	**1.21**

Source: Data Obtained through Analysis of Soil samples in RCRQA Lab, SKUAST-2014.

a negative deviations of –0.038 in altitudinal zone B, –0.012 mg/kg in altitudinal zone C, –0.054 mg/kg in altitudinal zone D, –0.082 mg/kg in altitudinal zone E and –0.076 mg/kg in altitudinal zone F (Table 15.5). The reason could be that organic matter and pH influence the concentration of iodine in the soils because OM binds up iodine ions in the soil but the increasing slope and coarser texture cause iodine ions flow and translocate easily during rainfall. The study area being formed during Orogensis of Himalayas and subjected to tremendous transformation both by natural and human activities. Extensive soil erosion in this mountainous region[24] and water leaching of some acid arenaceous soils low in organic matter increases the magnitude of iodine losses and reduces the intrinsic availability of soil selenium and zinc. High soil acidity strongly potentiates crop uptake of aluminium, iron and manganese.[25]

Concentration of Iodine in Drinking Water of Sample Villages

Analysis of Table 15.6 shows the concentration of iodine in drinking water in the area has been noted as 0.486 mg/L with negative deviation of –0.010 from control samples.

The concentration decreases from an average concentration of 0.516 mg/L in altitudinal zone A to an average concentration of 0.495 mg/L in altitudinal zone F. Average concentration of iodine shows positive deviations of +0.013 mg/L from control sample in altitude zone A but decreases with altitude to a positive deviation of +0.011 from control samples in altitudinal zone B, positive deviations of +0.005mg/L in altitudinal zone C, +0.001 mg/L in altitudinal zone D, but decreases to negative deviation of –0.050 mg/L in altitudinal zone E and –0.013 mg/L in altitudinal zone F (Table 15.6). Low

Table 15.6: Concentration of Iodine in Drinking Water of Sample Villages

Altitudinal Zone	*Sample villages*	*Water Sample Site*	*Concentration of Iodine with deviation from Control sample (mg/L)*	*pH*	*EC (ms)*
A 1600- 1750	Chatragul, Ajas, Shirhama, Naidhu	GWS3, BWS1, KWS2.BLWS4	0.516 (+0.013)	7.71	3.52
B (1750-1900)	Gund, Aragam, Aloosa, Shiltra, Kalamabad	GWS1, BWS2, BWS9, KWS7, KWS4	0.514 (+0.011)	7.72	3.74
C (1900-2050)	Khanan, Arin, Sumlar, Haril, Mawar, Inderdeji, Potwari, Wanpur	GWS4, BWS5, BWS4, KWS6, KWS11, KWS12 KWS13, BLWS3	0.456 (+0.005)	7.72	3.60
D (2050-2200)	Chitibani, Malangam, Waderbala, Monabal, Laeche, Potus	BWS3, BWS8, KWS5, KWS9, KWS3, BLWS1	0.511 (+0.001)	7.67	3.80
E (2200-2350)	Wangat, Waniarm, Mukam, Rishwari, Kandi, Walthur	GWS5, GWS6, BWS7, KWS10, KWS1, BLWS2	0.426 (–0.050)	7.72	3.06
F (2350-2500)	Chontiwaliwar, Kitsan, Zachaldara	GWS2, BWS6, KWS8	0.495 (–0.013)	7.42	9.25
G (2500 and Above)	Uninhabited				
Average	**32**	**32**	**0.486 (–0.010)**	**7.66**	**4.49**

Note: Figures in Parenthesis Represent Deviation from Mean of Control Samples.

Concentration of I in Control Water Samples

Control Soil Sample	*Con. of I (mg/kg))*	*pH*	*EC (ms)*
GCSWS	0.495	7.42	3.65
BCWS	0.511	7.66	6.02
KCWS	0.506	7.59	1.20
BLCWS	0.488	7.32	2.11
Mean	**0.500**	**7.49**	**3.24**

Source: Data Obtained through Analysis of Water Samples in RCRQA Lab, SKUAST-2014.

concentration of iodine in drinking water with a declining trend with altitude is because of deficiency of iodine in the bedrock of the study area which has a direct bearing on the quality of drinking water.[26]

Concentration of Iodine in Staple foods of Sample villages

Average concentration of iodine in the staple foods in the study area was 2.728 mg/kg with a considerable negative mean deviation of –0.172 from control samples. The concentration decreases from an average concentration of 3.075 mg/kg in altitudinal zone A to an average concentration of only 2.467 mg/kg in altitudinal zone F. Average concentration of iodine shows positive deviations of +0.175 mg/kg from control sample in altitude zone A but decreases to a negative deviation of –0.060 mg/kg from control samples in altitudinal zone B, –0.463 mg/kg in altitudinal zone C, –0.017 mg/kg in altitudinal zone D, –0.233 mg/kg in altitudinal zone E and –0.433 mg/kg in altitudinal zone F (Table 15.7). Low concentration of iodine in the staple foods with a declining trend with altitude is because of deficiency of iodine in the soils of the study area.

Dependency on Local Staple Foods

Since the study area is agricultural. dominant food crops grown in the area are rice in the foothills and maize in the sloppy areas. People were more dependent on local foods both cereals and vegetables. Analysis of data reveals that near about 37.75 per cent of sample households were more than 50 per cent dependent on local foods, 28.77 per cent of households were 35-50 per cent dependent on local foods and only 32.97 per cent of households were dependent on local

Table 15.7: Concentration of Iodine in Staple Foods

Altitudinal Zone	*Sample Village*	*Staple Food Sample Site*	*Concentration of Iodine*
A 1600-1750	Chatragul, Ajas, Shirhama, Naidhu	GFS3, BFS1, KFS2, BLFS4	3.075 (+ 0.175)
B (1750-1900)	Gund, Aragam, Aloosa, Shiltra, Kalamabad	GFS1, BFS2, BFS9, KFS7, KFS4	2.840 (–0.060)
C (1900-2050)	Khanan, Arin, Sumlar, Haril, Mawar, Inderdeji, Potwari, Wanpur	GFS4, BFS5, BFS4, KFS6, KFS11, KFS12, KFS13, BLFS3	2.437 (–0.463)
D (2050-2200)	Chitibani, Potus, Malangam, Laeche, Waderbala, Monabal,	BFS3, BFS8, KFS5, KFS9, BLFS1	2.883 (–0.017)
E (2200-2350)	Wangat, Waniarm, Mukam, Rishwari, Kandi, Walthur	GFS5, GFS6, BFS7, KFS10, KFS1, BLFS2	2.667 (–0.233)
F (2350-2500)	Chontiwaliwar, Kitsan, Zachaldara	GFS2, BFS6, KFS8	2.467 (–0.433)
G (2500 and Above)		Uninhabited	
Average	**32**	**32**	**2.728 (–0.172)**

*Concentration of I in Control Staple Cereal Samples.

Control Staple Cereal Sample	*Con. of I (mg/L)*
GCSFS	2.300
BCFS	3.100
KCFS	2.500
BLCFS	3.700
Mean	**2.900**

Source: Data Obtained through Analysis of Soil Samples in RCRQA Lab, SKUAST-2014.

foods by less than 35 per cent. There is a considerable variation in dependency on local foods in different altitudinal zones of the study area Dependency on local foods more than 50 per cent increases with altitude from 26.19 per cent of sample households in altitudinal zone A to 50.91 per cent of households in altitudinal zone F (Table 15.8).

Table 15.8: Dependency on Local Staple Foods

Altitudinal Zone	*Sample Village*	*No. of households Surveyed*	*Dependency on local staple foods with per cent to total*		
			Low (<30%)	*Medium (30-50%)*	*High (>50%)*
A (1600- 1750)	Chatragul, Ajas, Shirhama, Naidhu	546	211 (38.64)	192 (35.17)	143 (26.19)
B (1750-1900)	Gund, Aragam, Aloosa,Shiltra, Kalamabad	678	257 (37.90)	182 (26.85)	239 (35.25)
C (1900-2050)	Khanan, Arin, Sumlar, Haril, Mawar, Inderdeji, Potwari, Wanpur.	1026	390 (38.01)	269 (26.22)	367 (35.77)
D (2050-2200)	Chitibani, Malangam, Waderbala, Monabal, Laeche, Potus	638	221 (34.63)	165 (25.86)	252 (39.49)
E (2200-2350)	Wangat, Waniarm, Mukam, Rishwari, Kandi, Walthur	782	175 (22.39)	236 (30.17)	371 (47.44)
F (2350-2500)	Chontiwaliwar, Kitsan, Zachaldara	330	65 (19.70)	97 (29.39)	168 (50.91)
G (2500 & above)	Uninhabited				
Average	**32**	**4000**	**1319 (32.97)**	**1141 (28.77)**	**1540 (37.75)**

Note: Figures in Parenthesis Represent Percentage to Total.
Source: Data Obtained through Analysis of Soil Samples in RCRQA Lab, SKUAST-2014.

Use of Iodized Salt

Coverage under use of iodized salt was satisfactory as 98.90 per cent of the households surveyed were using iodized salt however a considerable variation in use of iodized and non iodized salt in different altitudinal zones of the study area was noted.

Use of non-iodized salt shows a slight increases with altitude from 0.00 per cent of sample households in altitudinal zone A to 3.94 per cent of households in altitudinal zone F. (Figure 15.5). Use of non iodized salt was not found in altitudinal zone A but a very less per cent of households (0.30%) in altitudinal zone B, 0.49 per cent in

Table 15.9: Use of Iodized Salt

Altitudinal Zone	*Sample Village*	*No. of Households Surveyed*	*Iodized Salt Used*		*Keeping of Salt Box*	
			Yes	*No*	*Open Lid*	*Closed Lid*
A 1600- 1750	Chatragul, Ajas, Shirhama, Naidhu	546	546 (100.00)	0 0.00	112 (20.51)	434 (79.49)
B (1750-1900)	Gund, Aragam, Aloosa, Shiltra, Kalamabad	678	676 (99.70)	2 (0.300)	290 (42.77)	388 (57.23)
C (1900-2050)	Khanan, Arin, Sumlar, Haril, Mawar, Wanpur Inderdeji, Potwari	1026	1021 (99.51)	5 (0.49)	329 (32.06)	697 (67.93)
D (2050-2200)	Chitibani, Malangam, Waderbala, Monabal, Laeche, Potus	638	628 (98.43)	10 (1.57)	319 (50.00)	319 (50.00)
E (2200-2350)	Wangat, Waniarm, Mukam, Rishwari, Kandi, Walthur	782	768 (98.20)	14 (1.80)	489 (62.53)	293 (37.47)
F (2350-2500)	Chontiwaliwar, Kitsan, Zachaldara	330	317 (96.06)	13 (3.94)	250 (75.75)	80 (24.25)
G (2500 & Above)	—		Uninhabited			
Average	**32**	**4000**	**3956** **(98.90)**	**44** **(1.10)**	**1789** **(44.72)**	**2211** **(55.28)**

Note: Figures in Parenthesis Represent Percentage to Total.
Source: Sample survey, 2013.

altitudinal zone C. There was noted an increase in use of non iodized salt in altitudinal zone D (1.57%), altitudinal zone E (1.80%) and altitudinal zone F (3.94%) (Table 15.9). The reason behind the use of non iodized salt in high altitude zones D, E and F was storage of non iodized salt for severe winter as rock salt.

Analysis of data reveals that majority of sample households were keeping lid of salt box closed (55.28%) however a significant number of sample households (44.72%) were keeping salt box open lid, keeping salt box open lid leads to loss of iodine from the salt and leads to iodine deficiency in the humans (Table 15.9).

Use of Purified Drinking Water and Methods of Purification

Use of purified drinking water was noted only in 15.40 per cent of the sample households in the study area and shows a slight decrease with altitude from 32.42 per cent of sample households in altitudinal zone A to 0.00 per cent of households in altitudinal zone F. Use of purified drinking water was found as 32.42 per cent in altitudinal zone A, 24.92 per cent in altitudinal zone B and 17.34 per cent in altitudinal zone C. However, there was drastic decline in the use of purified drinking water in altitudinal zone D (7.36%), altitudinal zone E (5.75%) and altitudinal zone F (0.00%) (Table 15.10). The reason behind the use of non-purified water in high altitude zones D, E and F was as water collected from *nallahs* was considered as the pure.

Analysis of data reveals that majority of sample households (47.88%) were using boiling as method of purification of drinking and only 7.64 per cent of households were using aqua guard/purit for purification of drinking water however a significant number of sample households (44.48%) were using traditional method of keeping water pots as stored for at least one night so that the suspended particles get settled at the bottom of water pot. There is a variation in both use of purified drinking water and methods of purification in different altitudinal zones (Table 15.10).

Spatial Pattern of Iodine Deficiency Disease (Thyroid)

Thyroid is a trace element disease caused by deficiency of iodine. The disease was found in all the altitudinal zones with certain variation with respect to the altitude and age-sex groups as is shown in Table 15.11. Variation in the percentage incidence of thyroid with

Table 15.10: Use of Purified Drinking Water and Methods of Purification

Altitudinal Zone	*Sample Village*	*No. of Households Surveyed*	*Use of Purified Drinking water*		*Methods of Purification of Drinking Water*		
			Yes	*No*	*Boiling*	*Sedi-mentation*	*Aquaguard/ Purit*
A (1600-1750)	Chatragul, Ajas, Shirhama, Naidhu	546	177 (32.42)	369 (67.58)	84 (47.46)	67 (37.85)	26 (14.69)
B (1750-1900)	Gund, Aragam, Aloosa, Shiltra, Kalamabad	678	169 (24.92)	509 (75.08)	86 (50.88)	70 (41.43)	13 (7.69)
C (1900-2050)	Khanan, Arin, Sumlar, Haril, Mawar, Inderdeji, Potwari, Wanpur	1026	178 (17.34)	848 (82.66)	73 (41.01)	98 (55.06)	7 (3.93)
D (2050-2200)	Chitibani, Malangam, Waderbala, Monabal, Laeche, Potus	638	47 (7.36)	591 (92.64)	32 (68.08)	14 (29.79)	1 (2.13)
E (2200-2350)	Wangat, Waniarm, Mukam, Rishwari, Kandi, Walthur	782	45 (5.75)	737 (94.25)	20 (44.44)	25 (55.56)	0 0.00
F (2350-2500)	Chontiwaliwar, Kitsan, Zachaldara	330	0 (0.00)	330 (100.00)	0 (0.00)	0 (0.00)	0 (0.00)
G (2500 & Above)	—			Uninhabited			

Note: Figures in Parenthesis Represent Percentage to Total.
Source: Sample Survey, 2013.

Table 15.11: Incidence of Iodine Deficiency Disease (Thyroid) by Age and Sex

Altitudinal Zone	*Sample Village*	*No. of Households Surveyed*	*Total Population of Households Surveyed*	*Number of Thyroid Cases with per cent to Total Population*	*Incidence of Thyroid by Sex with per cent total cases*	
					Male	*Female*
A (1600- 1750)	Chatragul, Ajas, Shirhama, Naidhu	546	3450	191 (5.53)	101 (52.87)	90 (47.13)
B (1750-1900)	Gund, Aragam, Aloosa, Shiltra, Kalamabad	678	3445	215 (6.24)	110 (51.16)	105 (48.84)
C (1900-2050)	Khanan, Arin, Sumlar, Wanpur Haril, Mawar, Inderdeji, Potwari,	1026	5785	416 (7.19)	186 (44.71)	230 (51.29)
D (2050-2200)	Chitibani, Malangam, Waderbala, Monabal, Laeche, Potus	638	4254	307 (7.21)	141 (45.92)	166 (54.08)
E (2200-2350)	Wangat, Waniarm, Mukam, Rishwari, Kandi, Walthur	782	4124	354 (8.58)	149 (42.09)	205 (57.91)
F (2350-2500)	Chontiwaliwar, Kitsan, Zachaldara	330	2072	222 (10.71)	95 (42.79)	127 (57.21)
G (2500 & Above)	—			Uninhabited		
Average	**32**	**4000**	**23130**	**1705 (7.37)**	**782 (45.86)**	**923 (54.14)**

Note: Figures in Parenthesis Represent Percentage to Total.

Source: Sample Survey, 2013.

respect to the altitude and soil class is due the variability in the iodine content present in the soil at a particular altitude determined by soil pH, organic matter and lifestyles that includes the nature of eating and drinking habits, methods of cooking etc. Difference in the percentage with respect to sex can be attributed to the relative differences in the lifestyles.

Conclusion/Suggestions

The present research work leads to the conclusion that Iodine content in the soils, drinking water and staple foods of sample villages was less than the mean of control samples with mostly negative deviation and generally decreases with altitude. It was also found that Iodine in soil has direct relationship with organic matter and clay and inverse relationship with pH. Iodine content in water samples under study showed a relationship with the iodine content in surrounding soils. Leaching and run-off play an important role.

Majority of sample households were more dependent on local foods. Dependency on local foods more than 50 per cent increases with altitude from 26.19 per cent of sample households in altitudinal zone A to 50.91 per cent of households in altitudinal zone F.

A very sizeable number of sample households were using non-iodized salt and a large percentage of households were found keeping salt box open and boiling water for drinking purposes that are the main causes of loss of iodine.

Prevalence of thyroid was very large. It was found that there is a slight general increase in percentage prevalence of thyroid with altitude. In altitudinal zone A and B, females were suffering from thyroid more than the males while the case was reverse in altitudinal zones C, D, E and F where more males than females were suffering from thyroid.

On the basis of inferences drawn from the present analysis, the following measures are suggested for improving the health status in this mountainous region.

(1) Full Coverage under use of Iodized Salt

There should be 100 per cent use of iodized salt by the population. Iodized salt should be kept in a salt box with a proper cover and lid of the salt box should be closed after every use of the salt. Keeping lid of saltbox open leads to the loss of iodine. Aqua guard or purit should be used for purification of drinking water.

(2) Change in Food Habits

There is a need of change in food habits. People should not remain more dependent on local products cultivated on soil deficit in trace elements but should make more use of more iodine rich foods.

(3) Soil Analysis and Change in Soil Management Practices

Soil tests should be carried out to assess the fertility and trace element status of soil for cultivation of crops. Soil management practices needs to be modified in order to minimize the risk of trace element deficiency in the soils.

(4) Mass Awareness and Full Involvement of the Community

No health promotion programme can be successful unless community for whom it is intended is aware about it. Awareness programmes needs to be organized in the sample villages to make the people aware about health promotion programmes.

Acknowledgements

The authors are highly thankful and indebted to University Grants Commission, New Delhi for providing financial assistance in the Project "Geo-chemical environment and related health problems in North Kashmir Himalayas". Present research paper is a part of it.

Notes

1. Adriano, D.C. (2001), *Trace Elements in Terrestrial Environments: Biogeochemistry, Bioavailability and Risks of Metals*, New York: Springer-Verlaug, Inc., 175 Fifth Avenue, USA, pp. 1-24.
2. Keller, E. (1999), *Environmental Geology*, New Jersey: Merrill Prentice Hall Upper Saddle River, pp. 314-316.
3. Oliver, M.A. (1997), Soil and Human Health: A Review, *European Journal of Soil Science,* Vol. 48, pp. 573-592.
4. Fishbein, L. (1986), Trace and Ultra Trace Elements in Nutrition: An

Overview, *Paper Presented at the IAEC Workshop on Carcinogenic and Mutagenic Metal Compounds in CH-1884, Villars-Surallon.*

5. Warren, H. (1991), Geology and health, In: R. Akhtar (Ed.), *Environment and Health: Themes in Medical Geography,* New Delhi: APH, pp. 297-313.
6. Pyle, G.F. (1979), *Applied Medical Geography,* Washington, D.C.: V.H. Winston & Sons, p. 88.
7. Learmonth, A.T.A. (1988), *Disease Ecology,* New York: Basil Blackwell Ltd., pp. 46-49, 76.
8. Hunter, J. and Akhtar, R. (1991), The Challenge of Medical Geography, In: Akhtar, R. (ed), *Environment and Health, Themes in Medical Geography.* New Delhi: Ashish Publishing House, pp. 1-37.
9. Lindh, U. (2005), Biological Functions of the Trace Elements, In: Selinus, O. (Ed.), *Essentials of Medical Geology*, Elsevier, pp. 115-160.
10. Dissanayake, C.B. (1990), Human Health Problems in Sri Lanka, In: R. Akhtar and Yola Verhasselt (Eds.), *Disease Ecology and Health*, Jaipur: Rawat Publications, pp. 75-90.
11. Akhtar, R. (1998), Cancer Ecology in Kerala, India, *Intern, J. Environmental Studies,* Vol. 55, pp. 345-355.
12. Dissanayake, C.B.; Rao, C.R.M. and Chandrajith, R. (2010), Some Aspects of the Medical Geology of the Indian Sub-continent and Neighbouring Regions, In Selinus, O.; Robert, B.; Finkelman and Jose, A. Centeno (eds.), *Medical Geology—A Regional Synthesis, Springer*, Netherlands, pp. 175-198.
13. Jeelani, G. (2010), Chemical and Microbial Contamination of Anantnag Springs, Kashmir Valley, *Journal of Himalayan Ecology and Sustainable Development,* Vol. 5, pp. 1-8.
14. Bunnell, J., *et al.* (2007), Medical Geology: A Globally Emerging Discipline, *Geologica Acta,* Vol. 5, No. 3, 2007, pp. 273-281.
15. Furley, P.A. and Newey, W.W. (1982), *Geography of the Biosphere: An Introduction to the Nature, Distribution and Evolution of the World's Life Zones,* Butterworth-Heinemann Ltd., pp. 35-101.
16. Jamescon, J.L. and Weetman, A.P. (2005), Disorders of the Thyroid Gland, In: Kasper, D.L., Braunwald, E. and Fauci, A.S. (eds.), *Harrison's Principles of Internal Medicine.* New York: McGraw Hill, pp. 2104-2127.
17. Akhtar, R. (1978), Goiter Zonation in the Kumaon Region, *Social Science Medicine,* 12, pp. 152-163.
18. UNICEF (2002), *Iodine Deficiency Disorders and Universal Salt Iodization: South Asia Priorities.*
19. Zimmermann, M.B., *et al.* (2009), The Iodine Deficiency Disorders, *Lancet,* 372:1251-1262.
20. Zargar, A.H., *et al.* (1996), Pattern of Salt Consumption and Awareness about Iodine Deficiency Disorders in Kashmir Valley, *IDD Newsletter*, 12(3), pp. 46-48.
21. Khan, M.S., *et al.* (2014), Prevalence of Goiter among Primary School Children of Kulgam District, Jammu & Kashmir, India. In: *Academic Medical Journal of India*, Vol. II(1), pp. 18-21.

22. Raza, *et al.* (1978), *The Valley of Kashmir, A Geographical Interpretation: The Land,* New Delhi: Vikas Publishing House, pp. 43-47.
23. Brady, N.C. (1990), *Nature and Properties of Soils*, New York: MacMillan Publishing Company, pp. 331-397.
24. Kanth, T.A. and Bhat, M.S. (1991), Soil Erosion Zones in Kashmir Valley, *Transaction Institute of Indian Geographers,* Pune: Department of Geography, University of Pune, 13, 12, pp. 141-149.
25. Mills, C. (1997), *Zinc in Human Biology,* British, Springer Verlaug Berlin Heialberg, pp. 2-25.
26. Jeelani, G. (2004), Effect of Subsurface Lithology on Springs of a Part of Kashmir Himalaya, *Himalayan Geology,* 25(2): 145-151.

PART III
Socio-cultural Aspects and Health

16

The Cultural Environment of Medical Geography in Rural Hindu, India

L. Schuyler Fonaroff and *Arlene Fonaroff*

That village India has serious population and health problems are well-known. What is not known are techniques for optimum use of health facilities in order to utilize the manpower which exists. Despite increased life expectancy (27 years in 1939 to 45 years in 1964), the general health of rural Indians is in a precarious condition, and constant vigilance must be maintained to protect populations from a wide range of endemic and epidemic infections which not only cause many deaths, but debilitate energy and shorten life span. Owing to the prevalence of a variety of endemic diseases, villagers often maintain *laissez faire* attitudes about their physical well-being and come to believe that the disease state is man's natural one. In all of these illnesses there is the problem of implementing known methods of control, either because of lack of funds and technical assistance or resistance of the population due to persistent traditional cultural habits and beliefs about disease causation and treatment. Even where facilities are available, people are not always ready to use them because of such beliefs.

Despite inter-regional differences within the subcontinent, several main themes seem to persist in public health planning and also in the subsequent cultural and ecological responses. The purpose of this chapter is to examine the socio-cultural parameters influencing the medical geography of some Hindu communities in rural India.

Reprinted after having been edited, from *Pacific Viewpoint,* 7, 67-84, 1966.

The Problem

According to the World Health Organiszation, public health services may broadly be considered as those activities directed toward the protection of health in a community. However, planning *per se* must not be an end in itself, rather the goal must be toward use of facilities and services by those for whom they are intended.[1] The World Health Organization has emphasized that people must achieve health through their own action and effort. Therefore, successful public health service is largely dependent upon working *with* rather than *for* people. Health must first become a valued community asset before people become competent in achieving it.

The basic assumption in all public health programmes is that health is a purchasable commodity and that given enough funds, the subsequent implementation and successful completion of a health programme is to be expected. Inherent in such a goal is the need for planned change. However, this change must be initiated within specific social and ecological environments. Ideally these environments form the framework for public health endeavours. Following this line of reasoning, it might be useful to construct a cultural map which, while not necessarily presenting the holistic sociological characteristics of a region, will portray the pertinent traits which impinge upon implementation of health services. Such analysis may validate the underlying notion that successful change in public health practices is dependent upon awareness of inter-cultural differences.

However, it is vital to recognize that cultural behaviour is only one of two inseparable components of the health environment, the other being the natural setting. An analysis of one without the other is recognizably incomplete. Therefore, effective analysis must concern itself not only with man's social habits, but these actions should be placed within a bio-geographical framework. Disease may be considered a maladujustment to the environment, to which numerous factors contribute, including those of environment, culture, vector and host. Disease, therefore, becomes an anthropo-geographical phenomenon.[2]

The interaction of this multifaceted phenomenon can be illustrated by malaria. For malaria control, it would be pertinent to have a knowledge not only of mosquito life history, but also of the mosquito's specific ecological relationship with the physical environment. Against this scheme, a montage of social factors must be made in terms of the life history of individuals and techniques used by them in living the natural landscape. Only this holistic view of man within the physical environment can offer a more realistic approach to community health planning.[3]

Natural Versus Supernatural

Disease in India may be considered in a general two-part classification: diseases of epidemic nature which may become endemic, such as malaria, smallpox, plague and tuberculosis; and diseases such as dysentery, fevers, and hookworm, which are endemic but at times may reach epidemic proportions. Interestingly, this division seems to correspond to one made by many Indian villagers. This distinction is not a consciously organised categorisation, but a response which appears to have developed out of traditional thought patterns about illness.

Diseases in the first category are those associated with the Hindu religion and occurrence arbitrarily seems to cross-cut caste organisation. Non-epidemic diseases fluctuate in occurrence and prevalence according to social level within the caste system, and beliefs about the nature and incidence of such illnesses are attributed to conditions within the physical and social environments, rather than the supernatural environment. Villagers' awareness about gastro-intestinal diseases shows that there are fallacious ideas about the causes of dysentery and hookworm. In many villages, most people feel dysentery results from eating bad, heat-producing foods which cause excessive internal heat. A rural sanitation survey in Singur showed that only 40 per cent of the villagers recognised that flies in contact with contaminated faeces spread this disease.[4] As a result, curative measures centre on strict control of diet.[5] A detailed set of beliefs exist concerning the effect of specific foods on the body. This hot-cold food classification is known from much of the world and is also prominent in Latin America.

In the case of hookworm, less than 20 per cent of Singur villagers understood that there was a connection between walking barefoot and contraction of the disease. Likewise, in malaria it becomes apparent that "cultural blindness" skews a group's view of the environment, so that in many rural areas of the world a simple mosquito-disease cause-effect relationship is a difficult perceptual problem.

The zone of causative agents of disease widens and often moves toward the supernatural as the length of illness progresses. After a fortnight, members of higher castes generally believe illness is associated with that body of beliefs which some have referred to as the "Hindu Great Tradition".[6] Lower castes are more concerned with a variety of spirits, supernatural forces, and local gods.

Health planners have become aware that in order to encourage villagers to expend efforts at disease prevention and treatment, it becomes vital to work within the existing religious and social organisation. Most field workers realise that the greatest success occurs when traditional beliefs are coupled with Western knowledge.

The pertinent socio-religious factors influencing health practices in Indian villages are those concerned with the hierarchical ordering of life and the fatalistic nature of Hinduism. These factors influence the individual's thoughts and activities both within his own group and extend on to the larger universe.[7] Every individual is not only a member of a joint family within the village community but a member of a caste group which has a wider territorial spread. This traditional hierarchical ordering based on the *Varna* system divides people into two major groups: the higher, twice-born castes composed of *Brahmans* (priests and learned men); *Kshatriyas* (rulers and warriors); and *Vaisyas* (traders); and occupational castes which can be divided according to work specialisations.[8] Regional and territorial units contain several of these socially autonomous castes, and occupation is traditionally ascribed by caste membership. Traditional rules also govern actions between each group in such relationships as methods of speech, interdining, sex, touchability, etc.

This view of hierarchical structuring is extended so that non-Hindus are also placed in a quasi-caste status which serves to maintain the basic structure. As a result, this provides a workable solution for Hindu-Muslim relationships at the village level, with each group maintaining prescribed rules of interaction. We might extend this principle further by saying that in new social contacts, all non-Indians are placed in similar fashion within the hierarchy. The quasi-caste status may account for acceptance or rejection of specific public health workers. It may therefore determine the permissibility of co-existing medical systems. It also poses problems because ensuing social behaviour does not readily lend itself to acceptance of universally prescribed solutions in such public health measures as village sanitation drives.

The hierarchical organising factor demonstrates the Hindu's central value of maintaining balance within the universe. Any imbalance creates disruption, and the notion of *Karma,* "acting rightly", as a modal behaviour pattern attests to the degree of Hindu prescription to a state of equilibrium. This also manifests itself in a great deal of fatalism and resignation toward predestiny. Fatalism becomes explicit, however, only after attempts are made at problem solving.[9]

Imbalance in this system results in overall disruption. In reference to health, illness results if the normal balance of the body is disturbed. The traditional medical practitioner, the *vaid,* pays great attention to season and climate, diet and temperament. He therefore is mindful of an holistic environment and deals with the interaction between man and society within the physical setting. Faulty diets, lack of harmony with the supernatural world due to activity of ghosts and general displeasure of deities are considered among the prime causes of disease.[10] For example, smallpox is believed to be caused by a variety of local goddesses. The notion of a two-factor complex of virus and host is totally foreign to villagers. Brahmans are entrusted with diagnosis and recommendation of cures. *Dharma,* the moral and cosmological order, makes it necessary to rigidly follow prescribed ceremonies to propitiate the responsible goddesses. For diseases resulting in large numbers of successive deaths, such as smallpox or plague, worship is regarded as the only remedy; with such actions as fasting, witchcraft and animal sacrifices to augment ceremonials. This set of beliefs necessarily conflicts with a germ theory of disease and resultant preventive and curative measures such as vaccination. Most villagers refuse inoculations because of these differences of belief in causative agent. It seems perfectly reasonable for a villager to refuse an injection where a scratch on the arm is supposed to prevent smallpox when his appraisal of the universe determines that "an epidemic is air which cannot be controlled except through great supernatural powers".[11] Further, it is rather presumptuous to expect outside forces to have more power than the local gods, goodesses, and spirits who hold high positions in the hierarchical scheme.

The distribution of smallpox is closely related to the vaccination status of a population. Thus, factors affecting vaccination have a direct bearing on the incidence, distribution and severity of the disease.[12] Overcrowded housing conditions and unsanitary surroundings which result in the spread of this disease are only of secondary importance if the population has been vaccinated or has gained a degree of immunity from previous attack. Periodic epidemics in large centres where the infection is endemic or re-imported are probably due to the fact that vaccination protection was not renewed. This is because in a large population there is always the possibility of an increasing number of individuals who have become susceptible to the disease.[13]

There is considerable variety in belief about the amount of illness which results from supernatural action, and considerable transfer of patients between the Western doctor and the local practitioner. There are several local practitioners available for each village: the shaman or *bhagat* who has powers to appease disease deities, the priest, the *vaid,* the *hakim* who prescribes native medicinal cures, and public health personnel. What is interesting to note is the role of these practitioners as innovators. It must be remembered that these men hold high caste membership (exclusive of public health personnel, in some instances) and in all likelihood not only have the most frequent contact with outside influences but the greatest propensity for appreciating the advantages of change. It is through the experience of elders and knowledge of specialists that the nature of folk medicine may become heterogeneous. This heterogeneity is kindled by increasing outside contracts, education, and the need to apply new techniques according to the severity of a given disease.[14] For example, if a village specialist is exposed to malaria suppressants and can personally experience positive results by taking these drugs, he might be tempted to add them to his repertoire of cures. His esteemed position helps to allay the fears of patients who place supreme trust in the doctor's cures. Sometimes faith and recourse to Western medicine are reported to be stimulated by chance, as in the case of an influential villager who had medical training and experience during the war and who dispensed modern drugs to his own and neighbouring areas.[15]

However, the Western drugs do not serve as substitutes for the old magico-religious system of cures. In rural Rajasthan, it has been noted that Western remedies were only one of several sorts of healing and were by no means the most popular.[16] Utilization of several alternative responses to a health problem is by no means restricted to developing countries, and the incorporation of folk and technical medical aids is common even in Western society. There is a dual tendency on the part of people to talk of the efficacy of certain Western medicine, but to practise indigenous treatment at the first sign of illness. Acceptance of Western drugs comes as a last resort, and there is a different expectation of results.[17] It has been found that while villagers demand immediate results from Western prescriptions, they do not impose this restriction on the assured native treatments.

Folk medicine is believed by its adherents to be the best, most complete and secure way of treating illness. Not to be minimized in this connection is the relationship between patient and doctor, where each has a specified role to play in relationship to the other; and the relationship between both doctor and patient together and the community at large.[18] In rural India, the indigenous doctor regards the patient as a living creature, a part of the social world, and he has a sympathetic attitude and includes the patient's family and friends in the circle of therapy. The patient and the community in return have a total belief in the efficacy of treatment, which may be more important than the treatment itself.[19] Modern foreign doctors, however, use mechanical methods and tend to isolate the patient from his social sphere. Efforts of the Indian Government have increased the number of native-trained personnel. Yet the need for more practitioners persists. Further, there is a tendency for trained personnel to seek posts in urban rather than rural areas.

In dealing with epidemic and endemic diseases, the beliefs and attitudes of villagers run counter to those of Westerners. This is demonstrated by the Orissa malaria eradication project. Though technically sound, the project was unsuccessful because of the disparity between Western-influenced concepts of public health and Orissa views about cause and prevention of malaria.[20] Many Oriyas felt that malaria might occur because of climatic and dietary factors, but the prime reason for the disease occurrence was believed to be due to an angered god, evil spirit or black magic. The disbelief that malaria is a mosquito-borne disease resulted in the rejection of some public health measures. While villagers were amenable to the use of drugs, they rejected and sabotaged DDT spraying. A questionnaire survey revealed two prime reasons for this :

(1) There was no idea of DDT benefits except that it was thought DDT killed all insects, which of course it doesn't. The advantage of mosquito eradication did not impress the villagers, since they did not believe mosquitoes had anything to do with malaria. Furthermore, bed-bug numbers increased and DDT had a bad smell.

(2) Spraying interfered with traditional plastering and painting of walls for religious ceremonies and aesthetic reasons. This occurred at least ten times a year on such occasions as festivals, marriages, deaths, births, and in cases of smallpox.

Dhillon and Kar think that these seemingly insurmountable differences might be alleviated if influential leaders were located and convinced of the programme's advantages. Frequently such men are the only bilingual speakers and are willing to hear new ideas. A UNESCO programme initiated radio broadcasts to villages in an attempt to increase health education. Organised group listening and discussion on programme advice resulted in an increase from 41 per cent to 65 per cent awareness that malaria was a mosquito-transmitted disease.[21]

The power of local leaders has long been recognised as a potent force in innovation. As early as 1912, organised Indian groups, composed of both men and women who " ... believe in self-help and discard the fatalistic view that malaria is unavoidable and an act of god", have attempted to influence villagers.[22] At that time, many villagers contacted by such groups believed that this disease was due to evening mists rising from water, especially stagnent water, and as a result felt there could be no remedy in areas where there were frequent flood threats. We are not informed of the teaching process, but the groups were able to convince villagers that the mosquito was indeed the disease vector, and they urged formation of village-level groups to prevent malaria by filling in swampy depression and oiling ponds; and to treat it by taking quinine. These methods had been prescribed by foreign health experts for years, but it was not until unofficial and unpaid people came to village homes that a change occurred. Eventually, this project became formalised under collaborative auspices of the Bengal Government and the voluntary agencies. It can be seen, then, that certain events within communities create a widespread readiness to learn.

Spatial distribution of malaria and programmes related to its control are also affected by the timing of activities in respect to the varying rhythm and pattern of village life. The effect of population movements on incidence depends greatly on whether the migration coincides with the transmission season. Whenever the two coincide, the incidence and severity of the disease increase. Family visits and pilgrimages for religious and festival occasions affect malaria occurrence. Such movements, even on a small scale, influence eradication programmes and pose difficult administrative and political problems. For example, in Mysore, when floating labour was employed on the Bhadra Project, a high parasitic rate of endemic malaria resulted. On the Jog Project, permanent immigrant labourers were screened and treated before employment. A low malaria morbidity resulted.[23] The interaction between the problems of labour and malaria have long been a scourge to India's development. In the 1920s, there was considerable hindrance to forest resource developments because of the disease. Tea, sugar, coffee and rubber industries suffered because of regional factors which contributed to high malaria incidence. Thus, the labour problem may be considered synonymous with the malaria problem in that the disease has been a major cause of both inefficient and deficient labour. During the 1920s, only 58-60 per cent of the usable areas in Central and Western Bengal were under cultivation, while in less malarious areas cultivation was at the 90 per cent usability level.[24] Over the years, malaria eradication projects have greatly improved this situation. In the 1950s, Mysore State showed a yearly increase of 15 per cent of cultivated rice acreage, with a crop production increase of 33 per cent.[25] Studies suggest that malaria control yields many times its cost in direct financial profit.[26]

It is obvious, as one Indian astutely noted, that in order to successfully conduct a mosquito eradication programme one must first learn to think like a mosquito. Vectors have fairly distinct ecological preferences.[27] The physical interaction between wind and altitude regarding temperature and rainfall is significant to mosquito behaviour. Generally speaking, areas located at or above 6,000 ft. are free of malaria. Local temperature governs the time required for the vector to become infected after absorbing the plasmodial meal. Rainfall is a prime factor both in respect to drought and downpour. Multiple breeding sites develop after excessive downpours. Droughts, on the other hand, create small depressions holding accumulations of stagnant water, providing a favourite breeding place for certain vectors. Vegetation, a natural product of rainfall, also is part of the malaria ecology. Bamboos and many epiphytes are favoured by tropical downpours and have physical structures which create receptacles whose conditions favour certain mosquitoes.

The vector's behaviour is also affected by house types and food preparation. Materials used in house construction, for example, determine the efficacy of spraying; while construction design can be related to the flight level and other flying patterns of the mosquito. Vectors can also be encouraged or discouraged depending on whether cooking habits produce indoor or outdoor smoke.[28]

The Socio-cultural Environment in Operation

So far we have considered the relationship between religious belief and efficacy of modern medical practices and the actual reasons for spatial distributions of certain diseases. We have also considered certain aspects of village social organisation, particularly family, caste and leadership patterns. It appears that the whole system is arranged to ensure that there is always someone on whom one can depend.[29] It has also been noted that in critical situations, social class, factionalism and group differences are forgotten in favour of rendering or receiving help.[30] The village conduct code obliges the medical specialist to help even when not asked, irrespective of caste position of patient. This type of dependency seems incompatible with Western notions of personal privacy, individual responsibility and interpersonal trust. Yet in order for any technical programme to be useful, it must overcome these disparities of viewpoint.

The first impression of village attitude towards outsiders is one of guarded behaviour and suspicion, and the corporate unity of a village finds its fullest expression when conflict develops with outsiders.[31] The group which has the most contact outside the village is the *Panchayat.* Recognising the esteem of this village council and its traditional role in enforcing social sanctions, the Indian Government has made it the official authority in domestic affairs. However, rather than utilise the traditional occupants of office, elected and appointed officials compose the group. Co-existing, however, with the *Panchayat,* is a traditional unit composed of the village hereditary headmen, headmen of all families and castes, and additional rich and/or influential persons. Needless to say, factionalism and power struggles are rampant in this system of dual control.

Despite this, a picture of corporate unity is placed before the outside world. The view blurs, however, when internal mechanisms of interdependence and integration are put to the test. In the area of public health this can be seen by examining attempts to initiate and maintain sanitary programmes.

Much has been written about the unhygienic nature of rural India: contaminated wells, poor or non-existent drainage systems, piled

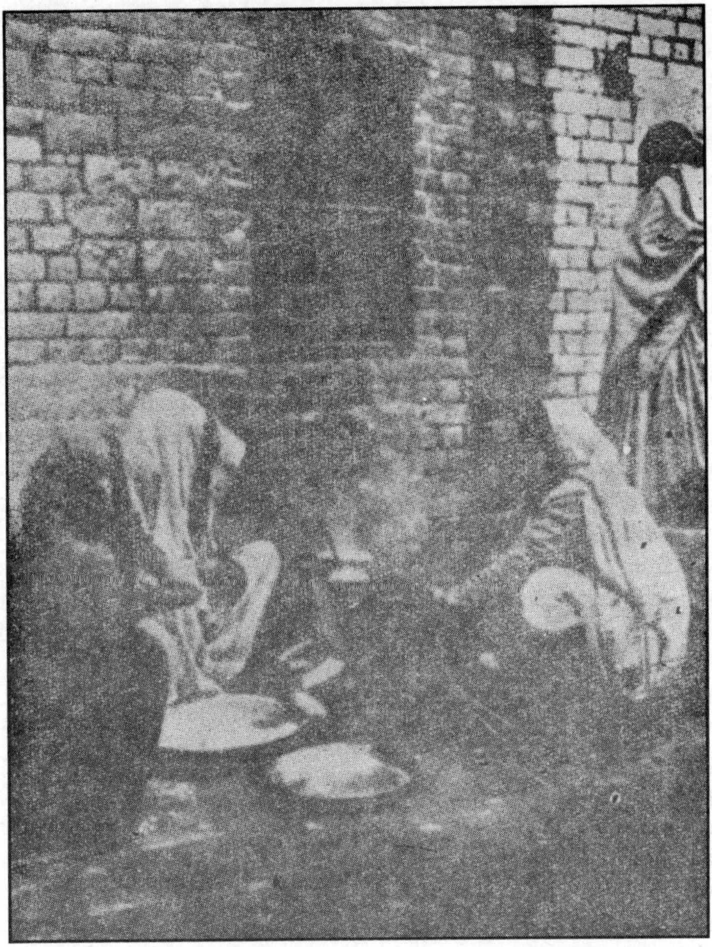

Fig. 16.1: Clothing, dietary habits and food preparation techniques at times are decisive in determining distributions of many diseases. Rickets and Osteomalacia, common in parts of the Punjab, are closely related to clothing and food habits. Indoor as versus outdoor cooking and eating habits also tend to modify the exposure the family presents to the insect-vector environment.

refuse and a general dirty, disarranged appearance. To promote consciousness of sanitation needs and practices, villagers have been encouraged to organise "clean your village drives", which in many situations have resulted in considerable success. However, inter-caste tensions within such projects have been detected, resulting in considerable problems.[32]

It may seem ironic that the caste structure, which exists in order to maintain ritual purity and to avoid ritual pollution, actually seems to perpetuate the antithesis of purity. Traditionally, low castes have always been expected to clean the village; specifically it is the responsibility of the untouchable sweepers. The social concept of distribution of manual labour operates as a deterrent in overall cleanliness campaigns. If high caste members were to clean streets they would face loss of prestige. However, the traditional obligation to maintain ritual purity does allow for overall inter-caste participation in certain activities, such as building wells and maintaining ponds and temples. The UNESCO radio education programme reached a village suffering from a Guinea worm attack and led to villagers realising that infected feet walking into a step-down well spread the infection.[33] This led to the conversion of step-down wells into a rope and bucket type and disinfection with chemicals. Sanitary measures which emphasize disinfection of wells meet with fair success, but intra-caste and inter-caste rivalries halt village-wide enforcement of paving lanes. In Gopalpur, officials recognised these forces and emphasized programmes which seemed to meet with the most receptivity among villagers.[34] They avoided community planned construction of a drainage system because it was recognised that inter-caste problems would interfere with completion. Recognition of factionalism within the caste, on the other hand, was used to public health advantage in Gopalpur. Knowing the trend for the educated families to provide the impetus for change, individual domestic groups were assisted in the construction of manure and soak pits. Families uneducated to the need for these pits joined in the effort only after educated groups were noticeably involved. Upper caste behaviour is frequently emulated by the lower caste. This principle can be extended to inter-caste dynamics, but Khare believes it necessary to plan not only for more intensive education, but for special, separate programmes geared to life values within the lower and higher castes.

Just as there appears to be discrimination in social relationships, some disease vectors also seem to discriminate in selection of their hosts. This discrimination is based on factors of the physical and social environment. Filariasis, for example, which is an insect-borne parasitic disease, occurs in many parts of India. An infected mosquito which breeds in ponds, swamps and rice fields, is not only active at

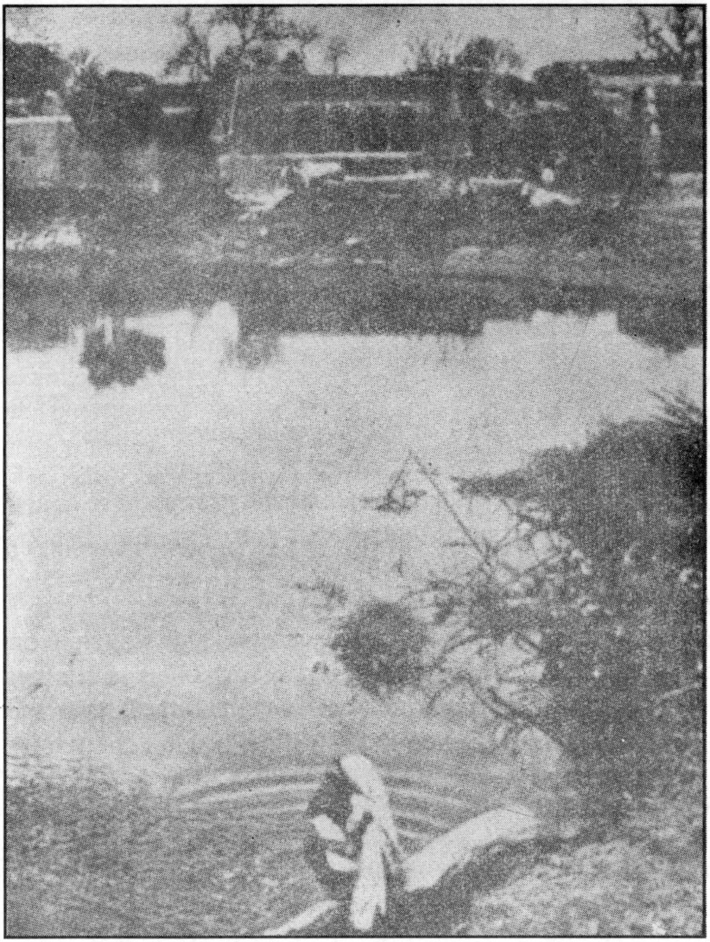

Fig. 16.2: Rankhandi Village Pond, water from such sources is used for cooking, bathing, and livestock watering. It is a constant source of gastro-intestinal infection and conveniently provides a local breeding area for insect-vector diseases such as Filariasis and Dengue Fever. Cholera also has many unexplainable seasonal characteristics and its endemicity may be perpetuated by such infected water sources.

night but also bites in daylight shade. The infected bites result in maturation of adult worms which live in lymph nodes, subcutaneous tissues or body cavities. Cultural factors such as social position, work practices, housing conditions and patterns of dress to a large extent determine the composition of the infected population, For example, high caste members who live in better constructed houses are likely to be bitten; occupational castes who work in rice fields stand a likely chance of infection; men, rather than women, are more susceptible because while working in fields or resting in the shade they wear less clothes and often strip to the waistst.[35] Cultural factors can also influence the spread and persistence of the disease. Boatmen plying numerous crafts, for example, from infected Malabar and other western coastal ports, brought endemic conditions to Saurashtra ports.[36]

The dominance of the physical environment, however, is the controlling factor in filariasis occurrence, and climate in particular appears to be the critical element in the density, longevity and biting activity of the mosquito.[37] Variation in temperature is directly related to the spread. Increase in mosquito population parallels increase in temperature, while humidity differences do not seem to produce noticeable effects. In Delhi between March and April, mosquito numbers decreased if the temperature went below 70 degrees and increased when above 100 degrees (at 80% relative humidity). The influence of climate can also be noted in movements between endemic and non-endemic areas. Exacerbation of symptoms occurred during and after the monsoon period. Improvement results in moving to a cold, dry climate where further infections cannot occur. Thus, it appears that endemicity results if breeding grounds are present with favourable climate and presence of the invertebrate host; while even if infection were introduced into an area with suitable breeding grounds, an adverse climate would hinder the spread of the disease.

Many village programmes, sanitation for example, are greatly deterred by the nature of the contact between outsiders and members of the village community. External influences for modernisation often initiate conflict between the traditional and superimposed political bodies, thereby threatening the stability of community life. Introduction of new and diverse occupations coupled with an emphasis on individualism places a serious threat on effective inter-caste co-operation. That is to say, inter-caste harmony was normally maintained through a symbiotic relationship, which now becomes threatened. Within the caste itself, active social resistance to sanitary programmes seems to occur where there is inter-caste insulation and mutual distrust. Passive resistance seems to be related to general educational backwardness and absence of initiative.

Both types of resistance must be channelled in a constructive way to aid villagers to act their own to achieve health.[38] Projects concerned with popularisation of sanitary means of excreta disposal face this very problem. Mukherjee estimates a maximum success target of 50 per cent in such projects.[39] He believes only 10 per cent of village families could easily be motivated to use latrines, with 15-20 per cent more families following once the example is set. Twenty per cent of the additional families would be difficult to motivate, but could probably be convinced to use latrines. Socio-economic status, literacy, influence of urban contact and age and sex are considered prime factors in this analysis.

In addition to these factors, social habits affect resistance to the use of latrines. For example, the widespread custom of promiscuous defecation results in a seeding of the soil with infective eggs and larvae of many parasites, while pollution of natural water bodies maintains such diseases as schistosomiasis. Some villagers disliked the idea of latrines because they felt them to be "unhygienic", harbouring bad odours, providing breeding places for flies and being difficult to clean. Villagers often feel constricted in an enclosed space and fearful that accidents will result should the pit collapse.[40] It is interesting to note that under 45 per cent of Mukherjee's sample made no connection between social barriers and *use* of latrines, although there was objection to use of the *same type* latrine for all. While 40 per cent of the sample were unaware that flies carried disease, 72 per cent broadly associated faeces and spread of gastro-intestinal infection. Despite the disadvantages cited by villagers, over 75 per cent said that they would use latrines if they were available at low cost. This seems to validate other observations that utility, convenience and availability play important parts in bringing new elements into village life.

The Land Use-disease Paradox—The Example of Scrub Typhus

Economic development must always be a consideration in disease occurrence. For example, scrub typhus is associated with the transformation of wasteland to usability. Maintenance of waste-lands by man is important in the creation of hyper-endemic foci. Subsequent use of wastelands to a great extent is responsible for the incidence of infections.[41]

There are four factors in this disease. The first is associated with a mite which exists on agricultural soil. When patches of cleared jungle are abandoned after temporary cultivation, the adult mite feeds on the juice of young grass leaves growing on abandoned areas. Secondly, the larval mite arrives *via* birds or rats who begin searching for food where man once lived. The larval mite then sucks the rickettsia from the rat's blood. Finally, man re-enters the scene and is bitten. Until man enters, a "silent zone of disease", as May called it, exists. When non-immune man enters and attempts to put the land to use again, the result is scrub typhus.[42]

Such cycles are characteristic of India. The current thorn-scrub vegetation of the Ganges-Jumna was once reportedly a dense forest. Scrub typhus was also experienced in Sumatra by the Goodyear Rubber Company after the 1923 slump in young rubber estates. When there is thorough cultivation of all available space, as is usually the case in high density population areas, few ecological niches remain for typhus.

Between the time of forest depletion and erosion, a situation occurs which breaks the countryside into a patchwork of vegetation units in various stages for cultivation. These conditions provide the ecological niches necessary for the dispersal and evolution of scrub typhus.[43] Control of this disease requires putting wastelands to use. This also requires termination of slash-and-burn agricultural techniques in order to prevent the development of grasslands which follow forest fires and interrupt the development of normal succession from scrub to secondary forest. This appears to be a paradoxical situation, since grass fires also temporarily dry the soil, making it unsuitable for the post-larval stages of the mite. Such situations complicate both effective public health control and land reclamation development programmes.

Conclusion

Unavailability of modern techniques is frequently responsible for survival of indigenous practices. To some extent these persist in order to maintain a state of equilibrium. Even if an individual is willing to give up old responses for new ones, a state of tension persists while old habits are being unlearned. During this interval, bebaviour can only be directed by bolding on to old, tested beliefs. It is during such a transitory state that Western public health measures must help ease anxiety by attempting to introduce change through already existing channels and with as much adherence as possible to the existing belief systems. Traditional behaviour toward officials in India has always been passive verbal acceptance followed by forgotten pledges. Thus, a "non-official" type of role behaviour should be established if change is to occur.[44] Obviously role behaviour serves important functions, but effective communication must recognise the cross-cultural variabilities of role relationships.

Misunderstandings result owing to false expectations on both sides of cross-cultural contact. As Carstairs learned, in order to be accepted as a practitioner he had to work within the prescribed physician's role for Rajasthani, and not London, society. Perhaps his most important lesson was an understanding that reassurance was of prime concern to the patient, for the practitioner speaks not only in terms of his skill in overt diagnosis and treatment, but with the authority of supernatural power.

Misunderstandings are also the result of differences in ideas about disease cause and cure. As certain diseases attributable to supernaturalism are controlled, it is believed that villagers will become less fearful of associated gods, and eventually this will result in a change in the belief system.[45] In the interim, for added security, villagers continue to use magico-religious techniques in order to propitiate causative agents, while simultaneously accepting certain modern medical treatments to ensure cure.

Misunderstandings, similarly, result because of planners' lack of awareness of varying cultural appraisals of resources. Perhaps this is the most long-lasting and difficult situation to alter. Blanket rules about land development without consideration of the numerous factors necessary to maintain regional unity may impinge upon the spatial distribution of certain diseases. In this connection, it has been suggested that there be a re-emphasis in considering problems of technological change and that in some respects rural areas "... are not so much underdeveloped as they are overdeveloped."[46] While this might be debatable, it appears that technological change not only adds a new dimension to existing landscape, but more often alters the already existing relationships between man and the environment by pressing techniques up to and beyond the point of an optimum utility. "In an overdeveloped area, too many techniques are too exhaustively applied to too many people and to too little land".[47]

Misunderstanding also results when there is lack of appreciation of existing conflicts within the village. This could lead to situations where expected results do not occur. Working through a village leader on one project might convince others to follow; while the same leader, because of caste membership, for example, will have no prestige power to convince followers in some other project. Not to be minimised is the individual's actions in terms of peer group reactions, for in tight-knit village India ostracism by the group is an expensive price to pay for attempting change. The breakdown of caste and family organisation is seemingly unpreventible with increasing outside contact. While it may be considered that such alteration could increase effective public health measures, it might be that an opposite effect would result because of the severity of inter-group factionalism.

Development projects in varying parts of the world are viewed largely as government drives rather than as movements of the people. In India, this results in a paradox: an expectation that the government should do things and a deep-seated scepticism when things are done.[48] This tends to round out the circle, for as noted at the outset, successful public health measures must be done with rather than for people.

Notes

1. W.H.O. *Expert Committee on Health Education of the Public,* pp. 4-6, Technical Report Series 89, 1st Report, Geneva, 1954.
2. May, J.M. (ed.) (1961), *Studies in Disease Ecology,* New York: V. Hafner.
3. Fonaroff, L.S. (1963), Malaria Geography: Problems and Potentials for the Profession, *Professional Geographer,* 15, 1-7.
4. Mukherjee, S. (1961), How to Popularise Latrines in Indian Villages, *Indian Journal of Public Health,* 5, 27-29.
5. Opler, M. (1963), Cultural Definitions of Illness in Village India, *Human Organization,* 22, 32-35.
6. Khare, R.S. (1963), Folk Medicine in a North Indian Village, *Human Organization,* 22, 36-40.
7. Opler, M. (1955), Foreword to Dube : *Indian Village,* IX, London: Routledge & Kegan Paul.
8. Dube, S.C. (1955), *Indian Village,* p. 35, London: Routledge & Kegan Paul.
9. *Ibid.,* p. 90.
10. Opler, M. (1963), *op. cit.,* p. 32.
11. Khare, R.S., *op. cit.,* p. 40.
12. Deutschmann, Z., The Ecology of Smallpox, p. 9 in J.M. May, *op. cit.*
13. *Ibid.*

14. Khare, R.S., *op. cit.*, p. 40.
15. Opler, M.E. and Singh, R.D. (1952), Economic, Political and Social Change in a Village of North-central India, *Human Organisation,* 11, 12.
16. Carstairs, G.M. (1955), Medicine and Faith in Rural Rajasthan, in *Health, Culture and Community* (Edited by Paul, B.D.), p. 112, New York: Russell Sage Foundation.
17. *Ibid.*
18. Loomis, C.P. (1960), Social Systems for Health, Chapter 6, in *Social Systems—Their Persistance and Change,* Princeton: D. Van Nostrand.
19. Mandelbaum, D.G. (1953), Planning and Social Change in India, *Human Organisation.* 12, 7.
20. Dhillon H.S. and Kar, S.P. (1963), Behavioural Science and Public Health, *Indian Journal of Public Health,* 7, 19-24.
21. Neurath, P.M. (1962), Radio Farm Forum as a Tool of Change in Indian Villages, *Economic Development and Culture Change,* 10, 279.
22. Blunt, Sir E. (1946), *Social Service in India: An Introduction to Some Social and Economic Problems of the Indian People,* p. 382, London.
23. U.S. International Cooperation Administration, Malaria Advisory Team, *Report on a Mission to India,* p. 129, January-April, 1957.
24. Sinton, J.A., What Malaria Costs India, *Record, Malaria Survey of India*, Vol. 5, 223-264 and 413-489, 1935-36, Vol. 6, pp. 91-169.
25. May, J.M., *op. cit.*, p. 215.
26. *Ibid.*
27. Learmonth, A.T.A. (1957), Some Contrasts in the Regional Geography of Malaria in India and Pakistan, *Transactions and Papers, Institute of British Geographers,* 23, 23-59.
28. May, J.M., *op. cit.* and Fonaroff, L.S., *op. cit.*
29. Marriott, McKim, Western Medicine in a Village in North India, in *Health, Culture and Community* (Edited by Paul, B.D.) *op. cit.*, p. 249.
30. Khare, R.S., *op. cit.*
31. Dube, S.C., *op., cit.*, p. 210.
32. Khare, R.S. (1964), A Study of Social Resistance to Sanitation Programmes in Rural India, *Eastern Anthropologist,* 17, 86-94.
33. Neurath, P.M., *op. cit.*
34. Khare, R.S. (1964), *op. cit.*
35. Keesel, J.F., *The Ecology of Filariasis*, pp. 54-66, in May, J.M. *op. cit.*
36. Raghawan, S. (1958), Climate and Filaria, *Bulletin of the National Society of India for Malaria and other Mosquito Borne Diseases,* 6, 143.
37. *Ibid.*, pp. 140-145.
38. Park, J.E. (1961), Human Factors in Rural Sanitation, *Indian Journal of Social Work,* 22, 196.
39. Mukherjee, S., *op. cit.*
40. Majumdar, N. (1961), Excreta Disposal in Rural India, *Indian Journal of Public Health.* 5, 32-34.
41. Audy, J.R., *The Ecology of Scrub Typhus*, p. 427, in May, J.M., *op. cit.*
42. May, J.M. (1950), Medical Geography : Its Methods and Objectives, *Geographical Review*, 40, 27.

43. Audy, J.R., *op. cit.*
44. Mandelbaum, D.G., *op. cit.*, p. 12.
45. Luchinsky, M.S. (1963), Problems of Culture Change in the Indian Village, *Human Organisation*, 22, 66.
46. Marriott, McKim (1952), Technological Change in Overdeveloped Rural Areas, *Economic Development and Culture Change*, 4, 261.
47. *Ibid.*, pp. 261-262.
48. Dube, S.C. (1958), *India's Changing Villages: Human Factors in Community Development*, p. 221, Ithaca: Cornell University Press.

17

Traditional Indian Medicine in Practice in an Indian Metropolitan City

A. Ramesh and *B. Hyma*

Introduction

Indigenous medical beliefs and practices have always been an integral part of many human cultures. A recent WHO Meeting on the Promotion and Development of Traditional Medicine observed that even though many health professionals and institutions often viewed traditional medicine "as a practice on the decline and of no importance" it is still important and has vitality.[1] Traditional systems of medicine continued to meet the health needs of most rural populations of the developing world and find patronage in urban areas as well.[2] WHO's recent Primary Health Care Strategy "Health for all by the year 2000" has recently attracted attention to the potential role traditional medicine can play and to revaluate its contributions.[3]

There are many reasons cited for the promotion and development of traditional medicine[4] : its approach is unique and holistic. It is culturally, socially and environmentally close to the people, that is, it is the people's own health care system and is accepted and utilized by them. It has a potential for wider application at low cost. It uses local resources (herbs, metals, minerals and so on), local technology and local labour. It is not dependent on alien technology, materials, expertise and knowledge. It is found particularly effective in dealing with many chronic ailments, allergic conditions, culturally linked

Reprinted from *Social Science and Medicine,* 15 D, 69-81, 1981.

psychosomatic diseases and illnesses. It is also recognized that the services of traditional healers and practitioners could be utilized with advantage at various levels of preventive and curative techniques in the health care programmes. It has the potential to contribute to scientific and universal medicine. Above all, WHO observes that "Its recognition, promotion and development would secure due respect for a people's culture and heritage".[5]

Research in traditional medicine has been heavily oriented towards medicinal plants. There is a need to investigate "the wider scope of traditional medicine as experienced in actual practice in the health care systems of various countries."[6]

Practitioners of traditional medicine represent a vast human resource outside the official health services.[7] It is well-known that many of the traditional medical practitioners of various categories (such as healers, herbalists, spiritualists, birth attendants or midwives) "have already undergone elaborate training in ancient systems of medicine that had evolved reliable methods of treatment and pattern of medications long before modern medicine came along. Other healers have had their skill handed down through generations—the distillation of a surprising degree of practical knowledge, skills and wisdom about the physical, mental and psychological ills of mankind".[8] Traditional medicine practitioners, both rural and urban, are of many grades and have various degrees of scientific knowledge, techniques and sophistication.

Collection and dissemination of information pertaining to traditional medicine is a complex task which is barely undertaken on a systematic scale. Scarcity of information and records about traditional medicine practitioners and their methods of practice is one of the major constraints in assessing their efficacy and formulating a definite policy by which they can be effectively integrated in national, state and regional health plans.[9]

To assess the effectiveness of traditional medicine in practice, this chapter concentrates its investigation in a metropolitan city of India where the traditional Indian medical systems continue to flourish. This study has restricted itself to examining the size, distribution and the current social, economic and political status and practice characteristics of traditional practitioners in the city of Madras, India.

A Note on the Traditional Medicine in India

In the history of medical systems in India, traditional medicine has not been static, but has continually evolved and progressed even in urban settings. In India there are two parallel systems of medicine, the modern system commonly referred to as allopathy and homoeopathy, and the Ayurvedic, Siddha and Unani system of medicine, commonly known as indigenous system. Naturopathy and Yoga also attract followers for their therapeutic values of the three indigenous systems of medicine, Ayurveda is used all-over the country.[10] Siddha is extensively used in the southern state of Tamil Nadu and in the neighbouring states.[11] The Unani system is used predominantly in areas of Muslim culture.[12]

On the basis of National Health Policy formulated in 1948, after the Independence of India, the Government is committed to promote and develop the indigenous system of medicine along with the modern medicine.[13] The Central Council of Research in Indian Medicine and Homoeopathy was constituted by the Government of India in 1969 with four sub-councils: (1) Ayurveda and Siddha, (2) Unani Medicine, (3) Homoeopathy, and (4) Yoga and Naturopathy.[14] This council has established minimum standards of qualification in Indian medicine and a curriculum for under-graduate and post-graduate education and training and the maintenance of a central register of practitioners.[15] It is observed by Charles Leslie that:

> The Ministries of Health in several states had Boards of Indigenous Medicine responsible for running government dispensaries, registering practitioners, and regulating school curricula. Companies with regional, and in some cases with national and international markets, manufactured Ayurvedic and Unani medicines which they advertised and distributed in a modern manner. National associations of practitioners sponsored conferences, published journals, and lobbied for legal privileges equivalent. to those of physicians trained in cosmopolitan medicine.[16]

The indigenous system of medicine is practised by a large number of hereditary medical practitioners and by persons trained in teaching institutions run by the State Governments and other approved bodies.[17] India now has a large number of qualified practitioners of integrated medicine and an estimated total of 7000-8000 professionally qualified practitioners of Ayurveda, Siddha, Unani and Homoeopathy are entering the profession every year.[18]

Carl E. Taylor has estimated that in India organized health services provide only 10 per cent of the medical care. Another 10 per cent is provided by qualified physicians in towns and cities. The balance is split between home medical care and indigenous practitioners."[19] Health coverage provided by IMPs (Indigenous Medical Practitioners—those who derive all or part of their livelihood as *Vaids*, practising Ayurvedic or Siddha System, as *Hakims*, practising the Unani system of medicine) needs to be intensively studied, seeking a detailed understanding of the IMPs' present contribution to urban as well as rural health services.

Though modern scientific medicine forms the basis for the development of the National Health Services in the country, ultimate objectives are to facilitate the integration and emergence of one system of medicine with its various sub-systems. Modern health care systems continue to expand and command people's respect, yet traditional systems are by no means on the decrease. However, it is still not very clear how the two approaches to medicine can be integrated or to what extent they can co-operate and interact.[20] In the search for effective ways either to integrate or develop these two systems, it becomes necessary to examine their competence and capacity, to serve and satisfy the basic health needs of the populations concerned and to be integrated into public health systems in primary health care.

Manpower development for training in traditional medicine is vast and complex, especially for a large country like India with its various systems of medicine practised in different regional and cultural settings. The inadequacy of our present understanding of indigenous medical processes at work at micro-level is quite obvious.[21] Collection of information, records, survey and assembly of factual data is far from complete at national, state or regional levels.

The Research Setting and Methods

This chapter is primarily concerned with some practical aspects of the persistence of traditional Indian medical practices (Ayurveda, Siddha and Unani) in the city of Madras, in the State of Tamil Nadu, India. This chapter investigates and presents a graphic outline of the services provided to the people by this parallel system of medicine. It considers the characteristics and the perspectives of the private registered practitioners within the system.

Madras is the fourth largest city in India with a population of nearly 3 million (1977 estimate), in which approximately 30 per cent live in 1200 slums and squatter settlements where the basic needs of these people are not fully satisfied. Madras is also one of the major centres of modern medicine in India, with its established medical schools, numerous hospitals (both private and public), nursing homes, clinics, dispensaries and medical practitioners (general and specialists, and so on). It is also one of the centres of traditional medicine where numerous Ayurvedic, Siddha, Unani and Homoeopatby practitioners, clinical and pharmacological research centres and other clinics and dispensaries (both private and public) are found scattered at various parts of the city.

These centres of traditional medicine, large and small, serve a significant majority of the city's population, and also draw a large number of patients seeking treatment from the immediate metropolitan region as well as from other parts of the State and out of the State. Unfortunately, very little published material has been available as to the number, distribution and growth or decline and socio-economic characteristics of practitioners of traditional system of medicine for this city. Very little is known about the way the two divergent approaches (modern medicine *vs.* indigenous medicine) to healing operate side by side in the same metropolitan setting. We seem to know even less about the reasons for the persistence of indigenous medical practices in the most expanding urban cultures, or about the structural accommodation which must be made in the urban environment with the advent of modern medical establishments and practices, and the people's health needs and behavioural responses to such rapid changes in the health care systems. Even though overall trends may appear to be moving towards adoption of modern scientific therapy in urban areas, general observations indicate that Indian systems of herbal medicine and practitioners are in no way diminishing in size in serving some of the basic health needs of the people in the city.

The chapter presents some discussion of the issues in the light of data and information obtained from the results of field questionnaires administered to private registered indigenous medical practitioners in the city of Madras over a period of 2 months in the summer of 1979. The results of the systematic interviews of practitioners are tabulated. The questionnaire evaluates the distribution, competence, capacity and effectiveness of these three systems in serving and satisfying the basic health needs of the city's population.

The following analysis is primarily concerned with the actual distribution and social characteristics of indigenous medical practitioners rather than the theoretical or developmental ideals. It offers a preliminary and tentative assessment and a few generalizations of our descriptive data and information drawn from a sample of 95 practitioners of a total estimated 957 registered practitioners of Indian indigenous medicine in the city. It was observed that there is no (official) complete record of registered practitioners of Indian medicine. Therefore, an attempt was made to compile two lists of registered Indian medicine practitioners from the following two major sources as suggested by the Director of Indian Medicine for the State, viz.:

(1) Office of the Registrar of Board of Integrated Indian Medicine.[22]
(2) The Indian Medical Practitioners' Co-operative Pharmacy and Stores Ltd. (known as IMPCOPS).[23]

Selection of Samples for the Study of the Spatial Aspects of the Socio-economic Characteristics of IMPs in Madras City

In the initial stage, all the 957 registered IMPs were located on a city map of Madras on the basis of addresses by postal service zones (Fig. 17.1). A spatial variation of the distribution of IMPs in Madras city was observed. A 10 per cent sample was drawn from a total of 957 estimated IMPs. Again a 10 per cent sample out of the total for each postal zone was drawn, in order to cover the entire city. Thus, a two-stage stratified random sampling method was adopted in order to conduct the detailed survey.

However, care was taken not to omit any postal service zone by choosing at least one practitioner, if the zone registers less than 10.

Spatial Distribution of IMPs in Madras City—A General Observation

A heavy concentration (more than 50 per cent of the total IMPs) has occurred in the old residential highly populated areas of the city followed by significant numbers clustered in the old commercial and

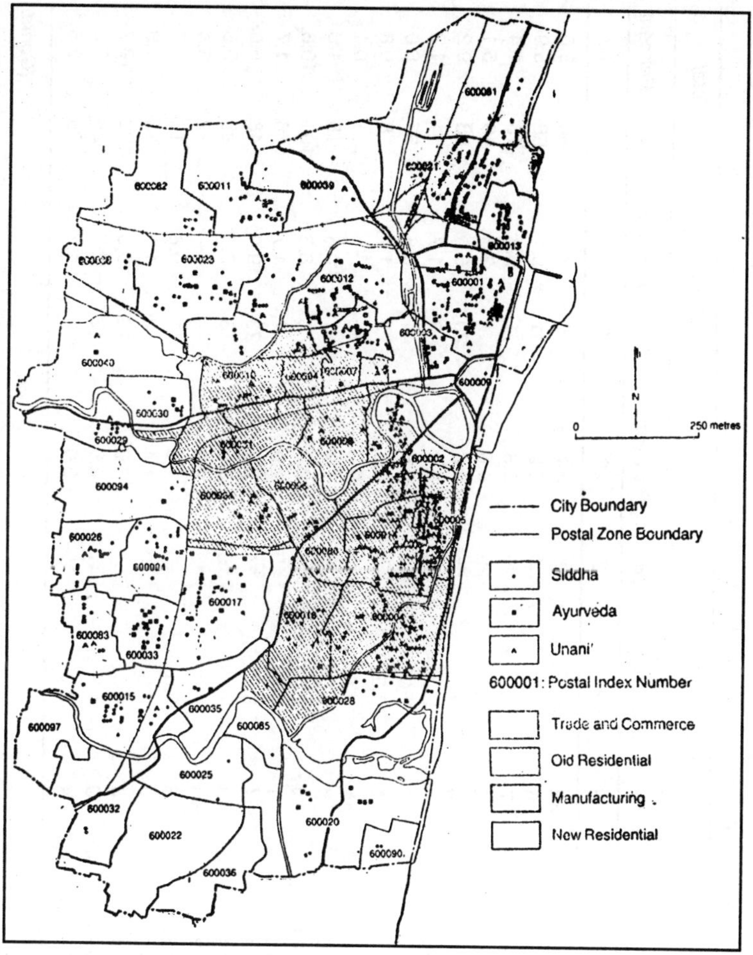

Fig. 17.1: Distribution of Practitioners in Traditional Medicine: Madras City

manufacturing sectors in the northern part of the city (Fig. 17.1). In the newly developed residential neighbourhoods (Anna Nagar, Ashok Nagar, Besant Nagar, Guindy, and Velacheri) their numbers are very low, below 0.1 per cent indicating a distinct spatial pattern of concentration in the diffusion of IMPs in Madras city (Table 17.1).

With regard to the three indigenous systems of medicine (*viz.*, Siddha, Ayurveda and Unani), it is observed that Siddha practitioners, numbering 635 out of a total of 956 IMPs, dominate the spatial pattern

Table 17.1: Practitioners of Indian Medicine, Madras City (Registered as of 1978)

Postal Zones (within Madras City limits)	*Pin code*	*Ayurveda*		*Siddha*		*Unani*		*Total*	
		No.	*Per cent*	*No.*	*Per cent*	*No.*	*Per cent*	*No.*	*Per cent*
1	*2*	*3*	*4*	*5*	*6*	*7*	*8*	*9*	*10*
George Town	600001	22	11.0	55	8.7	9	7.4	86	9.0
Mount Road	2	6	3.0	39	6.2	11	9.1	56	5.9
Park Town	3	7	3.5	5	0.8	1	0.8	13	1.4
Mylapore	4	16	8.0	29	4.6	4	3.3	49	5.1
Triplicane	5	13	6.5	55	8.6	20	16.5	88	9.2
Greams Road	6	4	2.0	5	0.8	2	1.7	11	1.2
Vepery	7	14	7.0	42	6.6	1	0.8	57	6.0
Egmore	8	1	0.5	5	0.8	2	1.7	8	0.8
Fort St. George	9	—	—	1	0.2	—	—	1	0.1
Kilpauk	10	6	3.0	8	1.3	1	0.8	15	1.6
Perambur	11 & 12	15	7.5	18	12.2	8	6.6	101	10.6
Royapuram	13	1	0.5	13	2.0	2	1.7	16	1.7
Royapettah	14	11	5.5	14	2.2	23	19.0	48	5.0
Saidapet	15	3	1.5	19	3.0	3	2.5	25	2.6
T. Nagar	17	14	7.0	18	2.8	—	—	32	3.4
Teynampet	18	5	2.5	10	1.6	1	0.8	16	1.7
Adayar	20	7	3.5	9	1.4	2	1.7	18	1.9
Washermanpet	21	9	4.5	81	12.6	12	9.9	102	10.7
Ayanavaram	23	9	4.5	17	2.6	3	2.5	29	3.0
Kodambakkam	24	4	2.0	19	3.0	2	1.7	25	2.6

(Contd.)

Table 17.1 (*Contd.*)

1	*2*	*3*	*4*	*5*	*6*	*7*	*8*	*9*	*10*
Kotturpuram	25	1	0.5	2	0.3	—	—	3	0.3
Vadapalani	26	1	0.5	11	1.7	2	1.7	14	1.5
Raja Annamalaipuram	28	3	1.5	8	1.3	1	0.8	12	1.3
Aminjikarai	29	3	1.5	11	1.7	1	0.8	15	1.6
Shenoy Nagar	30	2	1.0	7	1.1	—	—	9	0.9
Chetput	31	2	1.0	3	0.5	—	—	5	0.5
Guindy	32	1	0.5	1	0.2	—	—	2	0.2
West Mambalam	33	9	4.5	14	2.2	1	0.8	24	2.5
Nungambakkam	34	5	2.5	6	0.9	—	—	11	1.2
Nandanam	35	1	0.5	3	0.5	—	—	4	0.4
I.I.T.	36	—	—	2	0.3	—	—	2	0.2
I.C.F. Colony	38	—	—	4	0.6	—	—	4	0.4
Vyasarpadi	39	—	—	7	1.1	3	2.5	10	1.1
Annanagar	40	1	0.5	—		1	0.8	2	0.2
Tirvanmaiyur	41	—	—	1	1.2	—	—	1	0.1
Tondiarpet	81	—	—	14	2.2	2	1.7	16	1.7
Jawahar Nagar	82	1	0.5	9	1.4	1	0.8	11	1.2
Ashok Nagar	83	2	1.0	5	0.8	2	1.7	9	0.9
Flowers Road	84	1	0.5	1	0.2	—	—	2	0.2
Kottur	85	—	—	2	0.3	—	—	2	0.2
Besant Nagar	90	—	—	1	0.2	—	—	1	0.1
Golpalpuram	86	—	—	1	0.2	—	—	1	0.1
Total		**200**	**100.0**	**635**	**100.9**	**121**	**100.1**	**956**	**100.3**

Compiled from: IMPCOPS, Madras, 1979.
For location of postal zones, refer Fig. 17.1.

in Madras city (Table 17.1). This is again reflected in the very high concentration of Siddha IMPs in old residential areas. The Ayurveda practitioners (200) do not exhibit any definite pattern with regard to their spatial distribution. However, small concentrations are found in some old parts of the city. The Unani practitioners are concentrated in the same areas as *Siddha vaidyas*.

An Analysis of the Questionnaire Survey

In order to analyse in detail the spatial phenomena with regard to the IMPs in Madras, the sample practitioners (private and registered), 95 in all were interviewed by a detailed questionnaire. A total of 35 questions relating to the following 10 major socio-economic and practice characteristics were asked:

(1) System of practice;
(2) Practitioner's personal dimensions;
(3) Training background;
(4) Practice;
(5) Characteristic features of the patients seen;
(6) Diagnostic methods;
(7) Prescription of medicine;
(8) Procurement of medicine;
(9) Specialization; and
(10) Attitude and opinion.

The questionnaire contains a set of selected variables to describe the structure and characteristics of practice in this system. The interviews were conducted mostly in the Tamil language and where necessary in English by two of our graduate students. On an average, each interview took about an hour or so. In most cases no appointments were necessary to see the practitioners. The participation was voluntary. Most of them were pleased to respond to our questionnaire survey. They said it was the first of its kind they encountered and co-operated as much as they could.

System of Practice

Though there are three major types, Ayurveda, Siddha, and Unani, still a number of practitioners practised integrated medicine.[24] The survey showed that 36.4 per cent of the IMPs belong to Siddha system, followed by Ayurveda (36.4%), Unani (10.4%) and Integrated (20%) which clearly indicates the importance of Siddha and Ayutveda systems in meeting the basic health care needs.

Practitioner's Personal Dimensions

In order to clearly understand the structure, quality and function of a particular medical system, it is necessary to analyse the social characteristics of the practitioners such as sex, age, religion, language, general educational level, birthplace, father's occupation, and so on.

Practitioner's personal dimension shows some interesting characteristics. The bulk of them were male members. Only a handful of them were females in all the three systems. These few female practitioners are found to practice mainly integrated medicine specializing in gynaecology and obstetrics. It is interesting to note that practitioners of ancient Ayurveda and Siddha were traditionally males. It is reported, however, that a few females are now being trained in Ayurveda, Siddha and Unani Colleges. Unani medicine seems to be the domain of males.

Two-thirds of the practitioners interviewed were found in the age group between 40 and 60. It is interesting to note they were equally divided into the 40-50 and 50-60 age groups. The low figure in the age group between 20-40, clearly indicated that fewer practitioners have entered the profession in recent years in the city. It may be partly due to the closure in 1967 of the well-known institution of Indian Medicine which had offered L.I.M. (Licence of Indigenous Integrated Medicine) degrees, in Madras city since 1928.

Though most of the IMPs belonged to the Hindu religious community, a small proportion of them were Muslims. There were only two Christians who practised Indian medicine in our sample. Further, it can be pointed out that a fifth of the Muslims practised Siddha and Ayurveda systems rather than Unani which is favoured by Muslim culture.

About a third of the practitioners had college education. Thirty persons indicated that they had diplomas/certificates and practised Siddha or Ayurvedic medicine but received no formal education. The rest of the practitioners had 8-11 years of school education.

More than 50 per cent of the IMPs were born and brought up in Madras city itself, but of these the bulk of them practised Siddha medicine. About 16 per cent of the practitioners had rural background and another 10 per cent who came from outside the State of Tamil Nadu. It is interesting to note that most of the practitioners who came from outside the State are engaged in Ayurvedic practice, indicating that a strong base for Ayurveda exists outside the State of Tamil Nadu.

Nearly half of the practitioners interviewed entered the profession because of its tradition within the family. It was also observed that a small proportion (15%) of the practitioners have indicated that some of their relatives also practice Indian indigenous medicine.

Training Background of the Practitioners

About 34 per cent of the practitioners had their formal training (L.I.M. degree) from the former Government College of Indigenous Medicine, Kilpauk, Madras.[25] An equal number of people had their professional training outside the State of Tamil Nadu. A few others had some training either from the Venkataramana Ayurvedic College (private) or Siddha Institute (private) run by a well-known Siddha practitioner in the city who offered apprenticeship training and certificate for low income level groups under his guidance. Now, a state-run college of indigenous medicine at Palayamkottai in the Tirunelveli district in the south (established in 1968) has begun to produce a number of qualified Siddha practitioners.

The formal training from the former Kilpauk College in the city had helped a number of the practitioners in the city to engage successfully either in Siddha or Ayurveda or Unani with an integrated basis as L.I.Ms. and G.C.I.Ms. All the people interviewed were R.I.M.Ps. (Registered Practitioners of Indian Medicine). More than 50 per cent interviewed registered themselves between 1960-1978, which clearly indicates a growing interest in indigenous medicine. Overall, it can be said that great variations still exist in the training and standards of practice of Indian medical practitioners. The majority in practice seem to have had no formal schooling in indigenous medicine but one of apprenticeship to be an established practitioner. The duration of training is not uniform. About 41 per cent had 4-5 years of training in indigenous medicine. The duration of the apprenticeship varied generally from 3-5 years in most cases. It was also observed that most of the IMPs (more than 80%) were engaged in full-time practice. A very small proportion were found to be part-time and reported some other occupations such as tailors, potters, chartered accountants and other miscellaneous categories.

Practice

A small percentage of (10%) practitioners worked in more than two clinics in the city. It is also observed that most of the practitioners had not changed their location of practice since their registration, indicating either the stability of their practice or lack of other alternatives.

The location choice seems to be either older populated residential areas or economically viable areas. However, a quarter of the practitioners had their clinics in areas where they acquired them through hereditary practices. In general, the location choice exhibited a definite pattern. The high class and upper middle class neighbourhoods did not seem to attract the IMPs. Further, the middle income group were concentrated mainly in the residential areas in the old congested parts of the city. This is, however, not to say that the elites had no access to this health care system. Their case of mobility made it possible for them to select practitioners, clinics and dispensaries offering indigenous medicine.

More than 75 per cent of the practitioners worked like any modern medical practitioner in the city. About 50 per cent of them said that they take either one day or half day off a week and rarely any regular long vacations as such. It is hard to conclude as to whether they are too busy or have to work full-time to survive.

With regard to the number of patients seen, it was observed that about 50 per cent of the practitioners received about 5-20 patients per day. Only 10 per cent reported a high range between 20-40 patients per day. We suspect that some of these figures may be exaggerated by some of the IMPs. Casual checks with neighbours in the localities concerned somewhat confirmed this suspicion.

The general procedure (in contrast with modern medical practices) is to spend 10-20 minutes (25% of the practitioners) or 20-40 minutes (35%) per patient per day. In other words, this norm confirmed previous findings that "the more traditional and indigenous medical practitioner was in his approach to diagnosis and treatment, the more likely he was to spend more than 10 minutes with a given patient".[26]

Places of Practice—Some Characteristics

We were able to get a few details of the place of practice through our field investigators and by personal observations. These are summarized below:

Many of the practitioners with smaller practices lived in modest homes and some owned their own places. Few make home visits. Fewer than 10 of the most prominent men and women in the sample owned large homes, had a telephone and a car; and employed a nurse or other attendants. It was not possible to obtain an accurate or estimated figure of their annual income. Most of the IMPs were reluctant to report accurate earnings. About 50 per cent of those interviewed said they have at least one or more assistants. These assistants were found to be mostly males.

The Siddha practitioners largely catered to the low-middle income and low-income groups. The elites and upper middle class largely favoured Ayurveda. The Unani practitioners attracted mainly the Muslim population of the city. Some doctors in Ayurveda, Siddha and Unani seemed to have thriving excellent practices and command an immense reputation and popularity among the city's population. Others seem to have practices moderate to low in size.

Most of the practitioners run their clinics or dispensaries in their own homes. The clinics of these private practitioners varied considerably in their appearance. Most of them were small one-room places of simple appearance. They were sparsely furnished usually with a wooden table and two chairs, a long bench for patients to wait outside on the verandah. Most of them had a signboard (doctor's name and so on) on the main or easily accessible side street. Pictures of various Hindu deities were hung on the wall in a few clinics. Only two Siddha Vaidyas displayed signs of pictures of devils with horns outside their clinics on the road side. Women from low income groups seem to favour such clinics.

Some practitioners exhibited a framed diploma or certificate or their father's pictures. Very few instruments were kept except for an occasional stethoscope and a thermometer. Very few had wash basins. In some rooms medicine bottles were kept in open shelves. In others, they were neatly arranged in (glass of wooden) wall cupboards. Few had store rooms with stock of medicine. Very few clinics displayed any books, journals or magazines of Indian medicine. Many of the clinics were found to be badly maintained with poor ventilation, indicating either lack of taste, interest, indifference or financial inability of the practitioners in improving their set-up.

Characteristics of Patients

With regard to age or sex, there seems to be no definite pattern. Data from interviews with patients of practitioners, showed that 50 per cent of those interviewed were in the age group 20-50. A large number of housewives, and men in government services were met. A sizeable group of middle class people also attended the dispensaries run by these practitioners. At least 20 per cent of the patients said they had college education and 50 per cent of them have had no formal schooling. Most of the patients were drawn from within the city and from the immediate neighbourhood of practitioner's place of practice.

Most of the practitioners settled their fees with the patients at the time of each visit. A few of the patients received treatment on credit. Though most of the practitioners said that they do not collect money from the economically poorer sections of the community, the minimum charge for consultation ranged, between ₹ 2 to ₹ 5 per patient. 30 per cent of the patients interviewed said that it cost them less than ₹ 2 per visit. This indicated that the practitioners charge for their service on the ability of their clients to pay rather than conforming to fixed consultation fees. Most of the patients appeared statisfied with their practitioners and said they are warm and friendly and placed their confidence in them.

Diagnostic Methods

Few of the IMPs exhibited modern medical instruments such as stethoscopes, thermometers, blood pressure apparatus, syringes and needles. These were mainly used by those who practised integrated medicine. These practitioners also occasionally sent their patients for laboratory tests for blood, stools, urine and X-rays. About 30 per cent said they performed minor surgery like stitching, incising or dressing wounds, etc. A quarter would not treat any cases relating to minor surgery.

Most of the IMPs use physical examination such as viewing the patient's body (darsanam in Sanskrit), touching (sparsanam) and eliciting information by questioning (prasanam). It appeared that nearly 50 per cent of the practitioners use pulse rates, 32 per cent diagnose by eye examination and 25 per cent by examination of hair and ears. However, pathological methods of diagnosis seem to still play a less important role in their method of practice.

Prescription of Medicine

Less than 15 per cent of the practitioners said they prescribe Indian medicine as well as allopathy medicine. Nearly two-third of them said they prescribe only indigenous medicine. There were no responses from the rest. The prescription of medicine seems to be influenced to some extent by the hereditary formulae for preparing local herbs, powders, minerals, etc. and by local cultural knowledge and concepts related to the prevalent diseases in the area. Many methods and techniques employed are closely guarded secrets.

Procurement of Medicine

The medical resources of IMPs include a complex and wide variety of local herbs and minerals. Most said they obtained their supply from the local co-operative outlet, IMPCOPS. Few get their supply from other established popular outlets of private dispensaries of Ayurvedic, Siddha and Unani medicine in the city.[27] About a third said that they bought medicine from outlets operating outside the city. Further, it was found that only about a third prepared their own medicine out of raw-materials purchased from local and regional sources.

Specialization

There were some clear indications of the kinds of cases which the practitioners preferred to treat. However, 25 per cent of them would not treat any cases relating to the surgical side. Most of the practitioners were of the view that all types of diseases could be treated by indigenous medicine.

In the most commonly treated diseases noted in our survey, ailments like coughs, diarrhoea, dysentery, fever, indigestion, etc. have been given primary importance (by 80% of the practitioners) followed by skin disorders (45% of the IMPs treated these), ulcer (50%), nervous disorders (42%), rheumatism (24% and lung and bronchial ailments (24%). About 5-6 per cent of the practitioners claimed that they can treat specific cases like anaemia, arthritis, colics, cellulitis, dermatitis, diabetes, jaundice, obesity, rheumatism, sexual disorders, menstrual disorders, mental diseases, children's diseases, infertility, impotence etc.

There appears to be little formal specialization, in contrast with modern medicine. A handful of practitioners, however, claimed that they have developed special formulae in treating specific ailments like rheumatism, arthritis, children's diseases, skin diseases, etc. About 5 per cent claimed that they practised witchcraft and black magic. However, there are no clear records of potent medicines and their effects on patients. No written records nor files were maintained by the practitioners. Those few who did maintain some records were reluctant to produce them. So valuable information on types of diseases treated and the associated medicaments used is often lacking or unavailable to assess the efficacy of treatment.

Most of the doctors exhibited no interest in conducting clinical research in this method of practice.[28] However, by observing from long-term experience with their patients, some monitored the success of their particular medicine in treating specific ailments. Since only about 3 per cent of the practitioners said that they conduct research (mostly on pharmacological aspects) our conclusion on the lack of research activities in this field of medicine by private practitioners is fully justified.

About 60 per cent of the practitioners indicated that they do not have an affiliation with any of the professional organisations of Indian medicine in the city or outside the city. There seems to be little interaction between the individual private practitioners though many seem to know the existence of each other. However, an informal referral system does operate to some extent, especially between specialists of indigenous medicine. For example, about 25 per cent, mostly in Ayurvedic practice, said that they have some collaboration with others in the treatment of special disease. Reciprocal relationships among the private practitioners, and the local hospitals, and health care centres and clinics were almost non-existent.

Attitude and Opinion

Most of the practitioners seemed to have no definite opinion with regard to competition that exists between the various medical practices. Further, most of them (70%) indicated that they have no objections to their patients seeking other forms of medicine. Many would not make any specific recommendation and left it to the patient's choice. This analysis indicated that each system has a strong in-built structure of its own from the point of view of the patients as well. This is again reflected in the full satisfaction in their work (90%) and as well as their (80%) indication to continue in this profession.

Most of the practitioners were reluctant to give concrete suggestions with regard to the role played by the Government for supporting Indian medicine. Only 11 per cent responded with some comments such as "Government creates Siddha dispensaries by buildings and subsequently everything is closed because of want of doctors and poor planning" and "State Government is not helping the private practitioners" and "Tax incentives, job opportunities in public health services, etc., can be created."

The Concluding Discussion

This survey was carried out with an aim of ascertaining some of the strengths and weaknesses of traditional medical practices in an urban setting. Only a mixed assessment of practices can be presented at this stage.

The indigenous medical systems still remain a significant contributor to medical care of the people not only in rural areas but also in the cities. They seem to have survived in their present independent form, with each system retaining its own special features.[29] From our survey it is not possible to identify definitely or clearly whether a particular branch (Ayurveda, Siddha or Unani) of this system is able more effectively to meet the health needs of the population. All three seem to provide fairly satisfactory solutions for common local ailments. However, observations indicate that in Madras city, Ayurvedic institutions and clinics in general continue to enjoy more public support than Siddha and Unani. The proportion of the total urban population receiving Ayurvedic care has steadily increased as evidenced by an increase in the sale of its popular products as well as expansion of some of its dispensaries.

Constraints seen in the development of traditional medicine are discussed below.

Lack of standardised training and qualification of the practitioners is still evident, even though a large number are entering the profession every year. All grades and levels of training, with different knowledge, skills and sophistication of practice exist in the city. Most of the practitioners operate in isolation and their bargaining power is weak.

This may be partly due to their inability or failure to form effective associations or societies or to belong to those few in existence so as to improve the quality of their services as well as to protect their interests. The WHO recommends that the process of "encouraging the traditional medicine practitioners to form clubs or societies", can and "as a means of checking harmful practices eliminating quacks arid charlatans, assuring continuous informal education, cultural loyalty, and the conservation of high level of professional ethics and practice".[30]

Adoption of modern scientific and technical methods of practices is very incomplete. Even the lack of precision in diagnostic methods was observed. Techniques for preparation and preserving medical remedies are not standardized nor inspected closely. Absence of toxicological and pharmacodynamic analysis is noted except for those conducted on a small scale in a handful of government and private research clinics and laboratories.

There is no doubt that Indian medicine provides curative care of considerable significance to a wide range of urban population. Dunn pointed out that although a preventive perspective is strongly advanced in the classical Ayurvedic literature up to the present day, curative medicine seems to dominate the practices both from the point of view of practitioners giving and the patients receiving treatment.[31]

In this context, it would be useful to point out WHO's recent recommendation that as "In Mexico, priority is given to operational work which is oriented towards the validation or invalidation of popular medical (research) knowledge with the aid of scientific research. This approach permits close collaboration with the traditional healers themselves and to the community in general".[32] Removal of many of the obstacles in the development of indigenous medicine can also be achieved through public education by means of local journals, newspapers, seminars, conferences and through the use of mass media. Our field observations showed that just a beginning has been made in this direction. It is recognized that there is a great need for a multidisciplinary approach to the study of this system of medicine. Work teams should consist of anthropologists, botanists, chemists, geographers, pharmacologists, sociologists and the practitioners themselves—currently these professionals function in isolation.

Some other issues which remain unsolved can also be identified from our field research survey of the city of Madras.

The general register of all traditional practitioners is far from complete. A recent licensing campaign for registration has not met with much success. Low responses from the practitioners are evident and no strong action has been taken by the authorities to remedy the situation. Lack of specific field tests to evaluate their competence for legal recognition is also noticed. There is no indication of a census questionnaire to include traditional medical practitioners as a separate professional group.

Comprehensive information on the number of available manpower resources in the various types and categories of practitioners, their location, distribution, mobility patterns, and socio-economic characteristics is very important for planning and training programmes, if they are to be fully integrated into the overall health system.

Only lip service seems to have been paid to promoting the process of integration. Collaboration and co-operation between the two parallel systems has hardly begun. The WHO observes that training and re-training are necessary on both sides which will not only improve the status of IMPs among the health team members, but will help in "acquainting professional health personnel and students of modern medicine with the principles of traditional medicine in order to promote dialogue, communication and mutual understanding and eventual integration".[33]

Strengths of traditional medical practices based upon the materials gathered from this survey can also be pointed out.

In the informal sector of the city, many of the IMPs seem much more secure and confident and continue to offer a useful public service in the city. Though not all IMPs may be suited for integration into modern health care organizations, certainly a sizeable number may be eligible for incorporation.[34] Even where there is competition from modern practitioners in the same community, these IMPs are able to maintain stable practices and enjoy social prestige if not great economic prosperity.

A number of favourable factors support them: they charge less for their services; they are located in centres where effective demand for their service still exists; they provide many dietary prescriptions which are expected by people of Indian culture when they are ill.

All indications are that indigenous medical systems will probably continue to provide services as long as the central and state governments continue to sponsor the indigenous systems officially, and promote medical relief, education and training, and clinical and pharmacological research. At present indigenous medical services freely cut across all socio-economic groups as well as rural and urban areas. However, they still continue to occupy an insignificant position under the programmes for health planning in the states. The recent change in WHO policy orientation and consideration may also strengthen and protect the interests of indigenous medical systems.

From a survey of this kind, we can begin to learn much that will help us to propose and design a better health care network for both the rural and urban areas using all the alternatives available. Initially, a clear understanding of locally available medical practices is necessary before we even begin to start making suggestion and policy guidelines.

The possibility of bringing Indian medical practitioners into the national/regional/local health care programmes need to be continually evaluated especially in view of the shortages of trained health personnel to provide services for the development of rural as well as urban health care systems. For example, the Central and the State Governments in India, allocate funds to open up new clinics and dispensaries for IM, but they soon find themselves with no proper mechanisms for planning or co-ordination of activities for recruiting trained doctors and staff for this purpose. In some instances, the new buildings had to be closed or operated at a financial loss. The allocated finance often goes to waste for lack of manpower. Still there are many practitioners with little business as our sample survey indicates. Many of these people have no proper knowledge or easy access to information regarding various governmental programmes related to re-training and research.

Strong governmental commitment, support and planning for this system are still lacking. State aid to institution, dispensaries and private practitioners still remains a minor part of total health expenditures. The status of many of the private practitioners remain economically backward compared to allopathic doctors. Male domination to some extent may limit direct female access to health care in this system.

It seems to us that the first and foremost problem to which we must address ourselves is to see how we can make IM rapidly self-reliant and fully efficient; how to upgrade the quality of services provided by the private practitioners of this system; how to give them due recognition as respected members of the society; and how effectively to facilitate their participation and integration in national health care programmes.

The practical and survival value of Indian medical practitioners is certainly high. Thus given proper understanding, publicity and financial support, traditional systems of medicine can play a vital role in a country's health care delivery programmes, i.e. the capacity of health care can be considerably increased by the use of doctors trained in indigenous medicine. Understanding the complementarity of functions between the modern and the traditional medicine also awaits further exploration and research in the Indian urban setting.

This brings us to a final question as to whether one should advance the development of a dual health care system from which patients can select modern or traditional health services or an integrated system, where it is certain that traditional systems would occupy a subordinate role and lose their individual cultural heritage characteristics. This policy-implementation decision continues to pose a dilemma to many governments of developing nations.[35]

It is hoped that the findings of our preliminary investigation even in one Indian urban setting, will provide some guide for further understanding of the extent, durability and continuity of services provided by the Indian medical system and its contribution to the overall health care systems in operation.

Acknowledgements

We would like to express our deep appreciation and gratitude to four well-known, outstanding and highly respected practitioners of this profession, Dr. Kondal Rao, Dr. Ananda Kumar, Dr. B. Vaidyanathan and Dr. Neelavathy, without whose support, guidance and willingness to share their experience and knowledge as well as their excellent recommendation letter for this survey, we would not be able to gain easy access to IMPs in Madras city.

Special thanks to Dr. Kondal Rao who helped us in all stages of our research including the preparation of the draft of this paper with his critical comments. Deep appreciation goes to two graduate students, Sucharita and Sandhya, of Madras University, for conducting the field survey in a record period of 2 months; and to Dr. N. Sivagnanam, Department of Geography, Madras University, for generously assisting us in organizing and analysing our data.

Notes

1. World Health Organisation, The Promotion and Development of Traditional Medicine : Report of a WHO Meeting, Technical Report Series 622, 9, 1978.
2. Kurup, P.N.V. (1977), The Science of Life (Ayurveda), *Wld. Hlth.*, November, 12.
3. WHO, The Alma-Ata Conference on Primary Health Care, *WHO Chron.*, 32, 409, 1978.
4. Mahler, H. (1977), The Staff of Aesculapius, *Wld. Hlth.*, November 3, Kurup, *op. cit.*, (2), p. 15; WHO, *op. cit.*, (1), p. 13.
5. WHO, *op. cit.*, (1), p. 13.
6. *Ibid.*, p. 10; Bannerman, R.H. (1977), WHO's Programme in Traditional Medicine, *WHO Chron* . 31, 427.
7. Kurup, *op. cit.*, (2), p. 12; WHO, *op. cit.*, (1), p. 37.
8. Mahler, *op. cit.*, (4), p. 1.
9. WHO, *op. cit.*, (1), p. 37.
10. Ayurveda is the traditional Hindu system of medicine based on Vedic scriptures; it utilizes herbs, minerals and diet restriction in treatment of illnesses. Literature available on Ayurveda was found to be compiled some time during the fifth century B.C. Kurup, *op. cit.*, p. 15; Zimmerman, F. From classic texts to learned practices: methodological remarks on the study of Indian medicine. *Soc. Sci. Med.*, 12B, 97, 1978; Jaggi, O.P. *Indian System of Medicine. History of Science and Technology in India Series,* Vol. 4. Atma Ram, Delhi, 1976; Srinivasamurthy, G. *The Science and Art of Indian Medicine,* Theosophical Publishing, Madras, 1948.
11. Siddha systems of medicine in Tamil Nadu, an explanatory note: This system is considered as an independent entity. Its antiquity is well recognized. The exact period of its origin is not known (some claim that it existed before Vedic period). The therapeutics of Siddha medicine consist mainly of the use of metals and minerals, whereas in the earlier Ayurvedic texts, there is no mention of metals. It has, however, many similarities with Ayurvedic medicine. It uses also products of vegetable and animal origins. There were 18 Siddhas who were basically responsible for many branches of knowledge and their works were written in Tamil. There are at least about 500 works written and 3000 formulae. Initially, they were recorded on palm leaves. Many examples of palm leaf literature are still being transcribed and printed in Tamil. The exact figure of *Siddha Vaidyas* (practitioners) is not known. However, they are known to exist in thousands in the State of Tamil Nadu. For further reference, refer Ramamurthy, Iyer T.G. (1933), *The Gems of Siddha System.* Sri Vinas Press, Fort Erode, India, and Narayanaswamy, V. *Introduction to the Siddha System of Medicine,* Pandit S.S. Anandam (1975), Madras: Research Institute of Siddha Medicine, India.
12. The Unani system, also known as the Greek/Arab system of medicine, brought into India by the Muslim conquerors, has also been in use for

several hundred years. It uses herbs, minerals and metallic salts. Sanyal, P.K. (1964), *A Story of Medicine and Pharmacy in India.* Shri Amitara Sanyal, Calcutta; Bradenburg, D. (1977), The Unani Medicine: Traditional Therapeutics in India (German), *Medsche Mschr,* 31, 29.

13. National Health Policy objectives include provisions for the setting up of standardized education and training in all the Ayurvedic institutions and facilities for research, and training on scientific lines to absorb the practitioners of Ayurveda and Unani medicine into the State Health Organization, Keswani, N.H. (1969), Modern Medicine in Traditional Setting. In *Medicine and Culture* (Edited by Poynter, F.N.L.), p. 189. London: Wellcome Institute of the History of Medicine.
14. Through these four councils the Central Government is gradually or rather slowly promoting education and training (through established colleges or institutions or courses affiliated with the existing universities) in all the medical systems, clinical and pharmacological research (through support of private and public bodies and by establishing central and regional institutes of Indian medicine in the states) and establishment of special wings for Indian Medicine in new hospitals and starting new dispensaries. Cultivation of herbs in systematic fashion is also proposed under India's Sixth Five- Year Plan Programmes. See the Central Council for Research in Indian Medicine and Homoeopathy. Annual Report 1976-1977. Ministry of Health and Family Welfare, Government of India, New Delhi, 1978; Editorial. Ayurveda and Unani : massive support for research promised. *Herb. Cure (Hyderabad)* 3, 1, 1979.
15. Djukanovic, V. and Mach, E.P. (Eds.) (1975), *Alternative Approaches to Meeting Basic Health Needs in Developing Countries,* Geneva: UNICEF/ WHO Study.
16. Leslie, C. (1976), The Ambiguities of Medical Revivalism in Modern India, in *Asian Medical Systems: A Comparative Study* (Edited by Leslie C.), pp. 363-364, Berkeley: University of California Press.
17. Kondal Rao, Y. (1977), Drugs of Indigenous Origin and National Health Service, NIMA (*J. Natn. Integr. Med., Ass. India*) 19, 233.
18. WHO estimates that "There are about 5,00,000 practitioners of indigenous medicine in India, and their qualifications range from University doctorates, through certificates awarded in private schools, to skills and knowledge acquired after several years of apprenticeship to established practitioners. There are 108 colleges of indigenous medicine...." WHO, *op. cit.,* (1), p. 12; Kurup, *op. cit.,* pp. 14-15.
19. Taylor Carl E., The place of Indigenous Medical Practitioners in the Modernization of Health Services, In *Asian Medical Systems, op. cit.,* p. 286.
20. Djukanovic and Mach, *op. cit.,* p. 89, A full integrated type of training would adopt the essential principles of both indigenous system of medicine and modern medicine.
21. A few scattered case studies in India have been presented in the 1970s. Refer to : Alexander, C.A. and Shivaswamy, M.K. (1971), Traditional Healers in a Region of Mysore, *Soc. Sci. Med.* 5, 595; Bhardwaj, S.M.

(1975), Attitude Towards Different Systems of Medicine: A Survey of Four Villages in Punjab, India. *Soc. Sci. Med.* 9, 603; Bhatia, J.C., *et al.*, (1971), The Role of Indigenous Medical Practitioners in Two Areas of India, *Soc. Sci. Med.*, 5, 137; Bhatia, J.C., *et al.* (1975), Traditional Healers and Modern Medicine *Soc. Sci. Med.*, 9, 15; Chuttani, C.S., *et al.* (1973), A Survey of Indigenous Medical Practitioners in the Rural Areas of Five Different States of India, *Ind. J. Med. Res.*, 61, 6; Montgomery, E., Systems and the Medical Practitioners of a Tamil Town, in *Asian Medical Systems, op. cit.*

22. We discovered to our disappointment that this office could not provide us with an updated and completed list of practitioners. Our investigators were able to compile a rough list from raw information sheets furnished by this office. A total of only about 300 addresses could be obtained.
23. IMPCOPS—Indian Medical Practitioners' Co-operative Pharmacy and Society Ltd. This centre has been organized by the practitioners of Indian medicine by contributing to share capital. It has been in existence since 1944. From about 500 members, it has grown to have a strength of 8000 members with most of them coming from within the State of Tamil Nadu. The list of registered members provided us with addresses of members to about 957 in the city of Madras.

    IMPCOPS manufactures Ayurvedic, Siddha and Unani medicine numbering about 750 popular formulations. It has been recognized as an authorized supplier of Indian medicine by the Governments of Tamil Nadu and Andhra Pradesh. The profit motive is kept very low and its major objective is to supply quality medicines at a very reasonable costs. Large scale manufacture also ensures intensive and scrupulous measures to safeguard against adulteration, profiteering and peddling of spurious materials. IMPCOPS' aim is to place the IMPs as respected members of society and help them to continue to serve the people. It strives to supply pure, high quality drugs and medicinal concentrates. The preparation is carried out under expert supervision and in a hygienic environment. IMPCOPS is an institution in which all members are involved as producers, sellers and distributors and research workers. From IMPCOPS, *The Growth of IMPCOPS*, p. 5, Madras, 1978.
24. Integrated Medicine refers to students of indigenous medicine in well organized institutions who undergo training and practice in basics of modern medicine including surgical, obstetrical and medical legal work. The practitioners use modern drugs as well as indigenous medicine, and use modern diagnostic methods in their practice.
25. The Legal basis for the practice of Indian medicine: provision for the registration of medical practitioners of Madras dates from enactment of the Madras Medical Registration Act in 1914. The Act established a provincial medical council to register physicians and regulate their practice. Only degree and diploma holders from certain institutions were eligible for registration. "In 1933, the Madras Government issued rules to register practitioners of indigenous medicine. In the following years pressure

groups lobbied to change the rules to extend or further limit the legal status of physicians other than those trained in modern schools and to distinguish various grades of practitioners of IM. The rules changed back and forth, and the administrative interpretation and enforcement of them varied from year to year" (Edward Montgomery, 1976, pp. 276-277). However, in India, now each state has a Board of Registration for IMPs. In the state of Tamil Nadu, under the Act XXVII of 1956, two major categories (L.I.M., G.C.I.M.) and two classes, A and B of registration were, recognized. Under rules of registration of practitioners of Indian medicine issued in the year 1933, they include titles, R.I.M.P. and B.I.M.

Among the four major categories, changes continue to occur. For example, L.I.M. degree (Licence of Indian Medicine) was offered only between 1928 and 1967. Charles Leslie observed that "a prominent school in Madras offered programmes in Ayurveda, Siddha and Unani medicine. The school incorporated modern knowledge in curricula, offering basic science courses and clinical instruction in diagnostic teachniques and therapeutics of cosmopolitan medicine" (Leslie, 1976, p. 363). The capacity of the school was limited on an average to enrolling 120 students in Ayurveda classes, 15-20 students in Siddha and 5-6 in Unani medicine. The State Government closed this institution in 1967, for various reasons. Instead it opened a new Government College of Indian Medicine in a place called Palayamkottai in Tirunelveli district outside Madras city. This college is affiliated to Madurai University in the State. This college has offered B.I.M. (Bachelor of Indian Medicine) since 1968. It gives instructions in all the three systems; however a heavy bias towards instructions in Siddha medicine is reported. From 1978, this college was upgraded to offer post-graduate courses leading to M.D. (Master of Indian Medicine).

L.I.M., B.I.M. and G.C.I.M. (General Certificate in Indian Medicine) denote institutionally qualified practitioners based on years of training obtained in Tamil Nadu. On the other hand, R.I.M.P. denotes those traditional practitioners who have produced satisfactory evidence that they have been practising for 10 years or more, or for those who have obtained a certificate or diploma given by authorized Indian medical practitioners of IM under whose guidance they have undergone informal apprenticeship or training for a duration varying from 3 to 5 years.

It has been a common and accepted practice for some to acquire their professional training and skill through their forefathers or working as apprentices under hereditary practitioners. However, this picture is changing with the new regulations regarding registration and licensing and with the appearance of new institutions of learning and new curriculum development in the universities.

There are no Unani colleges as such in this State. There are two private Ayurvedic institutions in the State; the one in Madras city was started in 1905 and it has a college with a limited capacity of 12 students or so, and it offers instructions in Sanskrit only. It is affiliated with the University of Madras (from 1926) and this college was upgraded to give a degree in

"Bachelor of Ayurvedic Medicine and Surgery" (B.A.M.S.) from 1979-80 academic year.

Besides these, two classes of practitioners are maintained by the Registrar of Central Board of Indian Medicine in Madras city. *Class A* practitioners are those whose qualifications denote at least a minimum standard of professional training for undertaking medical, surgical (including obstetrics) and medico-legal work. *Class B* practitioners are those whose qualifications denote at least a minimum standard of professional training for undertaking medical work only.

26. Bhatia, *op. cit.,* (21), p. 146.
27. In the city, there are several popular pharmacies and dispensaries which sell Indian medicine directly to the public. Prescriptions are not needed for many of the popular remedies.
28. In the city, there are about four research centres of Indian medicine; two are sponsored by the Central Government; and two are seen as private institutes.
29. WHO, *op. cit.,* (1), p. 39.
30. *Ibid.,* p, 32.
31. Dunn, F.L. Traditional Asian Medicine and Cosmopolitan Medicine as Adaptive Systems, in *Asian Medical Systems, op. cit.*
32. WHO, *op. cit.,* (1), p. 29.
33. Bannerman, *op. cit.,* pp. 427-428.
34. Awasthi, P.N. (1977), Integrated Medicine under Janata Rule, *NIMA*, 19, 233.
35. Birchman, W. (1979), Primary Health Care and Traditional Medicine—considering the Background of Changing Health care Concepts in Africa *Soc. Sci. Med.,* 13B, 175; Dunlop, D.W. (1975), Alternatives to "Modern" Health Delivery Systems in Africa: Public Policy Issues of Traditional Health System, *Soc. Sci. Med.,* 9, 581.

18

Attitude Towards Different Systems of Medicine

A Survey of Four Villages in Punjab

Surinder M. Bhardwaj

Introduction

The role of indigenous systems of medicine is of considerable interest in India, not only because of its nationalistic overtones, but also because of the extreme shortage of medical manpower. The establishment of the Central Council of Indian Medicine in 1971 underscores this interest.[1] The community of scholars who participated in the Burg-Wartenstein Symposium have generated many fresh ideas on the study of Asian medical systems including those of India.[2] Taylor *et al.*, have suggested that in "theoretical analysis of social change, especially in the shift to modernity, medicine may be a more important index than has been realized".[3] In light of this, it seems useful to find out the attitudes of rural people towards indigenous and modern medicine.

This chapter reports and examines some findings related to the preferences of the rural people for indigenous and modern physicians and systems of medicine in four selected villages in Punjab and suggests certain conditions under which indigenous medicine may be preferred to modern by choice rather than by tradition.[4]

McKim Marriott in his study of a north Indian village several years ago asserted that the patronage of indigenous medicine surpasses

Reprinted from *Social Science and Medicine,* 9, 603-612, 1975.

that of Western medicine one hundredfold.[5] Oscar Lewis' observation on the concept of disease causation and cure in an Indian village near Delhi struck the same note. He made a general conclusion that the villagers prefer to resort to indigenous remedies.[6] Similarly, Fonaroff and Fonaroff pointed out that even where facilities are available people do not always use them due to persistent cultural habits and beliefs about disease causation and treatment.[7] More recently, Neumann *et al.*, on the basis of the Johns Hopkins University Rural Health Research Functional Analysis Study, pointed out that the government health services are utilized by only 10-20 per cent of rural people.[8]

While it is true that indigenous physicians still attract large numbers of rural people, evidence from some parts of India suggests that blanket generalizations about rural India as a whole need to be made with increasing caution. There are several reasons for this cautionary note. First, many extrapolations about rural India as a whole have been made on the basis of individual village studies. Secondly, there has been a tendency in the past to somewhat overemphasize the traditional elements of India with the result that attitudinal changes of the rural people toward modern medicine are not clearly appreciated. Thirdly, little attempt has been made to identify the conditions under which either an indigenous or a Western mode of cure is sought by the rural people. Finally, it could be erroneously assumed that indigenous medicine practitioners necessarily practice indigenous medicine.[9] In fact, as Leslie points out, a good deal of what is taught in indigenous medical institutions is borrowed from modern medicine.[10]

Assumptions of some scholars such as Fonaroff[7] mask the fact that attitudes toward a given system of cure may not be so much dependent upon tradition as on the expectancy of cure. Since a given individual could follow a "traditional" approach under one set of circumstances and take a "modern" course under others, there is the need to understand why rural people prefer indigenous systems of medicine on some occasions and the modern one under different conditions. T.N. Madan's seminal study showed that while the decision to choose a given system is dependent on many variables, effectiveness is the principle reason.[11] Madan also concluded that rural or urban origin of people had no significant bearing on their choice for the Western system of medicine.

Scope of Study

This study attempted to find out the type of medical practitioners and the system of medicine preferred by a sample of rural heads-of-households in four selected villages in Ropar District, Punjab. No claim is made that the results of the study have general validity for India as a whole.

Systems of Medicine in Punjab

Several "systems" of medicine are practised in Punjab, as in fact in India as a whole. They can be broadly grouped into the modern or "allopathic" system, and traditional or indigenous systems.

Practitioners of the allopathic (*angrezi*) system are called doctors. They practice modern Western system of medicine, but their competence varies widely. Most such physicians in rural Punjab are often poorly trained, except the ones that are appointed by the government in rural dispensaries or health centres. The indigenous (*desi*) medical systems fall into two chief types: the ancient *ayurveda* system of Hindu medicine and the *unani* (Ionian, Greek) system that came to India through Arabic-Islamic tradition.[12] In rural Punjab little distinction is made between these two systems although the practitioners of ayurveda are usually called the *vaidya* and those of unani as the *hakim.* Homoeopathy, a system of German origin, although popular in eastern India and represented by a few physicians in the urban areas of Punjab, is not popular in rural Punjab.[13]

Method of Study

Selection of Villages

In order to analyse the types of physicians and medicines preferred in rural areas, a survey of four specifically selected villages in Ropar District (Punjab) was carried out during summer, 1973. Three of the four villages were selected such that each had different type of medical practitioners; one with both allopathic and indigenous physicians, the second with only an *ayurvedic vaidya* and a third one with only a *unani hakim,* The fourth village was selected in which no physician existed at all. This selection by no means encompassed the entire spectrum of medical health facilities in the rural areas, but it provided the needed contrast for this study. The assumption underlying this selection was that where indigenous type physicians exist, people will more likely use indigenous rather than modern allopathic medicines. Thus, the following four villages were selected: Chamkaur Sahib, Rolu Majra, Lutheri and Chetamla (see Fig. 18.1. Map of the study area). Chamkaur Sahib has a Primary Health Centre (P.H.C.) with both indoor facilities for patients and outdoor dispensing of

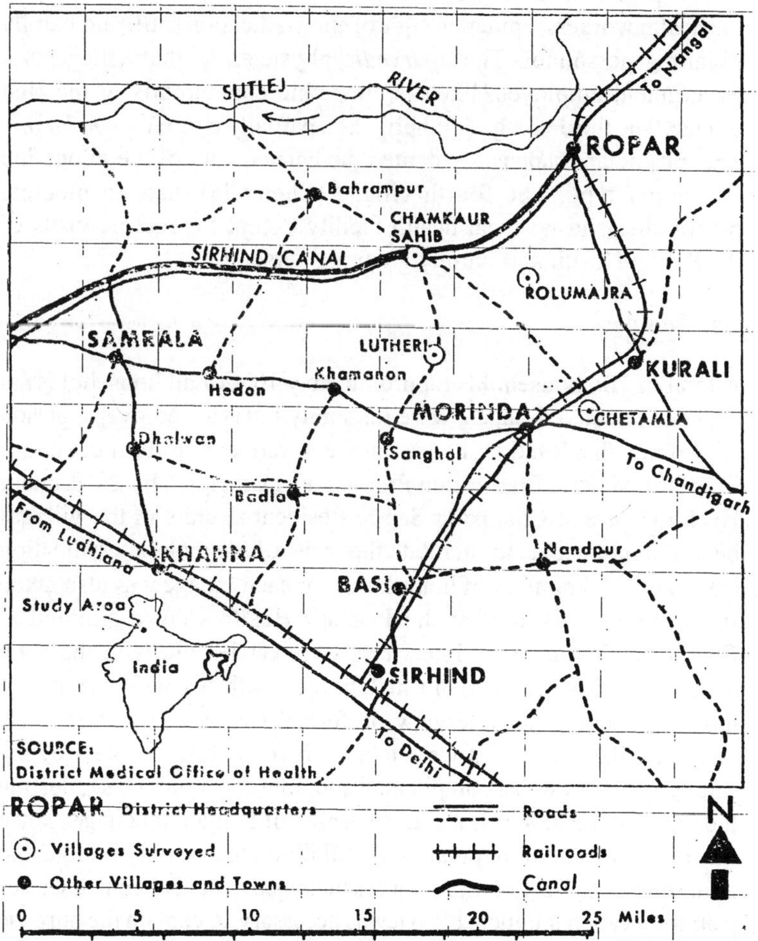

Fig. 18.1: Study Area.

medicines. The P.R.C. is staffed with two doctors both holding a degree in Medicine and Surgery. The Primary Health Centre provides basic preventive and curative services and has a Family Planning Unit. There are also two drug stores within the village, and two practising indigenous physicians. Thus, this village had what may in the context of rural Punjab be termed a "broad range" of medical and health facilities. Rolu Majra, the second village, has an *ayurvedic* dispensary. It has no other medical facilities except routine visits by the health workers, epidemic control and eradication staff, and Family Planning personnel. The *ayurvedic* physician in that village is a government employee, like his allopathic counterparts in the first village. The third village (Lutheri) has a partially trained *unani hakim.* This physician dispenses patented medicines, both of the allopathic and *unani* type. The fourth village (Chetamla), had no medical practitioner and no local health facility except for routine visits of the Public Health and Family Planning personnel.

The Sample

A total of 104 households (approximately 10% of all households) in the four selected villages, were randomly interviewed over a period of two months. Random house numbers were drawn from the house list of the Malaria Eradication Programme maintained by the Primary Health Centre at Chamkaur Sahib. Residential units in the villages bear a number so as to facilitate the visits of the malaria eradication staff. The total number of households for each village was also taken from the records kept at the Primary Health Centre situated at Chamkaur (Table 18.1). Interviews were carried out with the male head of the household or in his absence with his wife, widow or mother. Although an interview proforma was used, separate notes regarding the interviews were taken where necessary. Interviewing rural population was a complicated and time consuming task, despite the fact that the author is a native speaker of Punjabi language. Since the majority of adult population is still illiterate or barely literate and a substantial number of interviewees belonged to the Scheduled Castes (formerly called untouchables) it was necessary, to explain the purpose of survey at length in most cases. Lengthy, informal interviews were also carried out with the local physicians.

Table 18.1: General Data

Selected village	*Total number of households**	*Number of households interviewed*	*Per cent Households interviewed*
1. Chamkaur Sahib	620	48	7.4
2. Rolu Majra	156	19	12.2
3. Lutheri	150	20	13.3
4. Chetamla	129	17	14.7
Total	**1055**	**104**	**11.9**

* Unpublished data for 1973, courtesy of the medical officer in charge of the Primary Health Centre at Chamkaur Sahib, District Ropar (Punjab).

Data Analysis

The data derived from the household interviews were first cross-tabulated (Tables 18.2-18.9) in order to determine whether the type of physician and the type of medicine preferred by people significantly differ among: (a) the four villages, (b) the three main caste groups, (c) seven occupational groups, and (d) six categories of educational levels. In addition it was considered desirable (as will become clear in the sequel to explore whether the levels of education, and occupations significantly differ between caste groups and the four villages. These data are tabulated in Tables 18.10-18.12.

χ^2 was computed for each of the eleven above mentioned tables. It was necessary to collapse each table for χ^2 computation in order to meet the statistical requirements of this method. The results of these computations are listed under each table. Table 18.13 lists these results together for easy reference.

In addition to the above analysis, the places where the respondents purchased their medicines were identified by the frequency of their mention. Several respondents indicated more than one place where they usually purchased medicines. These data are mapped (Fig. 18.2) to bring out the need of rural. people to purchase medicines often from places other than their own village.

Preferred Type of Physician

Table 18.2 summarizes the response to the question: "If the need for the medicine arises in your household, who do you first go to ?" The question assumes that there is a "Threshold" for the "need" of

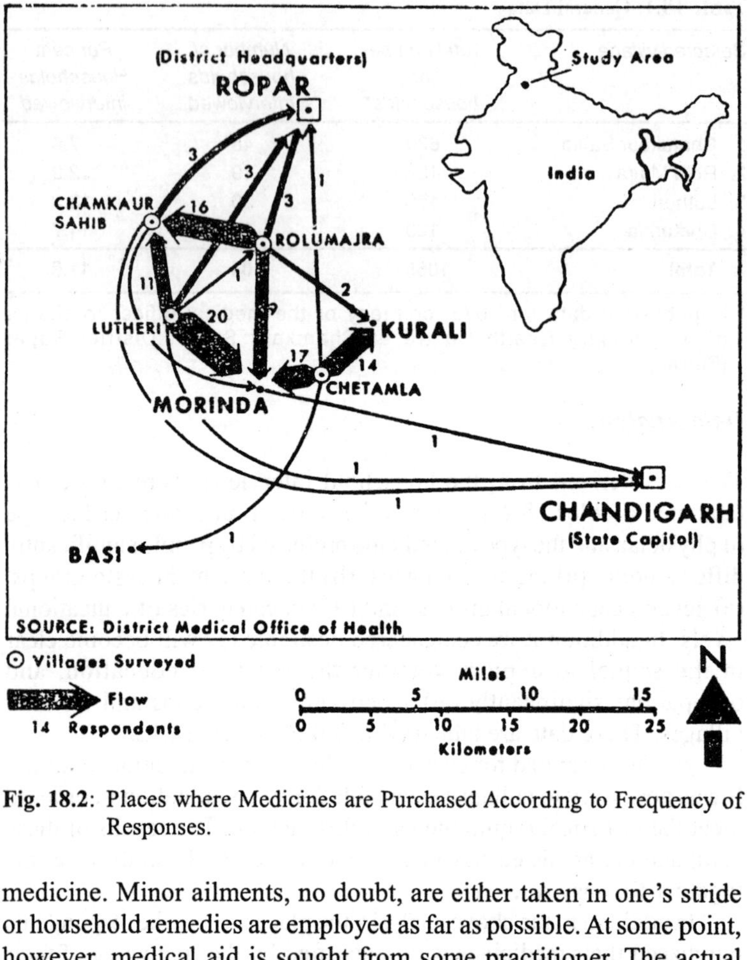

Fig. 18.2: Places where Medicines are Purchased According to Frequency of Responses.

medicine. Minor ailments, no doubt, are either taken in one's stride or household remedies are employed as far as possible. At some point, however, medical aid is sought from some practitioner. The actual choice to seek aid from an allopath, a *vaidya* or a *hakim* may depend upon a variety of factors such as the acuteness of a malady, accessibility to medical facility (both in terms of distance, time, as well as expenditure) chronicity of the disease, the status of a given member in the household, social relations with a physician, and the awareness about alternate facilities. From Table 18.2 the following observations may be made:

(1) The four villages studied are significantly disparate in their preference for the type of physicians: $\chi^2_{15}=38.848<0.005$.

Table 18.2: Type of Physician preferred by Village

Villages	*Number of households*	*Physician Preferred*				
		Vaidya	*Unani Hakim*	*Allopathi*	*Other*	*More than one*
Chamkaur Sahib	48	1	1	28	0	18
Rolu Majra	19	3	0	2	0	14
Lutheri	20	0	0	19	0	1
Chetamla	17	1	0	11	1	4
Total	**104**	**5**	**1**	**60**	**1**	**37**

$\chi = 38.848$. *d.f.* = 15, $P = 0.00105$. Contingency coefficient = 0.521.
Note: Table was collapsed before computing χ^2.
Source: Data collected by author, 1973.

(2) *Exclusive* patronage of a *vaidya* or *hakim* was very limited, whether or not such a physician was present in the village. Only 6 out of all the 104 households interviewed exclusively preferred an indigenous type of physician. None indicated exclusive preference for homoeopathic physician, even though homoeopathic is practised in many towns in the Punjab.

(3) Although allopathic doctors were exclusively preferred by more people than any other single type, over a third of the households had no specific preference for a particular type of medical practitioner: Even where a broad range of allopathic facilities are available (Chamkaur Sahib) about 37 per cent of the households indicated no exclusive inclination toward one type of physician. It seems that the expectancy of cure may be more important to people than the kind of physician.

(4) In the village (Rolu Majra) which has only an *ayurvedic* physician, only 3 out of 19 households showed a clear preference for such a type. A majority of households in that village indicated that they would visit different types of physicians depending on the disease. Since there is no other type of physician within the village, these villagers are compelled to seek medical aid at other places (See also Fig.18. 2.)

(5) The people of Lutheri village, which has a *unani* physician, overwhelmingly preferred an allopathic physician. This

resulted from the fact that even though the medical practitioner is theoretically *unani hakim,* most of the medicines he dispenses are of allopathic type. Thus, the people consider this physician to be an allopathic doctor irrespective of his formal (if partial) training in indigenous medicine. In addition, this village is only fifteen minutes bus-ride away from the government Public Health Centre at Chamkaur Sahib where allopathic doctors are available.

(6) Finally, the village in which no physician is available (Chetamla), the sample showed that people prefer to seek an allopath outside of their village. The map showing places where medicines are purchased (Fig. 18.2) emphasizes this fact.

It is clear then that given the need for professional medical aid, it is the "modern" doctor who is commonly preferred by the rural people although exclusive commitment to particular kind of physicians cannot be established. Our data do show that indigenous type of physicians command very limited *exclusive* patronage of patients.

Preferred Type of Medicine

In rural Punjab, as previously indicated, the term *desi* (literally "indigenous") normally includes both the *ayurvedic* and *unani* drugs, whether patented or generic. The *desi* medicines may be either bought under patented names or obtained from general merchants as household remedies. The term *angrezi* medicine connotes western (allopathic) drugs which bear modern anglicized nomenclature. The *angrezi* medicine is usually purchased under various patented names except in government dispensaries where mostly generic drugs are dispensed.

Table 18.3 summarizes the results of the question; "What type of medicine do you prefer?" On the basis of this question following additional observations can be made:

(1) The four villages show significant differences in terms of the type of medicine preferred; $\chi^2_{12} = 40.062 < 0.0005$.

(2) It is noteworthy that exclusive preference for *desi* medicines is extremely limited while preference for homoeopathy, is conspicuous by its absence. Thus, either *angrezi* medicine

alone or else a plurality of medicine types are preferred. Once again, the expected efficacy of the medicine rather than the system behind that medicine seemed to be of crucial importance to people. It appears to be no coincidence then that indigenous medical practitioners in the rural areas often store and sell several types of medicine, *desi,* as well as *angrezi.* This was true in the case of the indigenous physician at village Lutheri.

Table 18.3: Type of Medicine Preferred by Village

Village	*Number of households*	*Medicine Preferred*		
		Desi	*Angrezi*	*More than one*
Chamkaur Sahib	48	3	32	13
Rolu Majra	19	1	1	17
Lutheri	20	0	17	3
Chetamla	17	2	14	1
Total	**104**	**6**	**64**	**34**

$\chi^2 = 40.062$. *d.f.* =12 $P = 0.00020$. Contingency Coefficient = 0.527.
Note: Table was collapsed before computing χ^2.
Source: Data collected by author, 1973.

(3) Where both *desi* and *angrezi* medicines are equaily available (Chamkaur Sahib) most people tended to prefer the latter, but a significant number showed no particular commitment.
(4) Where only *desi* medicine was available in the villages (Chetamla) people generally go to the nearest place where *angrezi* rather than *desi* medicine is available (See also Fig. 18.2).

Social Characteristics and Physician/Medicine Preference

Three social characteristics of the rural population (caste, occupation and level of education) were examined for their possible bearing on the preference for physicians and medicines. The data are summarized in Table 18.4 through Table 18.9. In no case was the χ^2 value significant even at 0.05 level of confidence. This result indicates that the preference for types of physicians and medicines insignificantly dependent on these three major social characteristics of the population studied. Thus, the landowning castes who are also relatively wealthy,

Table 18.4: Type of Physician Preferred by Castes

Caste	*Number of households*	*Physician preferred*				
		Vaidya	*Unani Hakim*	*Allopath*	*Other*	*More than one*
Scheduled Castes (untouchables)	40	2	1	21	0	16
Jats (landowning)	35	2	0	22	0	11
Others	29	1	0	17	1	10
Total	**104**	**5**	**1**	**60**	**1**	**37**

$\chi^2 = 5.113$. *d.f.* = 10. *P* = 0.88327. Contingency Coefficient = 0.216.
Note: Table was collapsed before computing χ^2.
Source: Data collected by author, 1973.

and untouchables who are often abjectly poor almost equally preferred allopathic physicians and medicine. Conversely, the poor untouchables seemed no more prone to prefer indigenous physicians than the relatively wealthier *Jats* or other higher caste group. While inferences for India, obviously, are not intended from these limited data, we may at least suggest the fairly wide acceptability of modern medicine in the villages that were surveyed. When it comes to curative medicine in general, rural people are perhaps not as conservative as might be supposed basing one's judgement on the acceptability of Family Planning programmes. If anything, our data suggest the pragmatism of the rural population, irrespective of the social stratum to which they belong.

Discussion

This survey indicated that exclusive patronage of indigenous medicine and its practitioners is very limited and that people either prefer modern medicine or tend to keep their options open for a variety of available treatment. This study complements some of the observations made by T.N. Madan[11] in his study carried out in an urban setting. Expectancy of cure rather than the system of medicine seems implicit in the expressed preferences.

It was hoped that the expressed preferences about the type of physicians and medicine will be dependent on some of the major social characteristics of the rural population such as caste (Tables 18.4

and 18.5) occupation (Tables 18.6 and 18.7) and level of education (Tables 18.8 and 18.9). Since data about the income of rural people are extremely difficult to obtain and since occupation and caste are highly interdependent χ^2_{12}=94.736<0.001) it was hoped that the landowning (wealthier) caste group would show a different preference pattern than the poor untouchable. No such relationship however emerged in this study. The level of education is also highly caste dependent (χ^2_{10}=35.306<0.001, Table 18.10) and yet the preferences

Table 18.5: Type of Medicine Preferred by Caste

Caste	*Number of Households*	*Medicine Preferred*		
		Desi	*Angrezi*	*More than one*
Scheduled Castes (untouchables)	40	3	23	14
Jats (landowning)	35	1	22	12
Others	29	2	19	8
Total	**104**	**6**	**64**	**34**

χ^2 = 1.300. *d.f.* = 8. *P*=0.99456. Contingency Coefficient = 0.111.
Note: Table was collapsed before computing χ^2.
Source: Data collected by author, 1973.

Table 18.6: Type of Physician Preferred by Occupation

Occupation	*Number of households*	*Physician Preferred*				
		Vaidya	*Unani Hakim*	*Allopath*	*Other*	*More than one*
Farming	34	2	0	22	0	10
Agricultural Labour and Daily Labour	23	0	1	11	0	11
Handicraft	10	1	0	5	0	4
Trade-commerce	19	0	0	12	0	7
Transportation	4	0	0	0	0	2
Government and Professional Service	16	2	0	10	1	3
Total	**106**	**5**	**1**	**60**	**1**	**37**

χ^2 = 20.849. *d.f.* = 30. *P* = 0.89031. Contingency Coefficient = 0.409.
Note: Table was collapsed before computing χ^2.
Source: Data collected by author, 1973.

Table 18.7: Type of Medicine Preferred by Occupation

Occupation	*Number of Households*	*Medicine Preferred*		
		Desi	*Angrezi*	*More than one*
Farming	34	1	22	11
Agricultural Labour and Daily Labour	23	1	13	9
Handicraft	10	0	3	7
Trade—Commerce	19	1	14	4
Transportation	2	0	0	2
Government and Professional Service	16	3	12	1
Total	**104**	**6**	**64**	**34**

$\chi^2 = 21.380$. *d.f.* = 24. *P*= 0.61626. Contingency Coefficient = 0.413.
Note: Table was collapsed before computing χ^2.
Source: Data collected by author, 1973.

Table 18.8: Type of Physician Preferred by Level of Education

Level of education	*Number of Households*	*Physician Preferred*				
		Vaidya	*Unani Hakim*	*Allopath*	*Other*	*More than one*
Not literate	54	2	1	29	0	22
Primary school	17	1	0	11	0	5
Middle school	11	0	0	5	1	5
High school	12	0	0	8	0	4
College	9	2	0	6	0	1
Other	1	0	0	1	0	0
Total	**104**	**5**	**1**	**60**	**1**	**37**

$\chi^2 = 20.347$. *d.f.* = 25. *P* = 0.72760. Contingency Coefficient = 0.405.
Note: Table was collapsed before computing χ^2.
Source: Data collected by author, 1973.

were not apparently dependent upon level of education. Similarly, even though the villages are significantly disparate in their level of education (χ^2_{15}=26.506<0.05, Table 18.11) this is an insignificant determinant of preferences. These results suggest that other social dimensions need to be explored than those studied here. The implication that expectancy of cure may be important in preferences needs further research.

Table 18.9: Type of Medicine Preferred by Level of Education

Level of education	*Number of Households*	*Medicine Preferred*		
		Desi	*Angrezi*	*More than one*
Not Literate	54	4	32	18
Primary School	17	0	9	8
Middle School	11	I	8	2
High School	12	0	9	3
College	9	1	5	3
Other	I	0	1	0
Total	**104**	**6**	**64**	**34**

$\chi^2 = 6.091$. *d.f.* = 20. *P*=0.99836. Contingency Coefficient = 0.235.
Note: Table was collapsed before computing χ^2.
Source: Data collected by author, 1973.

Table 18.10: Level of Education by Caste Groups

Caste	*Number of House-holds*	*Level of Education*					
		Not Literate	*Primary*	*Middle School*	*High School*	*College and above*	*Other*
Scheduled Castes (untouchables)	40	31	4	3	2	0	0
Jats (landowning)	35	15	7	2	3	8	0
Others	29	8	6	6	7	1	1
Total	**104**	**54**	**17**	**11**	**12**	**9**	**1**

$\chi^2 = 35.306$. *d.f.* = 10. *P* = 0.00027. Contingency Coefficient = 0.503.
Note: Table was collapsed before computing χ^2.
Source: Data collected by author, 1973.

It is evident from Figure 18.2 that people of the three study villages (Rolu Majra, Lutheri and Chetamla) normally purchase medicines at places other than their own village. Where no medical facility or drug store exists (Chetamla) there is of course no choice but to make trips to places where needed drugs are available. But even in the villages where an *Ayurvedic* or *Unani* physician exists (Rolu Majra, Lutheri), the range of medicines available is small and thus the villagers have to procure drugs from outside sources. It may be noted that very few people of Chamkaur Sahib purchase medicines

Table 18.11: Level of Education by Villages

Village	*Number of House-holds*	*Level of Education*					
		Not Literate	*Primary*	*Middle School*	*High School*	*College and above*	*Other*
Chamkaur Sahib	48	20	9	7	10	1	1
Rolu Majra	19	11	4	1	0	3	0
Lutheri	20	12	2	0	1	5	0
Chetamla	17	11	2	3	1	0	0
Total	**104**	**54**	**17**	**11**	**12**	**9**	**1**

$\chi^2 = 26.506$. *d.f.* = 15. $P = 0.03440$. Contingency Coefficient = 0.451.
Note: Table was collapsed before computing χ^2.
Source: Data collected by author, 1973.

outside of their own village because of the existence of local drug stores; in fact many people from other villages buy the necessary medicines in this village. Further research is called for to determine: (a) the degree to which existing drug stores meet the needs of people in different villages; and (b) the cost and time implications of the necessity to purchase medicines from distant sources.

On the basis of our limited sample it would be absurd to make generalizations about an entire sub-continent. Unfortunately, such generalizations about India have been often made in the past. This study suggests that there may be many parts of rural India where a significant awareness about the modern system of medicine has occurred and villagers do not repose *exclusive* faith in the indigenous systems of medicine or their practitioners. However, to argue that rural people in a part of Punjab are more favourably disposed to modern medicine does not mean that their attitudes toward all aspects of modern curative and preventive medicine and family planning measures have undergone fundamental change. Observations of this study are pertinent only to the curative aspect of modern medicine. In this respect, the concepts of disease causation, though important in their own right, are less significant for the villagers than their beliefs regarding the expectancy of cure by preferring modern medicine over the traditional.

We must then pose the question as to why and under what conditions people prefer to use the services of allopathic doctors or use "*angrezi*" medicine. Also, under what conditions people might use the services of indigenous physicians (*vaidya* or *hakim*) or purchase indigenous (*desi*) medicines.

Our interviews with the physicians in the study area as well as interviews with the heads of households suggest that people still harbour some firm beliefs regarding the comparative curative aspects of indigenous and modern' medicine. In general, people associate modern (*angrezi*) medicine with quick cure in acute stages of most diseases. On the other hand, *desi* medicine is traditionally associated with slow cure and is presumed to be more effective in chronic diseases. It is very difficult at present to state precisely how these beliefs have become widespread, not only in the villages we studied, but also much more generally in the state of Punjab and possibly in other parts of India. Perhaps one of the reasons for the association of allopathic medicine with quickness of cure has had to do with the demonstrated success of a few very effective allopathic medicines such as quinine, *sulpha* drugs, and above all penicillin and related groups of broad-spectrum antibiotic "wonder" drugs. It was found in our study area that injections are considered superior to oral medication whenever this alternative is available. This preference for injections (colloquially called *sua,* i.e. the needle), it appears, may have come about due to the success of Cholera and Typhoid inoculation programmes and even more due to the use of penicillin for which injection is the normal mode of application. Thus, injection in general has come to be accepted as the more desirable method of treatment. Since, the practice of giving injections is mostly associated with modern medicine preference for allopathic doctors becomes understandable. Several individuals told us that when one is suffering, one needs quick cure and therefore, it would be unwise to use *desi* medicine, which is "slow" in its action. Also, since *desi* medicine in its traditional form is associated mostly with oral or topical mode of application and these modes are considered to be slow in their effectiveness, people tend to prefer allopathic medicine, particularly in the form of injections.

The positive inclination of the people toward injections may have been partly responsible for the adoption of this technique by several indigenous physicians also. Joshi[14] has rightly observed that "most of these (indigenous) practitioners use modern drugs including injectables freely." In one household it was found that the farmer had kept the hypodermic needle for the use of his family and friends for injecting penicillin whenever the need arose. It is not unusual that a farmer will request the doctor for the *sua* (injection). It is no wonder,

Table 18.12 : Caste Groups by Occupation

Occupation	*Number of Households*	*Caste*		
		Scheduled Castes	*Jats*	*Others*
Farming	34	2	28	4
Agricultural Labour and Daily Labour	23	21	2	0
Handicrafts	10	5	0	5
Trade—Commerce	19	5	0	14
Transportation	2	2	0	0
Government and Professional Services	16	5	5	6
Total	**104**	**40**	**35**	**29**

$\chi^2 = 94.736$. *d.f.* = 12. $P = 0.0000$. Contingency Coefficient = 0.690.
Note: Table was collapsed before computing χ^2.
Source: Data collected by author, 1973.

then that some *hakims* and *vaidyas* in the rural areas of the Punjab have adopted injection as one of their techniques. The *unani, ayurvedic* as well as the homoeopathic injections are now available in the druggists' shops. In general, the rural people tend to seek *angrezi* (modern) treatment rather than *desi* in the acute maladies. It should be pointed out, however, that many patented indigenous medicines are marketed with anglicized nomenclature and are packaged like the allopathic medicines. It is not therefore clear whether people consider the modernized indigenous drugs as different from allopathic drugs.

In the chronic cases, people try several remedies, but the patronage of indigenous physicians and medicine in these cases seems to be still widespread. This may depend on several factors such as the frequency with which medicines are needed, the cumulative cost of medicines, effort involved in procuring treatment and not the least, the nature of relationship between the patient, his family and the physician.

In the chronic diseases such as tuberculosis, the cure is likely to be slow no matter what system of treatment is used. Under this condition then, the allopathic (modern) system seems to have a less competitive advantage over the indigenous systems. Since there exists a pre-conception in the minds of most rural people that allopathic

Table 18.13: Summary of χ^2 Computation: Tables 18.2-18.12

Table No.	Row Variable	Column Variable	χ^2	d.f.	P.	Contingency Coefficient	Result
2.	Villages	Type of Physician Preferred	38.848	15	0.00105	0.521	Significant
3.	Villages	Type of Medicine Perferred	40.062	12	0.00020	0.527	Significant
4.	Caste	Type of Physician Preferred	5.113	10	0.88327	0.216	Not Significant
5.	Caste	Type of Medicine Perferred	1.300	8	0.99456	0.111	Not Significant
6.	Occupation	Type of Physician Preferred	20.849	30	0.89031	0.409	Not Significant
7.	Occupation	Type of Medicine Preferred	21.380	24	0.61626	0.413	Not Significant
8.	Level of education	Type of Physician Preferred	20.347	25	0.72760	0.405	Not Significant
9.	Level of education	Type of Medicine Preferred	6.091	20	0.99836	0.235	Not Significant
10.	Caste	Level of Education	35.306	10	0.00027	0.503	Significant
11.	Villages	Level of Education	26.506	15	0.03440	0.451	Significant
12.	Occupatlon	Caste	94.736	12	0.00000	0.690	Significant

medicine is less effective in chronic cases than *ayurveda* or *unani,* there seems to be a tendency to use the latter two types of medicines in such cases. Tied in with this pre-conception is the personal relationship between the patient and the physician, which assumes greater weight when the patient is suffering from a chronic ailment. In this case the indigenous physician, particularly if he is present in the village, may become important. Chronic maladies require protracted treatment, thus necessitating frequent patient-physician contact as well as increased cost of medicines. A system that can ease the patient-physician relationship as well as ensure low cost of medication can thus have a distinct advantage over the one that cannot. This may in part explain the still widespread use of indigenous mode of cure.

The indigenous physician, in addition, is usually a part and parcel of the rural social *milieu.* Even though his training in the diagnosis and treatment may not be modern, he enjoys a distinct social advantage. He usually enjoys the deference of the village community. Most often the indigenous medical practitioner does not charge any fee for his advice or for the occasional house call. He may, of course, compensate himself by charging a little more for his medicines, but even so, the indigenous medicines are substantially less expensive than *angrezi* medicines. The personalized treatment and generous doses of advice that the rural people are able to get from the indigenous physician is tantamount to the villagers being "obliged" to the physician. The reinforcement of this socio-medical reciprocity relationship appears to make the indigenous physician a vital part of the *rural milieu* wherein he commands respect. Such intimate social ties in the rural system can rarely be achieved by government appointed medical doctors (mostly allopathic) in the rural dispensaries, for at least two reasons. First, these physicians are subject to being transferred after a few years and thus never become part of the rural social system. Secondly, most government appointed doctors exude an elite behaviour, and tend to have less empathy with the rural people particularly those belonging to the lower castes. Therefore, such doctors are not considered to be very helpful for the treatment of chronic diseases. In several instances, the local druggist assumes greater importance as a "physician" for protracted illnesses than the local government appointed physician.[15]

A possible direction for further research may be toward a classification of common diseases into meaningful categories on the basis of culturally perceived degree of acuteness or chronicity. Such a classification would help identify groups of diseases for which either modern or traditional mode of remedy is sought by the rural people. This has obvious implications for planning a health care and delivery system which will be more responsive to the socio-cultural patterns in the rural areas. This approach could be also helpful toward formulating more realistic policies aimed at better utilization of indigenous medical manpower of India. The Central Council of Indian Medicine has clearly a significant role to play in this effort.

While it is true that in the past most people tended to associate modern medicine with culturally pre-conceived ill effects such as production of "heat" or dryness" in the body, such attitudes have apparently undergone substantial change. The probable causative factors of such change and the extent of change itself need fuller documentation.

From the viewpoint of social research on modernization there is need to identify and investigate the role of indigenous medicine organizations such as All-India Ayurved Mahamandal and the impact of major indigenous pharmaceutical establishments such as the Gurukul Pharmacy and Hamdard Dawakhana. In addition, the impact of the soldiers of Indian Armed Forces in bringing modern health ideas to the villages of Punjab cannot be neglected, particularly because Punjab has provided a large number of soldiers to the Indian army.

Limitations of the Study

Data were not collected for the income of households which could have illuminated the choice of physicians and medicine. However, in the rural areas, because of heavy dependence on agriculture, and traditional crafts such data are extremely difficult to collect and are likely to be unreliable. Such problems are less acute in studies related to urban populations. Direct questions were not asked in the questionnaire about diseases in the households for which medical aid was sought. Had such questions been asked, it is probable that preferences of physicians and medicine could be further clarified. Finally, the four specifically selected villages, do not exhaust the range of medical facilities available in rural Punjab. Future research should consider a larger number of villages in the sample so as to represent a greater variety of situations.

Conclusion

Four villages in the Ropar district of Punjab were selected to determine the type of physicians and system of medicine preferred by the rural people.

Statistically significant differences were found to exist among the villages in terms of the preference for different types of physicians and medicine on the basis of interviews with 104 randomly selected heads of households. Preference for indigenous physicians and medicines on an exclusive basis was found to be extremely limited. The rural people either tended to prefer modern medicine and physicians, or kept their options open depending upon their circumstances. These preferences, furthermore, were discovered to be insignificantly dependent upon the three main social characteristics (caste, occupation and level of education) of the rural population.

It is suggested that culturally relevant classification of diseases be developed to better appreciate the bases of preference of rural people for specific type of medical system. Forces that are bringing about significant changes in the attitudes of rural people toward indigenous medicine need to be fully explored along with the response of the indigenous medical systems to the impulses of modernity.

Acknowledgements

Encouragement to do this research in India came from Dr. A. Timmappaya, Director of the National Institute of Health Administration and Education, New Delhi; and Dr. Charles Leslie, Professor of Anthropology, New York University.

I wish to thank Dr. E.F. Bordne and the Department of Geography, Kent State University, for providing financial assistance through the James Beck Fund, which enabled me to carry out fieldwork in India. For many helpful comments and data processing I am thankful to Dr. Milton E. Harvey.

Notes

1. For details on the preparatory steps leading toward the establishment of Central Council of Indian Medicine see: Rajya Sabha, Parliament of India. *The Indian Medicine and Homoeopathy Central Council Bill, 1968: Report of the Joint Committee,* New Delhi: Rajya Sabha Secretariat, November,

1969; For an earlier comprehensive official report on the role of Ayurveda see: Government of India, Ministry of Health, *Report of the Committee to Assess and Evaluate the Present Status of Ayurvedic System of Medicine,* New Delhi, (n.d. ca. 1959).

2. Taylor, C.E., *et al.* (1973), Asian Medical Systems: A Symposium on the Role of Comparative Sociology in Improving Health Care. *Soc. Sci. & Med.*, 7, 307. This Symposium was held at Burg-Wartenstein in July, 1971.
3. *Ibid.*, p. 308.
4. The term Indigenous Medical Practitioner applies to persons practising full-time any type of curative medicine without a recognized qualification in modern medicine. This is the working definition used by National Institute of Health Administration and Education (India).
5. Marriott, McKim (1955), Western Medicine in a Village of Northern India, *Health, Culture and Community* (Edited by B.D. Paul) p. 241. New York: Russel Sage Foundation.
6. Lewis, O. (1965), *Village Life in Northern India,* p. 265, Random House, New York. (Originally Published by the University of Illinois, 1958).
7. Fonaroff, L.S. and Fonaroff, A. (1966), The Cultural Environment of Medical Geography in Rural Hindu India, *Pacific Viewpoint,* 7, 67.
8. Neumann, A.K., Bhatia, J.C., Andrew, S. and Murphy, A.K.S. (1971), Role of the Indigenous Medicine Practitioner in Two Areas of India: Report of a Study, *Soc. Sci. & Med.*, 5, 137.
9. Several scholars point out that the so-called indigenous medical practitioners employ a combination of traditional and modern remedies. See Bhatia, J.C., Vir Dharam, Timmappaya, A. and Chuttani, C.S. (1973), Indigenous Medical Practitioners and their Attitudes Toward the Proposed Rural Health Scheme, *Nat. Inst. Hlth. Admin. & Educ. Bill.*, 5, 302.
10. Leslie, C. (1973), The Professionalizing Ideology of Medical Revivalism, in *Entrepreneurship and Modernisation of Occupational Cultures in South Asia* (Edited by Singer, M.), p. 239, Dukel University.
11. Madan, T.N. (1969), Who Chooses Modern Medicine and Why? *Econ. & Pol. Weekly,* 4, 1475.
12. For a concise description of the *Ayurvedic* and *Unani* systems of medicine and historical sidelights see: Planalp, J.M. (1971), *Heat Stress and Culture in North India,* pp. 19-27. Natick (Massachusetts), U.S. Army Research Institute of Environmental Medicine.
13. The relative paucity of homoeopathic physicians in Punjab as compared with the Eastern Ganga Plain is evident from the *Directory and Who's Who of Homoeopathic Practitioners, 1970-71*, B. Jain Publishers, New Delhi. Also see: Institute of Applied Manpower Research. *Stock of Doctors of Non-Allopathic Systems of Medicine,* National Institute of Health Administration and Education, New Delhi, 1967.
14. Joshi, G.V. (1970), Presidential Address, *Indian Med. Ass. J.*, 54, 238.
15. The author has noted that in several larger villages the local druggist also prescribes medicines even though he may not be officially authorized to do so.

19
Geography of Traditional Medical Systems in India
With Special Reference to Jammu & Kashmir

Nilofar Izhar

In different societies and communities people had a wide range of choices in seeking health care.

The geographical pattern of medical systems is as diverse as their social and cultural pattern. The geography of medical pluralism in India especially the continued existence of different medical systems in the country is the reflection of cultural geography of India (Bhardwaj, 1980).

Health care in India presents a complex scenario that was shaped by colonial and post-colonial history and politics, and enhanced by a vibrant and thriving medical pluralism. Multiple medical systems such as bio-medicine, *Ayurveda*, *Unani*, *Siddha*, Homoeopathy, Naturopathy, Yoga and a variety of folk traditions, all contribute to provide health care in Indian present time (Sujatha and Abraham, 2012).

Commenting on the existence of medical pluralism, Banerji (1981) stressed that the interrelationship of the indigenous and modern systems of medicine in India are function of the interplay of social, economic and political forces in the communities.

In the context of India different traditional medical systems existed not only in the historical perspective, but still these traditional medical systems are practiced in different regions of the country. Data pertaining to the distribution of traditional medical practitioners obtained from Director General, Health Services, New Delhi for the year 2009 reveals that with the exception of Maharashtra the practitioners of *Ayurveda* system are dominant throughout India with its core area in northern India (Fig. 19.1). Homoeopathy was practiced in the north and eastern India. The distribution patterns of homoeopathic practitioners were clearly linked with the migration of Bengali physicians in the late 19th and early 20th centuries with their relative strength in the Ganges plain of northern and eastern India. Throughout rest of India, homoeopathy has limited distribution as indicated by Census data (Bhardwaj, 1980). However, analysis of data for the year 2009 reveals a different scenario of distribution of homoeopathic traditional practitioners in India, with major concentration in Maharashtra, West Bengal and Bihar.

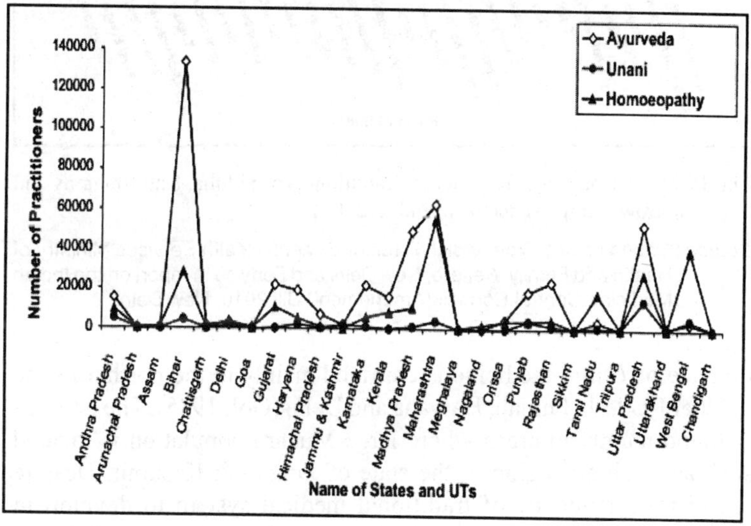

Fig. 19.1: Distribution of Registered AYUSH Practitioners in India (2009).

Source : Based on data from CBHI, Director General Health Services Ministry of Health and Family Welfare, New Delhi.

The *Siddha* system is largely confined to the southern state of Tamil Nadu. More than five thousands of practitioners of *Siddha* medicine are known to exist in Tamil Nadu. To some extent, they are also found in the neighbouring state of Kerala. Naturopathy is confined to southern states of Tamil Nadu and Andhra Pradesh (Fig. 19.2).

The distribution pattern of *Unani* system of medicine in India shows that with the exception of Andhra Pradesh in the south, the

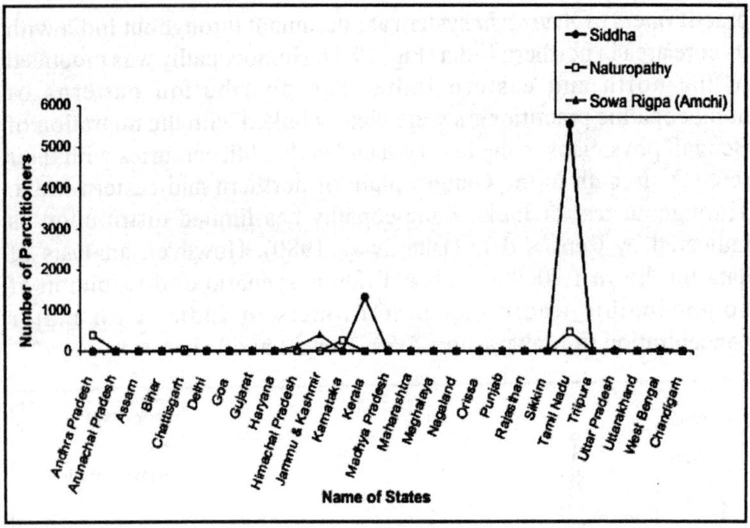

Fig. 19.2: Distribution of Registered Practitioners of Siddha, Naturophathy and Sowa Rigpa (Amchi) in India (2009).

Source : Based on data from CBHI, Director General Health Services Ministry of Health and Family Welfare, New Delhi and Forty sixth report on the Indian Medicine Central Council (Amendment) Bill 2010, New Delhi.

practice of *Unani* medicine is confined mainly to the northern state of Uttar Pradesh, Punjab, Haryana and Delhi (GoI, 1985). The practice is found mainly in areas where large Muslim population is located such as Kashmir region in the state of Jammu & Kashmir. Despite the historic tendency of traditional medical system to develop in certain regions, the analysis of recent data from Ministry of Health and Family Welfare (GoI, 2009) depicts a different pattern in the distribution of traditional Unani practitioners. The states of Bihar and Maharashtra also having high concentration of *Unani* practitioners (Fig. 19.1).

Some 400 practitioners of 'Sowa Rigpa' or '*Amchi*' system of medicine are practicing in Ladakh followed by Himachal Pradesh 120, West Bengal 50, Uttar Pradesh 40, Sikkim and Arunachal Pradesh 30 (GoI, 2009). Thus, people's preference for diverse system of medicine is the reflection of cultural diversity of India. At the same time, the indigenous medical knowledge goes into making of the health culture of a region.

Medical Pluralism in Jammu & Kashmir State

Throughout the State of Jammu & Kashmir there is an increasing pluralism in healthcare practices which indicate that the traditional medical system contribute significantly to the healthcare resources of the state, which comprises three distinct divisions, namely Jammu, Kashmir and Ladakh. Marked areal differentiation in the physical realms of these distinct regions resulted into great diversity in cultural and socio-economic condition of the population living in these areas. Each division has its own distinct characteristics as well as distinct system of traditional medicine.

Medical systems in the State of Jammu & Kashmir is as diverse as their physical and cultural realms. In addition to bio-medicine system, practitioners of traditional medical system such as *Vaid* (Ayurveda), *Hakeem* (Unani), *Amchi* (Sowa Rigpa), and a number of practitioners of folk traditions, all practice various forms of healing treatment. Thus, to gain relief from their sufferings people in these areas opt multiple systems of treatment for their ailments.

Jammu Region: The region is situated at an altitude between 300-3000 meters, having a warm tropical climate. Of the total population of Jammu more than two-third are classed as Hindus and majority of them live in south-eastern part of the region. Culturally, ethnically and linguistically they are closely related to the Punjabi speaking people in Punjab state. *Ayurveda* is dominant traditional system of medicine in Jammu region (Izhar, 1993).

As far as the transhumance communities of Jammu & Kashmir are concerned, Gujjar and Bakherwal community constitutes a sizeable population of the state. The Gujjar community of Kashmir has their own cultural and linguistic heritage. Bakherwals are the offshoots of Gujjar in Kashmir and both are nomadic tribes having some common enlightening cultural as well as linguistic inheritance. They are found at several places in Jammu & Kashmir and are mostly herdmen by occupation. It is estimated that 99.3 per cent of Gujjar and Bakherwal population in Jammu & Kashmir are Muslim. During their bi-annual seasonal migration people with their herd move vast distances in search of best pastures. About 90 per cent of Bakherwals are still nomadic, and oscillate between winter and summer pastures along with their flocks of sheep and goat (Magray, 2010). Bakherwals of Kashmir Valley are sheep rearers and with the change of season they move from Anantnag to Pahalgam up to the Amarnath cave and return with the onset of winter (Dhar, 2001).

While most of the Gujjar are opting a sedentary life still the older ones practicing the age old migratory grazing and a sojourn in Alpine pasture during summer (Misri, 1996). With the approach of colder weather they drive their buffaloes, goats and sheep down into the Himalayan foothills. During the migration Gujjar resort to several services and types of medical care. Along the way they purchase medicines from shopkeepers for various health problems. The Gujjar spiritual healer also travels among them, the holy exhalation of spiritual healer thought to have curative properties for different ailments. Gujjars wore protective amulets, so the person feels 'tashaffi' (psychological healing). Depending upon accessibility, they also consult a private allopathic practitioner or visit public health centre.

However, it is significant to mention the medical traditions of this transhumance community of Jammu & Kashmir whose medical healers consist of non-codified spiritual healers to highly codified practitioners of *Angrezi* system (Allopathic). Thus, the way 'they cope the sicknesses' and their 'health belief' indicate a 'health tradition' of turning towards different systems of medicine according to their accessibility and health care need. It also confirms that people belief and practice in the realms of disease and its treatment is very important to the overall health of a population.

The Kashmir: The valley of Kashmir is situated between 1800-4000 metres above the sea level on the northern border of Jammu. Srinagar is the summer capital of Jammu & Kashmir State. The majority of population resides in the lower reaches of valley. At present more than ninety five per cent of the population are Muslims. In the valley of Kashmir, *Unani* medicine exerts considerable influence on health belief and consequently contributes significantly towards healthcare system as Bhardwaj writes "*Unani* medical system dominates in Kashmir" (Bhardwaj, 1980). The findings of a study done by Nilofar Izhar (1993) also show that *Unani* medical practitioners are the major component of the indigenous medical manpower in the entire valley of Kashmir.

However, in the valley of Kashmir, the ratio of practitioners who were practicing *Ayurveda* and *Unani* system is changed due to the turmoil of 1990s. In fact the picture of medical pluralism has been drastically changed due to the disturbed conditions in the Kashmir

Valley which led to the migration of mainly Hindus to Jammu and other parts of the country.

An interview conducted at the Regional Research Institute of Unani Medicine Srinagar shows that almost sixty-eight per cent of patients were patronizing the clinic after going through the modern medical system. Twenty per cent of patients came directly and twelve per cent claimed previous treatment in another traditional medical setting. Lesser number turned to the *Unani* medicine after using other traditional medical system such as Homoeopathy and *Ayurveda* (Izhar, 1998).

Most of the practitioners of *Unani* medicine practicing in other towns of valley of Kashmir undertook medicine as "hereditary profession". The profession of their father were stated as '*Hikmat'*, or *'Pir'* or *'Imam mosque* and *Hikmat'* both. Having such a background of the practitioners, there is always a chance of fusion between '*Unani*' and 'Spiritual' system of medicine which certainly adds more fame, faith and respect in their status The percentage of *Unani* practitioners belonging to 'ageing group', i.e. sixty and above, is much higher in the other areas of Kashmir valley than in the urban Srinagar where comparatively more practitioners possess BUMS degree and belong to "younger age group". However, there are examples when an experienced *hakim* is much preferred by the people than degree holder young practitioner of *Unani* medicine. Thus, often an experienced older *Unani* practitioner with no formal qualification is consulted especially for some chronic ailments which in their opinion an allopath is unable to treat (Izhar, 1993). There is no denying the fact that in the villages and remote areas the traditional medical practitioners are fulfilling the healthcare need of the bulk of the population.

In addition to this, codified practitioners of *Unani* medical system of Regional Research Institute of Unani Medicine, Srinagar, claimed that over the years the institute has emerged as leading research centre of *Unani* medicine in the State of Jammu & Kashmir. The Institute made achievement in the successful treatment of some chronic diseases.

The mobile wing of the clinical Research Programme collect information in research cases and also provides free medicine to socially and economically weaker section of the society in rural as well as remote areas and urban slums near Srinagar. They also serve the people in the areas where healthcare facilities are either rare or none at all, since the possibility of coming across cases of common and chronic diseases are high in such areas. Despite the severe winters and disturbed conditions due to turmoil in the valley, the clinic was attracting large number of patients not only from Srinagar but also from other parts of the valley. Due to the presence of large number of patients sometimes the staffs of the clinic are compelled to open the OPD for longer hours (RRIUM Report, 2009).

The Ladakh: Highest among one of the three regions of Jammu & Kashmir and India's remote region (1,5000 ft. above sea level) is Ladakh. In the terrain of Himalayas, for centuries the only medical system which are accessible to the people has been the '*Amchis*', who are most sought after people. The *Amchi* system of medicine is known in Ladakh as 'Sowa Rigpa'. Although some people prefer to go to the few allopathic dispensaries of their region most of them still depend on these traditional healers who are in great demand in the region (Gohil and Chetan, 1987) especially in the remote and widely scattered populated mountainous terrains.

The *Amchi* system of medicine develops significantly due to the climate and cultural conditions of the region. Tradition has that this complex system of healing was approved by Buddha himself 2500 years ago. In *Amchi* system of medicine the cause of all sickness is in an imbalance in between these 'humors'—*rlug, mkris-pa* and *badkhan* (wind, bile and phlegm). The maintenance of good health depends upon the life sustaining forces within the body (LSTM, 2008).

Although, the use of Allopathic medicine has increased in recent decades it cannot treat the full range of health problems. *Amchi* medicine has effective remedies for the vast majority of Ladakhi's health problem such as respiratory problems caused by the high altitude and the smoke in their dwellings and partly by the salty, buttered tea they frequently drink and most important of all, astrology and centuries old rituals are used in conjunction with Amchi remedies so that patient experience psychological healing. Most Ladakhi villages are situated in remote places, few have road access. Thus, the indigenous knowledge of *Amchi* sustains the socio-cultural fabric of village life and is a trusted, effective and affordable system of healthcare (LSTM, 2008). Besides, providing the harmony of families, social relations, mental balance of individual. They are the main consultants for the community decision-making.

While surgery is not performed by these *Amchi* practitioners—in case of severe illnesses Ladakhis are sent whenever possible to doctors qualified in bio-medicine. Whenever they are required to stay in modern hospitals Ladakhis do not feel at ease. "When a rural Ladakhi goes to hospital the medical milieu is very foreign to him" (Doogue, 2004). Thus, this centuries old health system is not only vital to Ladakhis but also remarkable and irreplaceable part of their heritage.

Conclusion

To sum up, in India, multiple systemic approaches are found even in places where the best of biomedical facilities are available. In contrast to technology dominant modern medical system, proponent of traditional medical system claimed personalized, inexpensive, easy accessibility and holistic in nature.

Thus, the three geographical segments of Jammu & Kashmir State are inhabited by people of differing socio-religious backgrounds, lifestyle and ethnicity, a feature which could be unique in studying the adoption of different systems of medicine by these physically, ethnically and culturally distinct people.

Acknowledgements

I would like to express my deep appreciation and gratitude to well-known, outstanding and highly respected practitioner of Unani medicine Hakeem Mohammad Yosuf the Ex-Director of Regional Research Institute of Unani Medicine, Srinagar, Kashmir and the para-medical staff of the institute for support and willingness to share their experiences and knowledge with me. Without their support the interviews which I conducted in the OPD clinic of the Institute for weeks could not have been possible. A part of present study is taken from the project work assigned to me earlier by U.G.C., New Delhi under the scheme of U.G.C. Research Associateship and the CSIR's scheme of Research Pool Scientist.

References

Beals, A.R. (1976), Strategies of Resort to Curers in South India, In C. Leslie (ed.), *Asian Medical System: A Comparative Study*, Berkeley: University of California Press, pp. 184-200.

Bhardwaj, S.M. (1975), Attitude Towards Different System of Medicine: A Survey of Four Villages in the Punjab-India, *Social Science and Medicine*, Vol. 9, pp. 603-12.

Bhardwaj, S.M. (1980), Homoeopathy in India, In Giri Raj Gupta (ed.), *The Social and Cultural Context of Medicine in India*, Vol. 6, New Delhi: Vikas Publishing House, pp. 31-54.

Cant, S. and Sharma, U. (1999), *A New Medical Pluralism? Alternative Medicine, Doctors, Patients and the State*, London, UCL Press.

Dhar, B. (2001), "Anthropology and Transhumance", *Human Ecology*, Special Issue, No. 10, pp. 151-156.

Doogue, E. (2004), Ancient Amchi Medicine, *Himalayan Healer*, www.nomad srsi.org.

Gesler, W.M. and Kearns, R.A. (2002), *Culture, Place and Health*, London: Routledge Publications, p. 30.

Gohil, R.N. and Chetan, R. (1987), Nubra—An Oasis Beyond Desert, In Y.P. Pandey and S.C. Joshi (eds.), *Western Himalayan Environment: Problems and Development*, Vol. I, Nainital: Gyanodaya Prakashan, pp. 427-435.

GoI (1985), *Health Statistics 1985*, New Delhi: CBHI, Director General Health Services, Ministry of Health and Family Welfare.

GoI (2009), *Health Statistics 2009*, New Delhi: CBHI, Director General Health Services, Ministry of Health and Family Welfare.

Gupta, D. (1988), For a Sociology/Anthropology of Illness: Towards a Delineation of its Disciplinary Specificities, *International Sociology*, Vol. 3(4), pp. 403-13.

Hyma, B. and Paul, B.K. (1991), Geographic Research in Traditional Medicine, In Rais Akhtar (ed.), *Environment and Health: Themes in Medical Geography*, New Delhi: Ashish Publishers, pp. 221-244.

Hyma, B. and Ramesh, A. (1985), *Siddha* System of Health Care—A profile of Users in Madras City, India, *Trans. Inst. Indian Geographers*, Vol. 2, No. 1, pp. 17-39.

Izhar, N. (1990), Patient Origins and Usages of a Unani Clinic in Aligarh Town, India, *Social Science and Medicine*, Vol. 30, No. 10, pp. 1139-41.

Izhar, N. (1993), *Geographical Distribution of Traditional System of Medicine in Urban Srinagar-J&K*, Unpublished Monograph submitted to U.G.C., New Delhi, p. 78.

Izhar, N. (1998), Health Seeking Behaviour in Kashmir, *Geographia Medica*, RUX Editice, Perugia, pp. 385-390.

Janzen, J.M. (1978), The Comparative Study of Medical System as Changing Social System, *Social Science and Medicine*, Vol. 12, pp. 121-29.

Leslie, C. (1977), Pluralism and Integration in the Indian and Chinese Medical Systems, In D. Landy (ed.), *Culture, Disease and Healing: Studies in Medical Anthropology*, New York: MacMillan Publisher, pp. 511-517.

LSTM (2008), *Ladakh Society for Traditional Medicine: Perspective of Amchi Medicine, Conservation and Medicinal Plants*, Annual Report, Leh.

Magray, M.B. (2010), J. & K. Gujars: A Sedentrized Tribe, *Jammu Kashmir Newspoint*, 5th December.

Misri, B. (1996), Nomadic Graziers of Himalaya : The Gujjar of Jammu & Kashmir, In *Proceedings of the Second Meeting of the Temperate Asia Pasture and Fodder Sub-regional Working Group*, Dehra Dun, pp. 53-60.

Press, I. (1978), Urban Folk Medicine: An Overview, *American Anthropology*, Vol. 8, pp. 71-84.

Quaiser, N. (2006), Politics, Culture and Colonialism: Unani's Debate with Doctory, In Biswamoy Pati and Mark Harrison (eds.), *Health, Medicine and Empire, Perspectives in Colonial India*, New Delhi: Orient Longman Pvt. Limited, p. 317.

RRIUM (2010), *Report on Activities and Achievements*, Srinagar.

Scrambler, G. (2002), *Health and Social Change: A Critical Theory*, Buckingham: Open University Press.

Sujátha, V.A. and Abraham, L. (2009), Medicine, State and Society, *Economic & Political Weekly*, April 18, Vol. XLIV, No. 16, p. 35.

Turner, B. (2004), *The New Medical Sociology: Social Forms of Health and Illness,* New York: W.W. Norton & Company.

PART IV
Health Care

20
Inequalities in the Distribution of Health Care in India

Rais Akhtar and *Nilofar Izhar*

Health problems in a developing country such as India, are predominantly reflections of poverty. Substantial decrease of morbidity and mortality is more likely to be accomplished through an improved system for health including preventive services than from further advances in medical science. Indeed in the end such improvements are likely to result from all-round social and economic development, from structural change in the society of some kind. Therefore, the necessity of sufficient availability of health services such as hospitals, health centres, beds, doctors and other health personnel can hardly be overemphasized. The present health facility structure is inherited from colonial India. The colonial masters believed in selective development in order to serve their purpose.

Port towns were developed and the status of western type of health care was raised even beyond the need of the select population, and the hinterland was neglected in terms of everything. Later selected urban, industrial and hill resort centres were developed without any consideration of need based health planning.

As Radhika Ramasubban has rightly emphasised that "at all times the highest priority was the protection of the European population. Another was to ensure that disease and epidemics did not affect Britain's trade".[1] The Royal Sanitary Commission Report also states that "the main enemy of the British soldier in India was not the Indian enemy but disease."[2] Simultaneously, the indigenous or traditional system of medicine that used to serve the vast majority of the population was greatly discouraged and the western type of medicine introduced, that too in the selected places. Such process had led to enclaves of development in terms of health facilities, and it may rightly be said that health facilities are abundant where there is less need and *vice versa*.

Notwithstanding the fact that the country achieved independence more than three decades back, the gap between regionally developed and backward areas had widened. Benerji has rightly pointed out that:

> political economic forces play a dominant role in the shaping of the health services of a community, for instance, through decisions on resource allocation, manpower policy, choice of technology, and the degree to which the health services are to be available and accessible to the population.[3]

To quote Radhika Ramasubban,

> whenever there are cuts or readjustments in plan outlays, the health sector is among the first victims. Expediency rather than any well defined principles govern the laying down of priorities in the planning process, allocation of funds, planning of programmes, allotment of portfolios, and appointment and transfer of personnel.[4]

As regards the contribution of medical research towards the development of health services system, Radhika Ramasubban further states that "the medical research and development system is isolated from its users, the health services system. It has a poor record of producing results for the solution of local health problem. When results are achieved, they remain unutilised due to the limitations of the health services system".[5]

Ideally each village should have its own health centre or sub-centre, with staff and functions such as Fendall[6] has described. However, countries such as India cannot afford to provide health centres to each and every village. But a group of villages could be provided one health centre ideally located and also equipped with the specific health needs of the region. Unfortunately in India, ideal health planning has been replaced by political health planning or political epidemiology as Arthur Brownlea puts it. Political interference is evident in an example from Uttar Pradesh where primary health centres were being established at a density of one block (an administrative sub-divisional unit). However, in one block, there were two large villages and each was represented by a very strong and active politician of the ruling party. Which village was to get the health centre? Eventually, the block was subdivided into two blocks and a health centre established in each of the two villages. Thus, a policy is bent and locational "theory" and health care efficiency compromised.[7]

Without understanding the real meaning of development, one document published by the Ministry of Information, Government of India, says that "planned development of over two and a half decades has resulted in vastly improved health facilities".

The number of doctors and hospital beds have increased by more than two and a half times and that of nurses by more than five times. The number of medical colleges has increased from 30 before the First Plan to 106 at present. In rural areas there are about 5400 primary health centres and more than 39,000 sub-centres at present whereas none existed before 1951.[8] It may be asked as to where actually the increase in the number of health facilities took place? The answer is that the areas already served were further overserved. As regards the increase in medical colleges, it is a fact that the first choice of a present day medico is to go abroad or try to get an appointment in a well developed urban centre or to start private practice in a big town. How then will the vast mass of rural population be served by these medicos?

According to one report, "India is, in terms of absolute numbers, the world's largest donor of medical manpower. There is scarcely a recipient country in the world where there are no Indian physicians. In all, it is estimated that there are some 15,000 Indian physicians outside India".[9] In terms of an Indian estimate, it costs about US$ 9600 for the education of a physician, the 15,000 Indian physicians at present outside India represent a lost investment to India of US $144 million. There is no denying the fact that had they stayed, most probably they would not have got suitable employment and place of their liking, in view of the fact that at present physicians are needed mostly in un-attractive places such as rural areas, tribal areas and sometimes inaccessible hilly regions. As an Indian physician, quoted by the *New York Times* (24th March, 1974) puts it, "There is not even a hut in many villages to work from, there is no medicine, equipment is zero ...." In our opinion there is some exaggeration in the statement. However, the real significance of such economic losses lies in the fact that money spent on the education of these emigrant physicians would have been better spent on other forms of health personnel and health care.

There is a peculiar situation prevailing these days in India in terms of demand and unemployment of physicians. There is considerable unemployment of physicians.[10] On the other hand several hundreds of health centres and dispensaries located in unattractive rural areas are without doctors. During an investigation (1973-74) in the Kumaon Himalayas, the senior author noted that most of the physicians serving the rural areas of Naini Tal and Almora districts had been trying hard to get themselves transferred to a suitable place specially urban areas. According to them when a physician is punished by the higher authorities he is transferred to a remote inaccessible hilly area. Such an attitude has to be changed if the government is genuinely interested in attracting physicians to such difficult areas.

Establishment of Primary Health Centres and Sub-centres and the Achievements in Different Plan Periods

As has been stated that the health planners felt greatly satisfied to see the considerable increase in various components of health services, Table 20.1 shows that in the First Plan there were only 67 Primary Health Centres in the country. The number of PHCs rose to 5799 in early 1980. Similarly, there is a substantial increase in the number of beds, doctors and nurses between First and Fifth Plans. Table 20.2 reveals that the availability of beds, doctors and nurses is very close to the desired norms set by the Mudaliar Committee. However, as it has been stated that such an increase in the number of health facilities is creating more disparities between developed and underdeveloped areas.

Per capita Expenditure on Health

How could a balanced and uniform health care planning be carried out in the face of uneven expenditure on health in different states (Table 20.3). Table 20.3 highlights the variations in the per capita expenditure on health and family welfare in different states. The states of Uttar Pradesh and Bihar which consists about one fourth of the

Table 20.1: Establishment of Primary Health Centres and Sub-centres in India since First Plan

	PHCs	Sub-Centre
First Plan	67	
Second Plan	2565	
Third Plan	4919	22826
Fourth Five Year Plan	5283	33509
Fifth Five Year Plan	5400	38115
Sixth Five Year Plan as at 31.3.1980	5499	49323

Source: *Pocket Book of Health Statistics of India*, 1980, C.B.H.I., Directorate General of Health Services, Ministry of Health and Family Welfare, New Delhi, p. 75.

Table 20.2: Achievements in different Plan Periods (Medical and Public Health)
Achievements in Medical and Public Health, Progressive Total

Plan Period Position at the end of Plan		*Beds*	*Doctors*	*Nurses*
1st Plan (1951-56)		125000	65000	18500
2nd Plan (1956-61)		186000	70000	27000
3rd Plan (1961-66)		240000	86000	45000
4th Plan (1969-74)		282000	138000	88000
5th Plan (1974-78)		314000	170000	108000
6th Plan				
I. 1978-79 (likely achievements)		322000	178000	113000
II. 1979-80 (likely achievements)				
Poulation per unit	At the end of 1978-79	1991	3622	5673
	Desired norms as per Mudaliar Committee	1000	3500	5000

Source: *Pocket Book of Health Statistics of India*, 1980, C.B.H.I., Directorate General of Health Services. Ministry of Health and Family Welfare, New Delhi, p. 35.

country's population spend only about ₹ 5 to ₹ 8 per person per annum. Significantly, these areas also suffer with several types of communicable diseases, such as filariasis, *kala-azar* (*Visceral leishmaniasis*), leprosy and malaria and other waterborne diseases. Barring some districts of western Uttar Pradesh and southern Bihar, most of the area is backward both agriculturally and industrially. On

Table 20.3: Per Capita Expenditure on Health and Family Welfare

(in Rupees)

	1975-76		1976-77		1977-78	
	Health	*Family Welfare*	*Health*	*Family Welfare*	*Health*	*Family Welfare*
Northern Region	14.36	1.33	15.80	2.59	20.64	1.55
1. Himachal Pradesh	21.46	1.80	21.69	4.69	30.41	2.98
2. Bihar	5.25	0.79	5.76	2.09	6.94	0.93
3. Uttar Pradesh	5.48	1.25	5.75	2.21	8.11	1.33
4. Haryana	12.95	1.57	14.29	2.98	18.91	1.56
5. Punjab	18.80	1.68	16.78	2.65	20.95	1.42
6. Jammu & Kashmir	22.27	0.89	30.35	0.92	38.57	1.12
North-Eastern Region	37.76	0.60	41.05	1.21	48.72	1.00
7. Sikkim	34.89	0.17	54.24	0.93	68.50	1.54
8. Assam	11.36	0.90	11.05	2.06	12.24	0.93
9. Meghalaya	35.45	1.14	31.62	2.13	39.98	1.85
10. Manipur	24.44	0.74	18.70	1.54	22.98	1.51
11. Tripura	15.84	0.61	16.35	1.46	21.21	0.76
12. Nagaland	100.47	0.03	98.13	0.19	119.98	0.26
13. Arunachal Pradesh	41.90	0.02	57.31	0.22	56.15	0.17
Eastern Region	11.41	1.04	12.29	2.83	13.92	1.26
14. West Bengal	13.30	0.92	14.90	2.98	16.54	0.75
15. Orissa	9.52	1.17	9.68	2.69	11.31	1.78
Central Region	7.31	1.08	10.07	3.43	10.76	1.37
16. Madhya Pradesh	7.31	1.08	10.07	3.43	10.76	1.37
Western Region	13.62	1.35	15.84	2.59	18.37	1.76
17. Rajasthan	15.32	1.20	16.95	2.26	19.69	1.24
18. Gujarat	11.93	1.50	14.74	2.93	17.06	2.28
Southern Region	25.93	1.70	27.28	2.80	29.79	12.45
19. Maharashtra	14.83	1.44	15.08	2.44	16.88	1.13
20. Karnataka	11.85	2.27	12.09	3.79	12.64	2.08
21. Kerala	18.41	1.68	19.51	2.64	19.26	1.77
22. Tamil Nadu	12.17	1.43	15.63	2.77	14.73	1.52
23. Andhra Pradesh	9.85	1.33	12.00	3.17	13.49	1.71
24. Pondicherry	57.95	2.02	60.93	3.06	65.77	2.12
25. Goa, Daman & Diu	56.74	1.76	55.75	1.73	65.19	1.67

Source: Combined Finance and Revenue Accounts of the Union and State Governments in India for the years 1975-76, 1976-77,1977-78, *Pocket Book of Health Statistics 1980*, pp. 36-37.

the other hand, most of the states of the North-eastern region and Southern part of the country enjoy high per capita expenditure on health. During 1975-78, per capita expenditure on health in the North-eastern region ranges between ₹ 38 and ₹ 120 with highest per capita expenditure, i.e. ₹ 120 is recorded in Nagaland in the financial year 1977-78. Next to the North-eastern region, per capita expenditure on health is high in Southern region. Pondicherry and Goa, Daman & Diu States spent ₹ 66 and ₹ 65 respectively per person per annum during 1977-78. However, it should be noted here that Pondicherry and Goa reflect the colonial influence of French and Portuguese respectively. Besides these two states are at present governed by the Central Government. It is quite evident that imbalances are bound to occur in the face of wide disparities in the money spent on the health sector in different regions. According to Barrett, "these per capita figures do seem to show that there is an absolute minimum size for State Health Programmes such that the states with smaller populations tend to have the highest per capita figures.[11] He has rightly suggested that:

> If there were a real commitment to increasing the coverage of health care and to providing basic health care to disadvantaged groups, some form of analysis of health expenditure in terms of the type of care provided (such as primary, secondary and tertiary care) and its location (both geographic and social) is necessary. These data can then matched against rough estimates of the number of people who might be in need of such care.[12]

Distance and Health Care

Another important aspect in the study of health care geography, is the distance between a settlement and the health facility. A study conducted by the Registrar General's Office in connection with the infant and child mortality (Table 20.4) reveals that only about 41 per cent of villages and about 35 per cent of the total rural population of the country have access to the health facility within 2 kilometres of distance. On the other hand health facilities are available within 2 kilometres for about 84 per cent of the total urban population of the country.

Distribution of Hospital Facilities

An attempt has been made to map the pattern of hospital facilities in

Table 20.4: Per cent Distribution of Villages/Urban Blocks and Estimated Population by Type of Medical Facility and Distance

R/U/T Distance	*Per cent Villages/Urban Blocks having Medical Facility*	*Per cent Population having Medical Facility*
Rural within		
2 kms	40.9	35.3
2-5 kms	23.7	24.9
5-10 kms	20.5	23.7
10 kms +	14.9	16.1
Urban within		
2 kms	84.4	83.9
2-5 kms	13.0	13.6
5 km +	2.6	2.5
Total		
Within		
2 kms	56.5	44.1
2-5 kms	19.8	22.8
5-10 kms	13.5	19.7
10 kms +	10.1	13.4

Source: *Survey on Infant and Child Mortality,* Registrar General's Office, New Delhi, 1979.

India in the years 1957 and 1975. Figures 20.1 and 20.2 show the hospital/population ratio per million population. The index ranges between 5 and 35 and more hospitals per million of population. It can be observed from Figure 20.1 which shows the distribution of hospitals in 1957, that in general high population density areas of Gangetic Plains and north-western parts of the country lacked adequate hospital facilities in comparison to low population density areas. Barring tourist resorts such as Simla, Naini Tal and Darjeeling, most of the mountainous areas were not having adequate hospitals. Similar is the case with the tribal areas of Baster, Koraput and Araku valley where only 5-10 hospitals were available per million population. On the other hand, in some less populated areas of eastern Rajasthan and western Madhya Pradesh the index of hospital availability rose to 35. However, with the increase in population during 1957-75, the distribution pattern of hospital facilities in 1975 highlights imbalances in the growth of population and the growth of hospitals. For instance, the growth of hospitals was not coterminous with the increase in

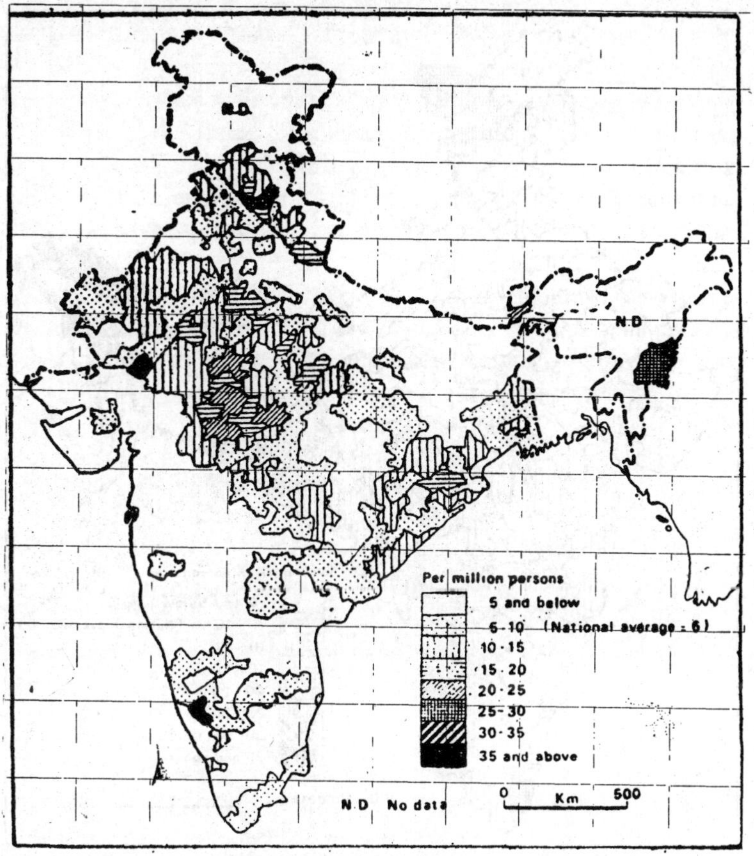

Fig. 20.1: India: Distribution of Hospital Facilities by District, 1957.

population in eastern Rajasthan and western Madhya Pradesh. Instead high hospital availability areas were scattered all-over the country. The low population density and a special preference to the north-eastern region and Ladakh area of Kashmir, resulted in the high availability of hospital facilities. Besides some areas with economic and strategic significance such as military centre of Gorakhpur and mineral rich and industrially developed areas of eastern part of the country shows comparatively high hospital facilities. Hospital facilities are also very high in the educationally and industrially developed Kerala State on the western coast. However, even after 18 years, in most of the high population density areas of the north, central,

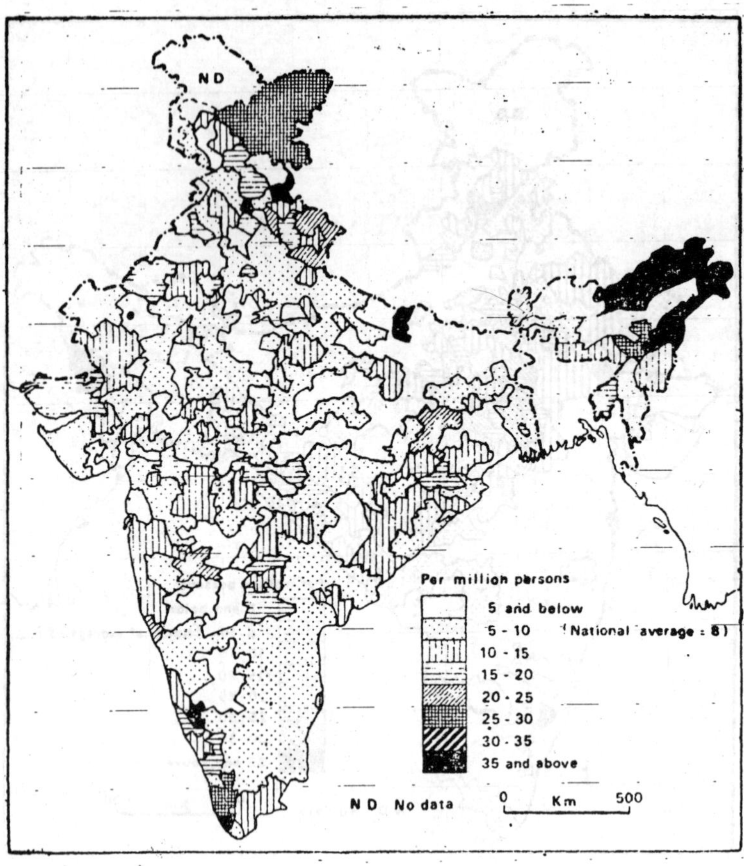

Fig. 20.2: India: Distribution of Hospital Facilities by District, 1975.

western and southern regions hospital facilities are utterly inadequate (well below national average), although the process of regional development touched almost all areas of development.

Distribution of Bed Facilities

Availability of beds is an important indicator of health services. The distribution pattern of beds is shown in Figures 20.3 and 20.4 for 1957 and 1975 respectively. It is evident from figure 20.3 that most of the districts in the north and in the south possessed less than 25 beds for 1,00,000 population. Districts with bed facilities ranging

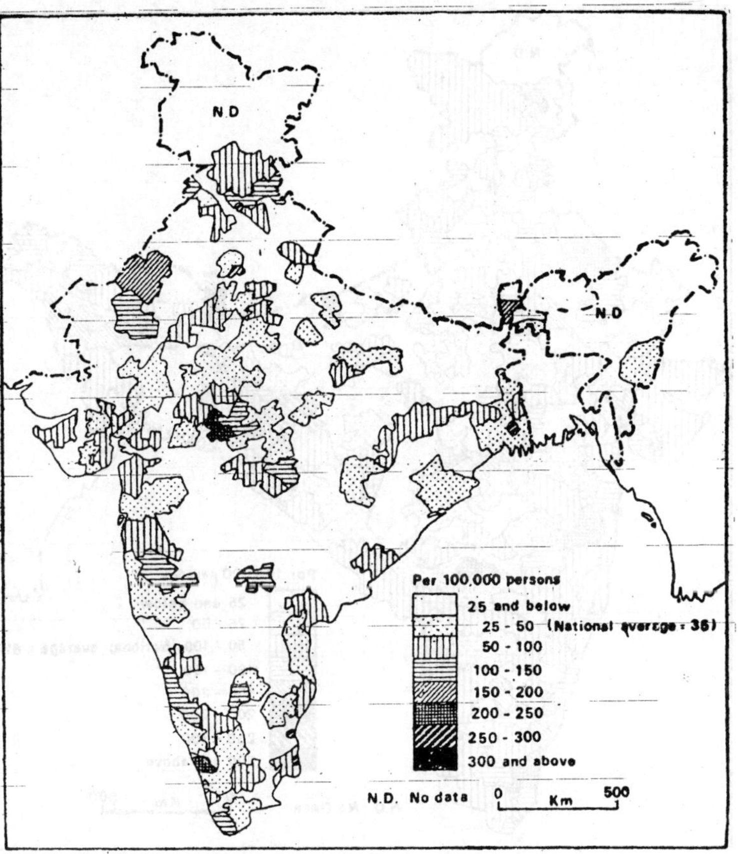

Fig. 20.3: India: Distribution of Bed Facilities by District, 1957.

between 50 and 150 per 100,000 population were widely scattered all-over the country. The northern areas of Himachal Pradesh and Punjab, some districts in western Rajasthan, Gujarat, western Madhya Pradesh, western Maharashtra and western coastal areas show high availability of beds in comparison to the high population density areas of the north-central and southern parts of the country. A look at the Figure 20.4 which shows the availability of beds in 1975, highlights the fact that barring some districts such as Gorakhpur and hilly districts of Uttar Pradesh, growth in the availability of beds in the last 18 years appeared in already developed areas. The areas with poor health

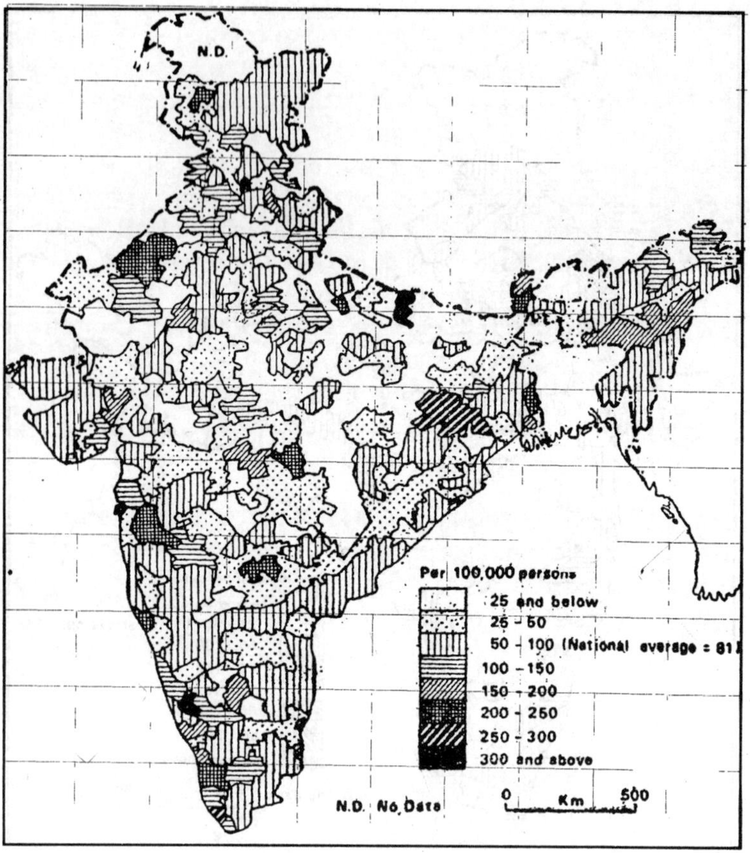

Fig. 20.4: India: Distribution of Bed-Facilities by District, 1975.

services were further neglected in terms of bed facilities. The increase in the number of beds was shared by the north-western, western coastal areas and the north-eastern region. Such distribution pattern is a clear indication of unsystematic health services planning in which the actual needs of the areas is often ignored.

Spatial Pattern of Health Care Delivery

The hospital/population and bed/population ratios have been computed in order to study the pattern of health care delivery by states in rural as well as urban areas.

Rural Areas

Table 20.5 pinpoints an important fact that apart from the disparities in the availability of hospital and bed facilities between rural and urban areas, imbalances are evident even in rural areas of different states. For instance, the hospital facilities vary between 0.4 hospital per million population in Bihar and 10 hospitals per million population in Punjab in the northern region. The availability of beds per 1,00,000 population also ranges from 2 in Bihar and 32 in Himachal Pradesh. On the other hand, hospital/population and bed/population ratios range between 2 and 60 and 3 and 131 respectively in the north-eastern region. Barring Assam, Meghalaya and Tripura hospital/population and bed/population ratios are adequate in the region in terms of all-India level. Largely underdeveloped central region is one of the most neglected areas as regard the rural health care facilities. The rural areas of southern states are comparatively better with Goa, Daman & Diu and Kerala states have 35 and 33 hospitals respectively per million population. The bed/population ratio in the southern region varies between 10 in Andhra Pradesh and 77 in Goa, Daman & Diu. The hospital/population ratio is considerably higher in island territories of Andaman & Nicobar and Lakshadweep with 112 and 63 hospitals respectively per million population—the highest in the rural areas in the country. Similarly, bed/population ratios of 328 and 157 in Andarnan & Nicobar and Lakshadweep respectively are highest in the rural areas.

Urban Areas

The hospital and bed facilities are unevenly distributed in urban areas too. There is a wide variation in the hospital/population ratio, i.e. 9 hospitals per million population in Chandigarh and 347 in Arunachal Pradesh. Similarly, the bed/population ratio varies considerably with the lowest 53 per 1,00,000 population in Dadra & Nagar Haveli/and 2580 in Arunachal Pradesh. After Dadra & Nagar Haveli/the lowest bed/population ratio is obtained in Madhya Pradesh (i.e. 169)—the largest state in terms of area and second largest in terms of population. The analysis of the data removed the impression that the health facilities are in abundance in highly urbanized and developed areas. As it is evident from the Table 20.5 that only 16 and 9 hospitals per million population are available in highly urbanized and developed

Table 20.5: Pattern of Health Care Delivery by State (Rural/Urban 1979)
Number of Hospitals per 10,00,000 Population
Number of Beds per 1,00,000 Population

	Rural		*Urban*		*Total*	
	Hospital	*Bed*	*Hospital*	*Bed*	*Hospital*	*Bed*
Northern Region						
1. Himachal Pradesh	7	31	132	967	16	97
2. Bihar	0.4	1	37	390	4	40
3. Uttar Pradesh	1	4	51	329	8	49
4. Haryana	0.7	4	43	369	8	69
5. Punjab	10	28	46	350	19	105
6. Jammu & Kashmir	0.5	2	38	452	8	85
7. Delhi	5	15	16	348	15	314
8. Chandigarh	—	—	9	481	8	435
North-Eastern Region						
9. Sikkim	21	80	51	1266	24	191
10. Assam	2	6	62	615	7	60
11. Meghalaya	1	3	81	877	13	130
12. Manipur	13	42	42	561	17	108
13. Tripura	3	8	62	599	9	70
14. Nagaland	60	131	97	862	64	204
15. Arunachal Pradesh	35	74	347	2580	47	167
16. Mizoram	20	109	79	890	27	198
Eastern Region						
17. West Bengal	3	25	23	333	8	101
18. Orissa	6	10	81	444	12	46
Central Region						
19. Madhya Pradesh	1	1	30	169	6	36
Western Region						
20. Rajasthan	1	3	43	339	9	63
21. Gujarat	2	8	106	408	31	120
Southern Region						
22. Maharashtra	3	13	56	400	19	134
23. Karnataka	2	11	26	381	8	101
24. Kerala	33	121	47	619	35	202
25. Tamil Nadu	3	13	22	289	9	96
26. Andhra Pradesh	5	10	52	348	14	76
27. Pondicherry	—	—	55	1129	23	475
28. Goa, Daman & Diu	35	77	212	1006	82	322
29. Dadra & Nagar Haveli Islands	—	—	13	53	13	53
30. Andaman & Nicobar	112	328	114	999	113	481
31. Lakshadweep	63	157	—	—	63	157

Source: Based on data collected from the *Pocket Book of Health Statistics of India*, 1980, C.B.H.I., Directorate General of Health Services, Ministry of Health and Family Welfare, New Delhi, pp. 60-70.

states of Delhi and Chandigarh respectively. On the other hand, the hospital/population and bed/population ratios are the highest in less urbanized and less developed Arunachal Pradesh of the north-eastern region.

Imbalances in Health Care in Rural/Urban Areas

In general, the hospital and bed facilities are comparatively adequate both in rural as well as in urban areas in the north-eastern region followed by southern region (Table 20.6). However, hospital and bed services are inadequate in Bihar, Uttar Pradesh, Jammu & Kashmir in the northern region. Hospital and bed facilities are utterly inadequate in the central region. Significantly, the indigenous system of medicine has also been encouraged in the southern states resulting in the highest ratio of traditional hospitals per million population.

Table 20.6: Pattern of Health Care Delivery by Region (Rural/Urban, 1979)
Number of Hospitals per 1,00,000 Population
Number of Traditional Hospitals per 10,00,000 Population
Number of Beds per 1,00,000 Population

Regions	*Rural*		*Urban*		*Total*		*Traditional Hospital*
	Hospital	*Bed*	*Hospital*	*Bed*	*Hospital*	*Bed*	
Northern	4	12	46	466	15	157	2.76
North-Eastern	19	45	103	1031	26	141	0.05
Eastern	4.5	17	52	388	30	73	0.30
Central	1	1	30	169	6	36	0.48
Western	1.5	5.5	74	373	20	91	1.46
Southern	13	41	60	528	25	182	3.29

Source: Based on Data Collected from the *Pocket Book of Health Statistics of India*, 1980, C.B.H.I., Directorate of Health Services, Ministry of Health and Family Welfare, New Delhi, pp. 69-70 and 73-74.

Distribution of Health Personnel

Table 20.7 provides a totally different picture of the availability of doctors and dentists in different parts of the country. Doctors as well as dentists are mainly concentrated in large urban centres. According to one report "the largest Indian cities are crowded with physicians. One source states that Bombay, Calcutta and New Delhi have physician/population ratios of an order of one physician per 500 people".[13] This is reflected in the population figures per doctor and

Table 20.7: Distribution of Health Personnel (Population per Doctor/Dentist by State, 1977)

	Doctor	*Dentist*
Northern		
Himachal Pradesh	6988	48129
Bihar	4666	626990
Uttar Pradesh	50[illegible]4	195938
Haryana	5776	65257
Punjab	2024	20393
Jammu & Kashmir	3709	—
Delhi	1400	13324
Chandigarh	810	8788
North-Eastern		
Sikkim	4558	—
Assam	2502	191462
Meghalaya	8333	—
Manipur	3800	—
Tripura	7192	—
Nagaland	3764	—
Arunachal Pradesh	3333	—
Eastern		
West Bengal	1732	83309
Orissa	3678	414483
Central		
Madhya Pradesh	6825	342028
Western		
Rajasthan	4362	—
Gujarat	2628	50376
Southern		
Maharashtra	1785	35646
Karnataka	4869	92123
Kerala	2656	57505
Tamil Nadu	3408	135129
Andhra Pradesh	2789	162652
Pondicherry	2603	—
Goa, Daman & Diu	1790	34678
Dadra & Nagar Haveli	7000	—
Islands		
Andaman & Nicobar	2321	—
Lakshadweep	2000	—

Source: *Pocket Book of Health Statistics of India*, 1978, Directorate General of Health Services, Ministry of Health and Family Welfare, New Delhi, pp. 56-57.

dentist which show that Chandigarh has the lowest number of population dependent on one doctor and dentist each. The West Bengal and Maharashtra states which comprise largest urban centres of Calcutta and Bombay respectively also have lower number of people being served by one doctor. The distribution of different types of health personnel is shown in Table 20.8. The number of doctors per 1,00,000 population is the highest in the eastern region followed by southern region. Dentist/population and homoeopath/population ratios are highest in the western and eastern region respectively. Southern region has adequate number of nurses and midwives in terms of population. Western region has the highest Auxilliary Nurse Midwife (A.N.M.)/population ratio. The highest health visitor/population ratio that is 2 per 1,00,000 population is obtained in the northern region. It is evident from the Table 20.8 that as regards the availability of health services is concerned, southern region is well off. The overall situation is utterly inadequate in the central region. Not only the general health facilities, but even highly specialized hospital facility is maldistributed.[14] For instance out of 18 hospitals equipped with the facility of open heart surgery, seven are located in only one state that is Maharashtra (5 in Bombay and 2 in Pune) in western India. Who are benefited? Of course the rich Indians and the Arabs utilize these facilities. Dissatisfied with the British hospitals, Arab patients now prefer to be treated for serious illness in India that too in Bombay.[15] The smaller state Kerala on the Western Coast with about 3.7 per

Table 20.8: Distribution of Health Personnel by Region, 1977

(per 1,00,000 Population)

	Doctor	*Dentist*	*Homeopath*	*Nurse*	*Midwife*	*A.N.M.*	*Health Visitor*
Northern	26	8	21	14	12	7	2
North-Eastern	18	6	5	13	10	10	0.23
Eastern	36	4	28	11	11	9	0·28
Central	14	3	16	15	15	12	1.13
Western	28	22*	6	16	12	14	1.20
Southern	35	14	17	37	39	12	1.22

*Data for Gujarat State only.

Source: *Pocket Book of Health Statistics of India*, 1978, C.B.H.I., Directorate General of Health Services, Ministry of Health and Family Welfare, New Delhi, pp. 52-57.

cent of the total population of the country (1981) gets two such hospitals while no facility of open heart surgery is available in north Indian state of Bihar with about 10 per cent of country's population. Uttar Pradesh (the largest state in terms of population) in the northern India with 16 per cent of the total population of the country, only one such hospital is provided. The vast areas of north-western and eastern India are completely neglected in the provision of open heart surgery. This is yet another evidence of wide disparities in the availability of health facilities in India.

Patterns of Growth in Health Care Delivery—1957-1975

Notwithstanding the fact that all the states could not be considered in the evaluation of the growth of health care delivery due to the problems related with the changes in the political boundaries, the patterns do reveal that sufficient growth both in the number of hospitals and beds took place in northern and southern regions (Table 20.9). The central region is completely neglected to the extent that hospital/population ratio which was 13 in 1957 fell to 9 in 1975. Growth rates in per cent for hospitals and beds range between 33 and 600 and 88 and 243 respectively in the southern region. In contrast there is a growth of only 9 per cent in the number of beds in the central region. Barring Andaman & Nicobar, the number of beds rose in all the states with the lowest 9 per cent increase in Madhya Pradesh and 567 per cent in Bihar, although in terms of bed/population ratio Bihar lagged behind. The hospital/population ratio also fell in Manipur, West Bengal and Rajasthan. Thus, with few exceptions the growth of hospital and bed facilities is recorded in most of the states, the increase is considerable in the southern and northern regions.

While talking about the pattern of the growth of health facilities, it should be noted that the growth of population is considerably lower than the health facilities. However, the uneven distribution of health facilities resulted in the wide disparities in different regions.

	Total of 1957	Total of 1975	Percentage Growth
Population	437202747	547949809	25
Hospitals	2265	6596	191
Beds	139862	460886	230
Doctors	88389	162814	84

From the above it can be seen that only 25 per cent population growth is recorded during 1957-75 while the number of hospitals, beds and doctors rose by 191, 230 and 84 per cent respectively.

Besides there are variations in the growth of bed and hospital facilities in different urban areas.

It may be pointed out that as regards the growth in the number of beds is concerned, Bombay recorded a highest per cent that is 134,

Table 20.9: Pattern of Health Care Delivery 1957 and 1975
Number of Hospitals per 10,00,000 Population
Number of Beds per 1,00,000 Population

	Hospitals		*Growth in*	*Beds*		*Growth in*
	1957	*1975*	*Per cent*	*1957*	*1975*	*Per cent*
Northern Region						
1. Bihar	1	4	300	6	40	567
2. Uttar Pradesh	5	8	60	23	39	113
3. Delhi	12	15	25	201	314	56
North-Eastern Region						
4. Manipur	27	17	–37	50	108	116
Eastern Region						
5. West Bengal	10	8	–20	70	101	44
6. Orissa	10	12	20	25	46	84
Central Region						
7. Madhya Pradesh	8	6	–25	33	36	9
Western Region						
8. Rajasthan	13	9	–31	39	63	61
Southern Region						
9. Karnataka (Mysore)	6	8	33	42	101	140
10. Kerala	5	35	600	59	202	242
11. Tamil Nadu (Madras)	5	9	80	51	96	88
12. Andhra Pradesh	5	14	180	30	76	153
13. Pondicherry	11	23	109	226	475	110
Islands						
14. Andaman & Nicobar	15	113	653	611	481	–21

Note: Several states in different regions have not been included due to the changes in the political boundary during 1957 and 1975, thus data is not comparable.

Sources: 1. *The Directory of Hospitals in India,* Directorate General of Health Services, Ministry of Health, New Delhi, 1959.

2. *Directory of Hospitals in India,* 1978, C.B.H.I, Directorate General of Health Services, Ministry of Health and Family Welfare, New Delhi, 1978.

Urban Centres	Beds per 1,00,000 Population		Growth Per cent	Hospitals per 10,00,000 Population		Growth Per cent
	1957	1975		1957	1975	
Bombay	128	300	134	11	10	–9
Calcutta	273	392	44	18	19	6
Delhi	161	266	65	9	12	33
Madras	301	438	46	9	11	22

the lowest being 44 in Calcutta. The growth in hospital facilities varies between 6 per cent in Calcutta and 22 per cent in Madras with Bombay reveals a downward growth.

As it has been already observed that there are wide imbalances in the distribution of health facilities between urban/ rural areas, the urban and rural shares in the population and health facilities have also been studied.

	Urban	Rural	All
Population*	20%	80%	100%
Hospitals**	74%	26%	100%
Beds***	87%	13%	100%
Doctors+	70%	30%	100%

Source: * 1971 Census population
** Data for 1975
*** Data for 1975
+ W.H.O. World Health of Statistics Annual Report, 1972, Vol. III, Geneva, W.H.O., 1976.

It is evident from the above that rural areas with about 80 per cent of the total population manage to get only one-third of the total hospitals, one-seventh of total beds and a little less than half of the total doctors in the country.

Conclusions and Suggestions

The study highlights that there are wide imbalances in the availability of health facilities in different regions, not only in rural/urban areas but even rural to rural and urban to urban variations are evident. Although considerable growth in health facilities is recorded, the uneven distribution has resulted in the disparities in their availability.

Regionally developed areas enjoy high per capita expenditure on health at the expense of rural and undeveloped areas. Villagers have to travel large distance in order to get health care, though villages constitute about 80 per cent of the total population. This is because the population of the areas has not been considered for the purpose of health planning and also the hospitals and health centres are not ideally located.

In order to provide better health care to the people, the disease structure of the area[16] and the health behaviour of the population have to be studied before making any decision of the amount and the type of health care for a region. It has been reported that there is a considerable increase in the incidence of cancer in Punjab and therefore, the region requires a number of cancer hospitals equipped with modern techniques of diagnosis and treatment.[17] Similarly, *kala-azar*, leprosy and filaria prone areas of eastern Uttar Pradesh and Bihar need hospital facilities to treat such health problems. Goitre in the *tarai* and mountainous areas and guinea worm disease in Rajasthan are particular examples in this context.

Health behaviour of a population in different parts has been studied by a number of scholars. Studies by Carstairs in rural Rajasthan[18], and McKim Marriott in a north Indian village[19] highlight the fact that it is no good to provide health facilities based on western medicine to those who have faith in traditional or folk medicine. Such health facilities remain unutilized. Similar evidences were found in Bhardwaj's study in rural Punjab[20] and by Bahuguna in the Himalayan villages.[21]

Besides the means of communications and transport are important to be considered as patients prefer easily accessible hospital or health centre for treatment. In another study,[22] the author found out that villagers in the mountainous area prefer to walk down 10-15 kilometres in the valley area to reach a health centre and do not utilize the facility located about 3 kilometres away from their home as it involves climbing up and down the high ridge. Similar is the case with the plain area. Patients travel longer distance where good transport facilities are available.

To sum up, the following aspects may be considered in order to provide better health care to the people:

1. Health planning should be based on population.
2. Traditional medicine be given importance.

3. Establishment of general as well as special hospitals in rural areas.
4. Compulsory service for doctors in the rural areas. Benefits in terms of money and position if serving tribal and inaccessible areas. Posting of a doctor in such areas as a punishment be stopped.
5. General 3 years medical course be introduced in order to avoid emigration.
6. Community health worker scheme is a good beginning. however, the selection procedure is biased in favour of the powerful group or the upper caste.
7. Hospitals and health centres be located centrally, particularly in rural areas though surely there has to be a trade-off between decentralization and the range of facilities provided.

Acknowledgements

Authors are deeply grâteful to Professor A.T.A. Learmonth of the Open University for his constructive suggestions. Also thankful to Professor N.R. Fendall of the Liverpool School of Tropical Medicine for his comments, although we do not agree to his opinion. We are deeply grateful to Prof. R. Mansell Prothero and the Leverhulme Trust for providing us opportunity to carry out this research work in Liverpool. Acknowledgement is also made of assistance regarding data and material received from the Director, Central Bureau of Health Intelligence, Ministry of Health and Social Welfare, New Delhi, and the Librarian, School of Tropical Medicine, Liverpool.

Notes

1. Ramasubban, R. (1982), *Public Health and Medical Research in India: Their Origin under the Impact of British Colonial Policy,* SAREC Report No. R4 : Swedish Agency for Research Co-operation with Developing Countries, Goteborg, 1982.
2. *Royal Sanitary Commission Report* (1859), Vols. I and II, 1863, p. 31.
3. Banerji, D. (1981), The Place of Indigenous and Western Systems of Medicine in the Health Services of India, *Social Science and Medicine,* 15A, 100.
4. Ramasubban, R., *op. cit.,* pp. 42-43.
5. *Ibid.,* p. 43.

6. Quoted from Gale, G.W. (1965), Some Factors Affecting Rural Health Services in Developing Countries, *The Lancet,* II, 697.
7. Brownlea, A. (1981), From Health to Political Epidemiology, *Social Science and Medicine,* 15D, 57-68.
8. Ministry of Information and Broadcasting, *India Annual, 1980,* p. 98, New Delhi.
9. Mejia, A. Pizurki, H. and Royston, E. (1979), *Physician and Nurse Migration: Analysis and Policy Implications,* p. 277. Geneva: W.H.O.
10. Seventy per cent Medical Graduates Unemployed in Bihar, *The Times of India,* 29th June, New Delhi, 1982.
11. Barrett, A. (1977), *An Introduction to the Health Planning and Budgeting Systems in India,* pp. 6-7, Discussion paper, Institute of Development Studies, Brighton: University of Sussex, December.
12. Barrett, A., *op. cit.,* p. 12.
13. Djukanovic, V. and Mach, E.P. (eds.) (1975), *Alternative Approaches to Meeting Basic Health Needs in Developing Countries: A Joint UNICEF/WHO Study,* p. 85, Geneva: W.H.O.
14. Open Heart Surgery in 18 Hospitals, *The Times of India,* 25th October, 1982, New Delhi.
15. The Arab Patients and the Indian Doctor, *The Times of India,* 20th June, 1982, New Delhi.
16. Diseases Prevalent among Miners, *The Times of India,* 27th April, New Delhi, 1982, Agate Workers Suffer from Lung Diseases, *The Times of India,* 6th May, 1982, New Delhi.
17. Cancer Incidence up in Punjab, *The Times of India,* 22nd February, 1979, New Delhi.
18. Carstairs, G.M. (1955), Medicine and Faith in Rural Rajasthan, In *Health, Culture and Community,* pp. 107-134 (Edited by Paul, B.D.) New York: Russel Sage Foundation.
19. Marriott McKim, Western Medicine in a Village of Northern India, in Paul, B.D. (ed.) *op. cit.,* pp. 239-268.
20. Bhardwaj, S.M. (1975), Attitude Toward Different Systems of Medicine: A Survey of Four Villages in Punjab—India, *Social Science and Medicine,* 9, 603-612.
21. Bahuguna, A. (1981), Attitudes of People Towards the Medical Care Amenities in a Mountain Environment—A Case Study of Two Villages in Garhwal, *Himalaya: Man and Nature,* July, 14-17.
22. Akhtar, R. (1978), Health Facilities in Almora District of Kumaon Himalayas. Also see, Spatial Distribution of Health Facilities in Rajasthan, *Geographical Review of India,* 40, 206-214.

21

A Simple Method of Obtaining a Health Hazard Index and its Application in Micro-regional Health Planning*

B.N. Mukherjee

Introduction

A simple procedure has been described in this chapter to solve the problem of identifying settlements or villages within a block or a district which are in need of extra health facilities. The advantages of this technique are that it is based on readily available data for different settlements, does not require the use of a computer, and provides a simple method of assessing the relative level of health need that is more objective than simple intuitive ranking. It should be noted that the term "health" is used in this chapter mainly to imply well-being, robustness, vitality and similar connotations.

* This chapter arises as a part of health planning exercises performed in connection with the activities of Central Research Cell of the Pilot Research Project in Growth Centres, a scheme administered by the Department of Community Development, Ministry of Agriculture, Government of India, New Delhi. The findings and views expressed in this chapter should not be construed as necessarily the same as those of the Government or any organisation with which the author is affiliated. The author assumes sole responsibility for all opinions, interpretations, and conclusions presented in this chapter. However, he is thankful to Mr. K.G. Krishna Murthy for his computational assistance and to Mr. K. Venkataramani and Mr. V.K. Agarwal for their help in processing some of the data reported here.

Reprinted from *Regional Studies,* **10,** 105-122, 1976.

This chapter does not concern itself with the planning of the details of a health services delivery system. Nor does it deal with the conceptual and operational problems of health and health services. The main purpose is to describe a rapid—approximate method of deriving a health hazard index from a simple weighing technique based on arbitrary assignment of weights to a set of health related variables. The health hazard index can be used for deciding which villages do require additional health care facilities. An attempt has also been made to show how factor analysis could be used as an alternative approach to solve the same problem. Instead of assigning arbitrary weights, one can determine the weights from the results of factor analysis and component analysis. Weights obtained from the use of factor analysis as well as component analysis have been compared to the arbitrary weights using data from twenty study areas. The *pros* and *cons* of factor analysis are also discussed in this chapter.

The Proposed Technique

Since one of the purposes of the health planning exercise was to identify the settlements where the status of health would need extra care, attempts were made to construct an index of health hazard by aggregating various health related indicators. Four sets of variables which were readily available for 20 different blocks covered under the Pilot Research Project in Growth Centres, Government of India, were chosen parsimoniously for the index construction. These are described below.

Variables used in the Index Construction

The following four sets of variables were identified for each village or settlement and used in the present study to establish the relative need for extra health services among the different villages.

(i) *Demographic Variables*
   - (a) Total number of women (1971 Census).
   - (b) Percentage of Female Literacy (1971 Census).

(ii) *Distance (Accessibility) Variables*
   - (a) Distance in km. to the nearest primary health centre (PHC) or hospital irrespective of whether the facilities are in or outside the block.

(b) Total distance in km. to the nearest railway station or a fast moving transportation system in wet season.

(c) Distance in km. to regular bus stop in wet season.

(iii) *Existing Health Care Facilities*

(a) Percentage of assisted birth (by doctor or at hospital).

(b) Total doctor's visit per 1,000 population.

(iv) *Present Health Problems*

(a) Death rate per 1,000 population.

(b) Infant mortality rate per 1,000 live births.

The nine measures described above were selected not only because they were readily available but also closely approximated the various information considered significant in measuring the relative need for health facilities. While it would have been possible to include other variables, the above were considered more or less sufficient and avoided the problem of duplication. For example, the medium *per capita* income of families in a settlement is positively correlated with percentage of female literacy in that settlement. As such, the former variable was not included in the analysis. Similarly, the number of children below 5 years old is highly correlated with the number of women in that settlement. As such, only one of the variables was considered sufficient for the analysis. The latter variable was finally chosen because it could be readily available from the 1971 Census data.

The Problem of Weighing

The main problem encountered in the formulation of a suitable index for solving the health facility location problem was the question of assigning relative weights to be given to the variables chosen for this purpose. In order to obtain a composite relative health hazard index, each variable ideally should receive no greater weight than its share of influence. Two criteria were adjudged important in this connection; the amount of influence a variable would have by itself and the extent to which it correlated with other variables in the set, thus introducing a built-in bias or overlapping influence.

A basic principle underlying the weighing system was that weights must be assigned to minimize overlapping influences. Factors which on conceptual grounds are supposed to be inversely related to the need for extra health facilities were assigned nagative weights. Examples of such variables are the: (a) percentage of assisted births, (b) percentage of female literacy in the settlement, and (c) total number of doctor's visit.

The weights arbitrarily assigned to the different variables are shown in Table 21.1.

Rationale for the Weights

The rationale for the weighing system adopted for the study and shown in Table 21.1 is explained as follows:

Table 21.1: Arbitrary Weights Assigned to Various Variables for Computing a Health Hazard Index

Sl. No.	*Variable*	*Weight*
(1)	Infant mortality per 1,000 live births	5
(2)	Total distance from the nearest PHC or hospital	5
(3)	Death rate per 1,000 population	4
(4)	Numbor of women, 1971 Census	3
(5)	Total distance to regular bus stop	2
(6)	Total distance to railway station during wet season	2
(7)	Percentage of assisted birth by doctor and/or hospital	–1
(8)	Total doctor's visit	–1
(9)	Percentage of female literacy	–2

Since the settlements which are presently far away from the existing health centres (mainly PHC or hospital) of that area need additional centres in their vicinity, variable No. 2 (Distance from the nearest PHC or hospital) received a weight of 5 points. In order to emphasize the health status of the community, infant mortality rate was assigned a weight of 5 points. The total death rate was adjudged the next most important factor determining the need for extra health facilities. So, this variable was assigned a weight of 4. Although indicators such as infant mortality rate (IMR), death rate are affected by purely demographic phenomena, still they directly reflect the health status. In addition, these indicators also suggest indirectly the level of possible utilization of health services. Since the possible utilization of health service is also a linear function of population size, the number of women in the age group 15-45 years was considered the next most important variable. A weight of 3 was assigned to the number of women in a settlement.

The two general distance variables, i.e. distance to regular bus stop and distance to major transport system during the rainy season, were given a weight of 2 each. Since female literacy is supposed to be positively related to maternal health child care and home sanitation (see Table 21.2), it appears reasonable to consider the settlements having a relatively higher percentage of illiterate females deserve a greater attention for health facilities than settlements where the percentage of female literacy is higher. For this reason, a negative weight of –2 was assigned to female literacy rate. Percentage of assisted births (by doctors and/or at hospital) and total number of doctor's visits to the settlement were considered as part of the existing health facilities. Thus, these two variables received a negative weight of one point each.

Calculation of a Health Hazard Index

The first step in the calculation of an index for health hazard is the ranking of all Number of settlements in the block (or district) for each of the characteristics (variables) listed in Table 21.1. If a particular variable is missing, an attempt is made to replace it by a variable which is supposed to be highly correlated with this variable.

In the actual assignment of rank for each settlement with respect to a given attribute (characteristic), the highest rank (the lowest positive integer, that is unity) is given to that settlement which scores highest on a particular variable. However, for all practical purposes, calculation of decile scores for each settlement with respect to each variable is considered satisfactory. Although the conversion of a raw score from the sample observations to a decile score results in some amount of information loss, the loss can be allowed in view of the gain in computational short cut.

The decile rank* corresponding to a raw score, when multiplied by 10, represents an approximate per cent of cases in a comparison

* Decile *points* and decile *ranks* are two different values. If lowest 10 per cent of the settlements have scores (on a particular variable) which are less than a particular value (point), that *value* is the 10th percentile, or the first decile point. Thus, a decile point is a value of the variable below which a certain percentage of cases fall, the percentage being taken in units of 10. Decile ranks are transformed values corresponding to the decile points and take the integer values ranging from 1 to 10. The median is the 5th decile (point). Any value equal to or below the median will have a decile score (rank) of 5 or below.

Table 21.2: Product moment Correlation between Two Mortality Variables and Certain Socio-Demographic Variables: by Study Area

Study Area	*Sample Size*	*Correlation between Infant Mortality and*		*Correlation between Death Rate and*	
		Female Literacy	*Female Population*	*Female Literacy*	*Female Population*
01 Andhra Pradesh	28	–0.05	–0.13	–0.12	–0.12
02 Assam	100	–0.20+	0.06	–0.28*	–0.14
03 Bihar	75	–0.21+	–0.03	–0.30*	–0.23*
04 Gujarat	48	–0.06	–0.09	–0.18	–0.25*
05 Haryana	127	0.00	–0.07	0.00	0.17
07 Madhya Pradesh	140	0.12	0.13	0.03	–0.03
08 Parbhani (Maharashtra)	185	0.06	0.05	0.06	0.09
09 Wardha (Maharashtra)	109	–0.11	–0.07	–0.27*	–0.05
10 Meghalaya	148	–0.11	0.05	–0.16+	–0.13
11 Mysore	76	–0.03	–0.19	–0.14	–0.32*
13 Pondicherry	82	–0.04	–0.03	–0.30*	–0.15
14 Punjab	163	0.11	0.16	0.02	–0.21*
15 Rajasthan	124	–0.03	0.01	0.07	0.14
16 Tamil Nadu	59	–0.14	–0.23*	–0.22*	–0.50*
17 Tripura	64	0.12	0.28*	–0.24*	0.13
18 Kadipur (Uttar Pradesh)	171	–0.04	–0.15	–0.03	–0.20
20 West Bengal	113	–0.11	0.08	–0.18+	–0.21*

* Statistically significant from a zero correlation at the 0.01 Level.
\+ Statistically significant from a zero correlation at the 0.05 Level.

group which achieved scores lower than the one cited in terms of multiples of 10. As the name implies, the decile system divides the distribution of scores into 10 parts, ranging from 1 to 10. Thus, if N is the total number of cases in the distribution then the first $N/10$ cases having the ranks of 1, 2, and so on are assigned a decile rank of 10. The next $N/10$ cases are given a decile rank of 9 and so on.

After all the raw scores are converted to decile ranks, it is necessary to check, at least roughly, the accuracy of this transformation. If the total number of settlements is equal to 10 or multiples of it, that is N=10K, then K number of observations will have a decile rank of 1, another K number will have a decile score of 2 and so on.

The procedure for obtaining a weighted health hazard index for each of the settlements is straight forward once the raw scores on each of the p number of variables have been transformed to decile scores. For each settlement, the decile score with respect to each variable is multiplied by the weight corresponding to that variable and the products are added to obtain a total health hazard index for that settlement. Thus, the weighted composite health hazard score, for ith settlement, say, Hi is given by the formula :

$$H_i = \sum_{j=1}^{p} W_j D_{ij} \ (i = 1, 2, \ldots, N \text{ and } j = 1,\ j = 1, 2, \ldots, p) \quad \ldots (1)$$

where W_j is the weight assigned to the ith variable in accordance with values shown in Table 21.1 and D_{ij} is the decile score of ith village on the jth variable. The H_i index represents each ith settlement's degree of health hazard and thus indicates some kind of relative need for extra health facilities.

Table 21.3: Illustration of the Calculation of Health Hazard Index for Bagh Bari Village, Panitola Block, Assam

Statistics	*Serial Number of Health related Variables (1)*								
	1	*2*	*3*	*4*	*5*	*6*	*7*	*8*	*9*
Raw scores = X_{ij}	250	071	7	179	2	3	25	0	21.22
Decile score = D_{ij}	9	5	-5	4	6	2	9	6	7
Weight = W_j	5	5	4	3	2	2	–1	–1	–2
Profit = $W_j D_{ij}$	45	25	20	12	12	4	–9	–6	–14

Sum of the Product = $\sum_{j=1}^{p} W_j D_{ij} = (45+25+20+12+12+4)–(9+6+14)$

Health hazard *index* = $H_j = 118–29 = 89$

It should be noted that H_i score represents an ordinal type of measurement. From the H_i scores, it is thus possible to obtain a priority listing of settlements in terms of their need for health facilities. A settlement scoring, say 170, however, does not necessarily have twice the hazard or need for health facilities as compared to another settlement having H_j of 85.

Health Hazard Index for Settlements of Panitola Block, Assam

In order to illustrate all the steps delineated in the preceding section, the data obtained for the Panitola Block, Assam will be used in this section. Table 21.1A in the Appendix displays the raw data of all the 98 settlements of this block on each of the nine health-rated variables already referred to. In Table 21.2 of the Appendix are given the corresponding decile scores for each of the settlements. Following formula (1), the H_i (health hazard index) scores for each of the 98 settlements are obtained. When i=1, the H_j score, for Bagh Bari (code 001) of Panitola Block is found to be 89 only. Table 21.3 shows the calculation.

After calculating all the 98 health hazard scores, one for each settlement of Panitola Block, these scores are re-ranked from high to low using integer number 1 through N, in case there is no tie. In the case of tie, the mean rank is assigned to each of the tied scores. The next score in the array receives the rank normally assigned to it. Thus, the rank of the scores, for example, 28, 22, 15, 15, 15, 7, 3 would be 1, 2, 4, 4, 4, 6 and 7.

The next step is to select the first K number (K<½N) of settlements which are on the high side of the health hazard and similarly, the last K number of settlements which have low health hazard index. These two groups of settlements are shown in Figure 21.1. Table 21.4 gives a listing of these two groups of settlements along with their corresponding health hazard index and relative rank. It is seen that so far as Panitola Block is concerned, the two groups of settlements shown in Table 21.4 differ distinctly in the expected direction in terms of death rate, distance from the nearest PRC and/or hospital, and to some extent in terms of visit of doctors. But the typology shown in Table 21.4 is not clear with regard to infant mortality rate (IMR). This is so because in Panitola Block, the infant mortality rate is reported to be very low as compared to other study areas. The mean IMR for Panitola Block is 130 as against 152 for Turkaulia Block, Bihar; 139 for Talala Block, Gujarat; 163 for Seloo Block, Maharashtra; 277 for Bishalgarh Block, Tripura; and 180 for Ghazipur Block, Uttar Pradesh, and so on. As a result of heavy concentration of low IMR scores shown by a large number of settlements of Panitola Block, the IMR does not differentiate the two extreme groups of settlements classified on the basis of health hazard scores. With regard to death rate or the distance to the PHC, the two groups are well differentiated as can be seen from Table 21.4. The typology shown in Table 21.4, therefore, not only provides a rough check on the accuracy of the calculation of the health hazard index but also shows how meaningfully the index serves the purpose of classification.

Table 21.4: Typology-based on Ranking in Terms of Health Hazard Index of First 20 Villages having Poor Status and Last 20 Villages of Panitola Block having almost Satisfactory Status

Code	Village Name	Health Hazard Index	Health Hazard Rank	Is PHC Distance more than 7 kms?	Is Infant Mortality Rate more than 125 ?	Is Death Rate more than 10?	At least one Doctor Visit?
098	Silikhaguri	159	01	Yes	Yes	Yes	No
029	Dharia Raitak	157	02	Yes	Yes	*No**	No
060	Nunpuria Kaiborta	152	03	Yes	Yes	Yes	No
081	Okanimoria Bengali	152	04	Yes	Yes	Yes	*Yes*
076	Nephaphu	150	05	Yes	Yes	Yes	No
079	Menpuria Bengali	148	06	Yes	Yes	Yes	No
094	Rangmala	139	07	Yes	Yes	*No*	*Yes*
002	Bans Bari	134	08	Yes	Yes	Yes	No
055	Khari Katia	134	09	Yes	Yes	Yes	*Yes*
050	Kamhato Habi Gaon	132	10	Yes	Yes	Yes	No
021	Charaichungi Gaon	131	11	Yes	Yes	Yes	No
072	Nadua Gohain Gaon	128	12	*No*	Yes	Yes	No
084	Pakharijania	127	13	Yes	Yes	*No*	No
031	Dighalibari	126	14	*No*	Yes	*No*	No
030	Dhekiajuri	123	15	Yes	Yes	*No*	*Yes*
014	Boragdhi	122	16	Yes	Yes	Yes	No
059	Luhali	122	17	Yes	Yes	*No*	No
089	Piparatali Gaon	119	18	Yes	Yes	No	No
058	Kumar Gaon	118	19	Yes	Yes	Yes	No

(Contd.)

Table 21.4 (*Contd.*)

078	Now Gaon	117	20	Yes	Yes	Yes	*Yes*
054	Kath Gaon	064	79	*Yes**	No	No	*Yes*
071	Murari Pathar	063	80	*Yes*	No	No	*Yes*
097	Sessakash Gaon	062	81	No	No	No	*Yes*
025	Chungi Chuck	061	82	No	*Yes*	No	No
045	Jugi Pathar	061	83	No	*Yes*	No	No
028	Dharia Gaon	058	84	*Yes*	No	No	No
049	Kailabari Gaon	058	85	No	*Yes*	No	No
039	Gandhia Naharam	056	86	No	No	No	No
073	Nadhua Grantgaon	049	87	No	No	No	No
043	Hatkhola Bengali Gaon	047	88	No	No	No	*Yes*
062	Merili Pathar	047	89	No	No	No	No
075	Nalanihola	046	90	No	No	No	No
005	Balijan Paniera	045	91	No	No	No	*Yes*
009	Betmela	044	92	No	No	No	*Yes*
051	Kanji Khowa Bengali	044	93	No	No	No	No
036	Dinjay Satra	043	94	No	No	No	*Yes*
023	Chetia Gaon	035	95	No	No	No	*Yes*
024	Chetia Pathar	035	96	No	No	No	*Yes*
065	Morankari	022	97	No	No	No	*Yes*
048	Kadamoni Gaon	009	98	No	No	No	No

* Italicised responses are indicative of incongruent situation.

The typology such as the one shown in Table 21.4 helps one in identifying settlements, if any, which might be near the primary health centre (PRC) or a hospital within 7 km. distance and still have a high health hazard index. For example, it is seen from Tables 21.4 and 21.1 that Naduajohain Gaon is not even 5 km. from the nearest PRC and yet, the settlement has relatively higher infant mortality and death rates than other settlements of Panitola Block. Identification of these types of anomalous elements encourages one to look into the motivational aspects of health services utilization.[1]

Use of Health Hazard Index for Planning Purposes

One important advantage in the classification of settlements in the high group on the basis of health hazard index is that it shows some spatial groupings in the block map (as displayed in Fig. 21.1). For a rational planning one may then determine the distances of the settlements falling in the high group from the nearest centre which

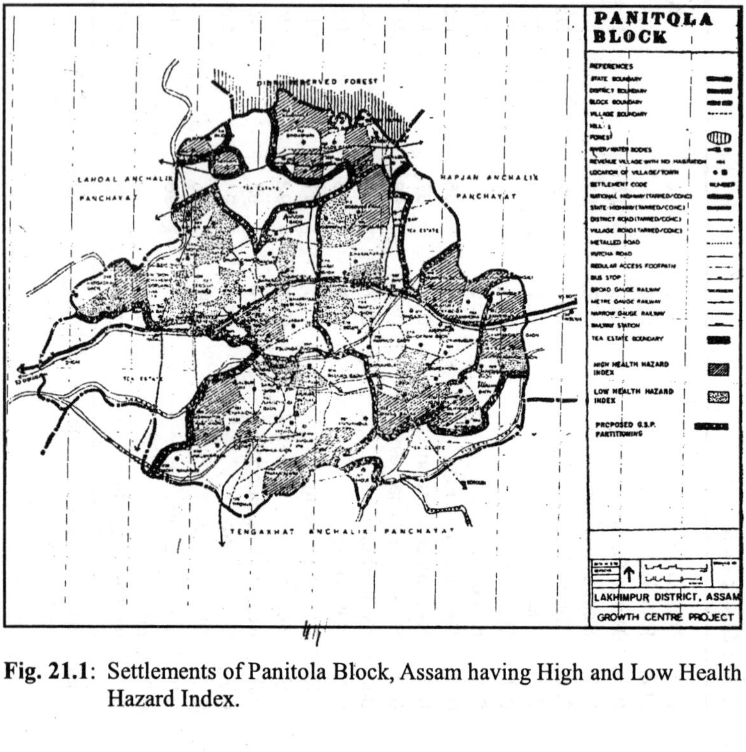

Fig. 21.1: Settlements of Panitola Block, Assam having High and Low Health Hazard Index.

may be existing or proposed under the General Settlement Plan (GSP). In the case of Panitola Block, it seems possible, for example, to partition the entire block into four sub-regions following a set-covering computer programme written in Fortran IV which determines the minimum number of centres and optimal spatial location for every given value of a maximum travel distance (*D* max.). This set-covering algorithm has been described by Banerji and Fisher.[2] Using a criterion of 10 km. maximum travel distance, it is found that in addition to the existing facility in Hatkhola Bengali Gaon (Code No. 43), three more facilities (centres) are required, namely, one each at Panitola (087), Buraguda (014) and Balijan Gaon (004). On the basis of this set-covering solution, the GSP partitioning of this Panitola Block into four sub-regions may be done, keeping in view the accessibility and other optimal utilization considerations. Such a partitioning has been attempted using thick broken lines in the block map shown in Figure 21.1. It is to be noted in this connection that instead of Balijan Gaon (004), Rangchangi Town (093) is probably more suitable for the location of a new facility both in terms of number of socio-economic institutions and populations. For thc same reasons, a new facility at Bindhakata (012) is more preferable to the location of Buragadha (014).

For the purpose of planning, information on the travel distance of the settlements falling in any particular sector from the new facility (centre) proposed within this sub-region under such a GSP partitioning should be also obtained and presented in a tabular form as in Table 21.5. Since both population and distance considerations are important for deciding the justification of having a new facility, it is desirable to include these information in table. Table 21.5 has been presented as an example in this context.

It is seen from Appendix A.1 that both Hatkhola Bengali and Panitola Town have some health care facilities. Therefore, there is no question of proposing any new health centres at these places. One can, however, recommend for the improvement in the quality of these existing centres. If any new health centres are to be constructed for the Panitola Block, then one should consider the feasibility of having these new centres located at Rangchangi Town (093) and Bindhakata (012). Both these proposed centres are identified as possible growth centres in the GSP. In terms of priority, probably the argument in favour of opening the centres first in Rangchangi Town and subsequently at Bindhakata is more convincing mainly in terms of

Table 21.5: Population and Distance of 20 Settlements in and Around Rangchangi Town, Panitola Block

Code	Settlements in and around Rangchangi Town	Distance from Rangchangi Town (km.)	Population (1971)	Total No. of Existing Institutoins*	Health Hazard Index
004	Balijan Gaon	4.0	254	6	117
021	Charaichungi Gaon	2.8	191	0	126
022	Charichungihabi	3.8	453	2	121
024	Chatia Pathar	5.2	520	4	035
033	Dikomnaharani	7.1	282	7	079
050	Kamhatar Habi Gaon	5.2	90	1	132
052	Kaphua Gaon	2.5	644	2	111
059	Luhali	3.3	746	3	122
061	Matai Khona	5.1	1176	3	094
064	Miri Hola	0.8	146	0	065
070	Murani Anguri	1.5	668	7	080
071	Murani Pathar	1.2	123	0	063
084	Pakharijania	4.2	722	5	122
088	Patlungmara	4.9	183	1	094
093	Rangchangi Town	0.0	547	7	073
095	Sarupathar	3.1	86	0	116
096	Sarupathar Gaon	2.3	74	1	097
097	Sessakash Gaon	4.1	234	3	062
100	Tipomia	4.4	689	3	106
102	Udalguri	3.5	490	5	076
	Average	**3.45****	**416†**	**3.00†**	**95.5††**

* Total number of various kinds of social institutions, such as, banks, dispensaries, schools, health centres etc. which are presently existing. The total is not weighted by the number of institutions under each category.

** Median.

† Arithmetic Mean.

†† Settlements having a high hazard index.

utilization prospects, spatial and population criteria. The average distance of all the 20 settlements in the south sub-region from the proposed Rangchangi centre will be about 4 km, as can be seen from Table 21.5. It will serve 20 settlements covering a total of 8320 people, almost one-sixth of the population of entire Panitola Block (excluding the inhabitants of the tea estates). Thus, the proposal of having a new sub-health centre at Rangchangi is not inconsistent with the minimum need approach. According to the minimum standard fixed for the

Fifth National Plan, there should be one public health centre for a block population of 80,000-1,00,000 supported by 8-10 sub-centres, each serving a population of 10,000. In addition to one primary health centre presently located at Kanjikhowa Bengali (Code 051), there are only two dispensaries and two hospitals in the entire Panitola Block excluding the various tea estates which are exclusively open to tea estate employees. The doctors at the tea estates are available to villagers of the adjoining villages only under exceptional circumstances and that too rarely for humanitarian reasons. The hospital located in Hatkhola Bengali (Code 043) is quite far from settlements near Rangchangi Town. Figure 21.1 also shows that compared to the other three sub-regions, the south sub-region of Panitola Block is, on the whole, at a greater risky situation so far as health hazard is concerned. As such it seems reasonable to propose tentatively for an upgraded type of new sub-health centre (SHC) in Rangchangi Town under the charge of a Medical Officer with provisions of at least 10 beds, adequate medicines and supporting staff. Such a sub-health centre* is likely to fulfil in general the health care need of the south sub-region of Panitola Block and in particular the six settlements situated near the Rangchangi Town which are found to score very high on the health hazard continuum, as can be seen from Table 21.5 and Figure 21.1.

Refinement in the Choice of Variables

Since analysis of household questionnaire data revealed that the number of women in the settlement has pretty low correlation with utilization of PRC, Hospital or SHC, the former variable was dropped from the weighing system and thus the calculation of health hazard index was based on eight variables. The weight for each variable remained the same as assigned before.

With the exclusion of the number of women variable, very little change, however, occurred with respect to the conclusion previously reached with regard to Panitola, Assam. The calculation of health hazard index on the basis of eight variables showed that out of the 20 settlements listed as hazard villages in Table 21.2, 18 have high health

* There is not a single sub-health centre (SHC) in the entire Panitola Block as on March 1974.

hazard index. Only two villages namely, Dighalbari (031) and Luhali (059) which had rank of 14 and 17 respectively obtained rank of 23 and 26 on the basis of the new 8 variable system. Under the new system, Luhali is replaced by Muluk Gaon (069) and a new settlement, Sarupathar (095) obtains a rank of 13. Thus, the conclusions arrived at with respect to the spatial conglomeration of health hazard area remains more or less unaltered on the basis of calculation made from 8 variables.

Application of Factor Analysis and Component Analysis

The technique illustrated above uses a procedure where an *arbitrary* system of weighing is involved in the calculation of a composite score. The problem of assigning weights to the various characteristics can also be solved by the application of factor analysis.[3] Factor analysis offers an objective solution to this problem because the factor loadings can be used as weights since "a loading is a weight for each factor dimension measuring the variance contribution the factor makes to the data vector".[4] In a sense, the factor loadings can be interpreted like correlation coefficients. Thus, if a particular variable has a loading of say, 0.90 on a particular factor (theoretical or hypothetical variable), then it can be said that the variable has a great deal of involvement with that hypothetical factor. Interested readers are referred to the discussion of the concepts, assumptions and applications of factor analysis appearing in Fruchter[5], Broadbent[6], and Rummel.[7] The application of factor analysis and the computational procedure involved in studying the comparability of the arbitrary weights used here in the calculation of the health hazard and factor loading are described elsewhere in detail.[8]

In an attempt to look more rigorously for patterns and relationships between groups of hazard-rated variables and groups of settlements, principal component analysis[9] was also performed. Principal component analysis is relatively a straight-forward method of transforming a given set of variables into a new set of composite variables or principal components that are independent of each other. The loadings (coefficients) on the first principal components can be viewed as mathematically unique weights. The use of these weights produces a set of linear composite scores which provide the single best summary of linear relationships exhibited in the data. The coefficients for the second principal component similarly provide the weights for computing the second best linear combination of variables under the condition that the second component is orthogonal (uncorrelated) with the first component and the second one must account for the proportion of variance in the data not accounted for by the first one.

The loadings (coefficients) on the hazard-rated variables for the first as well as the second principal components were compared in this study with the arbitrary weights shown in Table 21.1. For the purpose of examining the degree of congruence of two sets of scores, component scores obtained from the results of principal component analysis were compared with the composite health hazard scores.

The loadings from principal component analysis and factor analysis were derived using a computer programme without any *a priori* assumptions about the relationships between variables as in the case of arbitrary weights. However, in the case of factor analysis, the determination of communalities for different variables is one of the most ambiguous tasks in factor analysis. No such ambiguity is inherent in the principal component analysis. Therefore, both principal component analysis and factor analysis were used in this study for the factorization (decomposition) of the intercorrelation matrix and to derive the weights. "In component analysis, this factorization is unique, for the component coefficients have been chosen to partition the total variance orthogonally into successively smaller portions, and if the portions are distinct, only one set of coefficient vector will accomplish this purpose. This uniqueness of component coefficients is frequently overlooked by some investigators."[10]

Calculation of the Composite Score from Factor Weights

As mentioned above, the factor loadings of the different variables on the first principal-axis factor can be used as weights for corresponding variables for the purpose of obtaining a composite health need index. To determine the composite score for a particular settlement on the first principal-axis factor, the settlements data (after transforming the raw score data to standard scores such that the standardized data matrix, Z, of order $p \times N$ when post multiplied by its transpose, Z' and then divided by N will yield the correlation matrix, R, i.e. $ZZ'/N=R$) on each of the variables is multiplied by the factor weight for the variable given by the first column of factor loading matrix, A*. The sum of these weight-times-standard score products for all the variables yields a very gross estimate of factor scores.[+] Settlements showing high factor scores on the first principal-axis factor in this study will therefore represent those places which need extra health facilities.

Table 21.6: First Principal-axis Loadings for Three Different Study Areas

Variable	*Loadings on the First Principal-axis*		
	*Aska**	*Panitola*	*Suwana (Rajasthan)*
Infant mortality rate	0.81194	0.49303	0.00958
Distance to PHC	0.25921	0.23097	0.33934
Death rate	0.63927	0.89789	–0.14370
Number of women	—	–0.23576	–0.69592
Distance to bus stop	0.35266	0.02501	0.48478
Distance to railway station	0.39355	0.40502	0.47499
Percentage of assisted births	–0.08448	–0.04484	–0.31073
Doctor's visit	–0.31434	–0.11380	–0.53855
Female literacy rate	–0.02761	–0.44140	–0.25266

* Based on Eight Variables. Information on Number of Women was not Available for Aska.

---

* The factor matrix is a table with p number of rows aud r number of columns. In matrix notation, the reduced correlation matrix, R* which is a symmetric matrix of order $p \times p$ was decomposed as below:

$$R^* = O\wedge^2 O'$$
$$= O\wedge\wedge' O'$$
$$= A^* A^{*'}$$

where A* is a $p \times r$ factor loading matrix ($r<p$). $\wedge^2$ is a diagonal matrix of characteristic roots with a rank of r, and O is an orthogonal matrix, i.e. $OO' = Ip$. In the example under reference, i.e. Aska data, $p = 8$ and $r = 4$.

[+] To estimate the factor scores on the first four principal axis factor, it is recommended to use the following formula written in matrix notation:

$$F^* = (A^{*'} A^*)^{-1} A^{*'} Z = W Z$$

where $(A^{*'} A^*)^{-1}$ is a symmetric matrix of order four and inverse (reciprocal) of the matrix $(A^{*'} A^*)$. The r by p matrix (here $r = 4$ and $p = 8$) can be regarded as a weight matrix given by $W = (A^{*'} A^*)^{-1} A^{*'}$. The score of N settlements on the jth factor $j = 1, 2, \ldots, r$) can be then expressed as

$$fj' = wr'Z$$

where $W'j$ is simply the jth row vector of the weight matrix W.

In the actual calculation of factor scores for each of the 89 villages of Aska Block some departure from the above procedure was made for the sake of computational short-cut. Instead of using the standard scores, the decile scores already obtained were used. So the composite scores for each settlement is the sum total of products between the settlement's decile scores on a particular variable and the corresponding factor weight.

It may be first noted that the principal-axis factor weights compare well with the arbitrary weights as can be seen from Table 21.6. As such, the composite scores obtained through factor weights correspond fairly well the health index obtained by the arbitrary weighing device. The ranks in terms of both these composite scores were calculated along with the difference in the rank (*d*). From these results, the Spearman-Rank difference correlation, also known as rho coefficient, was calculated to examine the amount of correspondence between these two sets of rankings. For the Aska data, the rho correlation is found to be 0.902 which is statistically significant at the 0.001 level. Thus, the simple procedure of obtaining an index of health hazard proved to be quite efficient so far as the Aska study is concerned.

Comparison of Arbitrary Weights with Principal Component Weights

Thus, the analysis of Aska data indicates that the set of weights arbitrarily chosen for the proposed index of health hazard compares favourably with the weights derived objectively by the technique of factor analysis. In order to be further sure about this conclusion, an attempt was made to see the extent of comparability between the set of arbitrary weights and the objective weights derived from the application of principal component analysis.[11] For this purpose, the data from Panitola Block, Assam, was used. For a total of 98 settlements, the intercorrelations among the 9 health variables were obtained to form the matrix, R, which was then subjected to a principal component analysis. The intercorrelation matrix is shown in Table 21.7. The first principal component weights are also shown in the right margin of Table 21.7. The first principal component accounts for 27.01 per cent of the total variance. Following this analysis, scores for all the 98 settlements on the first principal component were obtained using a special computer programme written in Fortran IV for calculation of component scores.* The first principal component scores are shown in Table 21.8 along with the health hazard index for each of the 98 settlements of Panitola Block, Assam. As a measure of agreement between these two sets of scores, the Spearman rho correlation was computed which turned out to be 0.6932. Thus, it appears that the health hazard scores calculated from the weights chosen arbitrarily are not inconsistent with the first principal component scores derived from the weights chosen by the method of principal component. The conclusion is further confirmed by the calculation of first principal component of 89 settlement of Aska Block, Orissa. The Spearman rho correlation between first principal components (which accounted for 24.2% of the total variation) and health hazard index turned out to be 0.9018. A similar confirmation was obtained from the analysis of data for the Bisalgarh (Tripura) Block. The Spearman rho in this case was found to be 0.65 and the first principal component explained 35.35 per cent of the total variation. To demonstrate the justification of using differential weights instead of obtaining a sum of the decile or ranked scores, an additional exercise was performed using the Panitola data. All the 98 settlements of this Block were ranked according to the scores obtained on each of the nine variables. These rank scores for each settlement were summed and on the basis of these composite rank sum scores[12], the settlements were ordered from high to low. This ordering was then compared to the order given by the first principal component calculated from the 9 × 9 intercorrelation matrix. Agreement for Panitola data was quite poor, and this is indicated by a Spearman rho of –0.1683. For the Bisalgarh (Tripura) data, the coefficient turned out to be –0.0473.

Further Validation of the Arbitrary Weighing System

In order to examine the degree of correspondence between the arbitrary weights and the weights derived by the Principal Component

* For obtaining principal component scores on all the 9 components, the computing formula which gives the mathematically "unique" solution can be written as

$$F = A^{-1} Z$$

where F is a $p \times N$ matrix of principal components and A^{-1} is the inverse of the $p \times p$ matrix of coefficients, and Z is the $p \times N$ data matrix in standard score form.

Table 21.7: Product-moment Intercorrelations* among Nine Variables used for Index Construction in Panitola Study, Assam along with their Mean, Standard Deviation and Loading on the First Principal Component (N =98 Settlements)

Variable No.	*Variable Name*	*Serial Number of the Variable*									*Loading⁺ on the First Principal Component*
		1	*2*	*3*	*4*	*5*	*6*	*7*	*8*	*9*	
(1)	Infant mortality rate	1000	033	550	075	–005	051	041	–067	–197	0.567
(2)	Total distance in kilometres from nearest PHC/hospital	033	1000	035	–169	099	422	–029	–017	–038	0.444
(3)	Death rate per 1000	550	035	1000	–169	–058	074	093	–074	–282	0.665
(4)	No. of women, 1971	075	–169	–169	1000	037	–167	237	–159	116	–0.368
(5)	Total distance to regular bus stops	–005	099	–058	037	1000	195	–132	054	002	0.132
(6)	Total distance to railway station	051	422	074	–167	195	1000	–096	–089	–226	0.587
(7)	Percentage of assisted births	041	–029	093	237	–132	096	1000	–131	159	–0.184
(8)	Total doctor's visit	–067	–017	–074	–159	054	–089	–131	1000	143	–0.162
(9)	Percentage of female literacy	–197	–038	–282	116	002	–226	159	143	1000	–0.610
Arithmetic Mean		129.7	6.91	10.7	27.57	2.19	6.62	13.7	0.367	19.5	—
Standard Deviation		128.2	32.2	10.3	169.5	2.98	3.83	25.7	0709	13.3	—

*All decimal points have been omitted from the Correlation Coefficients shown in this table.
⁺Also known as Correlation Coefficients of the first principal component.

Table 21.8: Calculation of the Spearman Rank Order Correlation (rho*) between First Principal Component and Health Hazard Index both Calculated on the Basis of 9 Variables as well as 8 Variables for the Panitola Block, Assam

Place Code	*Component Score*		*Health Hazard Index*		*Ranked Component Score*		*Ranked H.H. Index*		*Rank Diff. (d)*		*(d)²*	
	Nine	*Eight*	*Nine*	*Eight*	*Nine*	*Eight*	*Nine*	*Eight*	*Nine*	*Eight*	*Nine*	*Eight*
001	0.815	1.116	089	077	47	46	56	51	9	5	81	25
002	1.093	1.396	134	116	37	37	08	11	29	26	741	676
003	0.586	0.632	071	056	54	72	42	70	18	2	324	4
004	3.008	3.362	092	083	04	04	54	72	50	38	2,500	1,444
005	–0.446	–0.397	045	024	92	94	91	91	1	3	1	9
006	1.481	1.495	100	091	26	32	42	32	16	—	256	—
007	0.260	1.069	109	082	72	47	30	44	42	3	1,764	9
008	1.517	1.763	101	092	24	22	38	31	14	9	196	81
009	–0.302	–0.096	044	026	91	92	92	90	1	2	1	4
010	0.523	0.930	100	079	59	53	43	48	16	5	256	25
011	0.255	0.590	070	046	73	75	73	79	0	4	0	16
012	1.621	1.948	106	094	21	16	35	28	14	12	196	144
014	1.132	1.687	122	101	35	26	16	20	19	6	361	36
015	0.517	0.779	086	068	60	64	59	59	1	5	1	25
016	0.387	1.259	103	073	65	43	37	53	28	10	784	100
018	0.421	0.902	089	065	64	58	57	64	7	6	49	36
019	0.126	0.229	069	051	79	84	74	76	5	8	25	64
020	1.020	1.055	110	098	38	48	28	24	10	24	100	576
021	2.640	2.761	131	125	05	05	11	08	6	3	36	9

(Contd.)

Table 21.8: (*Contd.*)

022	1.857	1.978	116	101	14	14	21	21	7	7	49	49
023	–0.575	–0.626	035	020	93	95	95	93	2	2	4	4
024	–0.018	–0.044	035	020	84	89	96	94	12	5	114	25
025	0.041	0.404	061	043	82	79	82	83	0	4	0	16
026	1.205	1.443	099	087	32	34	47	38	15	4	225	16
027	0.312	0.993	077	053	70	51	63	75	7	24	49	576
028	0.917	0.957	058	046	43	52	84	80	41	28	1,681	784
029	1.411	2.044	157	127	27	13	02	06	25	7	625	49
030	1.534	1.457	123	117	23	33	15	10	8	23	64	529
031	0.889	1.398	126	099	45	36	14	23	31	13	961	169
032	0.714	0.680	076	067	50	69	65	60	15	9	225	81
033	1.857	1.731	079	070	15	25	62	55	47	30	2,209	900
034	0.378	1.000	116	089	67	50	22	35	45	15	2,025	225
035	0.732	1.555	109	082	48	30	31	45	17	15	289	225
036	–0.811	–0.790	043	019	96	97	44	96	52	15	2,704	225
037	0.911	1.138	096	090	44	45	50	34	6	1	36	1
038	0.152	0.759	110	083	78	66	29	43	49	11	2,401	121
039	–0.259	0.160	056	029	90	85	86	89	04	23	16	529
040	1.689	1686	100	088	19	27	44	36	25	4	625	16
041	1.802	1.758	107	098	17	23	34	25	17	9	289	81
042	0.324	0.439	064	049	69	76	78	78	9	2	81	4
043	–0.887	–0.378	047	020	97	93	88	95	9	2	81	4
044	–0.162	0.628	066	039	88	73	76	84	12	2	144	4

(*Contd.*)

Table 21.8: (*Contd.*)

045	1.173	1.531	061	037	34	31	83	85	49	11	2,401	121
046	0.606	0.727	085	070	53	67	60	56	7	54	49	2,916
047	0.975	0.909	075	066	40	55	68	62	28	11	784	121
048	−1.427	−1.468	009	003	98	98	98	98	0	7	9	49
049	0.383	0.727	058	046	66	66	85	81	19	13	361	169
050	4.800	5.627	132	126	01	01	10	04	9	3	81	9
051	0.175	0.338	044	032	77	80	93	88	16	8	256	81
053	0.220	0.905	105	078	75	57	36	50	39	7	1,521	49
054	0.279	0.088	064	061	71	87	79	66	8	21	64	441
055	2.118	2.097	134	128	07	11	09	05	2	06	4	36
057	0.432	0.421	101	086	63	77	40	39	23	38	529	1,444
058	1.283	1.605	118	106	30	28	19	16	11	12	121	144
059	1.349	1.584	122	098	29	29	17	26	12	3	144	9
060	0.564	0.790	114	096	55	62	25	27	30	35	900	1,225
061	0.732	1.302	109	079	49	42	32	49	17	7	289	49
062	−0.171	0.305	047	023	89	82	89	92	0	10	0	100
063	1.660	2.244	075	045	20	09	69	82	49	73	2,401	5,329
064	0.324	0.057	065	062	74	88	77	65	3	23	9	529
065	−0.785	−0.746	022	013	95	96	97	97	2	1	4	1
066	0.535	1.183	115	085	58	44	24	40	34	4	1,156	16
068	−0.043	0.677	084	054	85	70	61	73	24	3	576	9
069	1.700	1.741	111	105	18	24	27	17	9	7	81	49
070	0.549	0.894	075	054	57	59	70	74	13	15	169	225

(*Contd.*)

Table 21.8: (*Contd.*)

071	0.376	–0.049	063	060	68	90	80	68	12	22	144	484
072	1.243	1.800	128	104	31	21	12	18	19	3	361	9
073	–0.106	0.156	049	034	86	86	87	87	1	1	1	1
074	0.072	0.305	077	059	80	83	64	69	16	14	256	196
075	0.054	0.408	046	037	81	78	90	86	9	8	81	64
076	3.670	3.880	150	141	02	02	05	01	3	1	9	1
077	0.181	0.595	074	056	76	74	71	71	5	3	25	9
078	2.090	2.125	117	111	09	10	20	15	11	5	121	25
079	1.809	2.277	148	127	16	08	06	.07	10	1	100	1
080	0.966	1.810	152	122	41	20	03	09	38	11	1,444	121
081	2.209	2.375	152	137	06	06	04	02	2	4	4	16
082	0.662	0.790	109	091	52	63	33	33	19	30	361	900
083	1.489	1.361	076	070	25	39	66	57	41	18	1,681	324
084	1.870	1.959	127	103	13	15	13	19	0	4	0	16
085	1.185	1.429	100	094	35	35	45	29	12	6	144	36
086	0.031	0.849	096	066	83	61	51	63	32	2	1,024	4
087	–0.670	0.314	100	070	94	81	46	58	48	23	2,304	529
088	2.053	1.943	094	088	10	17	53	37	43	20	1,849	400
089	2.104	2.057	119	116	08	12	18	12	10	0	100	0
090	0.562	0.906	092	071	56	56	55	54	1	2	1	4
091	1.115	1.378	088	067	36	38	58	61	22	23	484	529
092	0.438	0.911	096	075	62	54	52	52	10	2	100	4
093	–0.118	–0.085	068	050	87	91	75	77	12	14	144	196

(*Contd.*)

Table 21.8: (*Contd.*)

094	1.612	1.913	139	112	22	18	07	14	15	4	225	16
095	3.444	3.751	116	113	03	03	23	13	20	10	400	100
096	1.380	1.303	097	094	28	41	48	30	20	11	400	121
097	0.845	0.763	062	056	46	65	81	72	35	7	1,225	49
098	1.962	2.371	159	135	11	07	01	03	10	4	100	16
099	0.936	1.305	097	085	42	40	49	41	7	1	49	1
100	0.981	1.046	101	080	39	49	41	47	2	2	4	4
101	1.892	1.855	113	100	12	19	26	22	14	3	196	9
102	0.516	0.661	076	061	61	71	67	67	6	4	36	16

* Rho for nine variables $= 1 - \dfrac{6\Sigma d^2}{n - n}$

$= 1 - \dfrac{6(48116)}{941014}$

$= 1–0.3068$

$= 0.6932$

Rho for eight variables $= 1 - \dfrac{6\Sigma d^2}{n - n}$

$= 1 - \dfrac{6(25209)}{941094}$

$= 1–0.1607$

$= 0.8393$

Method after eliminating the number of women from the analysis, the intercorrelation matrix between eight variables for Bhoi Block, Meghalaya, was subjected to a principal component analysis and the weights turned out to be almost a monotonic function of the weights chosen arbitrarily (see Table 21.9).

The first principal component for the Meghalaya data, however, explains only 23.05 per cent of the total variation. The first principal component weights and the percentage of total variation accounted for by this component for other eight study areas, are shown in Table 21.10. It is seen from Table 21.10 that the first principal component explains about 22.30 per cent total variation in most analyses. Although this contribution of first principal component is not high enough, it did allow in most cases interpretation of the component when the loadings on the individual variables were inspected. It also allowed a comparison between the arbitrary weights and the principal component weights.

In the case of six study areas, the first principal component showed almost zero loadings on the mortality related variables. For these study areas, the weights on the second component were also selected for the purpose of comparing with the corresponding arbitrary weights. The second principal component weights are shown in Table 21.11 separately for the six study areas.

As a next step, the Spearman rho correlation between the first component scores and the hazard index calculated on the basis of eight variables was computed for Meghalaya and this turned out to be 0.8566.

The above exercise was undertaken for each of the 20 study areas covered under the Growth Centre scheme and except in few cases, the Spearman rho between the component scores and health hazard index turned out to be quite high as can be seen from Table 21.12.

Table 21.12 shows the Spearman rho correlation between health hazard index and first principal components when both these scores were computed on the basis of nine variables as well as eight variables, as has been done in the case of Panitola study (see Table 21.8). It is seen from Table 21.12 that in the case of 13 study areas, the magnitude of correlation is higher when eight variables are used rather than nine variables. Thus, the exclusion of number of women from the analysis appears to have increased the comparability of the arbitrary weights with the principal component weights.

Table 21.9: Product-moment Intercorrelations among Eight Variables used for Index Construction in Bhoi Block Study, Meghalaya, along with their mean, standard deviation and loading on the first principal component

(N = 148 Settlements)

Variable No.	*Variable Name*	*Serial Number of the Variable*								*Loading* on the First Principal Component*
		1	*2*	*3*	*4*	*5*	*6*	*7*	*8*	
(1)	Infant mortality rate	1.000	0.1641	0.3695	–0.0448	–0.1499	0.0303	–0.0402	–0.1092	0.417
(2)	Total distance from nearest PHC/hospital	0.1641	1.0000	0.1054	0.2205	–0.3574	–0.1245	–0.1284	–0.2930	0.685
(3)	Death rate per 1,000	0.3695	0.1054	1.0000	–0.0467	–0.0357	–0.0032	0.0299	–0.1614	0.386
(4)	Total distance to regular bus stop	–0.0448	0.2205	0.0467	1.0000	0.4967	–0.1809	–0.0823	–0.2032	0.325
(5)	Total distance to railway station	–0.1499	–0.3574	–0.0357	0.4967	1.0000	–0.0595	0.0038	0.3203	–0.212
(6)	Percentage of assisted births	0.0303	–0.1245	–0.0032	–0.1809	–0.0595	1.0000	0.1307	0.3203	–0.477
(7)	Total doctor's visit	–0.0402	–0.1284	0.0299	0.0823	0.0038	0.1307	1.0000	0.1915	0.382
(8)	Percentage of female literacy	–0.1092	0.2930	0.1614	0.2032	0.0634	0.3203	0.1915	1.0000	–0.727
Arithmetic Mean		168.0	2.83	17.3	10.7	70.6	4.8	0.3	18.60	—
Standard Deviation		174.0	1.72	15.5	13.2	13.2	32.1	12.7	1.3	—

*Also known as Correlation Coefficients of the First Principal Component.

Table 21.10: First Principal Component Weights* for 8 Health Hazard Variables along with per cent of total Variance Explained in each Case for Different Study Areas

Name of Variable	*First Principal Component Weights for Different Study Areas*							
	Panitola (Assam)	*Turkaulia (Bihar)*	*Seloo (Maharashtra)*	*Harihar** (Mysore)*	*Aska (Orissa)*	*Suwana (Rajasthan)*	*Namakkal (Tamil Nadu)*	*Bisalgarh (Tripura)*
Infant mortality rate	684	578	472	189	660	163	324	–030
Total distance PHC	357	–451	407	530	467	493	006	704
Death rate	727	509	511	497	666	025	513	381
Distance bus stop	093	484	684	564	580	727	814	516
Distance railway station	506	174	780	766	576	653	789	631
Percentage asst. birth	–442	–797	–372	–092	–142	–509	–558	–639
Doctor's visit	–271	–241	–136	–485	–376	–473	–304	090
Female literacy	–612	–586	–506	472	–096	–243	–746	–881
Percentage of total variance accounted	22.98	26.22	26.73	24.21	24.20	22.09	28.81	30.68

*Decimal points have been omitted in each case.
**Now Karnataka.

Table 21.11: Second Principal Component Weights* for Eight Health Hazard variables along with per cent of total Variance Explained in each Case for Different Study Areas

Name of variable	*Second Principal Component Weight for Different Study Areas*					
	Thaneshwar (Haryana)	*Sehore (M.P.)*	*Chamkaur Sahib (Punjab)*	*Kadipur (U.P.)*	*Ghazipur (U.P.)*	*Memari (West Bengal)*
Infant mortality rate	297	859	727	787	784	665
Total distance PHC	807	165	370	122	–018	273
Death rate	191	881	663	864	809	770
Distance bus stop	568	–038	354	066	065	348
Distance railway station	246	055	259	–65	062	144
Assisted birth	061	–207	071	–066	–448	–460
Doctor's visit	–119	–207	–103	576	–376	081
Female literacy	–464	161	–066	013	–003	–192
Percentage of total variance accounted	17.40	20.69	16.47	21.58	20.25	18.84

*Decimal points have been omitted in each case.

Table 21.12: Spearman rho Correlation between Health Hazard Index and Principal Component Scores: by Study Area

Code	Study Area		No. of settlements	Correlation between H.H. Index and Principal Component Scores (9 Variables)		Correlation between H.H. Index and Principal Component Scores (8 Variables)	
	Name of Block	State		1st Component	2nd Component	1st Component	2nd Component
01	Sattenapalli	Andhra Pradesh	27	0.3443	0.5556	0.4127	0.4280
02	Panitola	Assam	98	0.6932	0.1717	0.8393	0.1588
03	Turkaulia	Bihar	75	0.5316	0.1829	0.5180	0.4205
04	Talala	Gujarat	48	0.5134	0.2527	0.6674	0.4193
05	Thaneshwar	Haryana	127	0.5592	0.4324	0.5634	0.6775
07	Sehore	Madhya Pradesh	139	0.3898	0.8391	0.5560	0.7551
08	Basmath	Maharashtra	185	0.4255	0.4664*	0.4589	0.4227+
09	Seloo	Maharashtra	109	0.7209	0.3743	0.8528	0.2582
10	Bhoi	Meghalaya	148	0.7500	0.0571	0.8566	0.0026
11	Harihar	Mysore	76	0.7114	0.0267	0.8055	0.1311
12	Aska	Orissa	89	0.9018	0.0281	0.9018	0.0281
13	Pondicherry	Pondicherry	82	0.6853	0.1384	0.8887	0.0247
14	Chamkaur Sahib	Punjab	163	0.0141	0.6267	0.0019	0.8851
15	Suwana	Rajasthan	124	0.4310	0.6420	0.7253	0.4364
16	Namakkal	Tamil Nadu	59	0.6049	0.1181	0.7528	0.0335
17	Bisalgarh	Tripura	64	0.6467	0.6008	0.8196	0.4258
18	Kadipur	Uttar Pradesh	171	0.6272	0.4501	0.6259	0.6556
19	Ghazipur	Uttar Pradesh	207	0.0273	0.0273	0.0811	0.7040
20	Memari	West Bengal	113	0.5285	0.3048	0.2505	0.8830

* The correlation between the H.H.I. and third principal component for this study area turned out to be 0.6147.

\+ The correlation between the H.H.I. and third principal component for this study area turned out to be 0.6093.

Table 21.12 also indicates that the correspondence between the arbitrary weights and the *first* principal component weights is quite poor for three study areas, namely, Chamkaur Sahib (Punjab), Ghazipur (Uttar Pradesh) and Memari (West Bengal). In each of the above three cases, the first principal component was identified as the distance factor and the second component was interpreted as the mortality variable. Therefore, when the Spearman correlation was calculated between the *second* principal component and the health hazard index, the coefficients turned out to be quite high in each of the above three cases as is seen from Table 21.12. Thus, the Spearman correlations reported in Table 21.12 establish some degree of mathematical equivalence (except for a constant of proportionality) of two sets of weights.

Discussion

The results of the factor analysis reported in this chapter indicate clearly that the weights arbitrarily chosen for the proposed technique of computing a health hazard index, are generally not very different from the weights appearing as first principal-axis loadings. That there is a monotonic relationship between the arbitrary set of weights and the factor loading weights, has been demonstrated for the Aska (Orissa) as well as Bhoi Block data. It has been shown using Aska and Panitola data that the ordering of the settlements within each of these blocks in terms of the proposed health hazard index shows a good deal of agreement with the ranking of these settlements according to composite scores obtained from the principal-axis. weights or according to first principal components. When the units of measurement for each variable are fixed equal (by transforming the scores in standard form), the first principal-axis method has some interesting statistical properties. It minimizes the variance of the composite scores[13], minimizes the differences between the various scores received by a particular settlement[14] and minimizes the generalized variance for all settlements receiving the same score.[15]

Although the use of principal component analysis or the principal-axis method of obtaining factor scores on a general health hazard factor is much more sophisticated than the simple method of index construction proposed here the latter approach is quite flexible in certain ways. For example, deletion of a particular variable in the set of nine variables considered for the analysis will have no effect on the weights of other variables. In the factor analysis approach, the factor weights (loadings) are not invariant under inclusion of any new variable or deletion of some variables from the set.

Furthermore, the characteristic roots (eigenroots) and as such the factor weights are influenced both by the original selection of the variables (which cannot necessarily be a random sample of all the potential variables) and by the varying quality of the data used in the analysis. More importantly, when the sample size is very small, say less than 30, the intercorrelations on the basis of which a factor analysis is run, have high sampling fluctuations. As such, it is not desirable to run a factor analysis unless the sample size is moderately large, say 80 and above. Thus, if factor scores are required for indexing or classifying a small group of settlements (say 30 or less), then the factor analysis approach is not desirable. The method proposed here will be certainly a better alternative approach in such a case.

On the basis of the health hazard index, one can readily identify the first 20 or 25 settlements which are badly in need of additional health care facilities. As a matter of fact, one should choose the first *k* settlements which have high health hazard indices (first *k* rank) and similarly, the last *k* settlements, which are supposed to be relatively better in terms of health care facilities. These two groups of settlements can be plotted geographically on the block map as has been done in Figure 21.1 so that high incidence areas can be located. To check the meaningfulness of the health hazard index, some typology* such as the one shown in Table 21.4 should also be worked out. If the high ranking settlements (having the high health hazard indices) from some spatial clusters, then they should be grouped into sub-areas to ascertain the most appropriate locations where health care facilities should be provided to optimise their utilities. The locations thus determined are then checked up with the minimum standard (as fixed in the fifth plan) to set up a public health centre. Concurrently, or alternatively, one can also check how the locations of the recommended health centres are consistent with proposals for new roads, new schools, etc. If the proposed health centres are found to be located in the higher order centres as identified in the General Settlement Plan (GSP), then

* If information related to health status other than the ones listed in Table 21.1 are available such as some kind of health service utilization data for all settlements of a particular block, then a typology based on these additional data should be constructed. Such a typology will serve as a powerful means of establishing the validity of the health hazard index.

there is not much problem for reconciliation. If, however, the proposed health centres fall far away from the higher-level centres and also show inconsistency with other sectoral plans, then it becomes difficult in general to reconcile these inconsistencies. However, using the Integrated Area Plan (IAP) approach, one may resolve to a great extent some of the inconsistencies in the different sectoral plans as well as between the sectoral plans and the general settlement plan.

Despite these useful features, it must be pointed out that the proposed health hazard index does not satisfy the property of a ratio scale. It has only ordinal properties, i.e. we can only say whether the computed health hazard index is greater than or less than or equal to a given health hazard index. The index is also not entirely independent of technological change since by shifting the bus station or railway station, one can change the distance data shown in columns 5 and 6 of Appendix A1. The proposed Index is also not a direct measure of health status since no health care facility utilization data have been used. It only helps us in identifying settlements where people run the risk of health, but does not define their health need.

Notwithstanding these major weaknesses, the proposed health hazard index satisfies the following desirable properties of an "ideal" index number:

(a) The index is capable of detecting small differences as well as class boundaries, if they exist.
(b) The index number can be used to portray the frequency distribution of health hazards in order to permit a "health status" profile which can be constructed for grouping or sub-grouping of the various settlements of the block.
(c) The index is capable of measuring both individual settlements and blocks and of comparing the two.
(d) The index number permits inter-regional comparisons in terms of the median health hazard index.
(e) Although an ideal index should preferably vary from 0 to 100, the proposed health index varies from 19 to 206. However, the index* is equally sensitive and meaningful (in the ordinal sense) at the low as in the high end of the continuum.

* By adding 19 to the *Hi* score and then multiplying it by 0.444, the transformed *Hi* score varies in the range of 0-100.

(f) The proposed index appears to be normally distributed in the population of individual settlements within a moderately large size block.

(g) It permits the use of non-parametric type of statistical analysis. The index is capable of determining what is statistically significant change in the health hazard index and what is a change due to chance variation.

Other properties of the proposed index will be discussed in a subsequent paper. Current research effort is directed towards exploring the extent to which the proposed index is: (a) capable of operationalizing other concepts related to health hazard and (b) compatible with other methods of measuring health hazard, so that two or more measures may be used simultaneously to supplement each other.

It must be noted that in addition to the nine variables upon which the health hazard index is presently based, numerous other equally valid and reliable indicators could be incorporated into the Index. A few obvious examples would be: overcrowding rate per family, general morbidity indices, health expenditures *per capita,* number of physicians per 1,000 population, number of children below 5 years per woman in the settlement, air, land and water pollution in the settlement, as well as various types of socio-economic data connected with a family's utilization of primary health centres, such as migration status, level of satisfaction with PHC, average waiting time, religious affiliation and many other such variables analysed by Abernathy and Moore[16] as also by Deshaies and S. Eidman[17]. Unfortunately, quantified data on these variables have not been gathered so far and the whole index is presently based on readily available data. The data on which the proposed index is based are easily available for any settlement and were chosen for index construction on the basis of several criteria in addition to availability: scope, available at least yearly, timeliness (i.e. latest data not more than 2 years old), and their relevance to health. It must be admitted, that it is possible to develop a more adequate index of health need by considerable amount of conceptual and analytical work so that the perfected index will have sub-indices or "Problem Indicators", such as, Accessibility Problem, Motivational Problem, Facility Problem, Ecological Problem and so on. Such multivariate types of problem indicators will be ideal for health planning.

There are quite a few problems in measuring health status[18] but still a reliable and valid measure of health status must be developed both to aid in determining where and when the health services should be provided and to measure the impact of these services on the beneficiaries receiving them. The approach developed in this chapter is a modest beginning in this direction. It is expected that the crude index proposed here will stimulate further research aimed towards its purification.

APPENDIX

Table A1

Village code Settle-ments	Column No. Name of the Settlement	1 Infant Mortality Rate (1000 live births)	2 Min. Dist. to PHC/ Hospital (hecto-meters)	3 Death Rate 1000 Population	4 No. of women 1971	5 Total Dist. to reg. Bus Stop (Wet Season)	6 Total Dist. to Railway station (Wet Season)	7 Assisted Births by Doctor/ Hospital (per cent))	8 Total Doctor Visits per 100 Population	9 Percentage of Female Literacy 1971
2001	Bagh Bari	250	071	07	179	02	03	025	0	21.22
2002	Bah Bari	190	155	15	263	00	01	000	0	19.77
2003	Balijan Gaon	000	074	02	207	06	06	000	0	16.90
2004	Balijan Gaon	120	054	62	131	00	11	020	0	18.32
2005	Balijan Paniera	000	065	04	305	00	04	000	2	32.45
2006	Bambari	000	126	12	149	00	05	000	0	03.35
2007	Bamunia Hiloidhari	200	055	12	460	05	05	100	0	26.08
2008	Beteoni	133	035	28	130	03	03	000	0	06.92
2009	Betnela	029	027	06	293	00	04	002	1	25.93
2010	Bhardhara Bengali	188	021	09	335	05	05	000	0	21.19
2011	Bharalua	000	060	08	395	00	08	006	0	25.82
2012	Bindhakata	250	094	07	190	00	15	075	0	24.73
2014	Boragadhi	250	079	13	334	00	06	050	0	15.86

(Contd.)

Table A1: (*Contd.*)

		1	2	3	4	5	6	7	8	9
2015	Borbaribengali Gaon	143	041	10	300	01	05	000	1	17.33
2016	Boruahola	000	076	22	592	05	05	100	0	15.70
2018	Chakalivaria	148	042	07	425	04	04	003	0	16.0()
2019	Changmai Borupathar	100	032	08	271	00	07	000	2	25.83
2020	Changmai Gaon	111	118	06	168	05	05	000	0	26.03
2021	Charalchungigaon	250	084	20	090	00	11	000	0	01·11
2022	Charalchungihabi	091	086	11	221	03	11	000	0	02.71
2023	Chetia Gaon	000	042	02	224	04	04	000	2	35.71
2024	Chetia Pathar	000	045	03	252	00	06	020	2	13.49
2025	Chungarchuck	167	027	02	295	00	03	000	0	21.35
2026	Dangarchuck	200	039	22	190	03	05	010	1	16.31
2027	Deodhai	125	026	18	363	00	02	062	0	12.12
2028	Dharia Gaon	000	093	00	171	00	06	006	0	01.16
2029	Dharia Raitak	154	096	10	656	08	08	000	0	03.04
2030	Dhekiajuri	200	099	10	092	07	07	000	1	20.65
2031	Dighalibari	160	049	08	493	07	07	000	0	11.56
2032	Dihingia	000	107	03	153	04	05	000	0	20.26
2033	Dikomnahaani	000	091	00	142	04	16	000	0	01.40
2034	Dimarugurigaon	240	098	07	481	00	05	036	0	35.13
2035	Dinjaychapori	333	048	05	545	00	07	044	0	14.12
2036	Dinjoysaira	000	049	04	359	00	05	000	3	34.26

(*Contd.*)

Table A1: (*Contd.*)

2037	Dohotia	143	122	16	088	00	05	100	1	27.27
2038	Gahoriparn Gaon	150	085	07	522	02	10	050	0	46.36
2039	Gandhia Naharam	000	019	04	438	04	04	000	0	18.49
2040	Gereki Gaon	000	092	08	168	02	11	000	0	00.00
2041	Gerekinepali	000	104	08	146	02	11	000	0	00.00
2042	Hatigadhai Gaon	000	046	00	243	06	06	000	0	14.18
2043	Hatkhola Bengali Gaon	118	000	02	458	01	01	011	1	26.63
2044	Ieraigaon	000	023	18	461	00	06	100	0	21.47
2045	Jugipathar	143	034	06	375	06	11	004	0	08.26
2046	Jugipathar Gaon	000	096	09	213	00	03	000	0	16.43
2047	Kadamoni Gaon	000	129	03	133	00	06	000	0	16.54
2048	Kadamoni Gaon	000	030	00	051	00	01	000	0	68.62
2049	Kailabari Gaon	143	012	07	181	01	02	025	0	06.62
2050	Kambator Habigaon	667	072	55	045	00	11	000	0	00.00
2051	Kanjikhowabengali	000	000	02	173	01	04	000	0	01.73
2052	Kapahua Gaon	125	101	04	315	01	09	001	0	36.50
2053	Kaptanchuck Gaon	105	129	07	472	00	05	100	0	28.38
2054	Kath Gaon	000	076	07	062	04	06	000	1	37.09
2055	Kharikatia	167	107	25	103	08	08	008	1	19.41
2057	Kukurek Howa	000	101	07	200	07	07	000	0	43.00
2058	Kumar Gaon	333	042	15	194	05	05	000	0	25.25
2059	Luhali	133	074	08	371	12	12	000	0	24.79
2060	Marankari Gaon	154	106	08	265	00	04	000	0	35.47

(*Contd.*)

Table A1: (*Contd.*)

		1	*2*	*3*	*4*	*5*	*6*	*7*	*8*	*9*
2061	Matiakhona	167	072	03	546	00	07	000	0	09.34
2062	Merilipathar	100	035	05	401	00	03	010	0	23.69
2063	Mid Gaon	250	110	10	567	00	11	000	0	12.69
2064	Miri Hola	000	086	10	066	00	07	000	1	45.45
2065	Morankari	000	025	07	118	01	03	022	1	46.61
2066	Morchagaon	129	058	18	585	05	05	028	1	17.60
2068	Muddi Gaon	067	049	02	718	00	08	000	0	18.52
2069	Muluk Gaon	250	100	12	066	00	15	025	0	43.93
2070	Murani Amguri	091	079	04	337	00	10	036	0	27.29
2071	Marani Pathar	000	086	00	062	07	07	000	3	22.58
2072	Nadua Gohain Gaon	250	042	15	407	05	08	020	0	15.72
2073	Nadua Grant Gaon	000	060	06	223	00	04	040	0	27.35
2074	Na-gaon	067	066	06	267	02	02	000	0	27.71
2075	Nalanihola	083	032	08	159	02	03	066	0	20.75
2076	Nephaphu	400	098	28	112	00	15	000	0	00.89
2077	Niz-chabua	214	022	08	276	01	03	014	0	29.71
2078	Now Gaon	133	073	22	096	04	10	020	1	04.16
2079	Nunpuria Bengali	273	073	24	326	04	04	000	0	09.20
2080	Nunpuria Kalbortha	288	078	16	660	01	03	000	0	13.63
2081	Okanimoria Bengali	500	098	18	242	05	05	000	3	07.02
2082	Okanimoria Kachari	111	096	13	265	04	04	000	1	30.18

(*Contd.*)

Table A1: (*Contd.*)

2083	Pakharijan	000	094	04	109	00	15	000	0	17.43
2084	Pakharij ania	154	109	05	358	17	17	000	0	33.79
2085	Panimudi Gaon	273	060	13	106	03	03	018	0	18.86
2086	Panitola Gaon	278	044	06	550	00	01	030	0	19.81
2087	Panitola Town	218	049	14	726	00	00	023	0	45.04
2088	Patlingmara	000	080	10	076	00	15	000	0	00.00
2089	Pipartali Gaon	167	112	10	049	00	10	000	0	08.16
2090	Polonga Gaon	033	039	15	321	00	05	000	0	14.33
2091	Ra Dang	125	037	04	306	00	13	000	0	11.76
2092	Rajabari	167	029	17	350	02	06	013	0	34.00
2093	Rangchangi Town	000	094	03	271	00	06	000	1	39.48
2094	Rangmala	200	105	07	434	02	11	000	1	07.37
2095	Saru Pathar	500	064	46	039	00	05	000	1	00.00
2096	Sarupathar Gaon	000	072	13	034	05	05	000	0	02.94
2097	Sessakash Gaon	000	056	04	108	00	07	000	1	00.92
2098	Silikhaghri	167	114	28	353	00	06	000	0	12.18
2099	Tiahjali Gaon	333	022	12	161	01	01	000	0	13.66
2100	Tipomia	105	124	02	348	02	13	000	1	33.62
2101	Udalguri	200	090	12	061	04	10	020	1	11.47
2102	Udalguri	000	063	04	227	00	05	000	0	09.25

Table A2

Village code	*Settlement Name*	*Decile Scores for VariableNumbers* Health Hazard*										
		1	*2*	*3*	*4*	*5*	*6*	*7*	*8*	*9*	*Index*	*Rank*
001	Baghbari	9	5	5	4	6	2	9	6	7	089	056
002	Bahbari	8	1	8	6	3	1	1	1	6	134	008
003	Balijan Gaon	1	6	2	5	9	6	4	3	5	071	072
004	Balijan Gaon	5	4	10	3	2	9	8	6	5	092	054
005	Balijan Pantera	1	5	3	7	3	3	2	10	9	045	091
006	Bambari	1	10	8	3	2	4	2	2	2	100	042
007	Bamuntahiloidhari	8	4	7	9	9	5	10	8	8	109	030
008	Beteoni	6	2	10	3	7	2	1	1	2	101	038
009	Betmela	4	2	4	6	3	3	7	9	8	044	092
010	Bhardhara Bengali	8	1	6	7	9	5	3	3	6	100	043
011	Bharalua	1	5	5	8	4	7	7	5	7	070	073
012	Bindhakata	9	8	4	4	2	10	10	7	7	106	035
014	Boragadhi	9	6	8	7	4	6	9	7	5	122	016
015	Borbari Bengali Gaon	6	3	6	6	6	4	3	8	5	086	059
016	Borua Kola	1	6	9	10	9	5	10	8	4	103	037
018	Chakalivaria	6	3	5	8	8	3	7	5	5	089	057
019	Changmai Barupathar	5	2	6	6	3	7	4	10	7	069	074
020	Changrmai Gaon	5	10	4	4	9	5	3	2	8	110	028
021	Charaichungi Gaon	9	7	9	2	1	9	5	4	1	131	011
022	Charaichungi Habi	4	7	7	5	7	9	6	4	2	116	021

(*Contd.*)

Table A2: (*Contd.*)

023	Chetta Gaon	1	3	2	5	8	3	2	10	9	035	095
024	Chetia Pathar	1	3	2	5	3	6	8	10	4	035	096
025	Chungi Chuck	7	2	1	6	3	2	1	1	7	061	082
026	Dangar Chuck	8	3	9	4	7	4	7	9	5	099	047
027	Deodhai	5	1	9	8	4	1	10	7	3	077	063
028	Dharia Gaon	1	7	1	4	2	6	7	5	1	058	084
029	Dharia Raitak	7	8	7	10	10	8	5	3	2	157	002
030	Dhekiajuri	8	8	7	2	10	7	4	9	6	123	015
031	Dighalibari	7	4	8	9	10	7	5	3	3	126	014
032	Dihingla	1	9	2	3	8	5	3	2	6	076	065
033	Dikomnaharani	2	7	1	3	8	10	6	5	2	079	062
034	Dimaruguru Gaon	9	8	5	9	5	4	9	7	9	116	022
035	Dinjay Chapori	10	4	3	9	5	7	9	7	4	109	031
036	Dinjoy Satra	2	4	1	8	4	4	3	10	9	043	044
037	Dohotia	6	10	9	2	1	4	10	10	8	096	050
038	Gahoripam Gaon	7	7	5	9	7	8	10	7	10	110	029
039	Gandhia Naharani	2	1	2	6	8	3	2	2	6	056	086
040	Gereki Gaon	2	7	6	4	6	9	5	4	1	100	044
041	Gereki Nepali	2	9	6	3	6	9	5	4	1	107	034
042	Hatigadhai Gaon	2	4	1	5	9	6	4	3	4	064	078
043	Hatkhola Bengali Gaon	5	1	2	9	6	1	7	9	8	047	088
044	Jerai Gaon	2	1	9	9	4	6	10	8	7	066	076
045	Jugipathar	6	2	4	8	10	9	7	5	3	061	083

(*Contd.*)

Table A2: (*Contd.*)

		1	2	3	4	5	6	7	8	9		
046	Jugipathar Gaon	2	8	6	5	2	2	1	1	5	085	060
047	Kadamoni Gaon	2	10	2	3	2	5	3	3	5	075	068
048	Kadamont Gaon	2	2	1	1	1	1	1	1	10	009	098
049	Kailabari Gaon	6	1	4	4	6	1	9	6	2	058	085
050	Kamhtorhabi Gaon	10	6	10	1	1	9	5	4	1	132	010
051	Kanj ikhowa Bengali	3	1	1	4	5	3	2	2	2	044	093
052	Kapahua Gaon	5	9	3	7	6	8	7	5	9	101	039
053	Kaptanchuck Gaon	5	10	5	9	4	4	10	7	8	105	036
054	Kath Gaon	3	6	5	1	8	6	4	8	10	064	079
055	Khari Katia	7	9	10	2	10	8	7	9	6	134	009
057	Kukurekhowa	3	9	5	5	10	7	5	3	10	101	040
058	Kumar Gaon	10	3	8	4	9	5	3	2	7	118	019
059	Luhali	6	6	6	8	10	9	6	4	7	122	017
060	Marankari Gaon	7	9	6	6	3	3	1	1	9	114	025
061	Matia Khona	7	5	2	10	5	7	4	3	3	109	032
062	Merilipathar	5	2	3	8	4	2	7	5	7	047	089
063	Miri Gaon	9	9	6	10	5	9	5	4	4	075	069
064	Miri Hola	3	7	7	1	1	7	4	8	10	065	077
065	Morankari	3	1	4	3	5	2	8	9	10	022	097
066	Moricha Gaon	6	4	9	10	9	5	9	10	5	115	024
068	Mudoi Gaon	4	4	2	10	5	8	5	3	6	084	061

(*Contd.*)

Table A2: (*Contd.*)

069	Muluk Gaon	9	9	7	2	1	10	9	6	10	111	027
070	Muraniamguri	4	6	3	7	4	8	9	7	8	075	070
071	Murani Pathar	3	7	1	1	10	7	4	10	7	063	080
072	Naduagohain Gaon	9	3	8	8	9	8	8	6	4	128	012
073	Naduagrani Gaon	3	5	4	5	2	3	9	7	8	049	087
074	Na Gaon	4	5	4	6	7	1	1	1	8	077	064
075	Nalani Hola	4	2	5	3	6	2	10	7	6	046	090
076	Nephaphy	10	8	10	3	2	10	6	5	1	150	005
077	Niz Chabua	8	2	5	6	6	2	8	6	8	074	071
078	Now-Gaon	6	6	10	2	8	8	8	9	2	117	020
079	Nunpuri Bengali	9	6	10	7	8	3	2	2	3	148	006
080	Nunpuria Kaibortha	10	6	9	10	6	2	1	1	4	152	003
081	Okanimoria Bengali	10	8	9	5	9	5	3	10	2	152	004
082	Okanimoria Kachari	5	8	8	6	8	3	2	8	9	109	033
083	Pakharijan	3	8	3	2	2	10	6	5	5	076	066
084	Pakari Jania	7	9	3	8	10	10	6	5	9	127	013
085	Panimudi Gaon	9	5	8	2	7	2	8	6	6	100	045
086	Panitola Gaon	10	3	4	10	5	1	9	6	6	096	051
087	Panitola Town	8	4	8	10	5	1	8	6	10	100	046
088	Patlungmara	3	7	7	2	1	10	6	4	1	094	053
089	Pipartali Gaon	7	10	7	1	1	8	5	4	3	119	018
090	Polonga Gaon	4	3	8	7	4	4	2	2	4	092	055
091	Raidang	6	3	3	7	3	10	6	4	3	088	058

(*Contd.*)

Table A2: (*Contd.*)

		1	2	3	4	5	6	7	8	9		
092	Rajabari	7	2	9	7	7	6	8	6	9	096	052
093	Rangchagi Town	3	8	2	6	3	6	3	8	10	068	075
094	Rangmala	8	9	4	9	7	9	6	9	3	139	007
095	Sarupathar	10	5	10	1	1	4	2	8	1	116	023
096	Sarupathar Gaon	4	5	8	1	8	5	3	2	2	097	048
097	Sessakash Gaon	4	4	3	2	2	7	4	8	1	062	081
098	Silikhaguri	8	10	10	8	4	6	4	3	4	159	001
099	Tiahjalia Gaon	10	1	7	4	5	1	1	1	4	097	049
100	Tipomia	5	10	1	7	7	10	6	9	9	101	041
101	Udalguri	8	7	7	1	7	8	8	9	3	113	026
102	Udalguri	4	5	3	5	3	4	2	2	3	076	067
Arbitrary Weights for the Calculation of Health Hazard Index		5	5	4	3	2	2	–1	–1	–2		

*The names of these serially numbered variables appear in Table 3.

Notes

1. Malenbaum, W. (1973), Health and Economic Expansion in Poor Lands, *International Journal of Health Services,* 3, 161-171.
2. Banerji, S. and Fisher, H.B. (1973), *Hierarchical Location Analysis for Integrated Area Planning: Experiences of the Pilot Research Project in Growth Centres, India,* Central Research Cell, Growth Centres Project, New Delhi: The Ford Foundation.
3. Harman, H.H. (1967), *Modern Factor Analysis,* Chicago: University of Chicago Press.
4. Rummel, R.J. (1970), *Applied Factor Analysis,* Evanston: Northwestern University Press.
5. Fruchter, B. (1968), *Introduction to Factor Analysis,* New Jersey: van Nostrand.
6. Broadbent, T.A. (1962), *An Introduction to Factor Analysis and Its Application to Regional Science,* Working Paper No. 13, London: Centre for Environmental Studies.
7. Rummel, R.J., *op. cit.*
8. Mukherjee, B.N. (1973), *A Health Hazard Index: A Simple Technique for Identifying Settlements Which Needs Extra Health Services,* Central Research Cell, Growth Centres Project, New Delhi: The Ford Foundation.
9. Anderson, T.W. (1958), *Introductian to Multivariate Statistical Analysis,* New York: John Wiley.
10. Morrison, D.R. (1967), *Multivariate Statistical Methods,* McGraw-Hill, New York.
11. Anderson, T., *op. cit.,* Kendall, M.C., *A Course in Multivariate Analysis,* New York: Hafner, 1968. Morrison, D.R., *Ibid.*
12. Kendall, M.C., *Ibid.*
13. Horst, A.P. (1936), Obtaining a Composite Measure from Different Measures of the same Attributes, *Psychometrika,* 1, 53-60.
14. Edgerton, H.A. and Kolbe, L.B. (1936), The Method of Minimum Variation for the Combination of Criteria. *Psychometrika* 1, 183:187.
15. Wilks, S.S. (1938), Weighing System for Linear Functions of Correlated Variables when there is no Dependent Variable. *Psychometrika,* 3, 23-40.
16. Abernathy, W.J. and Moore, J.R. Jr. (1971), *Regional Planning of Primary Health Care Services,* Research Paper No. 1, Palo Alto: Graduate School of Business, Stanford University.
17. Deshaies, J.C. and Seidman, D.R. (1971), Health Information Systems, *Socio-economic Planning Science,* 5, 515-533.
18. Moriyama, Z.W. (1968), Problems in the Measurement of Health Status, in *Indicators of Social Change,* pp. 576-600 (Edited by Sheldon, E.B. and Moore, W.E.) New York: Russel Sage Foundation.

22
Regional Disparities in Health Care Delivery in Jammu & Kashmir State, India

Ishtiaq A. Mayer, M. Sabar and *Sheraz A. Lone*

Introduction

Regional disparities in socio-economic parameters are ubiquitous phenomenon in developed as well as in developing countries but in the later ones, the problem of disparities is in acute situation due to overwhelming backwardness and existence of few developed pockets at the cost of others.[1] This phenomenon of spatially imbalanced regional development within a country is becoming a serious problem for policy-makers and planners particularly because the actual purpose of development stands defeated or muted when a section of population remains deprived of its benefits.[2] There are poor regions possessing rich resources and rich regions having poor resources.[3] This phenomenon of imbalanced regional development has not only resulted in several social, economic and political problems but has also posed a serious threat to the health of the people. Such type of disparities at national, regional and local levels influences India as well.

Near about three-fourths of the population in India live below or at subsistence levels; thereby poverty and its impacts thereof; are real challenging issues to tackle with. In such a context human development and well-being, social security support for health, education, housing etc. becomes critical. No universally agreed upon definition of poverty has been established. People are considered poor when they cannot secure minimum standards of well-being are denied or severely restricted.[4, 5] Although there is general consensus among social scientists that well-being is multidimensional and poverty as a lack of well-being. In India people living below or at subsistence level spend up to 90 per cent of their income on food consumption to meet minimum nutritional requirements and health curative measures. Although India ranks one of the largest private health sectors in the world the public health services are very inadequate. The public curative and hospital services are mostly in urban areas and in cities where only 31.16 per cent of the 1.27 billion populations reside.[6] Rural areas have mostly preventive and promotive services like family planning and immunization. The private sector has a virtual monopoly and dominance over ambulatory curative services in both rural and urban areas. Hence, inadequate health care facilities are the main reasons for poor health status of the Indians.

Allopathy, ayurveda, homoeopathy, *unani, siddha*, among others, are different systems of medicine available in India. The public sector ownership of health care is divided between Central and State Governments. The Constitution of India has made health care services largely a responsibility of State Governments but has left enough control for the Centre to intervene with health and health care planning policies of states. Health services in India are provided to the community through a network of Sub-centres, Primary Health Centres (PHCs) and Community Health Centres (CHCs) in the rural areas and through Hospitals and Dispensaries and by others in the urban areas. The Primary Health Care infrastructure in rural areas has been developed as a three-tier system comprising of Sub-centres, PHCs and CHCs. The norms for establishing these are as under:

Table 22.1 Health Centres and Population Norms

Centre	*Population Norms*	
	Plain Area	*Hilly Area*
Sub-centre	5000	3000
PHC	30000	20000
CHC	120000	80000

Source: National Rural Health Mission.

The most important parameter of human development index is based on health status of the people of any region. The better health condition is maintained by balanced diet, clean and hygienic environment besides the appropriate health care and welfare measures,

Table 22.2: Numbers of PHCs with Doctors and without Doctor/Lab Technician/Pharmacist

State	*As on March 2010 Number of PHCs*								
	Total PHCs	*With 4+ Doctors*	*With 3+ Doctors*	*With 2+ Doctors*	*With 1+ Doctors*	*Without doctor*	*Without Lady doctor*	*Without Lab. Tech*	*Without Pharmacist*
Jammu & Kashmir	375	59	89	170	57	0	204	86	23
All India	23673	873	985	6073	14040	753	4408	7924	3825

Source: Directorate of Health Services, Kashmir, 2015-16, Srinagar.

which are mainly rendered by the government agencies particularly in developing societies like India. The health care services and facilities available in India are highly haphazard in nature which she has inherited from colonial times. Some areas have more health facilities, available than the need of that particular area whereas majority of the areas have more demands for services. Thus, there exist disparities not only in rural and urban areas but also within rural and urban areas of different states of India.[7] The situation of health care delivery in Jammu and Kashmir State is also reflected by such uneven distribution pattern. Rural population in the state is nearly neglected in terms of health facilities. In fact, there are only a few health care units with bed facility in rural areas in some divisions. The health institutions, which have bed facilities, are generally located at urban centres. Thus, the strong polarization of health services is in urban areas and in cities.

Table 22.3: Average Rural Area Covered by Health Institutions

Health Institutions	*Average Rural Area (sq. km) Covered by a Health Institution*		*Average Radial Distance (kms) Covered by a Health Institution*	
	J&K	*All-India*	*J&K*	*All-India*
Sub Centre	117.21	21.47	6.11	2.61
Primary Health Centre	591.67	139.40	13.72	6.66
Community Health Centre	2766.07	770.90	29.67	15.66

Source: NRHM Jammu & Kashmir, 2013.

State Profile

The State as a whole is the northernmost part of India. The Himalayan mountain ranges separate its three sub-units, The Jammu, The Kashmir and The Ladakh Division from one another.

Physiographically, the state has varied relief features. On the south, the Jammu Division is less undulating gaining height towards north and merging with plains in the south. This north to south inclination has been divided into three major topographical facets. This has been referred to three-storey house.[8] In the middle is the Kashmir Division thought to be geologically tectonic in origin,[9] having half-closed eco-system.[10] Here in the depressions where waters have accumulated the lakes have emerged. India's largest fresh water lake—

the Wular, is the typical relief feature of this area. Where the land has gained altitude, there the perpetual snowfields give birth to some of the world's largest glaciers only after Polar region.[11] Lastly, the Ladakh Division is topographically more complex and all of the geological series from Paleozoic to present period are almost encountered.

Altitude and prevailing winds have given entire Jammu & Kashmir State a marked variation in climate. The altitude varies between 304.8 meters to 8611.4 meters above sea level. The state experiences varied climatic conditions ranging from the tropical heat during summers in Jammu to semi-arctic type of climate during winters in Ladakh. In the middle, Kashmir Division has moderate climatic conditions. In fact, climatic variations are found even at micro level.[12]

These physical conditions become hindrance in expanding welfare measures including health services to all areas of the state and have created polarization of such facilities at selected areas.[13, 14]

Kashmir Division

Rural population in the division is nearly neglected in terms of health facilities. In fact, there are only a few health care units with bed facility in rural areas of the division. The health institutions, which have bed facilities, are all located at urban centres. Thus, the strong polarization of health services is in urban areas. There are 1354 medical institutions of all order in the Kashmir division, which include district hospitals, sub-district hospitals, primary health centres, allopathic dispensaries and sub-centres and other more than 200 founded and controlled semi-government health institutions. These institutions serve a population of 68,88,475 persons (54.92% to total J&K population) (Table 22.4). The institution/population ratio is 1:5088. However, the dispensary/population ratio is 1:63782 and PHC ratio is 1:32493. The bulk of health care institution, about 65 per cent is of the nature of health sub-centres, which do not possess any type of specialized health services and machinery and equipment. Another important indicator pertaining to health care is the availability of hospital beds. The bed/population ratio for Kashmir Division is 1:1424. This ratio decreases to 1:698 if the inclusion of other 3654 beds is considered with various PHCs as claimed by health department; however these exist only on papers and not exist in reality. The bulk of bed facility is available in Srinagar city. The norms of providing different orders of health institutions with bed facilities are bent in Kashmir division.

Table 22.4: Population Distribution in J&K

Sl. No.	*District*	*Total Household*	*Percentage of Household to Total Household*	*Total Population*	*Percentage of Population to Total Population*
		Kashmir Division			
1.	Anantnag	153640	7.25	1078692	8.60
2.	Budgam	103363	4.88	753745	6.01
3.	Bandipora	58392	2.75	392232	3.13
4.	Baramulla	152635	7.20	1008039	8.04
5.	Ganderbal	45361	2.14	297446	2.37
6.	Kulgam	73728	3.48	424483	3.38
7.	Kupwara	113929	5.37	870354	6.94
8.	Pulwama	86241	4.07	560440	4.47
9.	Shopian	44411	2.10	266215	2.12
10.	Srinagar	191678	9.04	1236829	9.86
	Total			**6888475**	
		Jammu Division			
11.	Doda	79636	3.76	409936	3.27
12.	Jammu	314199	14.82	1529958	12.20
13.	Kathua	119583	5.64	616435	4.92
14.	Kishtwar	45209	2.13	230696	1.84
15.	Poonch	90261	4.26	476835	3.80
16.	Rajouri	130401	6.15	642415	5.12
17.	Ramban	55490	2.62	283713	2.26
18.	Reasi	56689	2.67	314667	2.51
19.	Samba	65385	3.08	318898	2.54
20.	Udhampur	99240	4.68	554985	4.43
	Total				
		Ladakh Division			
21.	Leh	21909	1.03	133487	1.06
22.	Kargil	18338	0.87	140802	1.12
	J&K	**2119718**	**100**	**12541302**	**100**

Source: Census, 2011.

For example, district hospitals, sub-district hospitals and PHCs are to be provided with 100, 30 and 10 beds respectively. Such a policy is not followed in most of the districts of Jammu & Kashmir. The Srinagar district hospital has more than 150 beds whereas the district hospitals of Budgam and Pulwama have not been more than 50 beds in each. Only a few PHCs have bed facility as per prescribed norms. Most of such institutions have 3-4 beds or are without any such facility and does not qualify the desired norms of bed/population ratio as suggested by Mudaliar Committee. One of its causes is that most of lower order health institutions in rural areas are run in rented accommodations.

There is a great variation in terms of health care facilities across the various spatial units (Districts) in Kashmir valley. Out of total 1354 institutions, maximum number of health institutions were found in district Kupwara (243), Baramullah (196) followed by Anantnag (183) and lowest number of institutions was found in the districts of Bandipora (60), Shopian (62) and Srinagar (70). The institution/population ratio is highest in Ganderbal (1:2361), Kupwara (1:3582) and lowest in Srinagar (1:17669) and Bandipora (1:6537) while as population/bed ratio prevails highest in Baramullah (1:1863), Kupwara (1:1836) and Bandipora (1:1634) and lowest is found in Ganderbal (1:684), Shopian (1:1138) and Budgam (1:1169).

Jammu Division

The similar situation prevails in Jammu Division. Rural population in the division is nearly neglected in terms of health facilities. The health institutions, which have bed facilities, are all located at urban centers. Thus, the strong polarization of health services is in urban areas. There are 1594 medical institutions in the Jammu division, which include district hospitals, sub-district hospitals, primary health centres, allopathic dispensaries and sub-centres and other more than 200 founded and controlled semi-government health institutions. These institutions serve a population of 53,78,538 persons (42.88% to total J&K Population) (Table 22.8). The institution/population ratio is 1:3374. However, the dispensary/population ratio is 1:40138 and PHC ratio is 1:27028. The bulk of health care institution, about 66.88 per cent comprises of health sub-centres, which do not possess any type of specialized health services. Another important indicator pertaining to health care is the availability of hospital beds. Table 22.9 reveals that bed/population ratio for Jammu Division is 1:1166. The norms of providing different orders of health institutions with bed facilities are bent in Jammu division. For example, district hospitals sub-district hospitals and PHCs are to be provided with

Table 22.5: District-wise Health Care Facilities in Kashmir Division

District	District Hospital	Sub-District Hospital/ CHC	Primary Health Centre	Allopathic Dispensary	District TB Centre	Medical Aid Centres	Sub-Centres	Total Institute	Assistant Surgeon	Dental Surgeon	Specialists	Nurses/ FMPHW/ ANMS	Paramedics
Anantnag	1	6	27	14	1	11	123	183	69	28	4	65	214
Budgam	1	9	36	9	0	3	121	179	43	10	7	36	71
Bandipora	1	3	6	6	0	5	39	60	93	33	18	90	189
Baramulla	1	6	28	21	1	13	126	196	126	45	25	106	230
Ganderbal	1	4	29	4	0	4	34	126	45	18	4	29	58
Kulgam	1	2	19	9	0	5	70	106	50	27	5	74	179
Kupwara	1	7	31	8	1	41	154	243	109	27	14	236	317
Pulwama	1	3	21	17	1	6	30	129	76	19	12	76	105
Shopian	1	2	6	4	0	5	44	62	37	11	3	45	75
Srinagar	1	1	9	16	1	1	41	70	78	16	19	66	115
Kashmir Div.	**10**	**43**	**212**	**108**	**5**	**94**	**882**	**1354**	**726**	**234**	**111**	**823**	**1553**

Source: Directorate of Health Service, J&K, 2014.

Table 22.6: District-wise Institution/Population Ratio in Kashmir Division

District	*District Hospital/ Population Ratio*	*Sub-District Hospital/ CHC/ Population Ratio*	*Primary/ Health Centre/ Population Ratio*	*Allopathic Dispensary/ Population Ratio*	*District TB Centre/ Population Ratio*	*Medical Aid Centres/ Population Ratio*	*Sub-Centres/ Population Ratio*	*Population Bed Ratio*	*Total Institution/ Population Ratio*
Anantnag	1:1078692	1:179782	1:39952	1:77049	1:1078692	1:98063	1:8770	1:1444	1:5894
Budgam	1:753745	1:83749	1:20937	1:83749	1:0	1:251248	1:6229	1:1169	1:4211
Bandipora	1:392232	1:130744	1:65372	1:65372	1:0	1:78446	1:10057	1:1634	1:6537
Baramulla	1:1008039	1:168007	1:36001	1:48002	1:1008039	1:77541	1:8000	1:1863	1:5143
Ganderbal	1:297446	1:74362	1:10257	1:74362	1:0	1:74362	1:3541	1:684	1:2361
Kulgam	1:424483	1:212242	1:22341	1:47165	1:0	1:84897	1:6064	1:1538	1:4005
Kupwara	1:870354	1:124336	1:28076	1:108794	1:870354	1:21228	1:5652	1:1836	1:3582
Pulwama	1:560440	1:186813	1:26688	1:32967	1:560440	1:93407	1:7006	1:1515	1:4344
Shopian	1:266215	1:133108	1:44369	1:66554	1:0	1:53243	1:6050	1:1138	1:4294
Srinagar	1:1236829	1:1236829	1:137425	1:77302	1:1236829	1:1236829	1:30167	1:1412	1:17669
Kashmir Div.	**1:688848**	**1:160197**	**1:32493**	**1:63782**	**1:1377695**	**1:73282**	**1:7810**	**1:1424**	**1:5088**

Source: Compiled by Author.

Table 22.7: District-wise Medical/Paramedical Personnel in Kashmir Division

District	*Assistant Surgeon/ Population Ratio*	*Dental Surgeon/ Population Ratio*	*Specialists/ Population Ratio*	*Nurses/ FMPHW/ ANMS/ Population Ratio*	*Paramedics/ Population Ratio*
Anantnag	15633	38525	269673	16595	5041
Budgam	17529	75375	107678	20937	10616
Bandipora	4218	11886	21791	4358	2075
Baramulla	8000	22401	40322	9510	4383
Ganderbal	6610	16525	74362	10257	5128
Kulgam	8490	15722	84897	5736	2371
Kupwara	7985	32235	62168	3688	2746
Pulwama	7374	29497	46703	7374	5338
Shopian	7195	24201	88738	5916	3550
Srinagar	15857	77302	65096	18740	10755
Kashmir Div.	**9488**	**29438**	**62058**	**8370**	**4436**

Source: Compiled by Author.

100, 30 and 10 beds respectively. Such a policy is not followed in most of the districts of Jammu & Kashmir. The Jammu district hospital has more than 150 beds whereas the district hospitals of Kishtwar and Ramban have not been more than 50 beds in each. Only a few PHCs have bed facility as per prescribed norms. Most of such institutions have less than 3 bed facility. Barring Jammu and Udhampur, district of the division fulfils the desired norms of bed/ population ratio as suggested by Mudaliar Committee.

Table 22.8 reveals inter-district variations in both health institutions and the availability of beds in Jammu division. In district Doda, 163 institutions are rendering health serve to a population of 4,09,936 persons (3.27% to total J&K population). Thus, the institution/population ratio is 1:2515 whereas the bed/population ratio is 1:907. The total health institution in Jammu district is about (291) and institution population ratio is 1:5258. The highest institutions (district hospital, sub-district, PHC, Allopathic and dispensaries) observed in Rajouri District (268), institution population ratio is about 1:2397 and bed population ratio is 1:763 which shows highest health care facilities in terms of men and material in Jammu division. While as lowest institution population ratio found in Jammu district (1:5258) and bed population ratio is 1:1609.

Table 22.8: District-wise Health Care Facilities in Jammu Division

Sl. No.	District	District Hospital	Sub-District Hospital/ CHC	Primary Health Centre	Allopathic Dispensary	District TB Centre	Medical Aid Centres	Sub-Centres	Total Institute	Assistant Surgeon	Dental Surgeon	Specialists	Nurses/ FMPHW/ ANMS	Paramedics
1.	Doda	1	2	17	23	0	34	86	163	58	17	15	80	61
2.	Jammu	1	7	39	13	1	10	220	291	125	21	47	153	160
3.	Kathua	1	4	26	11	1	12	139	194	63	4	13	247	240
4.	Kishtwar	1	1	9	12	1	25	46	95	27	7	6	32	40
5.	Poonch	1	3	17	15	1	10	96	143	45	6	18	64	160
6.	Rajouri	1	8	30	20	1	13	195	268	45	14	24	80	137
7.	Ramban	1	1	11	10	0	17	39	79	33	7	11	38	59
8.	Reasi	1	2	13	9	0	9	65	99	38	6	6	41	62
9.	Samba	1	1	12	2	0	3	75	94	40	11	13	39	50
10.	Udhampur	1	1	25	19	2	18	102	168	51	19	20	86	102
	Jammu Div.	**10**	**30**	**199**	**134**	**7**	**151**	**1063**	**1594**	**525**	**112**	**173**	**860**	**1064**

Source: Directorate of Health Service, J&K, 2014.

Table 22.9: District-wise Institution/Population Ratio in Jammu Division

District	*District Hospital/ Population Ratio*	*Sub-District Hospital/ CHC/ Population Ratio*	*Primary/ Health Centre/ Population Ratio*	*Allopathic Dispensary/ Population Ratio*	*District TB Centre/ Population Ratio*	*Medical Aid Centres/ Population Ratio*	*Sub-Centres/ Population Ratio*	*Population-Bed Ratio*	*Total Institution/ Population Ratio*
Doda	1:409936	1:204968	1:24114	1:17823	1:0	1:12057	1:4767	1:907	1:2515
Jammu	1:1529958	1:218565	1:39230	1:117689	1:1529958	1:152996	1:6954	1:1609	1:5258
Kathua	1:616435	1:154109	1:23709	1:56040	1:616435	1:51370	1:4435	1:1216	1:3178
Kishtwar	1:230696	1:230696	1:25633	1:19225	1:230696	1:9228	1:5015	1:793	1:2428
Poonch	1:476835	1:158945	1:28049	1:31789	1:476835	1:47684	1:4967	1:1119	1:3335
Rajouri	1:642415	1:80302	1:21414	1:32121	1:642415	1:49417	1:3294	1:763	1:2397
Ramban	1:283713	1:283713	1:25792	1:28371	1:0	1:16689	1:7275	1:1192	1:3591
Reasi	1:314667	1:157334	1:24205	1:34963	1:0	1:34963	1:4841	1:1215	1:3178
Samba	1:318898	1:318898	1:26575	1:159449	1:0	1:106299	1:4252	1:1307	1:3393
Udhampur	1:554985	1:554985	1:22199	1:29210	1:277493	1:30833	1:5441	1:1374	1:3303
Jammu Div.	**1:537854**	**1:179285**	**1:27028**	**1:40138**	**1:768363**	**1:35619**	**1:5060**	**1:1166**	**1:3374**

Source: Compiled by Authors.

Table 22.10: District-wise Medical/Paramedical Personnel in Jammu Division

District	Assistant Surgeon/ Population Ratio	Dental Surgeon/ Population Ratio	Specialists/ Population Ratio	Nurses/ FMPHW/ ANMS/ Population Ratio	Paramedics/ Population Ratio
Doda	1:7068	1:24114	1:27329	1:5124	1:6720
Jammu	1:12240	1:72855	1:32552	1:10000	1:9562
Kathua	1:9785	1:154109	1:47418	1:2496	1:2568
Kishtwar	1:8544	1:32957	1:38449	1:7209	1:5767
Poonch	1:10596	1:79473	1:26491	1:7451	1:2980
Rajouri	1:14276	1:45887	1:26767	1:8030	1:4689
Ramban	1:8597	1:40530	1:25792	1:7466	1:4809
Reasi	1:8281	1:52445	1:52445	1:7675	1:5075
Samba	1:7972	1:28991	1:24531	1:8177	1:6378
Udhampur	1:10882	1:29210	1:27749	1:6453	1:5441
Jammu Div.	**1:10245**	**1:48023**	**1:31090**	**1:6254**	**1:5055**

Source: Compiled by Authors.

Ladakh Division

The situation in Ladakh Division is comparatively on higher side. Since the absolute number of people is low which reduces ratio of different health delivery parameters *vis-à-vis* population. Rural population in the division is nearly neglected in terms of health facilities. In fact, almost every health care unit is provided with indoor bed facility. However, maximum health institutions, which have bed facilities, are all located at Leh—the largest urban unit of Ladakh Division. Thus, the strong polarization of health services is in urban areas. There are 290 medical institutions in the Ladakh division, which include district hospitals, sub-district hospitals, primary health centres, allopathic dispensaries and sub-centres and other more than 100 funded and controlled semi-government health institutions like Amchi centres.[15] These institutions serve a population of 2,74,289 persons (2.81% to total J&K population) (Table 22.11). The institution/ population ratio is 1:946. However, the dispensary/population ratio is 1:16135 and PHC ratio is 1:17143. The bulk of health care institution, about 19.6 per cent is based on health sub-centers, which do not possess any type of specialized health services. Another important indicator pertaining to health care is the availability of

Table 22.11: District-wise Health Care Facilities in Ladakh Division

Sl. No.	District	District Hospital	Sub-District Hospital/ CHC	Primary Health Centre	Allopathic Dispensary	District TB Centre	Medical Aid Centres	Sub-Centres	Total Institute	Assistant Surgeon	Dental Surgeon	Specia-lists	Nurses/ FMPHW/ ANMS	Para-medics
1.	Leh	1	4	2	14	1	100	33	155	60	6	10	270	300
2.	Kargil	1	6	14	3	1	86	24	135	23	2	5	194	234
	Ladakh Div.	**2**	**10**	**16**	**17**	**2**	**186**	**57**	**290**	**83**	**8**	**15**	**464**	**534**

Source: Directorate of Health Service, J&K, 2014.

Table 22.12: District-wise Institution/Population Ratio in Ladakh Division

District	District Hospital/ Population Ratio	Sub-District Hospital/ CHC/ Population Ratio	Primary/ Health Centre/ Population Ratio	Allopathic Dispensary/ Population Ratio	District TB Centre/ Population Ratio	Medical Aid Centres/ Population Ratio	Sub-Centres/ Population Ratio	Population Bed Ratio	Total Institution/ Population Ratio
Leh	1:133487	1:33372	1:66744	1:9535	1:133487	1:1335	1:4045	297	1:861
Kargil	1:140802	1:23467	1:10057	1:46934	1:140802	1:1637	1:5867	361	1:1043
Ladakh Div.	1:137145	1:27429	1:17143	1:16135	1:137145	1:1475	1:4812	327	1:946

Source: Compiled by Authors.

hospital beds. Table 22.12 reveals that bed/population ratio for Ladakh Division is 1:327. The bulk of bed facility in the state is available in Ladakh district. In district Leh, 155 institutions are rendering health serve to a population of 1,33,487 persons (1.12% to total J&K population). Thus, the institution/population ratio is 1:861 whereas the bed/population ratio in the same district is 1:297. The total health institution in Kargil district is about 135 and institution population ratio is 1:1043 and bed population ratio is 1:361. Similarly, Table 22.13 reveals strong medical staff at various health institutions of Ladakh Division.

Table 22.13: District-wise Medical/Paramedical Personnel in Ladakh Division

District	*Assistant Surgeon/ Population Ratio*	*Dental Surgeon/ Population Ratio*	*Specialists/ Population Ratio*	*Nurses/ FMPHW/ ANMS/ Population Ratio*	*Paramedics/ Population Ratio*
Leh	1:2225	1:22248	1:13349	1:494	1:445
Kargil	1:6122	1:70401	1:28160	1:726	1:602
Ladakh Div.	1:3305	1:34286	1:18286	1:591	1:514

Source: Compiled by Authors.

Levels of Development in Healthcare Infrastructure

Health care in Jammu & Kashmir is deranged and is not up to the prescribed standards; as such it faces serious crises in cost, quality of care and equitable distribution and standards of service to the population as a whole. To present the disparity in health care infrastructure Z-score method has been applied to compute composite score of various health indicators like various tiers of health institutions and health personnel etc. on the basis of their relative strength as reflected in ratio (health facilities per 10,000 of population). It may be pointed here that higher the value of Z-score determines higher development in health care and lower the value of Z-score means lower health infrastructure in Jammu & Kashmir State (Table 22.14). Thus, there exist noticeable regional imbalances in health care facilities. The values of Z-score vary from 10.53 in Jammu district to 29.27 in Leh district. These values have been categorized in five ranges, i.e. very high development, high development, medium development, low development and very low development. Table

Table 22.14: Z Score of Health Care Facilities in Jammu & Kashmir

Sl. No.	District	District Hospital	Sub-District Hospital/ CHC	Primary Health Centre	Allopathic Dispensary	District TB Centre	Medical Aid Centres	Sub-Centres	Assistant Surgeon	Dental Surgeon	Specia-lists	Nurses/ FMPHW/	Para-medics ANMS	Aggregate Z Score
1.	Anantnag	–0.607	–0.307	–0.643	–0.645	–0.282	–0.391	–1.063	–0.826	–0.322	–1.470	–0.702	–0.364	–7.622
2.	Budgam	–0.607	0.307	0.364	–0.692	–0.725	–0.422	–0.287	–0.912	–0.995	–1.159	–0.756	–0.562	–6.446
3.	Bandipora	–1.109	–0.102	–1.080	–0.549	–0.725	–0.376	–1.310	1.299	2.678	1.142	0.103	0.177	0.148
4.	Baramulla	–0.607	–0.307	–0.511	–0.263	–0.282	–0.376	–0.881	–0.076	0.661	–0.164	–0.483	–0.307	–3.596
5.	Ganderbal	–1.109	0.410	2.509	–0.645	–0.725	–0.376	1.711	0.243	1.489	–0.910	–0.516	–0.369	1.712
6.	Kulgam	–0.105	–0.410	0.233	–0.263	–0.725	–0.381	–0.221	–0.162	1.644	–0.972	–0.185	0.063	–1.484
7.	Kupwara	–0.607	–0.102	–0.161	–0.836	–0.282	–0.200	–0.023	–0.076	–0.063	–0.724	0.343	–0.048	–2.779
8.	Pulwama	–0.105	–0.410	–0.117	0.167	0.161	–0.386	–0.584	0.059	0.092	–0.413	–0.350	–0.385	–2.271
9.	Shopian	–1.109	–0.102	–0.730	–0.549	–0.725	–0.345	–0.221	0.095	0.454	–1.034	–0.210	–0.204	–4.68
10.	Srinagar	–0.607	–0.819	–1.431	–0.645	–0.282	–0.438	–2.400	–0.838	–0.995	–0.786	–0.729	–0.564	–10.53
11.	Doda	–0.105	–0.410	0.058	1.409	–0.725	–0.014	0.522	0.120	0.454	0.582	–0.075	–0.457	1.359
12.	Jammu	–0.607	–0.410	–0.643	–0.884	–0.282	–0.407	–0.567	–0.605	–0.943	0.209	–0.505	–0.550	–6.194
13.	Kathua	–0.105	–0.307	0.101	–0.406	0.161	–0.345	0.770	–0.359	–1.357	–0.413	0.908	0.000	–1.352
14.	Kishtwar	0.899	–0.512	–0.030	1.218	1.047	0.115	0.341	–0.175	–0.115	–0.102	–0.336	–0.411	1.939
15.	Poonch	–0.105	–0.307	–0.161	0.215	0.161	–0.334	0.374	–0.457	–0.995	0.644	–0.347	–0.101	–1.413
16.	Rajouri	–0.105	0.307	0.320	0.215	0.161	–0.339	2.075	–0.752	–0.529	0.582	–0.383	–0.335	1.217
17.	Ramban	0.899	–0.512	–0.030	0.406	–0.725	–0.133	–0.683	–0.187	–0.374	0.707	–0.354	–0.345	–1.331
18.	Reasi	0.397	–0.307	0.058	0.119	–0.725	–0.293	0.473	–0.126	–0.684	–0.537	–0.365	–0.366	–2.356
19.	Samba	0.397	–0.615	–0.074	–0.979	–0.725	–0.396	0.935	–0.076	0.092	0.831	–0.403	–0.442	–1.455
20.	Udhampur	–0.105	–0.717	0.233	0.358	1.047	–0.277	0.093	–0.482	0.092	0.520	–0.241	–0.390	0.131
21.	Leh	2.657	3.687	2.859	–0.215	2.818	2.886	0.027	3.903	0.661	2.945	3.509	3.536	29.273
22.	Kargil	2.456	1.946	–1.124	3.462	2.375	3.227	0.919	0.390	–0.943	0.520	2.078	2.423	17.729

Table 22.15: Levels of Development

Sl. No.	District	Aggregate Score	Levels of Development
1.	Leh	29.273	Very High
2.	Kargil	17.729	
3.	Kishtwar	1.939	High
4.	Ganderbal	1.712	
5.	Doda	1.359	
6.	Rajouri	1.217	
7.	Bandipora	0.148	
8.	Udhampur	0.131	
9.	Ramban	–1.331	Medium
10.	Kathua	–1.352	
11.	Poonch	–1.413	
12.	Samba	–1.455	
13.	Kulgam	–1.484	
14.	Pulwama	–2.271	Low
15.	Reasi	–2.356	
16.	Kupwara	–2.779	
17.	Baramulla	–3.596	
18.	Shopian	–4.68	
19.	Jammu	–6.194	Very Low
20.	Budgam	–6.446	
21.	Anantnag	–7.622	
22.	Srinagar	–10.53	

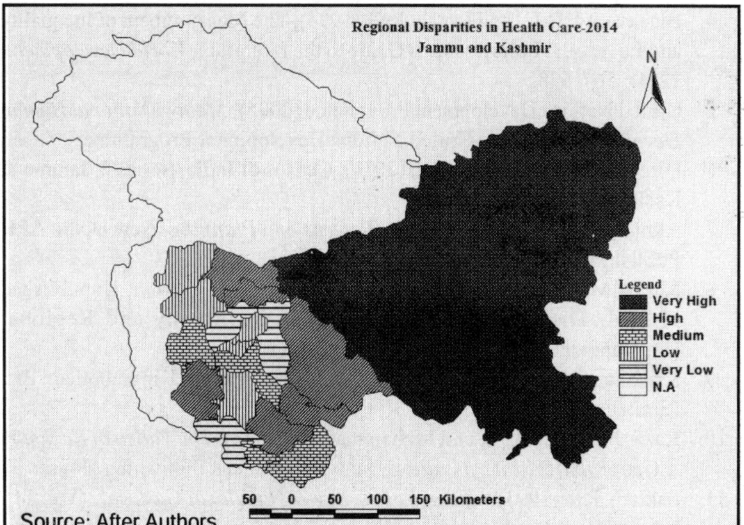

Source: After Authors.

22.15 reveals that Leh and Kargil districs possess very high level of development, while as six districts, *viz.* Kishtwar, Ganderbal, Doda, Rajouri, Bandipora and Udhampur fall in the high level of development. Ramban, Kathua, Poonch, Samba and Kulgam districts have medium level of health care development. The five districts namely Pulwama, Reasi, Kupwara, Baramulla and Shopian fall in the category of low level development. The remaining four districts fall in the category of very low development such as Jammu, Anatnag, Badgam and Srinagar. Srinagar and Jammu districts fall in low range of health facilities is attributed to high population numbers which lowers the ratio.

Notes

1. Sharma, and Kumar (1993), "Regional Disparities in the Levels of Socio-Economic Development in India", in Tripathi, R.S. and Tewari, R.P. (eds.), *Regional Disparities and Development in India*, New Delhi: Ashish Publishing House, pp. 61-80.
2. Shukla, A. (2000), *Regional Planning and Sustainable Development*, New Delhi: Kanishka Publishers, pp. 3-16.
3. Gulati, R.K. (1999), *Regional Disparities in Economic Development: Policies and Prospects for Balanced Regional Development*, Delhi: Deep & Deep Publications.
4. Blackwood, D.L., and Lynch, R.G (1994), The Measurement of Inequality and Poverty: A Policymaker's Guide to the Literature, *World Development*, 22(4), 567-578.
5. United Nations Development Programme (2005), *Malawi National Human Development Report*, United Nations Development Programme.
6. Directorate, Census of India, (2011), Census of India, Series 8, Jammu & Kashmir.
7. Akhtar, R. (2004), *Health Care Patterns and Planning*, New Delhi: APH Publishing Corporation, pp. 3-22.
8. Mir, A.M. (1982), *Regional Structure of Jammu Division*, Unpublished M.Phil. Dissertation, Department of Geography and Regional Development, University of Kashmir, Srinagar.
9. Krishnan, M.S. (1968), *Geology of India and Burma*, Higginbotham Pvt. Limited, pp. 522-523.
10. Raza, M., Ahmad, A., and Mohammad, A. (1978), *The Valley of Kashmir: A Geographical Interpretation*, New Delhi: Vikas Publishing House.
11. Saklani, P.S. (1993), *Geology of the Lower Himalaya: Garhwal*, (Vol. 14), International Books and Periodicals Supply Service.

12. Dar, R.A., Rashid, I., Romshoo, S.A. and Marazi, A. (2014), Sustainability of Winter Tourism in a Changing Climate Over Kashmir Himalaya, *Environmental Monitoring and Assessment*, 186(4), 2549-2562.
13. Mayer, A.I. (2007), *Medical Geography*, New Delhi: A.P.H. Publishing Corporation.
14. Akhtar, R. and A.Q. Khan (2004), *Spatial Organization of Health Care Facilities in Jammu and Kashmir*, New Delhi: A.P.H. Publishing Corporation, pp. 151-162.
15. Mayer, I.A. (2009), *A Geographical Analysis of Sustainability, Acceptability and Challenges of Amchi Medical Care System in Himalayan Region*, Ladakh, India, *Journal of Himalayan Ecology and Sustainable Development*, Vol. 4, pp. 77-87, Srinagar: University of Kashmir.

23
Medical Education, Doctors' Behaviour in India?
With Focus on Indian Doctors' Exodus

Rais Akhtar

Introduction—Historical Perspective

The unequal distribution of health care is a typical feature of developing countries including India. In these countries great majority of people suffer excess mortality and morbidity while in contrast the affluent enjoy a health status similar to that of most people in the developed world. Health services also show a lopsided pattern with expenditure primarily concentrated on sophisticated facilities in urban areas, leaving the rural majority practically un-served. The provision of a doctor is the most important component of health care facilities. However, rough estimates suggest that in India nearly 80 per cent of the doctor population work in urban areas which comprise about 25 per cent of the total population.

The amendment (1993) in the Consumer Protection Act, 1986* bringing private doctors also under the Act's purview has provoked loud protests from the doctor community. The focus of their protest is that there is a sacred tie between a doctor and a patient, and this relation will suffer with the implementation of this Act. Of course, there is a sacred tie between the two in many cases, but the large number of new generation doctors may not be practicing such medical

* Consumer Protection Act, 1986 (Amendment 1993) passed by the Government in 1993 is aimed at examining complaints against private doctors for negligence, if any.

ethics. There is a need to elaborate this dimension of medical ethics and the framework of a doctor in the Indian context with relevant examples.

It is an open fact that majority of Indian medical graduates either wish to emigrate or practice in urban areas. Therefore, one find it very difficult to understand as to why we still continue to train over 13,170 doctors annually in 165 medical colleges, at a cost of more than ₹ 1 million each.* These doctors, according to Antia (1989)[1], detest preventive and social medicine and the majority of whom wish to specialize in increasingly abstruse branches of curative medicine, more suited for those who migrate to the affluent countries or practice in affluent urban hospitals in the private sector . . . of the estimated three lakh allopathic doctors, over 70 per cent are at present working in the private sector and of these 80 per cent are in the urban areas, while 75 per cent of our population is rural. The reason for medicine being the students' first choice is not because of a sense of service to the people, especially the underprivileged, but because it ensures a lucrative practice with minimal risk and high social status. Hence, the rush for admissions, payment of capitation fees, opening of private medical colleges for those (affluent group) who cannot get admission into the highly subsidized government ones.

This argument by Antia can be substantiated by Table 23.1, which reveals that the majority of Indian doctors who went abroad for specialization belong to surgery and only an insignificant number, i.e. 45 belong to public health, which is so vital from the point of view of the Third World. This is clear evidence that majority of the doctors don't want to serve their own country and wish to remain in Western countries—United States and United Kingdom, where surgery and general medicine are more in demand than public health, while TB and chest diseases and pathology are more relevant in Third World countries.

Antia has also stated (1989), that:

> Maximising of monetary gain and overproduction of doctors has invariably led to corrupt practices like fee splitting, giving of unnecessary medicines and injections. The search for monetary gain has also led to the deliberate mystification of

* ₹ 39.69 is equal to USD 1 (in 1990), Current Exchange Rate is ₹ 66 equal to USD.

medicine. Patients are encouraged to seek the services of the doctors for every imagined illness and accept expensive and unnecessary investigations and therapies.

Banerji has rightly highlighted the crisis prevailing in the medical profession in India, which is, "manifested in the form of a sharp decline in the ethical standards in the practice of medicine".[2] He quoted examples of the deaths due to use of contaminated intravenous fluids in the prestigious J.J. Hospital in Mumbai and allegation of irregularities in the award of a doctoral degree in medicine to the daughter of the former Chief Minister of Maharashtra state. The Government of Maharashtra was forced to set-up two inquiry commissions (headed by Justice Lentin). These two commissions have highlighted the malpractices committed in the two premier institutions in the country, namely J.J. Hospital attached to the Grant Medical College and the quality of postgraduate medical examinations being conducted by the University of Bombay.

Table 23.1: Subject-wise Distribution of Indian Doctors Trained Abroad (1990-98)

Subject	*Total Number*	
	1990	*1998*
Surgery	1,601	1,678
General Medicine	1,187	1,216
Obstetrics/Gyanae	716	747
Paediatrics	414	443
Ophthalmology	297	306
Anaesthesiology	264	282
Pathology	89	100
Psychiatry	85	87
Radiology	75	78
Dentistry	65	66
TB-Chest Diseases	51	51
Medicine and Surgery	59	62
Public Health	45	45
Others	779	532
Total	**5,727**	**5,693**

Source: Health Information of India, Ministry of Health and Family Welfare, New Delhi, 1991, 1997 and 1998, p. 118.

Further examples of decline in medical ethics can be seen in the study conducted in Mumbai by R.S. Kumar, who uncovered some of the malpractices in the medical world. "If you visit a doctor for treatment of common cold for instance, you may be pumped with antibiotics, analgesics, vitamins, tonics and decongestants, when all it needs is steam inhalation at home and a couple of words of caution."[3]

Kumar quoted Pilgaonkar, a retired biochemist who had worked with the WHO, listing only 277 essential drugs and the country having no use for more than 1,000 formulations, even if multiple drug combinations for complicated diseases like tuberculosis are included. Yet the country has a floating market of 60,000 formulations, as drug stores stock many irrelevant medicines—a reflection of the patterns of demand created by the doctor-patient nexus. Kumar quoted one patient who revealed how he was lured into taking a blood test as well as an X-ray for a simple anaesthetic procedure. It is common knowledge that many practitioners are in collusion with agencies that own expensive equipments like computerized axial-tomography (CT) scans or laparoscopes who recommend patients to them for a commission from the organizations. The extent to which medicine is now viewed as a business is reflected in the rash of advertisements for diagnostic centres that have begun to sprout on the walls of the city and in trains and buses, as if the equipment were television sets or pressure cookers. Besides these, diagnostic centres in collusion with practitioners have been known to advise surgery, one more flourishing racket.[3a]

Besides, the scheme of importing high technology medical equipments donated through the American Association of Physicians of Indian Origin (AAPIO) in association with the Medical Council of India may add fillip to the trend to acquire inappropriate and unnecessary technology. This will only push up the cost of medicine not only in private institutions, but in public hospitals as well.[3]

According to Tinaikar (1992), over the last decade, the growth of high-tech, five-star hospitals on the one hand, and medical colleges which thrive on astronomical capitation fees, on the other, have substantially contributed to the steep fall in medical ethics and the commercialization of medical profession in this country. Most of these hospitals enjoy the status of public charitable trusts, and as research centres enjoy further rebates and tax concessions. Tinaikar suggests that it is the responsibility of the management of these hospitals to establish internal mechanisms of independent committees to investigate substantiated complaints from patients of overcharging or clandestine charging of fees, excessive or improper drugging, failure to disclose the condition of the patient or the result of diagnosis or the line of treatment, or the absence and "informed consent" and, above all, the use of patients for clinical research purposes.[4]

Such malpractices are not only confined to metropolitan cities, but are also increasing in smaller towns in India. One report suggests that private medical practitioners have never had it so good in Haryana, the state with the second highest per capita income in India. In Karnal, Hissar, Rohtak and elsewhere in Haryana, hysterectomy, cholecystectomy and appendesectomy clinics are seen everywhere.[5] A report on the flourishing of medical 'shops' in rural areas of Punjab reveals a grim story.[6] The number of non-qualified and uneducated 'doctors' have increased the past few years in the border district of Amritsar due to non-availability of medical facilities. In the garb of treating patients these quacks befool the poor and innocent villagers and make a fast buck. With majority of government doctors absenting themselves from duty in the remote areas, the people are left with no choice but to get themselves treated from these 'doctors'. These 'doctors' include graduates and undergraduates in humanities and sciences who worked as helpers to senior doctors in the cities; Registered Medical Practitioners (RMP); Ayurvedic and Unani physicians who worked as allopathic doctors; and mobile doctors who just carried with them a few medicines (used for all kinds of diseases), injections and a stethoscope. It has also been noted that these so-called doctors have liaison with private nursing homes operating in cities.

Easy money has resulted in the mushrooming of nursing homes and diagnostic centres set-up by not only doctors but quacks who are neither qualified nor hold any stake in the medical profession. The number of such centres has increased many folds with the introduction of computerized equipments which have become handy for the doctors to impress rural patients. In Delhi alone there are about 13,000 such nursing homes and diagnostic centres out of which only 1,000 are registered.

Doctor Dilemma

Table 23.2 shows the supply of doctors for the period 1950 to 1998. It is obvious that there has been more than a tenfold increase in the number of doctors. The latest figures reveal that India produces nearly 13,170 doctors a year. Contrary to this only about 9,000 nurses are trained, though even a rough estimate tells us that the actual need for nurses is over three times the number of doctors. As it is evident from the socio-political framework, the supply of doctors was deliberate. "The demand for medical education which led to the rapid expansion of medical colleges in the 1960s and early 1970s was in part fuelled directly by parents who saw the chances of emigration for their children."[7]

In 1986 alone 238 doctors left for abroad, more than 50 per cent to Arab countries, through Government of India's Foreign Assignment Section. However, large numbers of doctors who join foreign jobs are not covered under Government's Foreign Assignment Section.

Table 23.2: Number of Doctors, Medical Colleges and Annual Output of Doctors

	Doctor	*Medical Colleges*	*Annual Output of Doctor*
1950	65,000	30	950
1990	3,65,000	128	12,292
1998	5,03,900	165	13,170

Source: Ministry of Health and Family Welfare, New Delhi, and R. Jaffery (1988), *The Politics of Health in India*.

Doctor Shortage and Unemployment

On the one hand there is acute shortage of doctors particularly in rural and remote hilly areas; on the other hand, large numbers of doctors are unemployed and their number is on the increase. Table 23.3 shows the number of medical graduates and postgraduates on the live register of employment exchanges in different states and union territories. It is significant to note that the number of unemployed doctors is the highest in states with four metropolises namely, Delhi, Mumbai, Chennai and Kolkata. From the figure of nearly 25,612 unemployed doctors in 1986, the numbers rose to 31,360 in 1996 (Table 23.3). Despite the fact that nearly 50,000 Medical Graduates and 23,000 Post-Graduates are being produced in 362 medical colleges our large number of health centres and rural hospitals are running without doctors.[8]

In this context, the suggestion put forward by Gish needs serious consideration. According to him, "it may very well be that if the alternative of emigration is closed to these graduates many may then find their way into smaller and smaller population clusters."[9] Thus, there is urgent need to implement the parallel stream of medical practitioners to improve the health care system in rural areas.[10]

Table 23.3: Number of Medical Graduates and Postgraduates (1986-96)

States/Union Territories	*1986*	*1996*
Andhra Pradesh	1,894	5,067
Assam	138	105
Bihar	1,514	1,289
Gujarat	785	285
Haryana	405	607
Himachal Pradesh	113	507
Jammu & Kashmir	10	40
Karnataka	1,078	1,138
Kerala	1,492	3,764
Madhya Pradesh	1,133	858
Maharashtra	3,844	3,745
Manipur	45	132
Meghalaya	5	1
Orissa	528	1,825
Punjab	732	395
Rajasthan	673	2,382
Tamil Nadu	2,419	1,960
Tripura	17	85
Uttar Pradesh	1,814	1,110
West Bengal	2,145	1,221
Chandigarh	606	720
Delhi	3,873	3,561
Goa, Daman & Diu	113	146
Lakshadweep	7	6
Mizoram	4	17
Pondicherry	228	348
Total	**25,615**	**31,314**

Source : Health Information of India, Ministry of Health and Family Welfare, New Delhi, 1987 and 1997, Total in India, in 2012: Graduates-45,629, and Post Graduates-22,503.

Doctors in India: Working Conditions

Gish quoted one foreign returned doctor who wrote an article "Brain-drain in Medicine", published in the *Times of India* in November 1969, as saying,

> Today politicians and leader-writers never tire of repeating that there is a great need for doctors in rural areas (*TOI*, 2015) that while there may be one doctor for a thousand persons in the towns, there is often less than one doctor to a hundred thousand population in villages in the remote parts of the country. This is true and the need for medical facilities in the rural areas cannot be denied, but can one seriously expect a highly trained specialist or surgeon to go and settle down in a rural hospital? He has been trained, often at great expense to himself and the country, to perform a specialised task and his talents and skills would be completely wasted in a rural dispensary. Of the rural hospitals, the less said the better. The equipment is Victorian and often does not work. These hospitals lack laboratories and investigative facilities. The only way to get highly trained medical men to settle down in a rural area is to establish a University atmosphere of the kind which is found at the Christian Medical College in Vellore.[10, 11]

Another Indian physician, quoted by the *New York Times* (24 March, 1974) put it as, "there is not even a hut in many villages to work from, there is no medicine, equipment is zero. . . ." In my opinion there is some exaggeration in the statement. However, with such a lucrative framework in mind, it looks impossible to persuade urban doctors to settle down in rural areas. To quote Maru, "even in China where the government assigns jobs to every college graduate, and where dissenting leaders of the medical profession and the party were purged during the Cultural Revolution, it has not been possible radically to alter the distribution of high-level medical manpower in favour of the countryside"[12].

> It is obvious from the observations of doctors that the majority of them would not accept working in rural areas, and the available resources in the country cannot create Vellore-type atmosphere in our rural areas. It is worth noting that the vast majority of rural and urban population does not require specialized treatment though urban areas in India as in most developing countries are experiencing fast epidemiological transition similar to Western world. We in fact need a basic doctor who could treat the general communicable and water-borne diseases. Moreover, the present situation related to

the non-acceptance of rural jobs is against the accepted policy of the Government of India in respect of undergraduate medical education in the country. This policy clearly states "That the ultimate goal of medical education should be to enable its products to deal, in the most effective measures, with the health problems of the society." In view of this Bajaj has laid greater emphasis on the teaching of infectious diseases like amoebiasis. Nevertheless, the real significance of such economic losses lies in the fact that money spent on the education of these emigrant physicians or urban-based doctors would have been better spent on other forms of health personnel and healthcare.[13]

Election Promises

Notwithstanding the fact that the existing medical colleges in the country have not benefitted the majority of the population, especially in the rural areas, politicians are not tired of promising the opening up of new medical colleges during elections, obviously for gaining political support. The example of the State of Gujarat can be cited in this context.[14]

It is significant to note that Gujarat in 1989 had 613 unemployed doctors and certainly there was no need for an additional medical college to produce more doctors. Contrary to this, the state minister of health had announced in October 1989 that the Gujarat government has decided to open four new medical colleges with 50-seat capacity one each in Bhawnagar, Rajkot, Palanpur, and Surendranagar. According to the Gujarat government, the decision was taken in view of the shortage of doctors in the State. It is also evident from Table 23.3 that both Andhra Pradesh and Karnataka had a large number of unemployed doctors. Yet, both the State Governments had attempted to establish more fee-paying medical institutes. This had also contributed to the downfall of the two governments in late 1992. In the context of Gujarat, the decision to establish more medical colleges was taken by the state government, almost one month before the General Election in November 1989. In 1994, the Minister of Education in Gujarat had resigned due to the shifting of the location of one proposed medical college from his home constituency. This is a clear indication that the location of a medical college determines the influence of a politician.

Government Efforts

In 1990, the State Government of Uttar Pradesh (the most populous state of the country), finalized a new policy for transfer of doctors. According to it doctors will have to serve at a rural place for a period of three years. They could remain in a district for five years; specialized doctors could be posted for six years. In a division, comprising of 4-5 districts, a doctor could stay for not more than 12 years. However, lady doctors were exempt from these rules. A doctor who did not render services in rural or hilly areas for at least two years would not be entitled for promotion.[15] The policy has some rural focus and can benefit the people if implemented strictly. Nevertheless, in addition to promotion, some financial benefits to doctors serving in the rural areas would certainly go a long way in the successful implementation of this policy.*

In 1990, the Ministry of Health and Family Welfare, Government of India, proposed that it should be incumbent on all doctors to serve in rural areas before being awarded degrees. According to the then health minister, the situation in rural areas is truly dismal as of a total of 4.5 lakh doctors in the country, only 21,000 are working in villages, while the rural areas contain about 75 per cent of the total population. It has been pointed out that such proposal had been under discussion for quite some time, but has failed to take off because of stiff resistance from the medical fraternity.

Private Practice by Government Doctors

Doctors working in India remained seriously concerned with both private practice and urban preference. A large number of doctors in the state of West Bengal Health Service, agitated against enacting a

---

* The proposal of the Indian Health Ministry panel to create a parallel stream of a 3-year course of community health workers to improve the delivery of health care in rural areas, which generally suffer from basic communicable, nutritional and environment-based diseases is a welcome suggestion (Mudur, 2007). Similar proposal was suggested by the author 23 years ago in his joint paper (with Nilofar Izhar), "Inequalities in the Distribution of Health Care in India", in R. Akhtar and A.T.A. Learmonth (eds.), *Geographical Aspects of Health and Disease in India*, New Delhi: Concept Publishing Company, 1985, pp. 437-60.
Also see, R. Akhtar and N. Izhar (1986), "The Spatial Distribution of Health Resources Within Countries and Communities: Examples from India and Zambia", *Social Science and Medicine*, 22, pp. 1115-29.

legislation in 1990 making all teaching posts in medical institutions as non-practicing ones. They argued that the legislation would not stop private practice as teachers were the supporters of the Left Front Government and would continue their private practice. According to this report, some senior officers such as a vice-chancellor and some deans of medical faculties are engaged in private practice though officially debarred from doing so. In this context, it is interesting to note that a study carried out in 1991 decried private practice by doctors in medical colleges in India as it is the major reason for poor quality of their research output. The study conducted by the *National Medical Journal of India* (NMJI), aimed at assessing research done in India's 128 medical colleges over a nine year period.[16] The study noted that among the six institutions with highest publications, private practice is not permitted in five institutions.

Capitation Fee

Another serious problem is the establishment of private medical colleges. The criterion for admission in these medical colleges is mainly the paying of the capitation fee. Many such colleges have cropped up in Bihar and in the southern states. As a result, a large number of foreign students mainly from the Middle East and some from Africa, who cannot get admission in their own countries, and children of affluent parents (NRI) find their way into these medical colleges. These medical colleges not only run on the money they collect but have become a source of income leading to commercialization of medical education. According to Sinha "more and more medical colleges are being started every year and there is no way in which Medical Council of India can stop private medical colleges. Not only students with poor merit get entry into these private medical colleges but even the atmosphere is not conducive to medical education."[17] Interestingly, it was reported that the Indian Medical Association decided to start medical colleges in various parts of the country with an objective to provide quality education and eradicate several "unethical systems" prevailing in the medical education, including charging of capitation fee.[18] The intervention by the Supreme Court in the allotment of seats and fee structure in private medical colleges in Maharashtra will go a long way in streamlining the fee structure in medical colleges.

It is interesting to note that in 1990, a self-financing private medical college had started functioning at Vadakkankulam in south Tamil Nadu without the approval of the MGR Medical University, Medical Council of India or the state government. Similar self-financing dental colleges seemed to be suddenly mushrooming in the state. The Tamil Nadu Medical Students Association started an agitation against the establishment of these private medical colleges in the early 1990s. The association's argument was that the doctor-population ratio was actually in excess of the norms recommended by the Mudaliar Committee and that the students passing out of private medical colleges were not being properly trained due to the inadequate infrastructure. According to the association, the evil of capitation fee will vitiate all aspects of education and reduce medical and dental colleges into commercial establishments.[19] High capitation fees are one of the reasons that, as per *The Hindu* sources more than 9,000 Indians are enrolled in medical colleges in China as of 2013.[20]

The question is why India has failed to check the deterioration in medical education. The answer lies in the commercialization of medicine because of political patronage as discussed earlier.

To quote Madan,

> many of the newly opened medical colleges are, in the words of the President of the Medical Council of India, "monuments to political influence". The overproduction of doctors leads to unemployment since they are unwilling to serve rural areas despite the fact that large number of health centres in rural areas need doctors. Political support to the overproduction of doctors is evident from the fact that in India, as in Pakistan and Bangladesh, there are more doctors than nurses. Since the training of nurses has no material advantage, no private training centres are being established. Even the government is not keen in the establishment of new nurses training centres though there is acute shortage of paramedical staff in the country.[21]

Medical Education Abroad

Since the 1990s and immediately after the breakup of the Soviet Union, there has been a heavy rush of Indian students who seek admissions in medical colleges in Russia, Ukraine, Turkmenistan,

Kazakhstan. Thousands of students are being trained in these countries as well as in China, Romania, Bangladesh and Nepal. In several cases, even students of humanities and ineligible science students have been admitted in medical courses abroad.[22]

Medical Council of India, has taken a serious view of this, and in 2001 modified the Act, pertaining to medical education in foreign universities. The amended Act states that a person shall not be entitled to be enrolled on any medical register maintained by a State Medical Council or to have his/her name entered in the Indian Medical Register unless he/she qualifies the screening test in India prescribed for such a purpose. It is only after the successful qualification of the list that the foreign medical qualification is deemed to be a recognized medical qualification.

The Act further states that to be eligible to get admission and obtain medical qualification granted by any medical institution in any foreign country the candidate should obtain an eligibility certificate issued by the Council. Otherwise he shall not be eligible to appear in the screening test referred to in sub-section (Part III Section 4).

In the light of the above socio-economic and political framework of doctors, the policy-makers need to look into the system of present medical education in India. Establishment of medical colleges should be banned and all capitation fee colleges be closed down. Medical education should be available purely on merit. It may not be out of context to mention that majority of the doctors who completely ignore medical ethics might be coming from capitation fee based medical colleges. However, we need to research on this aspect before arriving at a definite relationship. Nevertheless, poor patients are being exploited. As regards private clinics and diagnostic clinics, it is suggested that all the private clinics be registered only when run by qualified persons. A policy should be evolved under which the distribution pattern of private practitioners is governed, whereby all the residential areas are benefited with the availability of private medical services. Thus, it was a timely decision by the government to bring the private medical practice under the Consumer Protection Act.

Contemporary Scenario

There are currently 362 medical colleges in the country that offer

45,629 MBBS seats and 22,503 Post Graduate seats between them. This makes India the largest producer of doctors in the world. In comparison, the United States only produces 18,000 doctors a year. The following figure shows the regional disparities in the availability of medical seats in different zones.[20]

Number of Medical Sets Across Zones

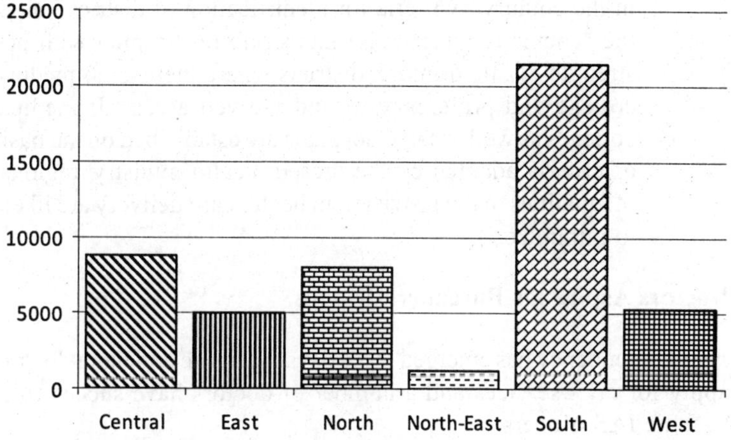

Source: Thomas Manuel, *The Wire* 28.8.2015.

The sad affairs of India's health care systems was highlighted by Andrew MacAskill and colleagues assert that "India's system for training doctors is broken. It is plagued by rampant fraud and unprofessional teaching practices, exacerbating the public health challenge facing this fast-growing but still poor nation of about 1.25 billion people.... In a four-month investigation, Reuters has documented the full extent of the fraud in India's medical-education system. It was found, among other things, that more than one out of every six of the country's 398 medical schools has been accused of cheating, according to Indian government records and court filings."[23]

Regional disparities and lack of accessibility to health care centres have now been understood by the Ministry of Health and Family Welfare. The increase in the number of medical colleges is not important but the location where the new medical colleges are being established. Identification of underserved areas is important, and the Ministry of Health and family Welfare's decision to establish 58 new medical colleges under a centrally sponsored scheme for

"Establishment of Medical Colleges attached with existing District/ Referral hospitals", The Health and Family Welfare Minister J.P. Nadda stated in a written reply in Rajya Sabha. The Minister stated that,

> "In the first phase, total 58 districts have been identified. This initiative would result in increase of 5,800 MBBS seats in the country." Criteria for identification of districts under the scheme are district hospitals/referral hospital with bed strength of 200 or more, districts where there is no medical college and preference to underserved areas.[8] If medical colleges as well as large hospitals are established on the basis of criteria adopted by the present health ministry, regional inequalities in the provision in health care delivery are likely to minimize.

Doctors Aspire for Bureaucratic Jobs

Another tendency has emerged these days that more and more doctors apply for civil services and a number of doctors have successfully become IAS officers.

As one of the Members of the UPSC PT Board, I have interviewed couple of doctors who want to serve larger society by becoming a Civil Servant, rather working as a doctor. A. Arun Thamburaj, a qualified doctor and an IAS topper from Tamil Nadu came sixth in the 2012 civil services examination, firmly believes that the "pen is mightier than the scalpel" in the service of people at least in India. Interesting several doctors have secure first position in UPSC Civil Services Examination. Shena Aggarwal, who holds an MBBS degree from the All-India Institute of Medical Sciences here, bagged the top slot in the 2011 Civil Services examinations.Before Shena Aggarwal, *Shah Faesal,* a *Kashmiri* doctor, hailing from Sogam village of border district Kupwara, *topped the* 2009 *civil services exams.* Another doctor IAS Nipun Jindal said, "The IAS was chosen for wider public platform. Here I will be able to serve the people in a better way as compared to medical profession. I want to improve upon the system in our country". An other doctor from Jammu & Kashmir stated that "Being a civil servant, I can be a 'doctor' for the whole society."

To a question about increasing number of doctors aspiring for civil services Roman Saini who was selected in 2013, replied, "First of all, very few doctors actually come to Civil Services. Every year about 55,000 MBBS students get their degrees. Yet only 50 get into civil services. Assuming 20 times of that number actually prepare and give the exam, only 1000 doctors try to change their field to Civil service every year. Now try to get the picture that a doctor giving this exam will give all the attempts possible. So, out of 4-5 batches of 2,50,000 doctors, only 1000 appear in this exam. This amounts to just 0.4 per cent totally refuting the argument that so many doctors come for IAS".

Despite the above the question remains if the increase in the number of medical colleges and the increase in the number of MBBS Seats, is going to benefit the country? I will assert NO. Government need to formulate policy to attract doctors to serve rural areas. "Attracting doctors to rural posts is an ongoing challenge for health departments across different states in India. One strategy adopted by several states to make rural service attractive for medical graduates is to reserve post-graduate (PG) seats in medical colleges for doctors serving in the public sector."[24] Even this provision may not be successful looking into the Gujarat scenario. Recent report from Gujarat stated that out of more than 4,300 MBBS students who passed out from state-run medical colleges between 2009 and 2014, only 530 served in government-run hospitals in rural areas for three years as per the bond they have to sign at the time of admission.

According to the data tabled in the Gujarat assembly recently, the state government has collected more than ₹ 15.68 crores from those MBBS students who have breached their bonds and opted out of this mandatory service in villages. As per the Gujarat government's rules, MBBS students of state-run colleges have to sign a bond at the time of admission, giving a promise that they would serve for three years in rural areas, failing which they have to pay ₹ 5 lakh.[25] The bond amount is too low, Government must collect total amount of money spent on MBBS Graduate. As stated in this chapter earlier regarding the politics of establishing medical colleges in Gujarat, this recent example from Gujarat is the reflection of our health policy paralysis and failure to utilize our precious health resource for the benefit of our rural hospitals in the country. Frankly speaking we do not produce doctors for the villages which comprise nearly 70 per cent of the total population in the country. There is urgent need to devise a new three years medical training programme similar to the Medical Assistant as is called in Vietnam and Ethiopia. Such medical assistant basically trained in communicable/infectious, and other environment and water-borne diseases, can serve better in our rural and inaccessible areas which are mainly affected by these diseases, rather than lifestyle based chronic diseases. We must also involve AYUSH physicians who can also serve in rural and inaccessible mountainous areas. We must also learn from China regarding Village doctors/barefoot doctors who have dramatically improved access to health care in China's rural communities over the last few decades.[26]

Acknowledgements

I am grateful to the Institute of Development Studies, University of Sussex, for awarding me visiting fellowship and enabling me to carry out my work on Politics of Health Care in India. I am also thankful to Dr. Malcolm Segall for his valuable comments.

Notes

1. Antia, N.H., "Poor Health: Who is to Blame?", *Economic & Political Weekly*, Vol. 14, No. 39, p. 2214.
2. Benerji, D. (1989), "Crisis in the Medical Profession in India", *Economic & Political Weekly*, Vol. 14, No. 20, p. 1091.
3. Kumar, R.S., "Health: Market for Outdated Technology?", *Economic & Political Weekly,* Vol. XXIII, No. 35, 1988, p. 773.

3a. ——— (1990), "The Great Medical Scam", *The Times of India*, 7 January.

4. Tinaikar, S.S. (1992), "Ethics in Medical Profession: Need for Prescription of Conduct", *The Times of India*, New Delhi, 26 October, p. 10.
5. H.T. (1993), "Doctors Thrive, People Suffer", *The Hindustan Times*, New Delhi, 1 September.
6. H.T. (1995), "Medical Shops Flourishing in Amritsar Villages", *The Hindustan Times*, 10 January.
7. Jaffery, R. (1988), *The Politics of Health in India*, Berkeley: University of California Press, p. 247.
8. *TOI* (2015), New Medical Colleges to come up in 58 Districts: Nadda, *Times of India*, December 16.
9. Gish, O. (1971), *Doctor Migration and World Health*, Occasional Papers on Social Administration, No. 43, London: G. Bell & Sons, p. 74.
10. Mudur, G. (2007), "Doctors Criticise Proposal for Community Practitioners in Rural India", *British Medical Journal*, 334: 12 (6 January).
11. Kalantri, S.P. (2007), (Editorial), "Getting Doctors to the Village: Will Compulsion Works"?, *Indian Journal of Medical Education*, No. 4.
12. Maru, R.M. (1977), "Health Manpower Strategies for Rural Health Services in India and China, 1949-75", *Social Science and Medicine*, Vol. 10, No. 11.

13. Bajaj, J.S. (1988), "Issues in Medical Education", *Indian Journal of Medical Education*, Vol. 17, No. 1.
14. HT (1989), "Four New Medical Colleges in Gujarat", *The Hindustan Times*, New Delhi, 22 October.
15. *TOI* (1990), "Rural Stint Before Degree", *The Times of India*, New Delhi, 16 September.
16. H.T. (1991), "Doctors' Private Practice Hampering Research", *The Hindustan Times*, New Delhi, 29 July.
17. Sinha, A.K.N. (1986), "Procedure and Policy of Medical Admission", *The Indian Journal of Medical Education*, Vol. 15, No. 1, pp. 65-68.
18. *TOI* (2005), "IMA to Start Medical Colleges", *The Times of India*, New Delhi, 9 May.
19. Ramachandran, T. (1990), "Row Over Private Medical Colleges", *Indian Express*, New Delhi, 24 March.
20. Manuel, T. (2015), "India Produces 50, 000 Doctors a Year. If Only Medical Education Were Better Regulated.", *The Wire*, August 28.
21. Madan, T.N. (1980), *Doctor and Society*, New Delhi: Vikas Publishing House.
22. H.T. (2008), "Aspiring Doctors Set Sight on Nepal, and Operation MBBS", *The Hindustan Times*, New Delhi, 8 June.
23. MacAskill, A ; Stecklow, S., and Miglani, S. (2015), Are India's Medical Schools Broken, *Reuters*, June 16.
24. Shroff, Z.C.; Murthy, S. and Rao, K.D. (2013), "Attracting Doctors to Rural Areas: A Case Study of the Post-Graduate Seat Reservation Scheme in Andhra Pradesh", *Indian J. Community Med.,* January-March, Vol. 38(1), pp. 27-32.
25. *Times of India* (2016), In Gujarat, only 530 Doctors Served in Rural Areas in 5 Years, April, 4.
26. WHO (2008), China's Village Doctors take Great Strides, *Bulletin of the World Health Organization*, Vol. 86, No. 12, pp. 909-988.

PART V
Contemporary Issues

24

Spatio-Temporal Variation of Air Pollution in Delhi

A Focus on Respiratory Diseases

Shyamoli Sen and *Nitasha Malhotra*

Increased concern over the adverse effects of air pollution on respiratory health of individuals has made it one of the leading issues in the public health scenario. Largest exposures to health damaging air pollution probably occur in the developing world, especially in urban areas. The global burden of disease (GBD) of the World Health Organisation (WHO) released in December, 2013 says air pollution is the sixth most dangerous killer in south Asia. Around 65 per cent of the air pollution deaths occur in Asia and close to quarter of this happen in India. Much of these health impacts are on respiratory health which seem to occur among the poorest and most vulnerable population as indicated by numerous researchers.

Long term exposure to harmful air pollutants increases the risk of respiratory illnesses such as asthma, allergies, chronic bronchitis and lung cancers. Children and the elderly are particularly vulnerable to these airborne toxicants due to their weak immunity status and it is generally found that these problems manifest themselves in a hyper-urbanized scenario like Delhi more clearly than other areas as is seen in the recent times.[1]

This chapter throws light on the aspect of air pollution and its spatial and temporal variations in Delhi within a specific time period. This attempt to study the spatio-temporal variation has been specifically done in order to examine the changing pollution scenario, whether good or bad within the specific time gap as this acts as a precursor in understanding the various respiratory diseases resulting from the adverse pollution scenario in the city.

Need for the Study of Air Pollution

Air Pollution is essentially an urban phenomenon as the processes of urbanization such as industrialization and vehicularisation are intimately related. Speedy and unplanned development of a city like Delhi gave an impetus to the process of urbanization and primacy. The high density of population in the city led to associated vehicular, industrial and domestic emissions affecting health of inhabiting citizens.[2] This adverse impact of air pollution impacted health in general and respiratory health in particular of Delhiites, which led to the need for the development of the concept of emission inventory, which provides a blueprint of the pollution burden on the health of human beings. Health impacts due to air pollution are estimated in terms of mortality and morbidity, which are derived from air quality data using dose-effect relationships. In principle, such relations are found through statistical comparison of death rates and morbidity in areas with different air quality problems. Globally, it is estimated that there are about 8 million deaths due to air pollution every year. Unfortunately, in India due to the constraint of lack of monitoring mechanism of spatial pollution data on day to day basis as well as limitations of time, there is no such data available at present. Nonetheless, it is a fact that without proper availability of pollutant exposure data, it is not possible to understand the impact of toxic exposure on respiratory health of individuals.

Furthermore, it is also pertinent to understand that why such a study is relevant in the context of a city like Delhi. After Independence, the city became a major centre of commerce, industry and education which resulted in the city sprawling in leaps and bounds over the years and thus it became a construction hub leading to indiscriminate emission of particulate matter coupled with a burgeoning rise in vehicular pollution causing maximum damage to respiratory health.[3] This pollution is thus a palpable manifestation of the intense pressure of urbanization.

The major polluting gases in the city are sulphur dioxide (SO_2), nitrogen oxide (NO_2), carbon dioxide (CO_2) and methane (CH_4). For the present study only the first two have been considered as one finds continuous monitoring of these gases by concerned authorities like Central Pollution Control Board (CPCB) and National Environmental Engineering Research Institute (NEERI). Apart from these two, the present research has also studied particulate matter as it is a crucial aspect from the respiratory health point of view. All these three pollutants taken together act as a direct potent force of altering respiratory health of individuals that plays the most crucial factor in the context of this study. Delhi is known as a "Particulate City", as a result of which study of particulate matter is of utmost importance in the context of the present research.

Air pollutants are classified as primary or secondary, based on their characteristics at the time of emissions and physical/chemical changes, they undergo while in the atmosphere. Primary pollutants are defined as those that are emitted into the atmosphere directly from the identifiable sources and remain scattered in the atmosphere in the same chemical form like particulates. Secondary pollutants are recognized as those which are formed in the atmosphere by the reaction among two or more primary pollutants like nitrogen dioxide. Sources of air pollutants can be point sources, line sources and non-point sources. The point sources include emissions from domestic sources and industrial sources, whereas, line sources include vehicular emissions and non-point sources include fugitive emissions, emissions from construction activities and from refuse burning. As mentioned earlier, this chapter deals with only those pollutants that have been continuously monitored over the years by authorities like CPCB and NEERI. The major sources are as shown in Table 24.1.

Table 24.1: Anthropogenic Sources of Major Greenhouse Gases

Pollutant	*Main Emission Source Categories*
Particulate Matter	Dispersion originated matter forms from breakdown of liquid or solid bulk material, i.e. by grinding, atomization, natural dispersion, wind erosion, etc. The condensation originated matter develops from a build up from molecular dimension after heating and cooling.
NO_2	Use of synthetic fertilisers, fossil fuel combustion, biomass combustion, soil and other agricultural emissions, nitric acid production.
SO_2	Fossil fuel combustion, biomass combustion, sulphuric acid production, inc, lead and copper smelting and cement manufacturing.

Source: Garg and Shukla (2002).[4]

Spatio-temporal Variation of Air Pollution from 2000 to 2008

The present research has studied the spatio-temporal variation of SO_2, NO_2 and SPM and RSPM over Delhi for the years 2000 and 2008 with the help of maps generated from CPCB monitored air pollution data (unit used is micrograms/cubic metre) from various monitoring stations of Delhi which has been shown in Tables 24.2 and 24.3. These two years have been randomly selected but the time gap of 8 years has been deliberately kept as this would provide a meaningful analysis of the temporal variation in Delhi. The monitoring stations also differ slightly over the two years as CPCB keeps changing its monitoring locations from time to time. Two maps have been generated each for 2000 and 2008 based on the CPCB monitored pollution data. The first map is for SPM and RSPM (in 2008, CPCB monitored only RSPM and SPM data was not monitored) and the second map is for SO_2 and NO_2 for both the years respectively.

In addition to the map-wise analysis of pollution scenarios of 2000 and 2008, it was felt that mere analysis of values *per se* do not reveal the actual picture as norms according to the National Ambient Air Quality Status (NAAQS) have changed during this time gap. It is therefore, this chapter has also analyzed the air quality with respect to the NAAQS based on a factor called the Exceedence Factor (EF). Exceedence factor is the ratio of annual mean concentration of a pollutant with that of a respective standard. In other words, the EF provides a clear idea about the degree of violation of stipulated norms set by NAAQS. The EF is calculated as follows:

EF = Observed Annual Mean Concentration of Criteria Pollutant/ Annual Standard for the Respective Pollutant and Area Class

The four quality of air pollution categories that can be assessed based on this EF criteria are:

Critical pollution (C) : when EF is > 1.5, **High pollution (H)** : when EF is between 1.0 – 1.5, **Moderate pollution (M)** : when EF is between 0.5 – 1.0; and **Low pollution (L):** when the EF is < 0.5

It is obvious from the above categorization, that the locations in

Table 24.2: Level of Air Pollution, National Ambient Air Quality Standards (NAAQS) and Exceedence Factor (EF) during 2000

Area	*SPM*	*NAAQS*	*EF*	*Air Pollution*	*SO_2*	*NAAQS*	*EF*	*Air Pollution*	*NO_2*	*NAAQS*	*EF*	*Air Pollution*
Nizamuddin	279	140	1.99	C	18.2	60	0.3	L	33.6	60	0.5	M
Ashok Vihar	306	140	2.18	C	11.6	60	0.1	L	27	60	0.4	L
Shahzada Bagh	342	360	0.95	M	17	80	0.2	L	41.4	80	0.5	M
Shahdara	282	360	0.78	M	17.7	80	0.2	L	26	80	0.3	L
Janakpuri	242	140	1.72	C	18.6	60	0.3	L	32.5	60	0.5	M
Siri Fort	225	140	1.58	C	15.9	60	0.2	L	24.6	60	0.4	L
Netaji Nagar	491	140	3.5	C	8.3	60	0.1	L	52.6	60	0.8	M
Najafgarh	671	360	1.8	C	14.8	80	0.1	L	57	80	0.7	M
Town Hall	590	140	4.2	C	14.3	60	0.2	L	64	60	1.06	H

Note: C-Critical, M—Moderate, H—High, L—Low.

Source: National Ambient Air Quality Status 2000, NAAQMS/2001-02, CPCB.

Table 24.3: Level of Air Pollution, National Ambient Air Quality Standards (NAAQS) and Exceedence Factor during 2008

Area	*RSPM*	*NAAQS*	*EF*	*Air Pollution*	*SO_2*	*NAAQS*	*EF*	*Air Pollution*	*NO_2*	*NAAQS*	*EF*	*Air Pollution*
Nizamuddin	200	40	5	C	5	50	0.1	L	42	40	1	M
Mayapuri	263	40	6.5	C	13	50	0.2	L	75	40	1.8	C
Shahzada Bagh	203	40	5	C	6	50	0.1	L	49	40	1.2	H
Shahdara	210	40	5.2	C	5	50	0.1	L	58	40	1.4	H
Pitampura	159	40	3.9	C	5	50	0.1	L	38	40	0.9	M
Siri Fort	215	40	5.3	C	5	50	0.1	L	49	40	1.2	H
Sarojini Nagar	180	40	4.5	C	5	50	0.1	L	69	40	1.7	C
Janak Puri	219	40	5.4	C	5	50	0.1	L	53	40	1.3	H
Town Hall	278	40	6.9	C	10	50	0.2	L	77	40	1.9	C

Note: C-Critical, M—Moderate, H—High, L—Low.
Source: National Ambient Air Quality Status 2008, NAAQMS/2009-10, CPCB.[5]

either of the first two categories are actually violating the standards, althougn with varying magnitude. Those, falling in the third category are meeting the standards as of now but likely to violate the standards in future if pollution continues to increase and is not controlled. However, the locations in Low pollution category have a rather pristine air quality and such areas are to be maintained at Low pollution level by way of adopting preventive and control measures of air pollution.

It is important to mention here that EF as a criteria to analyse the violation of pollution standards was used by CPCB for the 2000 data, however, the present research has employed the same method to analyse the 2008 data as well because of the fact that the use of a similar criteria to analyse the data for both the years would facilitate an ideal comparison.

Pollution Scenario in 2000

As discussed above, analysis of the pollution scenario has been made on the basis of maps generated from the CPCB data from different monitoring stations as given in Table 24.2 and EF valucs given in the said table.

SPM (2000)—The SPM values in Figure 24.1 have been indicated by proportional circles each of which corresponds to the location-specific data given in the above table. Out of the total of 9 monitoring locations, Shahzada Bagh, Shahdara and Najafgarh are industrial areas and the remaining 6, i.e. Nizamuddin, Ashok Vihar, Janak Puri, Siri Fort, Netaji Nagar and Town Hall are all residential areas. The map shows highest values at Najafgarh (671) followed by Town Hall (590) and Netaji Nagar (491). Najafgarh, on one hand has large tracts of land dedicated to agricultural activities including barren land as well while on the other a lot of this barren land is being converted to non-agricultural land uses which is leading to a spur in construction activities in this area. All these factors in conjunction with each other can be attributed to such high SPM levels. Contrarily, the lowest value is seen in Siri Fort which is about 225 micrograms/cubic metre.

As far as the EF is concerned, the three industrial locations of Shahzada Bagh, Shahdara and Najafgarh have little higher air quality standard than their residential counterparts as seen in the above table. If one looks at the EF and the resultant air quality, it is seen that barring Shahzada Bagh (0.95) and Shahdara (0.78), all other seven

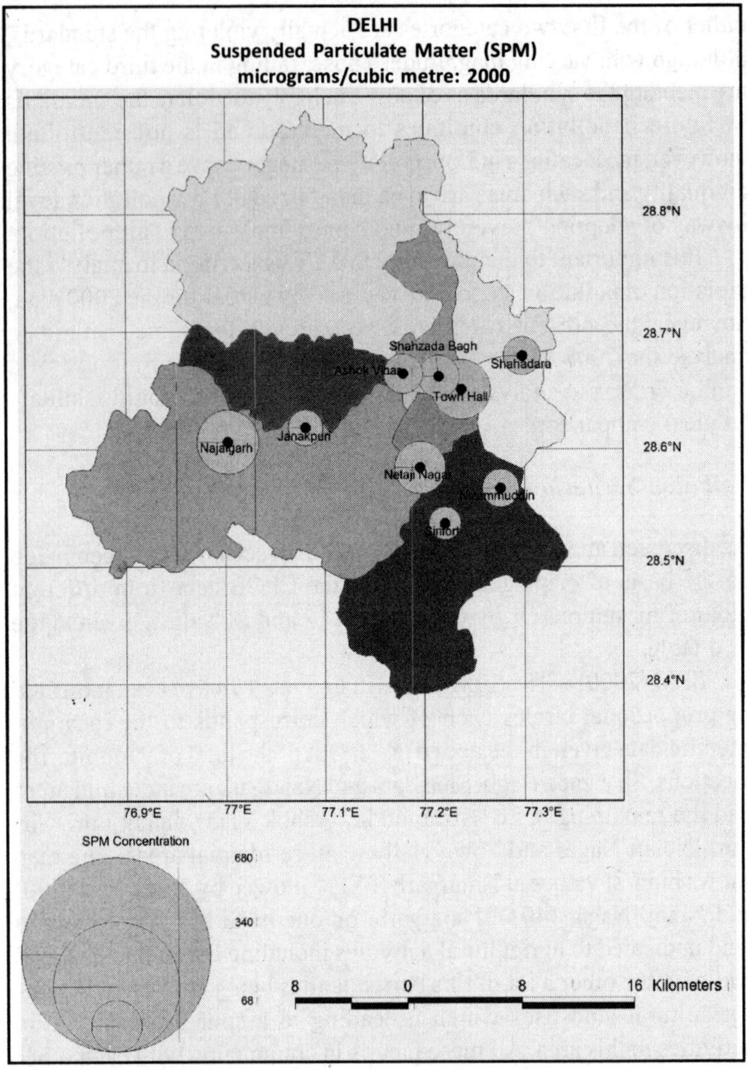

Fig. 24.1: Suspended particulate matter micrograms/cubic metre: 2000.

locations have critical pollution levels. It is noteworthy that since the last two to three decades, Delhi has been witnessing excessive construction activities which have resulted in such high levels of particulate matter in the ambient air. Furthermore, these construction

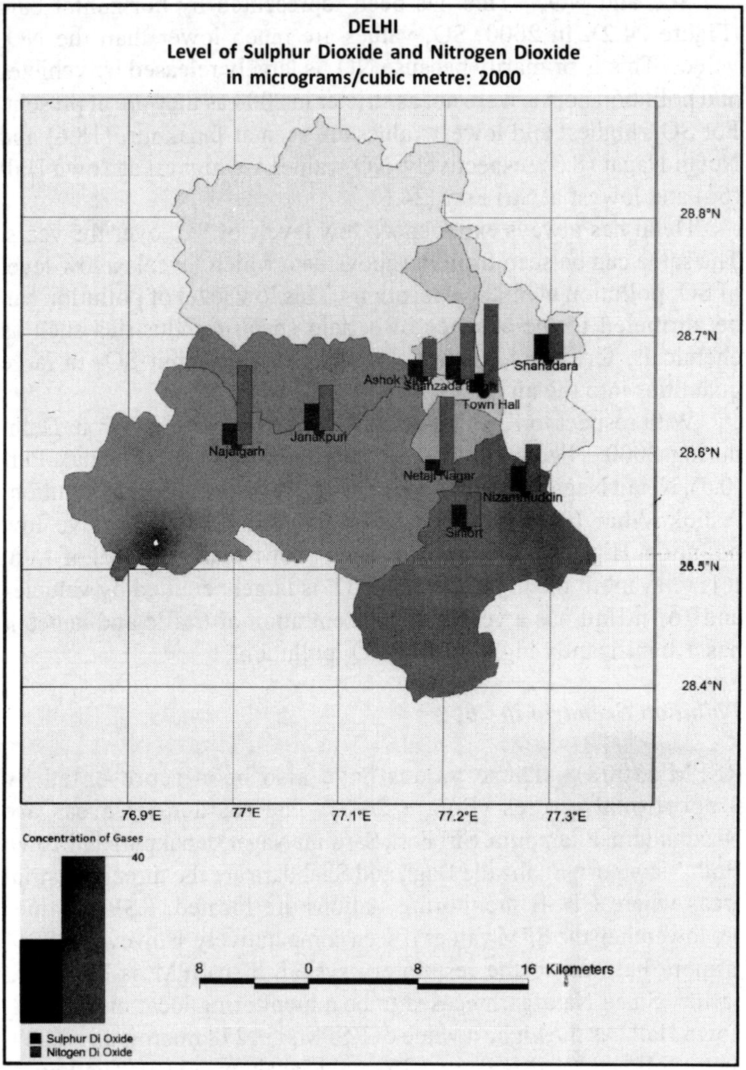

Fig. 24.2: SO_2 and NO_2 in Delhi: 2000.

activities are mostly concentrated in the residential areas of Delhi. Also, since Najafgarh although an industrial area, also houses large colonies and also has large tracts of agricultural land thus witnessed such critical levels of SPM pollution.

SO_2 and NO_2—This has been represented by horizontal bars (Figure 24.2). In 2000, SO_2 values are much lower than the NO_2 values. This is primarily because NO_2 is largely released by vehicles and pollution norms were not as stricter in 2000 as they are at present. For SO_2, highest and lowest values are seen at Janakpuri (18.6) and Netaji Nagar (8.3) respectively. NO_2 values are highest at Town Hall (64) and lowest at Siri Fort (24.6).

Delhi has always experienced low levels of SO_2 over the years. The same can be seen from the above data which reveals a low level of SO_2 pollution at all the 9 locations. This low level of pollution can be attributed to the absence of certain specific industries such as chemicals, fertilizers, leather etc. which usually emit SO_2 in large quantities into the air.

With respect to EF, NO_2 pollution was moderately high in Delhi during 2000. Nizamuddin (0.5), Shahzada Bagh (0.5), Janak Puri (0.5), Netaji Nagar (0.8) and Najafgarh (0.7) have moderate pollution; Ashok Vihar (0.4), Shahdra (0.3) and Siri Fort (0.4) have low pollution. High pollution is only seen in Town Hall at a level of 1.06. It is relevant to mention here that NO_2 is largely emitted by vehicles and Town Hall has a very high concentration of traffic and hence it has a significantly high level of NO_2 pollution.

Pollution Scenario in 2008

RSPM (2008)—These values have also been represented by proportional circles (Figure 24.3). The residential areas are Nizamuddin, Pitampura, Siri Fort, Sarojini Nagar, Janakpuri and Town Hall. Mayapuri, Shahzada Bagh and Shahdara are the three industrial areas where CPCB monitoring stations are located. RSPM values are lower than the SPM values if seen comparatively. However, RSPM is more harmful to the respiratory system than SPM as discussed earlier. Since Najafgarh ceased to be a monitoring location in 2008, Town Hall has the highest value of RSPM, i.e. 278 micrograms/cubic metre followed by Mayapuri (263) and Janakpuri (219). The lowest value has been recorded at Pitampura (159).

As far as EF of RSPM is concerned, situation is extremely grim. This is because one finds critical pollution levels at all locations and especially the worrisome locations are Town Hall (6.9) and Mayapuri (6.5). The lowest EF is at Pitampura which is 3.9 but is again much higher than the prescribed standard of 1.5 as discussed earlier.

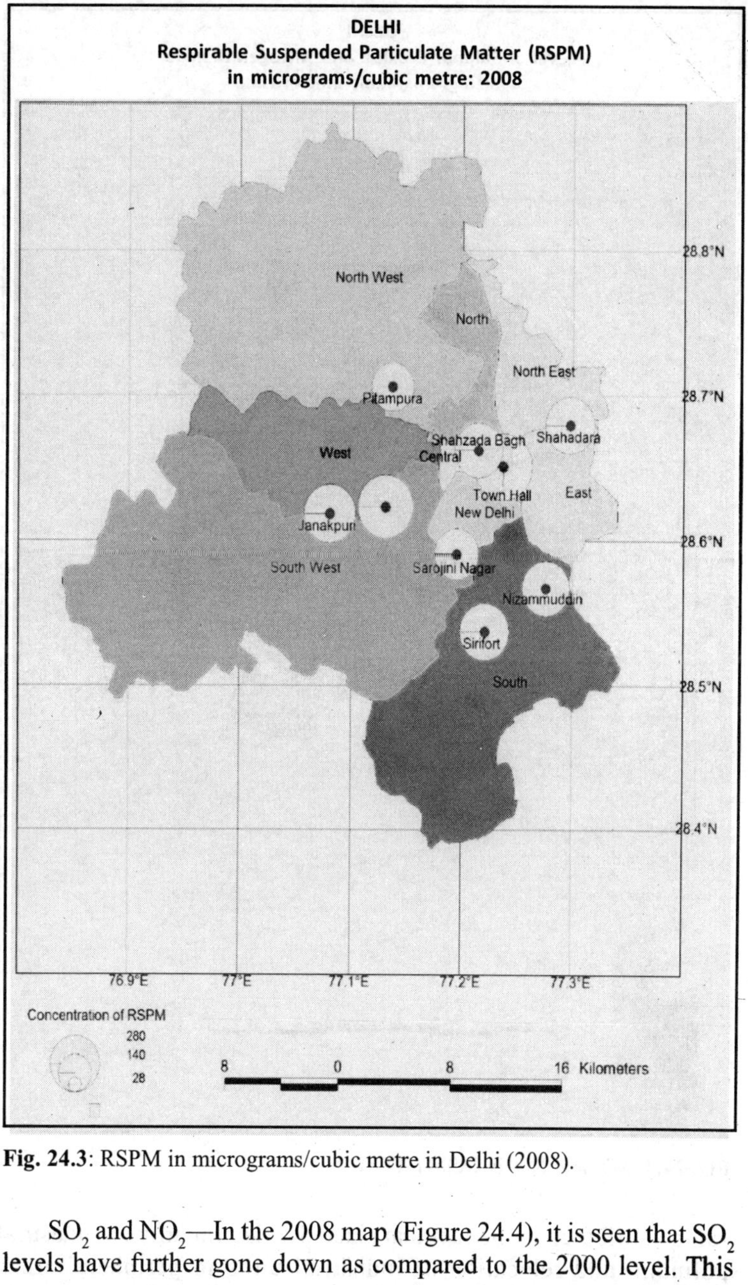

Fig. 24.3: RSPM in micrograms/cubic metre in Delhi (2008).

SO_2 and NO_2—In the 2008 map (Figure 24.4), it is seen that SO_2 levels have further gone down as compared to the 2000 level. This

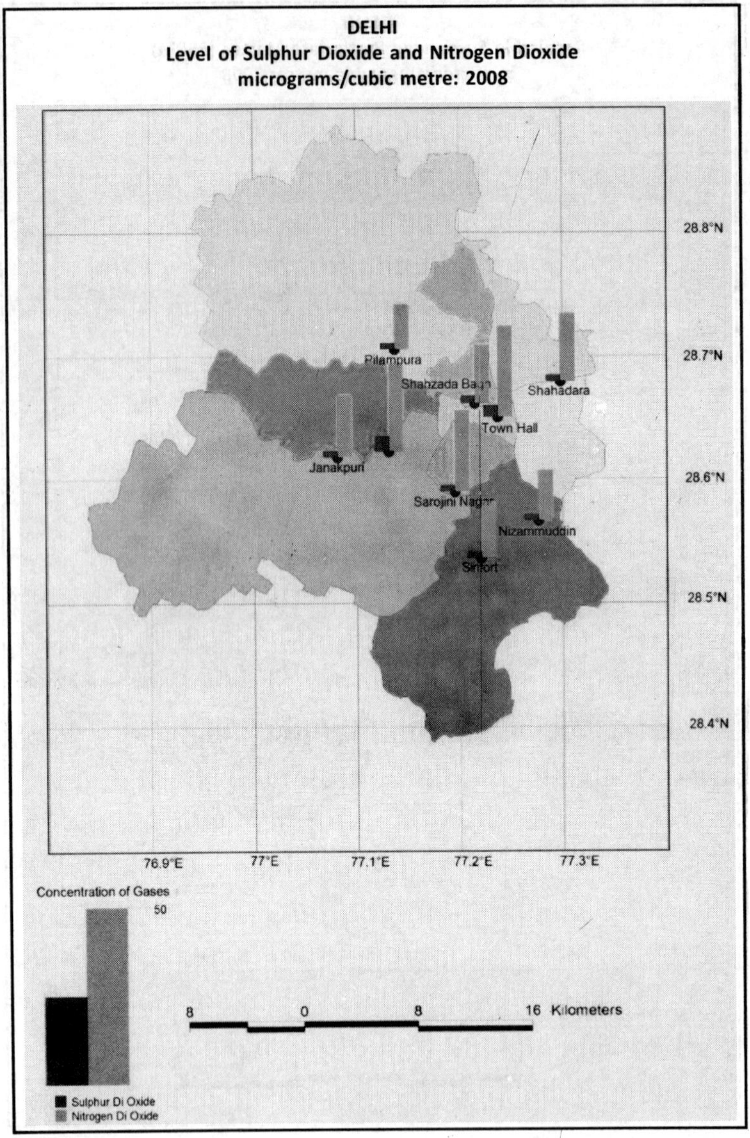

Fig. 24.4: SO_2 and NO_2 in Delhi (2008).

can be attributed to the fact that since SO_2 is primarily an industrial pollutant and relocation of industrial units to peripheral areas automatically reduced SO_2 emissions within the city. However, this declining trend is not seen in the case of NO_2. The highest and lowest NO_2 level is seen at Town Hall at 77 micrograms/cubic metre and Pitampura at 38 micrograms/cubic metre respectively. Such an appalling rise in NO_2 levels can be attributed to the ever-growing traffic congestion in the city in general and Town Hall in particular. It is interesting to note that Delhi adds more than 1000 vehicles every day to its roads.[5]

SO_2 values are highest at Mayapuri (13) followed by Pitampura (10). All other locations have less than 10 micrograms/cubic metre of SO_2. For EF values shown in Table 24.3, SO_2 levels are again very controlled even in 2008 as all locations exhibit low level of pollution.

All these locations have an EF level of SO_2 lower than 0.5. NO_2 levels are much higher than SO_2 levels. The highest is seen at Town Hall followed by Mayapuri at 1.9 and 1.8 respectively both having critical pollution. The lowest is seen at Pitampura at 0.9 which means it has moderate pollution. It is seen that all other locations have either moderate or high pollution. Higher levels of NO_2 can be solely attributed to vehicular emissions as NO_2 is primarily a vehicular toxicant. In a recently published article, it was seen that NO_2 concentration in 2012 in North Delhi, South Delhi and Central Delhi was 123.29, 199 and 140.5 micrograms/m^3 as against the ambient norm of 80 micrograms/m^3.

The PM10 concentration was 999.8, 621 and 436 micrograms/m^3 for these three locations respectively as against the ambient standard of 200 micrograms/m^3. Here, both the NO_2 and PM10 levels are way above the ambient standards. PM10 scenario is very worrisome since it has direct links with total pulmonary performance of an individual. Thus, it is evident that spatially as well as temporally, Delhi's pollution levels violate the stipulated norms as seen in the above figures.[6]

Respiratory Diseases Associated with Air Pollutants

According to the WHO Global Burden of Diseases Report 2010, nearly 6,20,000 premature deaths took place in India as a result of air pollution. Of all cities, experts feel that Delhi is the most vulnerable as it has the highest pollution level and has been held as one of the world's most polluted cities by global bodies including WHO.[3] The city seems to be paying an increasingly heavy price for its deteriorating air quality due to air pollutants generated by rising industrial activities, burgeoning vehicular population, increasing power generation and domestic emissions resulting in exposure of a large population segment. An average of 23 people die every day due to respiratory diseases in the capital, a number that has doubled in the past four years, data released by the Delhi government reveals. Doctors warn that worsening air quality, a major trigger for respiratory conditions such as chronic bronchitis, lung cancer and infections, may cause more fatalities in the coming years if appropriate measures are not taken. The latest statistical handbook, released by Delhi government shows respiratory diseases to be the fastest growing killer in a city where fatalities from most other ailments were declining.[7]

In a study of school children, it was examined how urbanisation, air pollution and environmental tobacco smoke causes and even triggers allergic respiratory disorders, especially asthma in school going children.[8] Results were based on a two-pronged approach, one on hospital based study and second on school based study of children.

It is certainly a challenge for medical experts and planners to control the respiratory ailments that are being experienced in all round the year indicating that Delhi's pollution scenario is grim and worrisome. The health effects caused in exposed population may not be directly due to affect of ambient concentration of pollutants, but rather based on the doses of pollutants received by respective receptor population. Air pollution damages the human respiratory system in various ways leading to further complications as is indicated in the Figure 24.5.

In India, Lvovsky et al., in 2000 reviewed the impact of particulate matter and discussed the issues relating to economic valuation of sickness and premature deaths due to outdoor air pollution. The pooled estimate of 0.84 per cent change in all-cause mortality relative to a 10 microgram/m^3 change in PM10 concentration was derived from a number of acute exposure studies. Similar to estimates of mortality, concentration-response functions were also derived for morbidity impacts such as respiratory hospital admissions, chronic bronchitis, cough, asthma etc.[9]

In another study, based on annual average concentration levels of PM10 and total city population in 2001, the number of cases of excess mortality and morbidity for Indian mega-cities, *viz.*, Delhi, Mumbai, Kolkata and Chennai were estimated.[10] It was observed from the figures that highest number of cases of excess mortality occurred

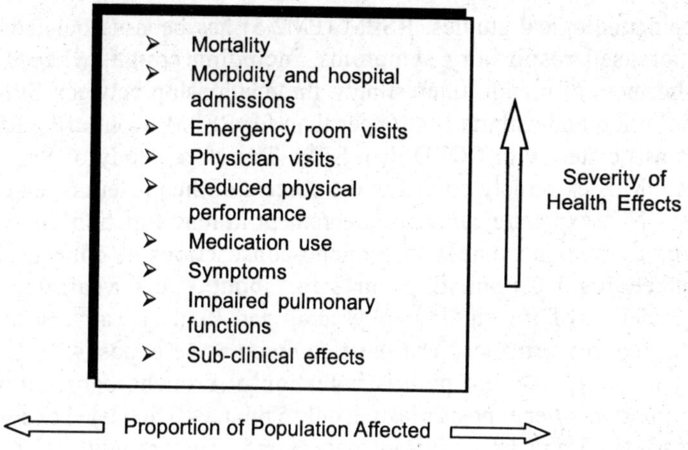

Fig. 24.5: Effects of Air Pollution on Human Health.
Source: CPCB, 2000.

in Delhi as compared to other metro cities. In fact, experts fear that in coming years, the heavy density of particulate matter in the city could cause havoc to the respiratory health of Delhiites.

Although all pollutants discussed above damage the respiratory health of individuals, however, different air pollutants pose different threats to the human respiratory system some of which are discussed in this section. Particulate air pollution result in changes in respiratory health status and depict several respiratory symptoms. Upper respiratory symptoms are stuffy or runny nose, sinusitis, sore throat, wet cough, etc. The lower respiratory symptoms include wheezing, dry cough, phlegm, dyspnea or shortness of breath, chest tightness and pain. The impaired lung function are the sensitive indicators of acute exposure of particulate air pollution. Asthma, allergies and bronchitis are other manifestations of health damaging effects of particulate pollution. Therefore, particulate matter in ambient air is associated with decrements in lung function as particulates enter the lung directly without being impeded by the nasal cavity owing to their small range of size. Thus, comparatively, RSPM is smaller in size than SPM and is not impeded by nasal cavity as a result is more damaging in general. An association between SPM air pollution and pulmonary function reduction has been reported in several epidemiological studies. RSPM (PM2.5) has been associated with increased respiratory symptoms, including cough, wheeze and shortness of breath. Interestingly, the relationship between SPM air pollution and asthma is stronger than for RSPM. Contrarily, RSPM is associated with COPD than SPM. Therefore, study of SPM and RSPM is extremely crucial in the context of the present research.

NO_2 exposure can cause decrement in lung function, increased airway responsiveness to broncho-constrictions at concentration exceeding 1.0 ppm. Exposures for about 3 to 4 years leads to incidences of bronchitis, emphysema, edema and have adverse effects on lung performance. The most common acute exposure to SO_2 at concentration >=0.4 ppm is induction of broncho-constriction in asthmatics after exposure lasting only 5 minutes. High level exposures leads to chronic bronchitis incidences and even morbidity effect. The children, elderly, smokers and those with chronic respiratory difficulties are most vulnerable group of population.[11] In other words, long term exposures to health damaging pollutants can also reduce life expectancy of individuals by complete alteration of the lung function caused by diseases like COPD, which when diagnosed at a later stage proves fatal in most cases.

Since the last two decades, researchers are examining the effects of urbanisation on global climate change and climatic parameters of the city of Delhi. In fact, large cities like Delhi can modify some of the climatic parameters in their immediate vicinity, resulting in a relatively small-scale but important variation in climate, which is called a 'microclimate'. Delhi is a classic example of such formation of a microclimate wherein due to excessive energy use and due to vehicularisation and other urban processes, there has been uncontrolled emission of Greenhouse Gases (GHGs) like CO_2, SO_2, NO_2, etc. as a result of which the surface air temperature is 15° C, which is 3° C above normal. This is an indication of the problem of climate change in the city.[12] Therefore, uncontrolled emission rates of GHGs automatically leads to uncontrolled pollution in the atmosphere coupled with particulate pollution. In addition, another important facet of pollution which forms part of temporal variation and which solicits great attention from researchers is seasonal aspect of Delhi's pollution, although the present research is not analysing data from a seasonal point of view. However, it is worth mentioning that from Delhi's point of view, pollution touches an extreme level in the months of November to January, i.e. the winter months leading to a spurt in asthma and bronchitis cases, which is relevant to the present topic in general. This rise in pollutant levels is particularly appalling in case of SPM and RSPM. Many studies have been conducted throwing light on this issue. Most have attributed it to the typical winter phenomenon of inversion of temperature and absence of winds and rainfall which fails to disperse the pollutants from the air and as a result forms a thick envelope of haze near the ground reducing visibility to 400 metres on an average. For instance, in a 4 year study conducted by School of Environmental Studies, Jawaharlal Nehru University has concluded that the blinding haze that chokes the city in winters is primarily composed of SPM and 80 per cent of this particulate matter is from natural sources and is even worsened by vehicular emissions. Another important source could be the smoke resulting from the burning of agricultural waste in Punjab and Haryana which quickly moves towards Delhi and forms a thick envelope of smog around the city. Moreover, this smog contains SPM which is not able to escape or settle down and remains suspended and causes severe respiratory problems during the winter months. In general, the winter months experience high levels of SPM and RSPM than SO_2 and NO_2 than other months (CPCB, 2008). It is thus Delhi hospitals experience a spurt in respiratory cases by 25 to 30 per cent due to the cold weather coupled with high particulate suspension in the air. It is noteworthy that although summers also have high levels of pollution, but it is not threatening to health since winds and occasional rainfall prevents the dust to remain suspended in the atmosphere.

To estimate health damages associated with air pollution in developing countries, policy-makers are often forced to extrapolate results from studies conducted in industrialised countries. However, such extrapolation may not always hold true since particulate pollution levels in developing countries are higher than their developed counterparts. In addition, in developing countries, people die at younger ages and from different causes than industrialised countries implying that such extrapolation of impacts of air pollution may be misleading. In such a similar study, a comparative analysis of pollution deaths was undertaken between Delhi and few US cities. These results revealed that 70 per cent of all deaths in US occur after the age of 65. In case of Delhi, over 70 per cent of all deaths occur before the age of 65, with over 20 per cent occurring before the age of 5. In another study in 1991 wherein data was obtained from the New Delhi

Municipal Corporation of Delhi (NDMC) region of Delhi which houses a large concentration of Delhi's premier hospitals and accounts for one-fourth of the total 60,000 deaths in the city on an average, it was seen that about 20-25 per cent of medically certified deaths are attributable to causes associated with air pollution. Therefore, such studies are indicative of the fact that estimation of health impacts relating to air pollution are not feasible, unless researchers focus their attention on emission inventory and exposure statistics.

In *conclusion*, it can be said that barring SO_2, all the other pollutants analyzed in the above discussion exceeded the ambient air quality standards set by CPCB in both the analyzed years. It is seen that value wise, figures may have marginally declined from 2000 to 2008 barring NO_2, but in reality, pollution scenario has become more critical in 2008 than 2000 since the NAAQS have also become stricter in 2008 as compared to 2000. Another noticeable fact is that spatially, Town Hall is the most vulnerable location on the pollution front since it has been maintaining its criticality from 2000 to 2008. This is followed by Mayapuri in 2008 and Najafgarh in 2000 both serving as hub of urban processes such as industrialization, construction activities and vehicularization.

Moreover, SPM and RSPM levels are comparatively much higher than SO_2 and NO_2 in Delhi's atmosphere. This has a direct relationship with respiratory health scenario of individuals residing in Delhi as particulate matter is most significant determining the morbidity and mortality profile of humans in most of the respiratory diseases. These diseases include chronic respiratory diseases like asthma and allergy, respiratory emergency room visits and hospital admissions due to aggravated asthma and bronchitis, acute respiratory symptoms due to decreased lung functions etc.[9]

Finally, pollution scenario during the winter months leading to the increased incidences of the aforementioned respiratory health problems is certainly a matter of grave concern for all, which is a matter of ongoing research. Since measuring individual exposures is not a practicable exercise, it is assumed that the subjects or inhabiting citizens have certain exposures to the worsening air pollution scenario as discussed above as they happen to be residents of Delhi for a considerable period of time. But, the threats of air pollution does not end here. The most frightening impact of this preventable disaster could come from lung cancer as several pollutants contain chemical carcinogens such as benzene, form-aldehyde and polycyclic hydrocarbons. These may act as slow poisons and may certainly add to the burden of cancer in the society. Therefore, it is felt that Delhi needs to initiate urgent steps to control the burgeoning pollution in the form of stringent emission norms and lifestyle modifications.

Notes

1. Yaari, E., *et al.* (2009), "Genetic Environmental Interactions in Asthma and Allergy: A Study in a Closed Population Exposed to Various Environments", *Annals of Allergy, Asthma and Immunology,* Vol. 102(3).
2. CPCB (2000), *National Ambient Air Quality Status 2000*, NAAQMS/2001-02, CPCB.
3. *Times of India* (2014), "Air Pollution Affecting even Foetal Growth", *Times of India,* December 5.
4. Garg, Amit and P.R. Shukla (2002), *Emissions Inventory of India*, New Delhi: Tata McGraw Hills.
5. CPCB (2008), *National Ambient Air Quality Status 2008*, NAAQMS/2009-10, CPCB.
6. Mail Today (2012), "Delhi Witnesses 30 per cent Rise in Respiratory Diseases due to High Pollution and Chill", *Mail Today*, January 6.
7. *Times of India* (2012), "23 Delhiites Die Everyday due to Respiratory Ailments", *Times of India,* November 21.
8. Paramesh, K., *et al.* (2002), "Environmental Factors and Respiratory Diseases", *Accessed* at www.worldjournal.org.
9. Lvovsky, K., *et al.* (2000), "Environmental Costs of Fossil Fuels: A Rapid Assessment Methods with Application to Six Cities", *The World Bank Environment Department Papers,* No. 78, October, Washington DC., USA.
10. Nema and Goyal, *et al.* (2006), "Understanding Urban Vehicular Pollution Problem *vis-à-vis* Ambient Air Quality—Case Study of a Mega City (Delhi, India)" in *Environmental Monitoring and Assessment* (2006); 119, Springer.
11. World Bank (2003), *For a Breath of Fresh Air: Ten Years of Progress and Challenges in Urban Air Quality Management in India 1993-2002*, Environmental and Social Development Unit, SE Asia, World Bank.
12. Kumar Bhuwan and R.B. Singh (2003), *Urban Development and Anthropogenic Climate Change, Experience in Indian Metropolitan Cities*, New Delhi: Manak Publications.

25

Gynaecological Morbidity

A Neglected Health Issue among Married Women in Western India

Anita Bhargava and *Anuradha Banerjee*

Introduction

Gynaecological diseases cover a wide range of chronic conditions that have substantial impact on women's reproductive health. Gynaecological morbidity is defined as structural and functional disorder of the genital tract not related to pregnancy, delivery and puerperium.[1] Gynaecological morbidity, caused by Reprodcutive Tract Infections (RTIs), have serious implications on women's health for instance undiagonosed infections caused due to improper use of contraceptive methods, IUD insertion and female sterilisation process in a perilous environment results in irreverisble impact on reproductive health. The three different types of reproductive tract infections that cause gynaecological morbidity among women are endogenous and iatrogenic in nature. Endogenous infections resulting from the overgrowth of organisms normally present in the reproductive tract (such as candidiasis and bacterial vaginosis) and iatrogenic infections related to medical procedures (such as menstrual regulation, abortion or IUD insertion). Hence, gynaecological morbidity varies from menstrual disorders, cervical cell changes, genital prolapse to appalling Sexually Transmitted Diseases (STDs) including Gonorrhoea, Chlamydia, Syphilis, Trichomonas and HIV infections.

According to World Health Organisation (WHO) estimates, STD alone cause at least 250 million new infections each year, including 120 million cases of trichomoniasis, 50 million cases of Chlamydia,

30 million cases of genital warts, 25 million cases of gonorrhoea, 20 million cases of herpes, 3.5 million cases of syphilis, and two million cases of chancroid.[2] The estimates clearly points out that sexually transmitted diseases among women are less likely to be symptomatic, they cause serious long-term consequences due to the lack of timely diagnosis. Moreover, STDs can easily infect women than men through an infected partner.[3]

In developed countries, since the problems are identified at early stages, the diagnosis and treatment of gynaecological morbidity is done easily. Such a timely intervention reduces the risks and lives of several women. However, in developing countries, gynaecological morbidity, other than sexually transmitted diseases, is diagnosed with relatively lesser. Women suffering reproductive tract infections in particular, may have an impact on ability to conceive as they prevent chances of pregnancy. Apart from health degradation, Gynaecological morbidities caused due to STDs/HIV in particular, are controlled by '*Culture of Silence*' that women internalise either due to shyness or due to fear of reporting which in turn develop distrust against her by family members. Hence, to preserve family prestige and congenial relations with in-laws ties, women do not seek treatment until the infections become perilous and affect her daily routine.

Etiology of gynaecological morbidity varies from region to region and across the sections of the society. As the literature suggests, women from deprived and poor living conditions combined with lack of hygiene and sanitation are at higher risks of the exposure. Gynaecological morbidities are common among women in the reproductive age groups in association with other risk factors such as low socio-economic status, educational attainment, knowledge and awareness, personal hygiene and sanitation, social environment, exploitation and abuse in forms of sexual/domestic violence, sexual behaviour of women as well as their intimate sexual partners.[4, 5, 6]

Three profound studies carried out in each of the selected states in the present study, highlighted the scenario of gynaecological morbidity. The study carried out in Rajasthan states that women's consider particular symptoms which men do not experience as women's illness. The illnesses, as reported in the study, are largely attributed to iatrogenic factors as plausible factors.[7] In a study carried out in Gujarat, it was found that women associated the gynaecological problems with dietary habits—eating food enriched with hot spices and chillies lead to such illnesses. The findings reflect the level of awareness and lack of knowledge among women.[8] In the study carried out in Maharashtra, it was observed that more than 80 per cent of women were suffering from one or multiple gynaecological problems, but very few sought treatment. Women were found severely anaemic, resulting into scanty bleeding during menstruation. Women reported menstrual discharge, vaginal itching, and pain during intercourse, urinary tract infections with backache and uterus prolapsed (which they referred as something coming out from below).[9]

Study Setting

The region of western India is comprised of the bigger states of India. Gujarat and Maharashtra, on one hand, are the most flourishing states in terms of urban-economic growth while Rajasthan, on the other side, is characterised by larger proportion of rural population and ranks near the bottom of many demographic, health and development indicators. However, the pace of urbanisation is clearly visible in all the three states. Sadly, in different set-ups, all the three states ranks low on almost all indicators related to women's health. Except metropolitan districts of Maharashtra and Gujarat, women's health status is a matter of concern in others parts of the states. A large proportion of women in Maharashtra lives in urban slums located at worst conditions of living such as dumping grounds, near sewerage, railway tracks and so on and their reproductive health conditions are equally degraded. A large section in these slums is the migrant population from states like Uttar Pradesh, Bihar, Madhya Pradesh and other states of the country.

Largely, women of all the three states are illiterate. The median age of their marriage is 15 years and has more than three children. Among the three states, women from Rajasthan ranks extremely low on women's autonomy in terms of decision-making, freedom of movement and control over money. However, the conditions of women in Gujarat are relatively better as various studies evince women's autonomy and freedom of movement. The prevalence of either clinically diagnosed or self-reported symptoms of gynaecologic morbidity is high among Indian women ranging from 46 per cent to as high as 92 per cent depending on the population studied and the morbidity criteria used.[10]

Methodology

Data

The data for this study is obtained from RCH-3 (Reproductive and Child Health). The RCH-3 has collected information from a nationally representative sample of 7,20,320 households, 643,944 ever-married women of the age group of 15-49 years of age. The survey adopted multi-stage stratified sampling covering 99 per cent of country's population from 50 census villages in rural areas and urban from each district of 28 states and six Union Territories based on Population Proportion Size (PPS) sampling.[11] The survey provided immense information on various demographic parameters such as family planning, maternal and child health, reproductive health of ever-married women and adolescent girls and so on. In women questionnaire, questions on gynecological household were asked to women who have given birth in the three years prior to the survey. Women were asked if in the preceding three months, they had experienced itching or irritation, boil/ulcer around vulva or severe pain in lower abdomen not related to menstruation. Women were also asked if they experienced pain while urination or defecation, swelling in the groin, painful blister like lesions in and around vagina, low backache, pain during sexual intercourse or blood after sex when not menstruating. In addition, questions were asked related to menstrual problems experience in preceding months.

Statistical Analysis

In this chapter, 94,369 women aged 15-49 years who were asserted married status at the time of survey from Gujarat, Rajasthan and Maharashtra, were considered. Although, only currently married women are not sufficient to cover all women, these women provide an scope to understand the prevalence of gynaecological morbidity because women living in married status have higher chances of exposure against reproductive health problems propelled by many factors.

The statistical techniques largely comprised of bi-variate and multi-variate analyses. Cross-tabulation is used to depict distribution of various indicators across the selected states cross-sectioning to rural and urban residences such as self-reported symptoms of gynaecological morbidity, menstrual problems and reproductive tract infections (RTIs). A logistic regression model is fitted with a binary outcome, categorised as one "if woman experienced any of the symptoms of gynaecological morbidity", and zero "if no morbidity was reported" is used in order to estimate the net impact of independent variables on the probability of risk or likelihood of getting morbid. The determinants used in the regression model were—age groups categorised into seven groups, keeping 25-29 years as reference category, educational attainment categorised into higher (reference category), none, primary and secondary, religion divided categorised into Hindu (reference category), Muslim and Others, Caste divided into General (reference category), Scheduled Caste and Scheduled Tribe, Status of Women divided into rich (reference catetory), poor and medium, prior obstetric history bifurcated into no (reference catetory) and yes, current family planning use categorised into other modern methods (reference category), none or traditional and female sterilisation/IUD and place of residence bifurcated into urban (reference category) and rural.

Ethical Statement

The data set of District Level Household Survey is used in the present study which is conducted by the nodal agency, IIPS (International Institute for Population Sciences) and funded by Ministry of Health and Family Welfare (MoHFW), Government of India (GoI). IIPS and MoHFW have approved the questionnaires used to collect the data from the wide sample after informed consent, across the country. The authors were not involved at either stages of the data collection or later stages.

Results

Profile of Women in Western India

From the available data, it was found that 75 per cent of women were from rural while 25 per cent of women resided in urban residence during the period of survey (Table 25.1). Out of 75 per cent, 44 per cent of women reside in rural Rajasthan followed by 32 per cent in Maharashtra and remaining was observed in Gujarat.

Table 25.1: Percentage Distribution of Women in Three States of India, 2007-08

State	*Type of Residence*				*Total*	*Per cent*
	Rural	*Per cent*	*Urban*	*Per cent*		
Rajasthan	31046	44	7751	33	38797	41
Gujarat	16749	24	6236	26	22985	24
Maharashtra	22945	32	9642	41	32587	35
Total	**70740**	**75**	**23629**	**25**	**94369**	**100**

Source: Computed from RCH-DLHS-3, 2007-08.

Similarly, out of 25 per cent, 41 per cent of women reside in urban parts of Maharashtra followed by 33 per cent in Rajasthan and 26 per cent in Gujarat. Around 51 per cent Scheduled Castes have been observed in rural residence while 49 per cent household are located in urban residence. It is notable that since the data is skewed, the proportion of women remained slightly high in rural residence.

Table 25.2 shows the percentage distribution of the women in rural and urban residence according to some selective characteristics. The age-group distribution clearly indicates the concentration of married women in the age groups of 25-29 and 20-24 years. Women are observed more in urban residence in these age groups as compared to their rural counterparts. Overall, Maharashtra has a larger concentration of women in these two age groups. However, it is notable that since the data is skewed, the proportion of women remained slightly high in rural residence.

More than 60 per cent of women in the sample practice Hinduism in all the three states with a major concentration in rural Gujarat (94%) followed by Rajasthan (93.6%). Nevertheless, women following Islam religion are seen in urban Maharashtra and Rajasthan. Women practicing various other religions are concentrated relatively more in rural Maharashtra followed by urban Rajasthan. Notably, a large proportion of women are from Scheduled Caste in all the three states. The higher concentration of Scheduled Tribe women is observed in rural Rajasthan and Gujarat. However, women are in considerable proportion in urban Maharashtra. Significantly, women of general category are observed low in all the three states.

Since, these states are better off in socio-economic development, largely, women showed secondary level of education attainment. However, a significant proportion of higher level of educational attainment is visible in urban Gujarat and rural Maharashtra. Overall,

Table 25.2: Distribution of Respondents based on Selective Characteristics

Background Characteristics	*States*						*Total*
	Rajasthan		*Gujarat*		*Maharashtra*		
	Rural	*Urban*	*Rural*	*Urban*	*Rural*	*Urban*	
Age in Years							
15-19	6.4	3.6	4.6	1.7	9.3	4.6	6.1
20-24	19.3	16.3	17.7	15.1	19.9	16.7	18.3
25-29	19.9	19.6	19	19.5	18.7	19.3	19.3
30-34	18.2	18.5	18.9	18.4	16.9	19.8	18.2
35-39	16.3	17.6	16.3	17.3	16.4	17.8	16.7
40-44	15.1	17.9	18	20.8	13.9	15.3	16
45-49	4.8	6.6	5.5	7.2	4.9	6.5	5.4
Total	**80.0**	**20.0**	**72.9**	**27.1**	**70.4**	**29.6**	**100.0**
Religion							
Hindu	93.6	78.9	94.0	83.3	88.5	69.3	88.1
Muslim	5.2	16.7	4.7	14.9	3.7	20.9	7.9
Others	1.3	4.4	1.3	1.7	7.8	9.7	4
Total	**80.0**	**20.0**	**72.9**	**27.1**	**70.4**	**29.6**	**100.0**
Caste							
Scheduled Caste	82.4	97.4	76.6	94.5	81	94.6	84.3
Scheduled Tribe	17.6	2.5	22.6	3.7	18.6	4.3	15.2
General	0.1	0.1	0.7	1.7	0.5	1.1	0.5
Total	**80.0**	**20.0**	**72.9**	**27.1**	**70.4**	**29.6**	**100.0**
Educational Attainment							
No Education	0.2	0.1	0.1	0.1	0.1	0	0.1
Primary	48.1	22.2	32.8	16.4	27.9	16.8	28.4
Secondary	48.5	60	63.6	66.8	69.6	71.3	64.2
Higher	3.2	17.7	3.5	16.3	2.3	11.9	7.3
Total	**80.0**	**20.0**	**72.9**	**27.1**	**70.4**	**29.6**	**100.0**
Wealth Index							
Poor	48.4	6.3	28.3	2.4	35.7	3.6	30.7
Middle	44.1	33.6	56	27.7	53.5	35.5	45.7
Rich	7.5	60.1	15.7	69.9	10.8	61	23.7
Total	**80.0**	**20.0**	**72.9**	**27.1**	**70.4**	**29.6**	**100.0**

Source: Computed from RCH-DLHS-3, 2007-08.

the rural and urban residences of Rajasthan evince low level of educational attainment.

The distribution of wealth index presents a very interesting picture. The poor women are observed in rural Rajasthan and Gujarat. However, they are significantly concentrated in urban residence of Maharashtra. The middle class women are distributed proportionately in all the three states. The rich class women are observed in a significant proportion in rural and urban Gujarat and Maharashtra. Such a complex settings of the women's characteristics has made this study very interesting.

Awareness of RTIs/STIs among Women

Awareness of RTIs/STIs among women is presented in Table 25.3. As an overview, the level of awareness is found low among women across all the three states.

Table 25.3: Awareness of RTIs/STIs among Women by their Age Groups in Three States of India, 2007-08

Age in Years	*Type of Residence*	*States*			*Total*
		Rajasthan	*Gujarat*	*Maharashtra*	
15-19	Rural	6.7	4.0	7.9	6.6
	Urban	2.8	0.7	2.9	2.3
	Total	5.7	2.5	6.0	5.3
20-24	Rural	20.7	16.5	21.2	20.3
	Urban	16.6	13.0	14.3	15.0
	Total	19.7	14.9	18.6	18.6
25-29	Rural	21.1	21.3	21.1	21.1
	Urban	20.9	22.0	20.5	21.0
	Total	21.0	21.6	20.9	21.1
30+	Rural	51.5	58.3	49.8	51.9
	Urban	59.7	64.3	62.3	61.6
	Total	53.6	61.0	54.5	55.0
Total	**Rural**	**74.5**	**55.0**	**62.4**	**68.0**
	Urban	**25.5**	**45.0**	**37.6**	**32.0**
Total		**100.0**	**100.0**	**100.0**	**100.0**

Source: Computed from RCH-DLHS-3, 2007-08.

The proportional difference between rural and urban residences has affected the distributional pattern as well. The awareness level increases as the age increases. In the age-group 15-19 is lowest as compared to other age groups. Women in the older age groups, on the other hand, showed substantial awareness. In context of state comparison, women from younger age groups in Maharashtra have awareness more than Rajasthan and Gujarat. However, in the older age groups women from Gujarat have better knowledge than women from other two states. As literature suggests, level of awareness among women is largely controlled by their sources of information. Women are found more aware if they are exposed to information spread through mass media particularly television and radio. In addition, it is observed that infected cases living in the community causes awareness as people can see an eye-evidence. In such ways, their misconceptions also overcome. Apart from it, women's peer group

Table 25.4: Knowledge of Modes of Transmission of RTIs/STIs among Women in Three States of India, 2007-08

Type of Residence	*States*			*Total*
	Rajasthan	*Gujarat*	*Maharashtra*	
Unsafe Delivery				
Rural	23.2	29.5	21.4	23.8
Urban	33.6	36.2	19.5	31.5
Total	**26.0**	**32.7**	**20.6**	**26.3**
Unsafe Abortion				
Rural	19.0	22.8	14.6	18.9
Urban	28.4	33.1	16.5	27.2
Total	**21.5**	**27.6**	**15.4**	**21.6**
Unsafe IUD Insertion				
Rural	13.0	24.1	14.0	14.7
Urban	24.4	34.7	16.1	25.4
Total	**16.1**	**29.0**	**14.8**	**18.2**
Unsafe Sex Homosexuals				
Rural	12.5	15.6	12.2	12.9
Urban	21.5	21.8	13.7	20.0
Total	**14.9**	**18.5**	**12.8**	**15.2**
Unsafe Sex with Multiple Partners				
Rural	56.4	63.2	72.1	59.5
Urban	64.1	72.4	74.2	68.2
Total	**58.5**	**67.5**	**73.0**	**62.3**
Unsafe Sex with Sex Workers				
Rural	35.7	33.5	22.6	33.6
Urban	40.1	42.7	22.5	37.3
Total	**36.9**	**37.8**	**22.5**	**34.8**

Source: Computed from RCH-DLHS-3, 2007-08.

play vital role in spreading information. Incorrect information leads to misconception while correct information allows women to understand and adopt preventive measures against it.

Knowledge of Modes of Transmission among Women

A wide variation of response is seen when women were asked about modes of transmission of RTIs/STIs and the results are presented in Table 25.4. Most of women from all the three states believed that the RTIs/STIs spread due to unsafe sex with multiple partners (59.5% in rural and 68.2% in urban) followed by unsafe sex with sex workers (33.6% in rural and 37.3% in urban).

Unsafe sex with homosexuals (12.9% in rural and 20% in urban) and unsafe delivery (23.8% in rural and 31.5% in urban) are the reasons, on the other hand, which are reported low by women from all the three states.

Despite both the events are related to them, yet poor knowledge of women is seen with regard to unsafe IUD insertion and unsafe abortion. However, states-wise, women from Gujarat have shown substantial reporting with regard to other reasons.

Menstrual Problems

Around 20 per cent of the married women have reported the occurrence of one or more symptoms of menstrual problems during the preceding three months prior to the survey. With more than 70 per cent of women in Rajasthan and Gujarat, the most commonly reported problem was painful periods in all the three states. Irregular periods were another commonly reported problem which was observed significantly in Gujarat and Maharashtra. A significant proportion of women from Rajasthan have reported frequent or short periods, which means their menstrual cycle was less than 28 days.

Another considerable proportion of women in Rajasthan (16 and 12%) have reported prolonged bleeding followed by experience scanty bleeding by women from Gujarat and Maharashtra. Women from Rajasthan have reported symptoms of excessive bleeding during menstrual periods followed by 10 per cent women from Maharashtra who have reported the same. A substantial percentage of women from the three states have reported the symptoms of no periods and menstrual-inter-menstrual bleeding from all the three states. Overall, it can be concluded that women from Gujarat have experienced lesser problems as compared to other two states.

Table 25.5: Women Reported Menstrual Problems during Past Three Months

Menstrual Problems	*States*						*Total*	
	Rajasthan		*Gujarat*		*Maharashtra*			
	Rural	*Urban*	*Rural*	*Urban*	*Rural*	*Urban*	*Rural*	*Urban*
No Periods	7.7	7.2	9.0	6.6	2.4	2.0	5.8	4.4
Painful Periods	73.9	70.9	70.3	60.4	69.4	63.3	71.2	64.4
Frequent or Short Periods	14.5	15.3	9.6	10.8	4.5	4.1	9.3	8.5
Irregular Periods	16.5	17.7	25.2	34.2	26.4	30.6	22.5	28.5
Prolonged Bleeding	15.9	12.3	6.9	6.2	6.9	7.9	10.2	8.5
Scanty Bleeding	6.8	7.0	11.5	11.0	24.6	20.1	15.2	14.6
Menstruation-inter-menstrual Bleeding	4.6	4.6	5.2	5.4	2.8	3.4	4.0	4.2
Blood Clots/ Excessive Bleeding	13.1	11.7	8.0	7.5	10.9	10.2	11.0	9.9

Source: Computed from RCH-DLHS-3, 2007-08.

Self-Reported Symptoms of RTIs

Table 25.6 shows the distribution of symptoms of Reproductive Tract Infections (RTIs) among women who reported the occurrence during the preceding three months of the survey. The symptoms of reproductive tract infections, in the survey were asked for those occurred outside the pregnancy and its outcome.

As an overview, the self-reporting of symptoms was less by women from all the three states. The results indirectly reflect the "culture of silence" which has been discussed earlier. Nevertheless, wet stain was reported by most of women from both the states as well as both the residence. Women have also experienced foul odour discharge discomforting situations. To avoid stains appear, they have to change their wearing many times a day. Low backache is another problem which most of women experienced particularly in their later ages and women who have reached menopause. Other reported problems were severe abdominal pain, urinary problems and vaginal itching and irritation. As a remark women report such problems after sexual relations with their intimate partners. Lowest reported symptoms were swelling in the groin, painful blisters or lesions, and

Table 25.6: Self-reported Symptoms of Reproductive Tract Infections (RTIs)

Reproductive Tract Infections (RTIs)	*States*						*Total*	
	Rajasthan		*Gujarat*		*Maharashtra*			
	Rural	*Urban*	*Rural*	*Urban*	*Rural*	*Urban*	*Rural*	*Urban*
Vaginal Itching/ Irritation	6.2	4.1	5.9	5.0	5.8	5.7	6.0	5.0
Boils/Ulcers/Warts	1.6	0.9	2.5	1.6	2.1	1.7	2.0	1.4
Severe Abdominal Pain	5.8	4.0	5.6	3.2	5.9	4.2	5.8	3.8
Urinary Symptoms	3.1	1.9	2.8	1.5	3.6	2.7	3.2	2.1
Swelling in the Groin	0.8	0.4	0.8	0.5	1.2	1.1	0.9	0.7
Painful Blister like Lesions	0.5	0.3	1.0	0.4	1.9	1.1	1.1	0.7
Low Backache	10.8	8.5	12.2	10.0	13.6	10.2	12.0	9.6
Pain during Intercourse	2.4	1.4	2.3	2.0	3.5	2.7	2.8	2.1
Bleeding (Non-menstrual) after Intercourse	0.3	0.2	0.4	0.2	0.6	0.3	0.4	0.2
Wet Stain	92.8	90.8	90.9	88.3	82.6	76.5	90.1	85.4
Foul Odour Discharge	39.0	31.5	34.2	26.8	26.3	22.6	35.2	27.4

Source: Computed from RCH-DLHS-3, 2007-08.

bleeding after sexual intercourse. State-wise, lowest percentages of women are observed in urban Rajasthan and Gujarat. Swelling in the groin and painful blister like lesions are other two symptoms that are observed low among women.

Vaginal Discharge Experienced by Women

Though perilous white discharge is largely reported (90.3% in rural and 90.5% in urban), but self-reporting is not sufficient to conclude that women were suffering from vulnerable white discharge (Leucorrhoea). Around 91.4 per cent of rural women from Rajasthan from both the residences have reported perilous white discharge.

Other perilous coloured discharge like yellowish is reported by 2.2 per cent women in total out of which 2.3 per cent of women were in Rajasthan, 2.1 per cent women were from Gujarat and two per cent were from Maharashtra. Medically, yellow discharge is found highly associated with obstetric fistula caused due to unsafe delivery. Among three states, Rajasthan's proportion is higher in home deliveries attended by untrained attendants (*dais*), the results can easily be correlated. On the other hand, blood stained discharge is usually caused due to unsafe sex with multiple partners and urban areas of Maharashtra such as Mumbai and Pune have higher concentration of sex workers and therefore, 2.3 per cent of women reported the problem, which is highest among the three states.

Table 25.7: Women Experienced Vaginal Discharge in Three States of India, 2007-08

Colour of the Discharge	*States*			*Total*
	Rajasthan	*Gujarat*	*Maharashtra*	
Non-Perilous				
Rural	4.2	9.2	3.9	5.1
Urban	4.0	9.2	4.0	5.2
Total	**4.1**	**9.2**	**3.9**	**5.1**
Perilous				
White				
Rural	91.4	86.3	90.8	90.3
Urban	91.8	86.4	91.4	90.5
Total	**91.5**	**86.3**	**90.9**	**90.3**
Green				
Rural	0.2	0.3	0.3	0.2
Urban	0.1	0.2	0.2	0.2
Total	**0.2**	**0.3**	**0.3**	**0.2**
Yellowish				
Rural	2.2	1.9	2.0	2.1
Urban	3.1	2.8	1.9	2.6
Total	**2.3**	**2.1**	**2.0**	**2.2**
Blood Stained				
Rural	1.7	1.8	2.7	2.0
Urban	1.1	1.3	2.3	1.5
Total	**1.6**	**1.7**	**2.6**	**1.9**

Source: Computed from RCH-DLHS-3, 2007-08.

Table 25.8: Odds Ratios (95% Confidence Interval) from Logistic Regression Analysis Examining the Association between Gynaecological Morbidity and Selected Characteristics of Women

Characteristics	*Odds Ratio*
Age groups	
25-29 ®	1.0
15-19	0.87*
20-24	0.90*
30-34	1.07
35-39	1.02
40-44	0.89*
45-49	0.65*
Educational Attainment	
Higher ®	
None	1.13**
Primary	1.42
Secondary	1.45
Religion	
Hindu	
Muslim	1.378**
Others	1.061
Caste	
General ®	
Scheduled Caste	0.75*
Scheduled Tribe	0.72*
Status of women	
Rich ®	
Poor	1.25**
Medium	1.23
Prior obstetric complication	
No ®	
Yes	1.14**
Current Family Planning Use	
Other modern methods ®	
None/traditional	1.08**
Female sterilization/IUD	1.09**
Place of residence	
Urban ®	
Rural	1.134

® reference group; *p<0.1; **p<0.05.

Determinants of Gynaecological Morbidity

Table 25.8 shows the results of logistic regression analysis assessing the association of selected characteristics with gynaecological morbidity.

The model is run to a binary outcome, categorised as *one* if women have reported for the symptoms gynaecological morbidity and *zero* if no morbidity was reported during preceding three months to the survey. The model included associative factors that are either categorical or mutually exclusive and collected in the survey. The model controls for age groups, educational attainment, religion, caste, wealth index and place of residence representing the socio-economic status of women. Most of the variables that were included in the model showed significant association with gynaecological morbidity. Most notably, level of educational attainment played a vital role in the occurrence of gynaecological morbidity as women with no or low level of education (odds ratio, 1.13) appeared with higher likelihood of morbidity. However, women with minimum level of education are significantly more likely to report symptoms. Women in the age groups of 30-34 and 35-39 years (odds ratio, 1.07 and 1.02) have showed higher likelihood of the morbidity as compared to the reference age group. For each additional age group, the likelihood has reduced significantly.

Compared with women who practice Hinduism, women from other two religions are more likely to have symptoms of gynaecological morbidity. The caste groups have not shown any significant association with gynaecological morbidity among women. The status of women is another important controlling factor that has shown strong association with the symptoms of morbidity as women from poor and middle class were significantly more likely to report gynaecological morbidity.

Relative to women have not reported any prior obstetric complications, experienced women showed 14 per cent higher chances of reporting symptoms of gynaecological morbidity. Those women who reported that they had been sterilised or using IUD as a family planning methods were significantly more likely to have gynaecological morbidity. On the other hand, women who did not practice any method or use traditional method to prevent pregnancy showed higher likelihood of gynaecological morbidity. Finally, the reporting of the symptoms is significantly controlled by the place of residence of women. The rural women are 13 per cent more likely to report gynaecological morbidity compared with the reference group.

Table 25.9 shows the treatment seeking behaviour of women for vaginal discharge. It is notable, except vaginal discharge, treatment seeking behaviour of other symptoms of gynaecological morbidity was not collected. Therefore, apprehension regarding treatment-seeking behaviour and women's perception is drawn based on the present analysis. Out of total women in the collective sample of the present study, only 40 per cent of women have consulted or sought treatment for vaginal discharge. The present analysis shows the source of consultation or sought treatment of those 40 per cent women.

Table 25.9: Treatment for Vaginal Discharge sought by Women of the three States

Source of Treatment	*States*							
	Rajasthan		*Gujarat*		*Maharashtra*		*Total*	
	Rural	*Urban*	*Rural*	*Urban*	*Rural*	*Urban*	*Rural*	*Urban*
Private	37.1	51.9	67.6	85.2	76.0	86.8	59.1	76.5
Government	42.1	28.9	23.1	6.0	19.9	6.0	29.2	12.6
Others	6.0	7.3	8.4	7.7	2.9	6.3	5.2	6.9
Traditional	14.8	11.8	1.0	1.0	1.1	0.8	6.5	4.0

Source: Computed from RCH-DLHS-3, 2007-08.

The analysis also unravelled the societal taboo related to such problems on which women could not talk openly. From the analysis, it is very clear those women either from urban or rural residence, majorly preferred treatment at private hospitals. Overall, 59 per cent of the total rural women have sought treatment from private hospitals as compared to government counterparts. Similarly, 76 per cent of the total urban women have sought treatment from private hospitals whereas only 13 per cent of the urban women preferred government services.

However, Gujarat and Maharashtra showed comparatively higher percentages of women from both the residences who sought treatment at private hospitals as compared with women from Rajasthan. The government services to sought treatment are rather observed in a greater proportion in Rajasthan. The poor status of women seems to be the factor that acts as constraint to women to seek treatment from private hospitals. The utilization of traditional methods evinces the poor status of women in Rajasthan.

Women have also sought treatment from places like clinics, dispensary, medical shops and others in a substantial percentage. However, the substantial percentages are also observed high in Rajasthan as compared with other two states. Such a skewed distribution clearly evince that women, rarely, undergo any medical examination prescribed by specialists. Due to such a lack of exposure, the problems tend to get severe in advance stages.

Discussion

Conceptualizing gynaecological morbidity and its association with factors of varied dimensions from the data based on only self-reporting or perception remained quite complex. However, the analyses carried out with the variables in the present study have provided relevant scenario of gynaecological morbidity and related aspects from RCH-DLHS-3 data. The results of the present study corroborated finding of research studies done in past from developing as well as developed countries emphasising various issues related to gynaecological morbidity. The findings of the present study evince that gynaecological morbidity is a matter of concern among women from Rajasthan and Maharashtra. For instance, various studies have talked about the negligence of women towards their health and cited associative factors attached to it. Sexual health primarily remains unconcerned by women because of shyness and sensitivity attached with it. As an overview, culture of silence dominates women restricting them to speak about it. Excluding metropolitan cities, the rural women in Maharashtra also lack the freedom of movement and discomfort in talking about the symptoms of gynaecologic morbidity with strangers (interviewers during the survey). However, in urban areas, gynaecologic problems due to sexually transmitted diseases (STDs) and HIV is highly prevalent as compared to the other factors. Unsafe sexual behaviour (extra-marital relations, commercial sex workers and others) often leads to high risks of gynaecologic morbidity among spousal partners.

A number of studies emphasis women's autonomy as an important factor that withholds the authority of movement in order to seek treatment. Few other studies have documented the socio-economic status of women that plays important role in seeking treatment of symptoms of gynaecological morbidity. Generally, women in rural areas are less likely to report the gynaecological problems either due to lack of awareness or discomfort in reporting. The results from Rajasthan majorly support the facts discussed here. In addition, the conservative society and women themselves are not willing to reveal such health problems.

However, since urban women possess relatively a higher autonomy, better socio-economic status, education and therefore the reporting of gynaecologic problems are also high as compared to their rural counterparts. Moreover, in urban areas, women have better exposure to various sources of mass media disseminating information on reproductive health. In case, found positive with the problems, women seek treatment from either public or specialist (gynaecologist/obstetrician) in private hospitals.

Despite relevant findings drawn for western India, there are several limitations of the present study. Foremost among all, is the reliance on women's self-reporting of gynaecological morbidity which was the outcome variable of the study. Various previous studies have shown that there have been low levels of correspondence between women's own reports of gynaecologic symptoms and the same diagnosed through laboratory tests or clinical examining. For instance, the symptoms of vaginal discharge or pain during sexual intercourse and other infections generally are obtained through client's histories that are based on women's reports. Secondly, women tend to recall only those symptoms that have been imprinted on their mind as a bad or life threatening experiences.

The second potential limitation is the lack of information on several such variables that have direct linkages or relation with the occurrence of symptoms for example domestic violence or sexual assault are the brutal experiences of women that leads to gynaecologic morbidity and questions on such sensitive issues are not covered in the survey. Previous studies suggest that strong normative support for violence against females exists in Indian societal setting[2], possible reducing the stigma attached to domestic violence and therefore the social desirability bias that would lead to underreporting. In addition, the levels of domestic violence have remained unclear, as they tolerate physical beating, abuse and forceful sexual intercourse silently. Forced sex, medically proven, leads to vaginal trauma, through direct physical force or lack of lubrication that increases the risk of STI transmission.[3]

Although, their level of awareness has been asked through several questions but their own experience of HIV/AIDS or STDs have not been collected.

Another important limitation is that the questions related to gynaecologic morbidity were asked to only those women who had given birth to in the three years preceding to the survey and occurrence of symptoms only three months preceding to the survey. Generally, the chances gynaecologic problems remain high among those who had delivered recently because of the obstetric complications. The female sterilization (IUD insertion) and prior obstetric history have the potential contribution of iatrogenic factors to gynaecological morbidity. Although the analysis controlled for the obstetric complication, the information is available only for the last birth. Since women would have been suffering from obstetric history or multiple factors, such information are not covered in the survey.

Nevertheless, the present study provided an open and better understanding of the factors associated with gynaecological morbidity that makes it a neglected issue among women. The results of the study demonstrate the need of address and recognition of reproductive health of women who are unable to seek health care services because of multiple restricting factors. It also insights the need to address the root causes of gynaecological morbidity and ways to prevent in future. Awareness among illiterate women should be brought through expansion of sources of information in rural areas particularly. Several studies suggested incorporating domestic violence support services into existing sexual and reproductive health care services to reduce the risks. Lastly, conclusion can be drawn based on the assumption that education is required at both the ends in order to transform the negligence into a need and hence securing future of women.

Notes

1. J.C. Bhatia, J. Cleland, L. Bhagavan and N.S.N. Rao (1997), Levels and Determinants of Gynecological Morbidity in a District of South India, *Studies in Family Planning*, 28(2), 95-103.
2. WHO (1990), Sexually Transmitted Diseases Increasing by 250 Million New Infections Annually, *Press Release*, Geneva, Switzerland.
3. F.A. Althaus (1991), Reproductive Tract Infections and Women's Health, *International Family Planning Perspectives*, 17(4), 145-150.

4. R. Stephenson, M.A. Koenig and S. Ahmed (2006), Domestic Violence and Symptoms of Gynecologic Morbidity Among Women in North India, *International Family Planning Perspectives*, 32(4), 201-208.
5. S.C. Kalichman, *et al.* (1998), Sexual Coercion, Domestic Violence and Negotiating Condom Use among Low-Income African Women, *Journal of Women's Health*, 7(3), 371-378.
6. J.C. Campbell (2002), Health Consequences of Intimate Partner Violence, *Lancet*, 2535(9314), 1331-1336.
7. Oomman N. (2008), "Examining Determinants of Gynaecological Morbidity from Women's Perceptions in Rural Rajasthan", *Reproductive Health in India: New Evidence.* (Ed.), Koenig, M.A, Jeejeebhoy, S., Cleland, J.C. and Ganatra, B., Jaipur: Rawat Publications.
8. Joshi, A., Dhapola, M. and Pelto, P.J. (2008), "Gynaecological Problems: Perceptions and Treatment-seeking Behaviour of Rural Gujarati Women", *Reproductive Health in India: New Evidence.* (Ed.), Koenig, M.A., Jeejeebhoy, S., Cleland, J.C. and Ganatra, B., Jaipur: Rawat Publications.
9. Char, A. and Vaidya S. (2008), "Gynaecological Morbidity among Women Seeking Sterilisation Services in Rural Maharashtra", *Reproductive Health in India: New Evidence*, (Ed.), Koenig M.A, Jeejeebhoy S., Cleland J.C. and Ganatra, B., Jaipur: Rawat Publications.
10. S.J. Jejeebhoy and R.J. Cook (1997), State Accountability for Wife-beating: The Indian Challenge, *Lancet*, 349 (suppl.1), 10-12; S.L. Martin, *et al.* (1999), Domestic Violence in Northern India, *American Journal of Epidemiology*, 150(4), 417-426
11. International Institute for Population Sciences. District Level Household and Facility Survey, Reproductive and Child Health 3 (DLHS-RCH-3), 2007-08, (2009), Mumbai: International Institute for Population Sciences (IIPS).

26

Geoecology of Cataract Blindness in India

Nitasha Malhotra

Blindness is both a medical and social problem of considerable significance. This impairment may lead to partial or complete dependency of the affected people for the rest of their lives. This kind of impairment affects not only the person concerned but also their families on whom they are dependent. Increased dependency makes these people economically non-productive—a great stress on the staggering economy of the developing nations. It also has several social and psychological ramifications. It causes lot of physical and mental stress on individuals who are affected by it. It is also the leading disability in the world, with India alone accounting for one third of the total blindness in the country.[1]

A review of the literature on the etiology of different kinds of blindness points to the fact that the underlying factors for blindness are related to social, cultural, environmental and economic factors, thus making it a problem for geographic investigation. Blindness in different regions of the world varies by different types and associated causes. Higher prevalence of a particular type of blindness in a particular area can be related to various parameters such as climatic conditions, lifestyles, nutritional status of the population, access to health care delivery and so on. All these factors individually or cumulatively play a major role in different regions in the world.[2]

It is important to examine questions pertaining to blindness such as the **prevalence** (in terms of distribution and causes) of blindness in the world. What are the factors that are responsible for its high incidence in certain parts of the world? Who are the people who are affected and where do they live? Why is the problem more acute in the developing, tropical countries with India alone accounting for the largest number of blinds in the world? The answers to the above quest leads us to another aspect of geographic research pertaining to **geoecology and epidemiology** of blindness in areas endemic to it. The emphasis lies on understanding the various ecological domains, which may have a direct or indirect influence on high incidence of blindness in India. In keeping with the objective of this study, it is important to first understand the prevalence of blindness in the world as a whole followed by its high incidence in certain parts of India.

Prevalence of Blindness in the World

Global Pattern

Key Facts

- 285 million people are estimated to be visually impaired worldwide: 39 million are blind and 246 million have low vision.
- About 90 per cent of the world's visually impaired live in low-income settings.
- 82 per cent of people living with blindness are aged 50 and above.
- Globally, uncorrected refractive errors are the main cause of moderate and severe visual impairment; cataracts remain the leading cause of blindness in middle- and low-income countries.
- The number of people visually impaired from infectious diseases has reduced in the last 20 years according to global estimates work.
- 80 per cent of all visual impairment can be prevented or cured.

According to WHO estimates there are 39.36 million totally blind in the world of which nearly 8 million are in India alone thus accounting for nearly 20 per cent of the world's blind population. It is pertinent to mention here that if the cases of low vision and visually impaired are also taken into consideration, then 285 million people are affected by visual impairment on a worldwide basis (Fig. 26.1). Blindness is of various types but the most common type is cataract blindness accounting for more than 50 per cent of total blindness in the world. Cataract blindness has higher incidence in the Third World countries most of which are located in the tropical zone. Different regions in the world exhibit different kinds of blindness. Examples of some regions in the world associated with different types of blindness are given below:

- In **East Africa** river blindness and blindness due to nutritional deficiencies and measles amongst children are the most important causes.
- In **South East Asia** including India, blindness is mainly attributed to the development of cataract amongst the aging populations. Cataract blindness is a disease of the tropical countries. There is a substantially large population suffering from this kind of blindness that is related mainly to the aging process. Besides cataract, infections of the eyes and trachoma are also major causes of blindness in the tropical lands.
- In **the developed world**, cataract blindness is well under control because of better health care delivery system. Here macular degeneration of the eye and diabetic retinopathy are the leading causes of blindness.

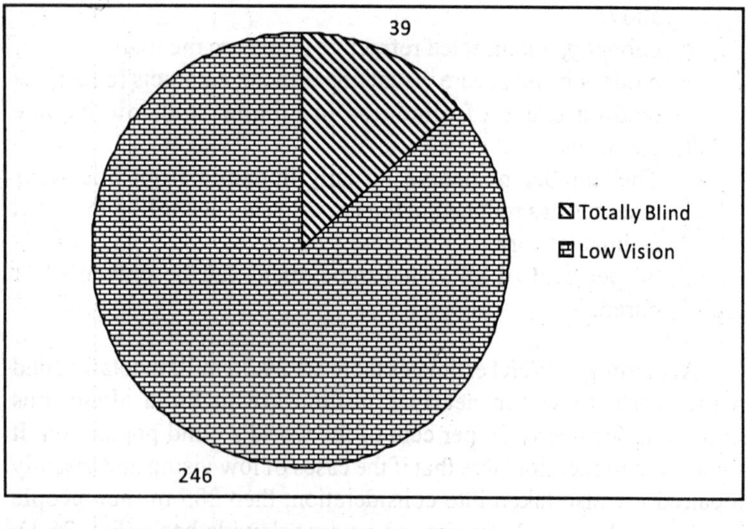

Fig. 26.1: Global Estimates of Blindness (in millions).

Source: www.who.int.org[3]

There are two recent studies estimating the prevalence of blindness and vision loss. One was published by the World Health Organisation Prevention of Blindness and Deafness Programme (WHO PBD) and the other by an expert group as part of the Global Burden of Diseases, Injuries and Risk Factors Study (GBD). The salient features of these two studies are:

- Both studies update the previous estimates by the World Health Organisation (WHO) released in 1995, 2002, and 2004. These estimates provide point prevalence estimates globally and for each of the WHO regions. They also estimate the major causes of vision loss.
- The two studies differ in their analytic approaches, however.
- Therefore, the studies give different results for the estimates of global blindness and visual impairment.

The key findings of both studies are presented in Table 26.1. It is worth noting that both studies cite the need for better data, particularly a greater number of regular, nationally-representative surveys that use standardized methodologies as defined by the WHO and that report results disaggregated by age and gender. There is also a need for studies to include near vision, which is so important for people's daily lives at home and at work.

Table 26.1: Comparative Analysis of WHO PBD and GBD Findings

	WHO PBD	*GBD*
Global Prevalence Blindness a Visual Impairment	Total: 285 million Blind: 39 million Low Vision: 246 million	Total: 223.4 million Blind: 32.4 million Moderate and severe visual impairment (MSVI): 191 million 95 per cent uncertainty intervals: 29.4–36.5 million blind,174-230 million visually impaired
Burden by Gender		Women represent 60.0 per cent of blindness and 57 per cent of MSVI
Burden by Ages	≥ 50 years represent 82 per cent of blindness and 65 per cent of VI	≥ 50 years represent 84.6 per cent of blindness and 77.5 per cent of MSVI

(*Contd.*)

Table 26.1 (*Contd.*)

Other Key Findings	The principal causes of blindness are: • Cataracts (51%) • Glaucoma (8%) • Age related macular degeneration (5%) • Childhood blindness and corneal opacities (4%)	A dramatic decrease (approximately 18 million cases of averted blindness) in the global age-standardized prevalence of blindness and MSVI for adults aged 50+ years: • 1990: 3.0% (2.7%–3.4 per cent)

Source: www.who.int.org

Regional Burden of Blindness

On a global scale, there are widespread regional disparities as is seen in Table 26.2. Since WHO is the chief collector and custodian of health data including that of blindness in the world both globally and

Table 26.2: Number of Visually Impaired and Corresponding Percentages of the Global Impairment by WHO Region and Country, 2010

WHO Regions	*Total Population (in millions)*	*Blindness*	*Low Vision*	*Visual Impairment*
		No. in millions (Per cent)	*No. in millions (Per cent)*	*No. in millions (Per cent)*
African Region	804.9	5.888 (15)	20.407 (8.3)	26.295 (9.2)
American Region	915.4	3.211 (8)	23.401 (9.5)	26.612 (9.3)
Eastern Mediterranean Region	580.2	4.918 (12.5)	18.581 (7.6)	23.449 (8.2)
European Region	889.2	2.713 (7)	25.502 (10.4)	28.215 (9.9)
South Eastern Asian Region (excluding India)	579.1	3.974 (10.1)	23.938 (9.7)	27.913 (99.8)
Western Pacific Region (excluding China)	442.3	2.338 (6)	12.386 (5)	14.724 (5.2)
India	1181.4	8.075 (20.5)	54.544 (22.2)	62.619 (21.9)
China	1344.9	8.248 (20.9)	67.264 (27.3)	75.512 (26.5)
Total	**6737.5**	**39.365 (100)**	**246.024 (100)**	**285.389 (100)**

Source: WHO, 2010.[4]

regionally, the analysis can be done on the basis of WHO regions as other estimates have been found to be not very scientific and robust.

Table 26.2 indicates that the majority of blind population resides in India and China, i.e. 20.5 per cent and 20.9 per cent. This is the precise reason why WHO has put forth separate for these two countries. Besides these two countries, African region, Eastern Mediterranean region and South East Asian region show high percentages of blind population.

People suffering from visual impairment per 100 population is an interesting measure to gauge the prevalence rate on a regional scale. WHO has been calculating this kind of data in the last few years (Fig. 26.2). The map clearly indicates that the continents of Asia and Africa have a much higher prevalence rate than other places like Americas or Europe. In Asia, the countries lying in the lower half of the continent and in Africa, the North Eastern side is worst affected. This aspect can be clearly attributed to the fact that these are first tropical countries receiving abundant sunshine and second both these areas have low income economies which are perennially poverty stricken and suffering from problems of malnourishment and undernourishment. Both these factors play a key role in prevalence of blindness as a whole.

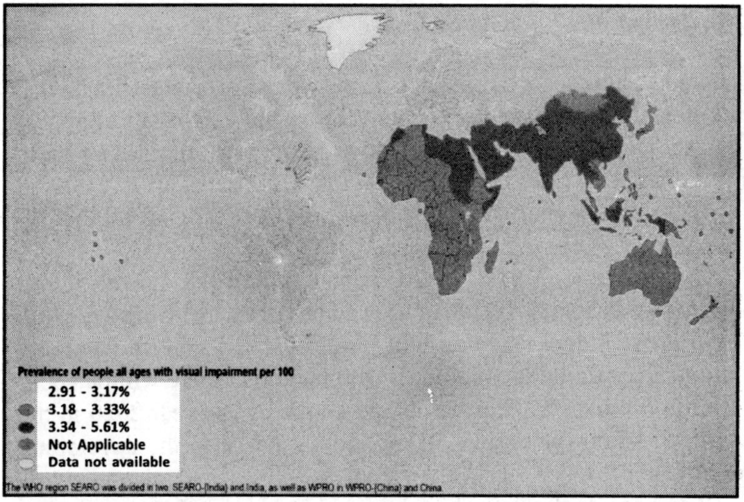

Fig. 26.2: Global Prevalence Rate of Visual Impairment, 2010.

Source: WHO, 2010.

Distribution of Blindness by Age

Blindness is most prevalent in the age group of 50 and older as shown in Table 26.3.

Table 26.3: Global Estimate of Number of People Visually Impaired by Age, 2010

Ages	*Population (in millions)*	*Blind (in millions)*	*Low Vision (in millions)*	*Visually Impaired (in millions)*
0 – 14	1848.50	1.421	17.518	18.939
15 – 49	3548.2	5.784	74.463	80.248
50 and Older	1340.80	32.16	154.043	186.203
All Ages	**6737.50**	**39.365**	**246.024**	**285.389**

Source: WHO, 2010.

It is as high as 86.69 per cent of the total blind population. This is a fairly high percentage of population and this can be attributed to senile cataracts which commonly afflict the aged population. This is followed by the age group of 15-49 years which accounts for 14.69 per cent of the blind population in the world. The age group of 0-14 years accounts for the smallest proportion of blinds, i.e. 3.6 per cent.

Distribution of Blindness by Cause

The three main causes of blindness in the world are cataract, trachoma, and glaucoma that together account for 62 per cent of all blindness as is shown in Fig. 26.3. The relative importance of each of these three diseases varies greatly by region because of differences in demographic structures disease incidence and availability/ accessibility of eye-care services.

According to World Development Report 1998, prevalence of blindness was highest in India followed by Africa and China in 1998. The present Indian situation will be discussed in the forthcoming sections. According to WHO, it is estimated that there will be about 54 million blind people aged 60 and above by the year 2020 in the world, of whom more than 50 million would be in the developing countries.

The pace of demographic changes has been and is expected to continue to be faster in the developing countries as death rates are declining faster with rapid improvements in medical facilities. The

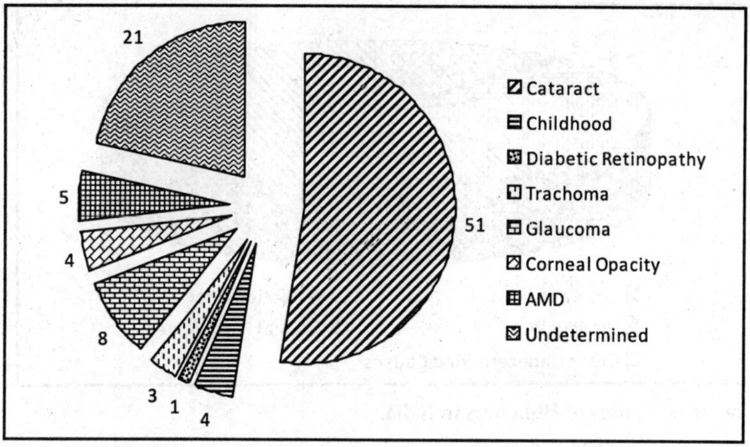

Fig. 26.3: Global Causes of Blindness as Percentages of Global Blindness, 2010.

Source: WHO, 2010.

life expectancy in these countries is also increasing at a faster rate as compared to the developed world. In these countries, the projected increase of the aged population in the period 1980 to 2020 is likely to be 356 per cent. Therefore, the prevalence of blindness in senile population is definitely on the rise with their numbers increasing so rapidly.

Prevalence of Blindness in India

It is noteworthy that the scourge of blindness has assumed alarming proportions in some of the developing countries like India according to WHO estimates. Most of the blindness (cataract) occurs inevitably due to the aging process of the body. However, this aging process may start at different age for different individuals depending on the kind of environment in which an individual is living. According to WHO reports, the reason for high incidence of cataract blindness in these countries is because the aging process starts at a much earlier age due to geographical reasons.[5] The Indian situation is no different. India accounts for one-fifth of the total blindness in the world. It is an enormous problem in India in terms of both economic loss and social burden. At present there are nearly 8 million blind eyes in the country and about 62.6 per cent of this is because of cataract. Other reasons are refraction error (19.7%), glaucoma (5.8%), corneal

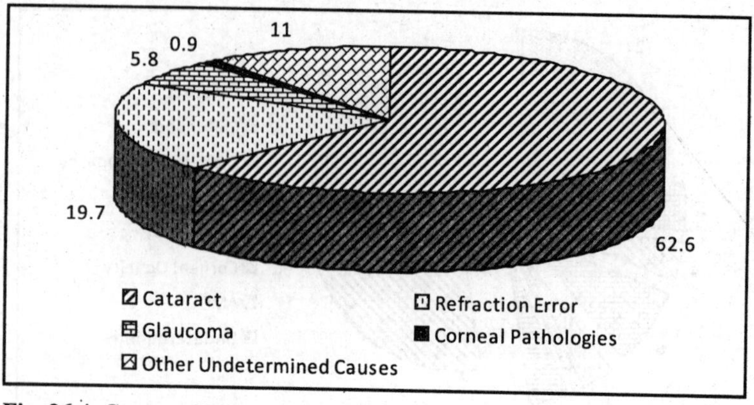

Fig. 26.4: Causes of Blindness in India.

Source: Vision 2020 India.org[6]

pathologies (0.9%) and other undetermined causes (11%). It is estimated that nearly 30,000 blinds are added every year.

Fortunately, cataract blindness is curable and eyesight can be restored in 90 per cent of the cases that are operated (Kupfer, 1998). The technique of the cataract operation has improved tremendously over the years and the success rate is very high.

The present annual level of performance of cataract operation is in the order of 1.6-1.9 million. To clear the backlog of cataract cases by the year 2000 and to tackle the rising incidence, 5 to 6 million cataract operations annually will have to be performed (vision 2020 India.org). India, a vast tropical country has a wide range of variation in climate and relief. In various parts of the country one comes across adverse environmental factors, varied social and cultural patterns, illiteracy, superstitions, taboos, poor sanitation and low personal hygiene. No wonder, many diseases occur in high proportions in our country.

Although the problem of blindness in India has always been acute going by the absolute number of blind, in the country, little effort had been made by the Government to collect spatial and temporal data so that the actual magnitude of different kinds of blindness could be determined. Before independence blindness data for different regions was made available by the Census of India 1891. Age-specific data is another important measure for introduction of interventions in this area. Fig. 26.5 shows that about 1.99 per cent of the population is

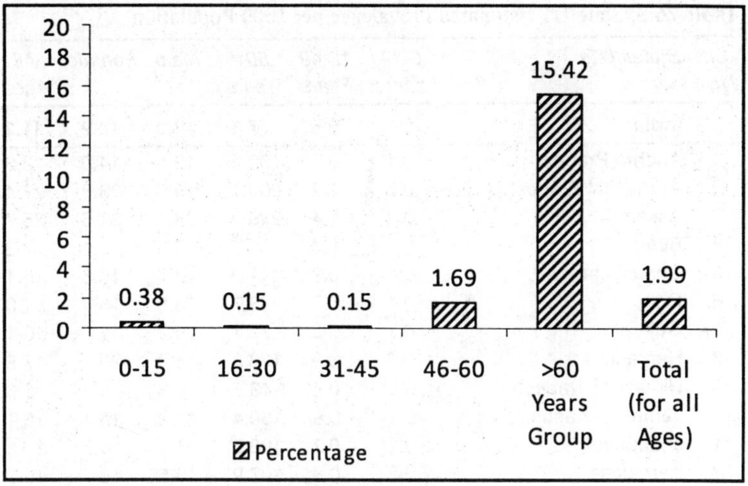

Fig. 26.5: Age Distribution of Blinds in India, 2011.

Source: Borker, 2011.[7]

blind out of the total population. To break this proportion into age-wise data, the maximum number of blinds, i.e. 15.42 per cent in the country fall in the >60 years group, which again reflects the dominance of cataract blindness that is directly related to older age. This is followed by 46-60 years group, 0-15 years and 16-30 and 31-45 years.

A state-wise analysis reveals that the maximum number of blind persons/1000 population is seen in Assam (28.7) closely followed by Arunachal Pradesh (21.4). Uttarakhand and Kerala show the minimum number of blinds at 5.3 per 1000 population. As far as age-wise analysis is concerned both Assam and Arunachal Pradesh have the highest number of blinds in almost all categories.

Cataract Blindness in India

Blindness due to cataract presents an enormous problem in India not only in terms of human morbidity but also in terms of economic loss and social burden. About 62.6 per cent of blindness in India is due problems relating to cataract. The annual incidence of blindness is about 3.8 million. The present level of performance is in the order of about 1.6-1.9 million cataract operations. In order to tackle the rising incidence, 5 to 6 million operations will have to be performed annually.

Table 26.5: State/UT Estimated Prevalence per 1000 Population

Sl. No.	*States/UTs*	*0-14 Years*	*15-49 Years*	*50+ Years*	*Male*	*Female*	*All Ages*
	India	**0.1**	**0.6**	**77.3**	**10.2**	**12.2**	**11.2**
1.	Andhra Pradesh	0.1	0.7	89.2	12.4	14.3	13.3
2.	Arunachal Pradesh	0.2	1.2	209.1	19.3	23.8	21.4
3.	Assam	0.3	1.4	236.9	26.1	31.5	28.7
4.	Bihar	0.1	0.4	55.6	6.6	8.1	7.3
5.	Chhattisgarh	0.1	0.8	111.2	13.7	16.6	15.1
6.	Goa	0.1	0.7	98.7	13.6	15	14.3
7.	Gujarat	0.1	0.5	72.1	9.2	11	10.1
8.	Haryana	0.2	0.9	133.8	15.8	20	17.8
9.	Himachal Pradesh	0.1	0.4	43.7	6.3	6.8	6.6
10.	Jammu & Kashmir	0.1	0.9	130.4	14.2	16.1	15.1
11.	Jharkhand	0.1	0.7	100.6	11.9	14.7	13.3
12.	Karnataka	0.2	0.8	107.9	15.5	18	16.7
13.	Kerala	0.1	0.2	27.8	5	5.5	5.3
14.	Madhya Pradesh	0.1	0.6	80.1	9.9	12	10.9
15.	Maharashtra	0.1	0.4	57	8.2	9.8	8.9
16.	Manipur	0.1	0.7	105.1	12.3	13.7	13
17.	Meghalaya	0.05	0.4	73.4	6.6	7.3	7
18.	Mizoram	0.1	0.4	70.3	6.8	7.8	7.3
19.	Nagaland	0.1	0.5	91.1	9	10.8	9.9
20.	Orissa	0.1	0.6	84.6	12.2	14.2	13.2
21.	Punjab	0.1	0.5	63.5	8.5	10.6	9.5
22.	Rajasthan	0.1	0.8	109.5	13.1	16.1	14.6
23.	Sikkim	0.05	0.3	60.2	5.6	6.7	6.1
24.	Tamil Nadu	0.1	0.3	38.3	6.8	7.9	7.3
25.	Tripura	0.1	0.4	56.6	6.8	7.7	7.2
26.	Uttar Pradesh	0.1	0.5	66.3	7.9	9.9	8.8
27.	Uttarakhand	0.04	0.3	39.5	4.7	5.9	5.3
28.	West Bengal	0.1	0.5	76.2	10.1	12.3	11.2
29.	A&N Islands	0.1	0.5	117.9	9.1	11.8	10.3
30.	Chandigarh	0.1	0.4	94.1	8.2	11	9.5
31.	D&N Haveli	0.1	0.5	89.6	8.5	9.4	8.9
32.	Daman & Diu	0.1	0.5	80.8	9.6	10.5	10.1
33.	Delhi	0.1	0.5	102.5	9.5	11.9	10.6
34.	Lakshadweep	0.04	0.3	43.2	5	5.5	5.3
35.	Puducherry	0.1	0.4	51.3	7	7.6	7.3

Note: Estimates are based on various surveys conducted by the National Programme for Control of Blindness (NPCB).

Source: Centre for Chronic Disease Control, National Commission on Macroeconomics and Health (NCMH) Background Papers—Burden of Disease in India, 2005 (Latest).[8]

Available data shows that there is a decrease in the prevalence of cataract blindness above 50 years of age from 7.6 per cent in 1989 to 5.3 per cent in 2001. In estimating the cataract blindness rates at different time periods, age-specific prevalence rates in the 1989 and 2001 surveys were used to estimate the number of cataract blind in the country over the period 2005-2020. Prevalence of cataract blindness in 2001 in the 50+ population was as follows:

- 50-59 years – 1.85 per cent
- 60-69 years – 5.63 per cent
- 70+ years – 13.3 per cent

Computing the age-specific prevalence rates of cataract blindness, it was observed that over the period 1989-2001, there was a 32 per cent reduction in the prevalence of cataract blindness at age 50-59 years, 54 per cent reduction at ages 60-69 and 22 per cent reduction at ages 70+ years over a one-year period. It has been assumed that this trend will continue till 2020.[9]

It is pertinent to mention here that cataract blindness is an imposing health challenge in the country. In spite of this fact research in this field on a spatial scale is still in its nascent stage. This kind of a research requires involvement of dedicated researchers including doctors, statisticians, social scientists and also government patronage so that effective data is generated which can help in planning effective interventions and strategies to deal with the problem. One such study was undertaken in the past and some major findings of this 1986-87 NPCB Survey Report were as follows:

- Females were found to be afflicted more compared to males. 160 females as against 142 males among every 10,000 people of that sex examined.
- Scheduled Castes had the highest prevalence of blindness of 200 persons among every 10,000 Scheduled Caste people examined.
- Pockets like inaccessible tribal areas and periods of famine/ drought/floods, etc. are associated with high prevalence of vitamin A deficiency.
- Northern and western parts of the country have higher prevalence of both cataract and trachoma which may be

attributed to geographical conditions such as high temperatures, less cloud cover, drought prone, reducing vegetation cover etc. Cataract prevalence is found to be high in Jammu & Kashmir, Rajasthan, Madhya Pradesh, Uttar Pradesh, Maharashtra, Andhra Pradesh, Tamil Nadu and Orissa.

According to this survey report, the major causes responsible for high prevalence of cataract in the country are:

1. Increasing life expectancy
2. Significantly more people in the risk group (>40).
3. Poor access to eye care facilities
4. Misconceptions about cataract surgery
5. Compromised water quality and environmental conditions
6. Lack of effective eye health education programmes

Cataract, which is the major cause of blindness both in the world and in India is curable by a simple operation in which the affected lens in the eye is either removed or replaced by an artificial lens (IOL surgery). Even though there are a large number of trained ophthalmic surgeons in the country, they are grossly underutilized because of the poor infrastructural facilities, their concentrations in the big cities, poor accessibility to health care delivery system in the vast rural and remote areas of the country.

Lack of knowledge and concern on the part of large number of people about the nature and cause of blindness and possible preventive measures add another dimension to the problem. There is widespread ignorance among the people even about simple eye-care, the role of nutrition, personal hygiene and prompt treatment. The progression of lens opacities is very variable. Some patients develop a mature cataract within a short period after the initial opacities are noticed. The exact etiology of cataract is not clear. UV radiation is the most commonly stated cause but available evidence is not sufficient proof. Similarly, dehydrational cases associated with repeated episodes of diarrhoea early in life exhibit high incidence of cataract blindness. Other factors may include exposure to domestic smoke from biogas fuels, nutritional status, smoking, diabetes and deficiency of antioxidant vitamins.

Comparison of Climatic Elements with Prevalence of Cataract Blindness in India

In this section the prevalence of cataract blindness in the country is compared with certain climatic elements which are likely to influence the distribution of blindness especially cataract.

Annual sunshine hours are highest in north-western part of the country (Rajasthan and southern part of Haryana) extending in the form of a belt towards the south-eastern drier parts across the Deccan Plateau and including large parts of Telangana in Orissa and Andhra Pradesh. These are highly drought prone, critical or vulnerable zones of the country where annual precipitation is highly variable and unpredictable. The cloud-cover is very less for most part of the year. Persons working outdoors for most part of the day are exposed to UV radiation, dry and dusty weather conditions, which can harm unprotected eyes considerably. Thus, geographical conditions seem to influence early development of cataract blindness in these pockets of the country. Some of these parameters are discussed below:

(a) *Temperature*—Generally speaking temperature is highly correlated with evaporation. Temperature varies from season to season and also depends on the cloud-cover in a particular area. Evaporation is higher when temperatures are high and cloud cover is low. Evaporation is more during summer months when the sun is strong.

(b) *Humidity and Wind*—In areas with low humidity evaporation is faster because the air has more water holding capacity. Besides wind also plays an important role. Humid air is constantly replaced by dry hot air leading to more evaporation. Moisture availability is also seasonal. More moisture (water) is available during the summer monsoons, which brings rains to almost all parts of the Indian subcontinent. However, there is great variation in the amount of rain received in different parts. The pockets of high annual evaporation include the north-western part of the country, which includes the dry, sandy, savannah type plains of Haryana and eastern Rajasthan, the Thar Desert of western Rajasthan. Another region where annual evaporation exceeds 250 cm lies in the leeward side of the Western Ghats, which includes the Chota Nagpur Plateau, Southern part of Bihar and some parts of Orissa.

Cataract is a condition when a normal transparent lens of the eye becomes opaque (clouded) thus blocking out the light and interfering with normal vision. A normal lens in the eye allows the light rays to pass through, and focuses a clean image on the retina and enables us to see. A cataract is neither a film nor a new growth. It is neither an infection nor a contagious disease. Cataract blindness is also referred to as senile cataract because it develops with age. Societies, which age faster, develop cataract at a much earlier age than others. In most patients, it is just a normal age related change of lens, analogous to graying of hair. Cataract is one of the leading causes of reversible blindness in India. In 95 per cent of the patients, it is just a normal age related change of lens, analogous to graying of hair. The distribution of this kind of blindness in the country through several surveys and experience of doctors in the field has shown that certain areas in the country are endemic to cataract blindness. These areas are characterized by particular geographic conditions (physical, social, economic and cultural), which seem to influence the early development of cataract. Several ophthalmologists have theoretically realized the importance of investigating the environmental, social, cultural and demographic factors leading to early cataract formation in many regions of India.[10] They have, however not been able to do much empirical work in this field especially in India where the problem of senile cataract is most serious. The etiology and geoecology of cataract blindness can be understood better by using a geographical perspective as well. The possible relationships of cataract formation through the above dimension are given below:

- High incidence of cataract is witnessed in regions where cloud cover is low or sunlight hours are more. This is because ultra-violet radiation (UVR) leads to early development of cataract.
- Cataract is also common in areas where people consume hard water and consume large quantities of yogurt.
- The rural areas have higher prevalence of blindness about 57 per cent more than the urban areas.
- Poverty, low income and illiteracy are also seen to be highly associated with this disease. These factors have an indirect effect as these may lead to deprivation of proper health care facilities, healthy living conditions and healthy food.

- Various ethnic and cultural groups tend to have different food habits and living styles, which over the years get manifested into genetic cause of cataract blindness. The literature survey has shown that genetic cause is the most predominant amongst all the risk factors since all the environmental factors together get manifested into these. Certain communities are more prone than the others.

Besides genetic reasons, history of high blood pressure and diabetes has also been associated with cataract blindness. Gastro-intestinal infections result in malnutrition, acidaemia, uraemia and dehydration. These cause certain chemical changes in the body, which facilitates the development of cataract.[11] There is also an association between cataract and low consumption of proteins and antioxidants such as Vitamin C and E.[12] Cataract blindness is a multifactorial disease and its etiology can only be understood by applying a disease ecology approach, which may help to find solutions to the problem in a more scientific and holistic manner.

Geo-Ecology of Cataract Blindness in India

Possible Risk Factors for Cataract Development

The high prevalence of cataract blindness in certain parts of India may be attributed to the interplay of various ecological parameters, which together create conducive conditions for the same. These ecological parameters have complex relationship with each other and it becomes difficult to isolate certain exposures from the influence of other exposures. The interaction with the environment is dynamic and ever changing.

Different researchers have given different models for analytical work on multifactorial diseases. One such model was given by Briggs, Corvalan and Nuriman in 1996. This model is called THE CAUSE-EFFECT FRAMEWORK, which can also be applied to the study of cataract. This framework helps to identify driving forces, pressure conditions, state, exposure levels, effects and action plans associated with a particular disease. This model for cataract blindness is given in Table 26.6.

In order to understand the exact role played by the different factors, there is need to develop a geo-ecological model (Fig. 26.6).

Table 26.6: The Cause-Effect Framework Model

DRIVING FORCES	⟹	➤ High population growth ➤ Poor economic growth ➤ Low levels of technology
PRESSURE	⟹	Driving forces imposes different kinds of pressure conditions: ➤ Environmental—high UV radiation, cloudless skies, lack of vegetation, deforestation ➤ Social—population pressure, culture, traditions, lifestyles ➤ Economic—due to poverty and occupations
STATE	⟹	These are conditions to which people are exposed in a particular milieu.
EXPOSURE	⟹	Actual amount of exposure which is dose related and varies from person to person
EFFECT	⟹	Exposures have a wide range of health effects. High exposure to UV radiation with low means of protection due to poverty, ignorance and poor diets may lead to early aging, which in turn leads to cataract development.
ACTION	⟹	After identifying the important links between different aspects of development, environment and health so that effective strategies may be formulated to control and prevent adverse health effects.

Senile cataracts are of known etiology. Few epidemiological studies of this common and heterogeneous condition have identified several factors associated with an increased frequency of lens changes. Some of these studies are listed below:

1. In 1998 Ughade, Zodpey and Khanolkar associated age-related cataract in central India with 21 risk factors. Of which low socio-economic status, cheap cooking fuel, history of diarrhoea, smoking, diabetes, low body mass index and heavy alcohol consumption were significantly influencing early cataract development.
2. Madan Mohan, Angra and Sperduto earlier conducted such a study in 1989 in which cataract blindness was studied in relation to several factors.
3. Outside India similar risk factors were identified by Chylac and Leske (1991) in U.S.A. and McCarty and Taylor (1999) in Australia.

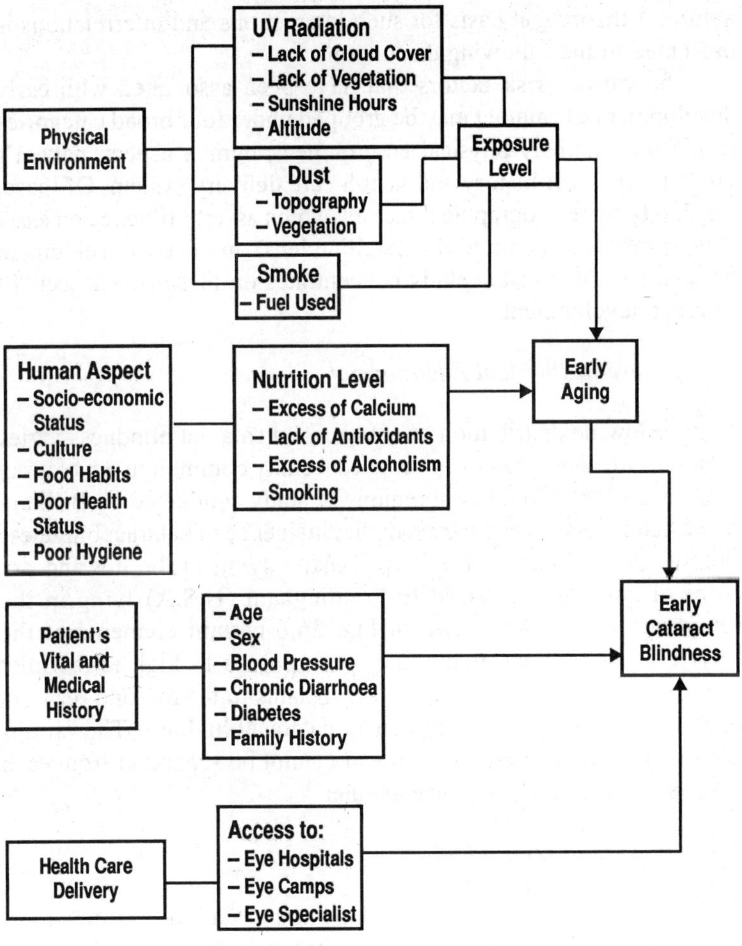

Fig. 26.6: Geo-ecological Model for Cataract Blindness.

Although most of the earlier studies recognize the contribution of such factors in influencing early development of cataract, few scholars have attempted a holistic treatment. Even health organizations like the WHO are advocating the use of this approach while formulating action programmes for the elimination of chronic diseases having multifactorial causation. The ecological and ecosystem perspective appears to be more appealing for nutrition analysis than the piecemeal approaches because of their holistic and integrative nature. A theoretical basis for such interactions and interrelations is presented in the following discussion.

The various risk factors that have been associated with early development of cataract may be grouped under four broad categories (Fig. 26.6), namely physical environment, human aspect, patient's vital and medical history and health care delivery system. Of these, the first two are geographical factors, which assert influence on early aging process (oxidation of crystalline lens) and early development of cataract. The present study concentrates on these two aspects of cataract development.

1. Exposure to Physical Environment

The worldwide distribution of cataract and cataract blindness varies widely, with senile cataracts being especially common in developing countries located in tropical regions. A study conducted by Brilliant and Chatterjee (1983) reported higher incidence of cataract blindness (almost three times) in the Punjab plains lying in the hot and dry tropical zone as compared to Framingham (U.S.A) lying in the temperate zone.[13] As shown in Fig. 26.6 certain elements of the physical environment determine the exposure to high ultra-violet radiation, dust and smoke which are irritants to the eye and result in early aging and early development of cataract blindness. The various elements of the natural environment cannot be separated from each other since they influence one another.

(a) Exposure to UV Radiation

There is evidence to suggest that exposure to radiation from almost all regions of the electromagnetic spectrum is capable of damaging the lens in the eye.[14] This is of particular concern because the eye as the skin is exposed to a wide spectrum of natural and man-made radiant energy. The risk of lens damage from ionizing and infrared radiation is well-known, but recent attention has focused on the cataractogenic potential of ultraviolet light and microwave radiation.

Ultraviolet light (that part of the electromagnetic spectrum between 100 and 400 nanometers) is a prominent component of solar radiation and is artificially produced for a variety of industrial and medical purposes. UVR (ultraviolet radiation) above 295 nanometers readily penetrates the cornea and efficiently absorbed by the lens.

Laboratory studies have shown that exposure to sunlight near ultra-violet light results in chemical and physical changes in lens protein and alterations in lens epithelial cells. Photochemical processes involving oxidation of tryptophan is related to cataract development.

In the case of Himalayas, there are four variables operative with respect to ultraviolet radiation.[14]

- *Effect of altitude*—It has been calculated that at 2000 mts, the ultraviolet flux may be 60 per cent greater than at 2000 mts. for the same duration of sunlight much more UV exposure is experienced at high altitudes than at sea level.
- *Duration of sunlight*—The regression of sunlight hours on altitude suggests that at 2000 mts, the average village in this study would receive about 8.5 hours of sunlight as compared to 12 hours of sunlight at sea level. This reduction of nearly 30 per cent in sunlight hrs. partially offsets the gain in UV radiation associated with increasing altitude.
- *Latitude*—The higher peaks of the Himalayas are directly north of the plains further from the equator. The effect of latitude is a little difficult to ascertain in the presence of other variables.
- *Cloud cover*—There are fewer clouds over the unobstructed plains while more clouds accumulate over the hills and mountains. This is likely to widen the gap between radiant energy reaching hill villages and plain villages. This could be one of the reasons for low incidence of blindness reported in the north- eastern states of India where the terrain is hilly and skies remain cloudy for most part of the year.

(b) Exposure to Dust

Some studies in the past have also associated early cataract blindness with dusty conditions.[15] Constant exposure to particle matter is common where sand blasting is common. Dusty conditions also prevail in arid areas where strong dusty winds raise dust from the ground into the atmosphere especially in the summer season.

(c) Exposure to Smoke

Here too the smoke particles cause the eye to have acute redness and dryness, which leads to early development of cataract. The ICMR study conducted by Mohan (1989)[17] found higher instances of cataract blindness amongst women exposed to smoking *chulhas* (stoves) and using cheap firewood for cooking due to economic reasons. Likewise in many other Indian studies have proved that use of cheap cooking fuels such as cow dung or wood leads to an increased risk of cataract.

Smoking is associated with cataract in a big way. It is believed that substances in inhaled cigarette smoke are carried internally to the eye and may cause the damage. It is felt that a similar pathway may be operating in the case of smoke inhaled from cheap cooking fuels. Smoking and tobacco chewing appear to induce oxidative stress and have been associated with both diminished levels of antioxidants, ascorbate and carotenoids and with enhanced cataract at a younger age.[16]

Exposure has two dimensions—level and duration. Many environmental factors produce effects only after a long period of exposure. Many hazards (for e.g. radiation, noise) have a cumulative effect.[17] For these hazards, the past exposure levels and the exposure duration are more important than the current exposure level.

2. Human Aspects

Literature survey of several studies on cataract blindness confirms the role of human factors (Fig. 26.6) to be equally important in the development of cataract in an early age. Human factors differ considerably from region to region especially in the case of developed and underdeveloped parts of the world. People belonging to developed economies, leading affluent lifestyles and maintaining a proper nutrition status are less exposed to the vagaries of the natural environment. Some of the human factors such as socio-economic status, health and hygiene levels of individuals, lifestyle, food habits, cultural practices and so on directly and indirectly influence the nutritional level of the affected populations which in turn influences the age of development of cataract.

(a) Nutrition Status

Nutrition level of the person plays a very important role in the development of cataract. Cataract formation like other age related symptoms are a result of oxidative stress. The lens has a very interesting structure. The lens fibers are continually replenishing throughout life. The lens actually grows. Its surface keeps getting compressed into the interior and new lens fibers grow outside. Once the lens fiber reaches its full length it begins to lose all its organelles, its mitochondria, its nucleus, its enzymes. So, it is very vulnerable to any damage to its structure. The lens proteins have a certain size and there is accumulation of sulphur-hydrogen group at the center. With increased oxidation the S-H group drops its hydrogen and one gets S-S linkages with the increase in accumulation of these in the lens, it begins to turn opaque and a cataract is formed. UV radiation exposure actually accelerates the process of oxidation within the lens. Therefore, UV radiation along with poor nutritional status enhances the development of cataract formation. Foods, which are antioxidant, are fresh vegetables and fruits with Vitamin A and E (these get destroyed on cooking). Intake of these in regular diet is quite essential to reduce oxidative processes taking place in the body.

(i) *Role of vitamins and antioxidants:* Several recent scientific studies have shown that intake of large quantities of antioxidants slow down the aging process in the human body. They develop a natural defence mechanism by which the body is able to overcome the oxidative stress.

Previous studies have reported a relationship between nutritional status and cataract. There was an increased risk of cataract formation with low frequency of protein consumption. The proportion of insoluble protein in the lens of undernourished patients was significantly increased compared to well nourish patients while the total proteins remained unaltered, suggesting an increased insolubilization process. Patients with higher nutritional level have less risk of cataract development. Consumption of vitamins C, B and E along with luteins and carotenes have a protective effect as far as cataract is concerned. Some studies have also shown associations of mineral consumption with cataract development.

(ii) *Role of calcium* (*milk*): In 1935, Mitchell and Dodge reported that diets rich in lactose or galactose caused rapid and massive opacification of rat lenses. The sugar alcohol products accumulate in the lens since they are not efficiently metabolized and have relatively slower rates of diffusion out of the lens than the parent sugars. This accumulation in turn causes hyper tonicity and osmotic swelling which if sustained will bring about rupture of the fiber cells. Communities, which are more dependent on milk and milk products (curds, curd milk and other milk products), are at a higher risk as far as lens opacities are concerned. This has been proved to some extent in a study that was conducted in Punjab by Chatterjee, Milton and Thyle, "Prevalence and etiology of cataract blindness in Punjab" in 1979.

Some established facts about nutrition status and cataract development are summed below:

1. In general, the higher the nutritional level of an individual lesser the risk of cataract.
2. There is significant positive correlation between antioxidant levels measured as AO3 (referring to composite levels of vitamin C, vitamins E and luteins) and protection against various types of cataracts. Intake of carotenes (vitamin A) also prevents fast progression of cataract in human lenses.
3. There is also significant association between cataract and low frequency of current use of proteins.
4. High risk of cataract has also been associated with deficiency of vitamin B complex (riboflavin).
5. Higher intake of galactose (milk and milk products such as yogurt) is also positively associated with lens opacities. High intake of calcium leads to opacification of lens. This has been proved in a study conducted on the milk drinkers of a village in Punjab.
6. Deficiency of riboflavin leads to cataract formation. Riboflavin deficiency is not uncommon in alcoholics. Young people with senile cataract are often alcoholics.

(b) Patient's Vital and Medical History

Besides the above geographical factors there are several personal and medical parameters, which may cause development of cataract (Fig. 26.6). These have been discussed below:

(i) *Age*—The close association of cataract blindness with increasing age has been well documented in most studies. It is well established that cataract formation is a function of age. This fact has been proved by various cataract studies conducted all-over the world irrespective of geographical conditions. It is well documented that senile cataract may serve as a marker for generalised tissue aging, since structural changes occurring in the protein of the lens during cataract formation are similar to those which occur elsewhere as part of the aging process.[18] The geographical factors in tropical countries like India, which lead to early ageing processes and therefore early development of cataract. It is estimated that a delay in cataract formation of about 10 years would reduce the prevalence of visually disabling cataract by about 45 per cent. According to Kupfer, C. (2000) such a delay would enhance the quality of life for much of the world's older population and substantially reduce the economic burden due to cataract related disability and cataract surgery.

(ii) *Sex*—Data from both Framingham Eye Study and Model Reporting Area for Blindness Statistics have shown that women over 65 years of age have higher rates of cataract blindness than men do. In the National Health and Nutrition Examination Survey for U.S.A. (1981) lens opacities were significantly more common in women than men. However, not many studies on the etiology of cataract blindness have shown any association of cataract with sex. However, a particular sex in a region may be more exposed to certain externalities for instance Ultra-violet radiation, dust and smoke. In such a case, this particular sex may have a higher or an earlier development of cataract.

(iii) *Medical factors*—When sugar levels are elevated in the human body, glucose is converted by aldose reductase (enzyme which metabolizes aldose) into sorbitol; the accumulation of sorbitol has been shown to damage the lens. A long-standing clinical impression has been that cataracts are more frequent and occur earlier in diabetics than non-diabetics.[19] However, numerous clinical and epidemiological investigations have reported conflicting results.

The effects of excessive sorbitol and fructose in the diabetic lens result in increased quantities of Na+ ions (sodium) within the lens and subsequent loss of K+ ions, amino acids. The sodium ions draw water making the lens hydrated. This ruptures the lens fibers causing vacuolation in the lens cortex leading to opacity. The rate of cataract progression depends on the glucose levels in serum the higher the glycerine, the faster the cataracts become mature. In the Framingham and Edinburgh studies high systemic blood pressure was associated with the presence of senile cataract. The contribution of genetic factors to senile cataracts also cannot be refuted. There are numerous reports of families with high cataract prevalence. Concordance of expression for cataract has been reported in monozygotic twins. Some studies suggest an association between cataract and genetically determined enzyme deficiencies

The Need for Integrated Policies, Strategies and Action

The reasons for early cataract development are highly complex and multifaceted. The health or medical sector alone cannot address this problem on its own. New and innovative approaches are needed to integrate and operationalise effective action to tackle this problem. This effective action may incorporate—

- Action on the driving forces through policy development and implementation. This may include policies on population control, poverty elimination, literacy, arid-land management and land use management.
- Action on the pressures on environment through socio-economic development, improvement in quality of life, afforestation, soils conservation and sound agricultural practices.
- Action on the state of the environment through improvement in local participation in sanitation, sewage disposal, protection of flora and fauna for the protection of desert ecology, safe drinking water and use of non-polluting alternate sources of energy such as solar energy, biogas or LPG.
- Action on human exposure through education on personal protection and initiative such as protecting oneself from direct solar exposure and smoke, eating a diet which is protective and delays the onset of cataract
- Action on the effect, i.e. extending the right kind of medical aid to cataract prone areas that is beneficial to all sections of the society. Efforts must be made, by a centralized body, for equitable distribution of foreign and government aid to combat the growing scourge of cataract blindness in India.

In order to find solutions to environmental health problems, interventions often corrective or remedial may be implemented at the source itself. The most effective long-term interventions aim to eliminate or reduce the effects of "driving forces" or "pressures" that produce the hazard.

Action on the driving forces, pressure and state of the environment eliminates the root causes of the problems associated with health-environment relationship. Actions on the specific exposures resulting in specific effects call for reactive approaches pertaining to the disease itself. Thus, a broad array of activities is clearly needed to solve the health-environment—development problems facing us today.

This type of blindness affects the aged population, which is growing in numbers all-over the world with increasing life expectancy. More and more people are added on to the existing number of blind year after year. This is largely due to the degradation of environment, population pressure, climatic conditions and related geographical problems.[20] Blindness has been mentioned as a major public health challenge and a debilitating factor for large elderly and other productive groups, but has not drawn much attention in social research and in health policies as it deserves. Blindness is also the leading disability faced by mankind and there is a need for understanding its etiology from the point of view of social scientist. All epidemiological studies on cataract blindness so far have adopted clinical approach because medical practitioners have conducted them. This is perhaps the reason why the programmes and policies adopted to overcome this growing scourge have not shown the desired results. There is need to adopt a disease ecology approach to identify the major factors which make a particular region endemic to a particular disease like cataract blindness. If in that particular region certain intervention policies are implemented to improve the geographic and social environment, it would help to find a more permanent solution to the problem.

Notes

1. Foster, A. (2000), "Vision 2020; The Cataract Challenge", *Commun Eye Health*, 13: 1-3.
2. Taylor, H.R., Keefe, J.E. (2001), "World Blindness : A 21st Century Perspective", *Br. J. Ophthalmol.*, 85: 261-6.
3. www.who.int.org, www.cbhidghs.nic.in, www.vision2020.org
4. World Health Organisation, Global Data on Visual Impairments 2010, Who/Nmh/Pbd/12.01.

5. Kupfer, C. (1984), "The Conquest of Cataract—A Global Challenge", *Trans Ophthalmol Society*, U.K., 104: 1-10.
6. Vision2020india.org.
7. Borker, Sagar (2011), "Epidemiological Study of Prevalence and Causes of Visual Disability in a Rural Community", *Journal of Indian Academy of Geriatrics*, 7.
8. Centre for Chronic Disease Control, National Commission on Macroeconomics and Health (NCMH), Background Papers—Burden of Disease in India, 2005.
9. Murthy, G.V.S., *et al.* (2008), "Current Status of Cataract Blindness and Vision 2020: The Right to Sight Initiative in India", *Indian Journal of Opthalmology*, November-December 56(6), 489-594.
10. Dhir, S.P. (1967), Detels R.; Alexander E.R., "Environmental Factors in Eye Diseases", *Am. J. Ophthalmol.*, July.
11. Chatterjee, G.C. (1976), "Nutritional Problems of India", *Science and Culture*, 42: 3-7.
12. Taylor, A.; Jacques, P.F. and Epstein, E.M. (1995), "Relations among Aging, Antioxidant Status and Cataract", *American J. Clinical Nutr.*, 62: 1439-1447.
13. Brilliant, L.B. (1983), "Associations among Cataract Prevalence, Sunlight Hours and Altitude in the Himalayas", *American Journal of Epidemiology*, 118(2): 250-264.
14. Mohan, M.; Sperduto, R.D.; Angra, S.K. (India), (1989), "US Case Control Study of Age Related Cataracts"; *Arch. Ophthalmol.*, 107: 670-676.
15. Ughade, S.N.; Zodpey, S.P. and Khanotkar, V.A. (1998), "Risk Factors for Cataract: A Case Control Study", *Indian J. of Ophthalmology*, December, 46:4, 221-27.
16. Taylor, H.R. (1999), "Epidemiology of Age-Related Cataract", *Eye*, June, 13: 445-448.
17. World Health Organization, "Global Initiative for the Prevention of Avoidable Blindness", WHO/PBL/97.61; Geneva: WHO, 1997.
18. Medding, D.R., Hertzman, C. (1998), "Socio-economic Status, Mortality and the Development of Cataract at a Young Age", *Social Science and Medicine*, June.
19. Leske, M.C., Chylack, L.T. Jr. (1991), "The Lens Opacities Case-control Study Risk Factors for Cataract", *Arch. Ophthalmol.*, 109: 244-251.
20. Akhtar, R. (1980), "Environment, Agriculture and Nutrition in Kumaon Region", (New Delhi : Marwah Publications).

27

Incidence of Kidney Disease in Kaviti and Kanchili Mandals of Uddanam Region

Srikakulum District of Andhra Pradesh State, India

M. Ganga Raju, Raju Rao, G., B. Visweswara Reddy, Demudu, G., Tamminaidu, G., Lalitha, K., Kakani Nageswara Rao, and *B. Hema Malini*

Disease in living beings mostly spread through food and drinking water. Of which, drinking water plays a major role as it influences the quality of the food. A safe drinking water is one that cannot harm the consumer which is free from pathogenic agents, harmful chemical substances, and pleasant taste and usable for domestic purposes[1]. Groundwater is superior to surface water but sometimes it contains high quantities of minerals and also contaminated with pollutants due to anthropogenic activities such as urban, industrial and agriculture.

Several investigations proved that excess concentration of minerals consumed through water and food effects human health. In USA and Europe, 2000 cases of methaemogolobinaemia and 7-8 per cent of infant deaths were reported due to excess concentration nitrates in drinking water[2] and incidence of gastric cancer in Colombia and Italy.[3] Similarly, overdose of fluorine causes chronic toxicity in human beings, which manifests significantly on dental and skeletal tissues and results in the incidence of dental and skeletal Fluorosis.[4] Water contaminated with insecticides and pesticides is responsible for liver, kidney diseases especially in the rural areas where agriculture is the main occupation. Some studies revealed that there is a link between chronic kidney ailments and pesticide residues in vegetables. Widespread use of the pesticide namely triple super phosphate, diammonium phosphate, rock phosphate and urea are suspected to be the reason for the high incidence of chronic kidney diseases.[5-6]

Since two decades an ailment which is different from normal Chronic Kidney Disease (CKD), has surfaced inflicting thousands of people in rural and dry agricultural regions of North central Sri Lanka with unknown etiology[7-8], along the Pacific coast of North central America and north coastal regions of Andhra Pradesh in India.[9] Medical communities named this mysterious disease as Chronic Kidney Disease with unknown etiology (CKDu). According to WHO, in Central America region, CKDu was spread in six countries along the Pacific coast for about 1126 kms and caused death of 2800 persons each year between 2005 and 2009. Of late, some parts of India, which is agriculturally potential brought into light for the incidence.[10] More or less similar type of disease occurred in China as nephropathy[11] and as Balkan endemic nephrophathy in Serbia, Bulgaria, Romania, Croatia and Bosnia.[12-13]

Globally, common CKD is an uniformly distributed disease which causes by infections and diseases like longstanding diseases like diabetes, hypertension, etc., and sometimes with the past history of glomerulonephritis.[14–17] However, unlike normal CKD, the new form of CKD with unknown etiology (CKDu) confines in specific geographical regions which are agriculturally fertile and experience prolonged dry and drought conditions and its incidence not linked with diabetes and hypertension. CKDu is a disease with slow progression, irreversible nature and mostly surfaced in the second decade of life and asymptomatic until its advance stage.[16] In CKDu the damage is to tubules and interstitium of nephrons rather than blood vessels of the kidney as in the case of CKD.

So far the causative factors for the incidence of CKDu are not yet identified except put forwarding probabilities. In agricultural regions where hot and dry conditions prevail, farmers work for long hours as a result they are subjected to extreme physical exertion, heat stress and dehydration.[18] In addition, their exposure to agrochemicals by consuming contaminated water makes them vulnerable to CKDu. Several investigations in the CKDU affected areas, indicated that the toxins in the environment which implicate kidney damage include heavy metals like cadmium, arsenic, lead, gold, platinum, silver, thallium, antimony uranium, and fluoride,[14, 19-20] air pollutants, algal toxins produced by in contaminated foods, tobacco chewing and smoking, and agro chemicals.[10-14, 21-24] Some studies indicated that accumulation levels of heavy metals in agricultural region depends on the type and quantity of fertilizer used in the cultivation and fertilizers such as rock phosphate, diammonium phosphate and triple super phosphate may contribute heavy metals to the soil as well as water in the agricultural fields.[6] Hence, incidence of CKDu linked with the hydrochemistry of the drinking water.[25] Further, use of aluminium utensils for household works like storing water and cooking create toxic compounds when it reacts with fluoride and harmful health hazard.[26-27] In addition, snake bites, ayurvedic medicines, aristolochic acid, nephrotoxic medications, country made alcohols[29] infectious diseases and genetic susceptibility are also considered as contributors for kidney damage.

India is one of the three major countries registering CKDu and it is second major disease (16.0%) after diabetic nephropathy (31.3%) and the incidence is highest in the southern parts of country.[10] Two regions namely coastal Uddanam in Srikakulam district and Chimakurthy mandal (30-40 km inland) in Prakasam district of Andhra Pradesh State are the identified regions of CKDu in south India.[29] World Health Organization has identified that Uddanam region as one of the three regions in the world with maximum concentration of CKDu cases. Around 4,000 villagers have died of renal failure in the last decade and almost a third of the population in Uddanam region suffers from CKDu.[29] Thereby, Uddanam became hot spot region of CKDu and drawn the attention of national as well as international medical communities to carryout investigations to find actual etiological causes for the disease. Five mandals namely Vajrapu Kotturu, Mandasa, Kaviti, Sompeta and Kanchili are together known as 'Udyanavanam' (Garden) due to rich growth of greenery. The CKDu sufferers of Uddanam region are mostly farmers of paddy crop and other plantation crops like coconut, jackfruit and cashew. The general pathology is chronic tubulointerstitial nephritis. This pathologic diagnosis in CKDu attributed to occupational and/or environmental exposures.

According to Raju and his associates,[30] the percentage of affected persons in Kaviti, Kanchili, Sompeta and Ichchpuram region are 5.91 per cent, 4.99 per cent, 1.52 per cent and 1.33 per cent respectively. They found that hypertension and diabetes are not responsible factors for the incidence of CKDu in this region. For the present study Kaviti mandal has taken as a study area as it shows highest percentage of incidence to understand the pattern of disease occurrence both demographically and spatially.

Study Area

Kaviti is located in the northern most coastal part of Uddanam region approximately between 18°56' and 19°04' N latitudes and 84°36' and at 84°44' E longitudes covering an area of 148 km^2 with an elevation of 41 m above mean sea level in Srikakulam district of Andhra Pradesh (Fig. 27.1). The Kaviti mandal is surrounded by Ichchapuram on the north, Kanchili and Sompeta mandals on the south, Orissa State on the west and Bay of Bengal on the east. Total population of the mandal is 70,945 with 33,590 male and 37,355 female population. It has total 111 villages and 21 panchayats. The sandy and red loams of Kaviti mandal support paddy cultivation and abundant spread of plantation crops namely coconut, cashewnut, jack and mango.

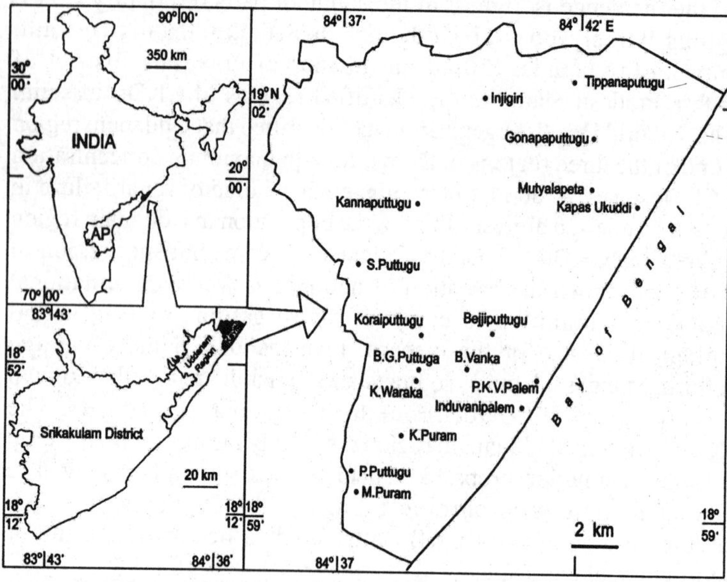

Fig. 27.1: Location Map of Kaviti Mandal in Srikakulam District of Andhra Pradesh.

The study area experiences mean annual temperature of 27.0° C. The temperature of the hottest month is 33.8° C and coldest month is 20.5° C. The annual rainfall of Kaviti mandal is 1161 mm. The region experiences semi-arid climate.

Data Collection and Methodology

Out of 111 villages of Kaviti, data on CKDu cases were collected from 28 villages through intensive door to door field survey during the period between 2007 and 2009 where ground water consumption is predominant. Table 27.1. and Fig. 27.2. shows the number of CKDu cases in 28 villages of Kaviti mandal.

Table 27.1 reveals that a total of 59 cases were identified in the mandal. Maximum cases were reported from B.G. Puttuga village (16) followed by K. Varaka with 5 cases and Bejji Putuga with 4 cases. In the remaining villages the incidence ranges between 1 and 2.

Table 27.1: CKDu cases in Kaviti Mandal (2007-2009)

Sl. No.	*Name of the Village*	*Total*
1.	Korrai Puttuga	2
2.	B.G. Puttuga	16
3.	Donka Puttuga	1
4.	Karapadu	2
5.	Dugonaputuga	2
6.	Silagam	1
7.	Kojjiria	1
8.	Borivanka	1
9.	Belagam	2
10.	Bingiputtuga	1
11.	Tungana	2
12.	Yealamanchiputtuga	1
13.	Korai Puttuga	2
14.	K. Varaka	5
15.	K. Tottidi Puttuga	2
16.	Tottidiputtuga	1
17.	Parri Puttuga	1
18.	Lolla Puttuga	1
19.	Bairagi Puttuga	1
20.	Kottaveedhi	1
21.	Muni Puttuga	2
22.	Jagati	1
23.	Landri Puttuga	1
24.	Govinda Puttuga	2
25.	Borra Puttuga	1
26.	Bejji Puttuga	4
27.	Hatti Puttuga	1
28.	Makalla Puttuga	1
	Total	**59**

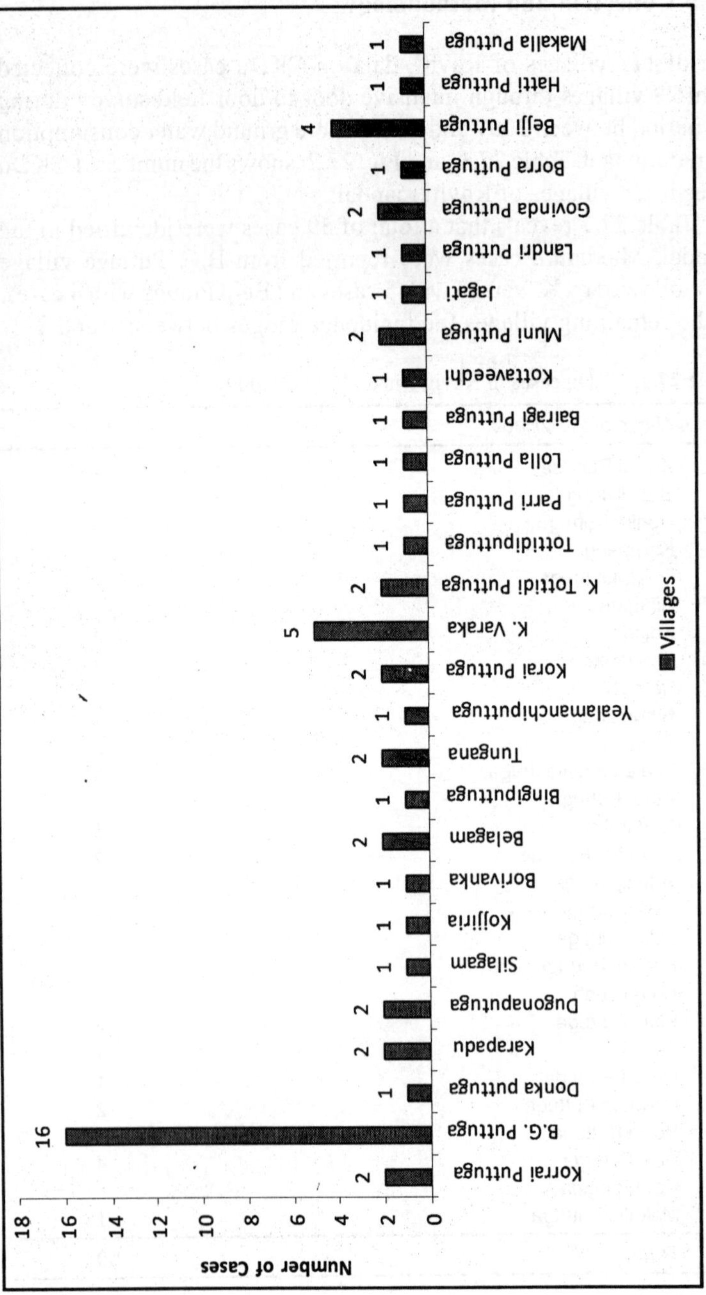

Fig. 27.2: Village-wise Incidence of CKDu in Kaviti Mandal during 2007-2009.

Fig. 27.2. illustrates the village-wise incidence of disease with maximum incidence in B.G.Puttiga followed by K.Varaka and Bejjiputtuga.

Age-wise Incidence

In general, it was observed that in several CKDu affected regions, the farmers in the middle age group who work in paddy fields and other agricultural activities are prone to the disease as they are exposed high levels of soil, water and other environmental hazards.[8] In Srilanka and some other CKDu affected regions most of the affected patients are in the age group between 30-60 years. Thus, age-wise analysis of incidence of CKDu is essential to understand which age-group is more prone to the incidence. Table 27.2 and Fig. 27.3 shows age wise incidence of CKDu in Kaviti mandal.

Table 27.2: Age-wise Incidence of CKDu in Kaviti Mandal (2007-2009)

Ago Group	*Male*	*Female*	*Total Cases*
0-10	1	0	1
11-20	2	0	2
21-30	5	4	9
31-40	**12**	**7**	**19**
41-50	**16**	**2**	**18**
51-60	5	3	8
61-70	1	1	2
71-80	0	0	0
Total	**42**	**17**	**59**

In the case of Kaviti the affected persons are in the age group between 21-50, who work in the paddy fields and other plantation crops. However, high incidence associated with 31-40 and 41-50 age groups with 19 cases and 18 cases respectively followed by nine cases in the age-group 21-30. Very low incidence was observed in the age groups of 0-20 and 51-60 and 61-70. This shows that highly vulnerability of the disease occurs in the farmers in the age between 21 and 60 years.

Gender-wise incidence

In CKDu affected agricultural regions elsewhere in the world disease

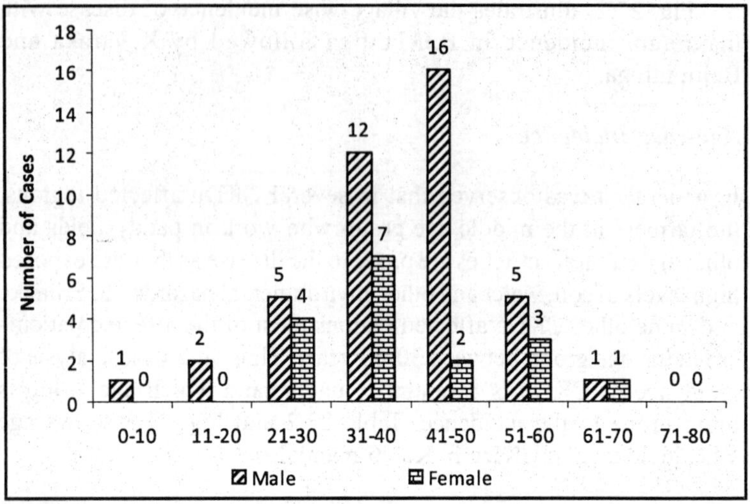

Fig. 27.3: Age-wise Incidence of CKDu in Kaviti Mandal during 2007-2009

incidence is more in males rather than in females. This is because the males are mostly farmers and exposed to agro-chemicals and other toxins used in the cropping. In addition, the farmers mostly drink chemically contaminated water in the agricultural fields itself. Another probability is due to long exposure to hot environment they need to drink more water to avoid dehydration. But the farmers due to work pressure drink less water. This type of negligence in the working environment leads to the dehydration which increases susceptibility to the disease. On the other hand, females who are engaged in the domestic activities rather than in farming with less exposure to outdoor environment and consume water from the wells are less vulnerable to CKDu disease. Fig. 27.4. and Table 27.3 provides gender-wise incidence of CKDu cases in Kaviti mandal during the study period.

Table 27.3 reveals that during 2007-2009, a total of 59 cases were reported in the mandal. Out of which 42 are men and 17 women. The analysis revealed that the incidence is mostly associated with male population rather than female. This is due to the fact that the main occupation in Kaviti mandal is agriculture and farmers are associated with the environment where soil and water are contaminated with fertilizers which ultimately effect the kidneys. Maximum of 16 CKDu cases were reported from B.G. Puttuga village. Out of which 12 are male and 4 females. K.Varaka and Bejji Puttuga

Table 27.3: Gender-wise Incidence of CKDu in Kaviti Mandal (2007-2009)

Sl. No.	*Name of the Village*	*Male*	*Female*	*Total*
1.	Korrai Puttuga	0	2	2
2.	B.G. Puttuga	12	4	16
3.	Donka Puttuga	0	1	1
4.	Karapadu	1	1	2
5.	Dugonaputuga	0	2	2
6.	Silagam	0	1	1
7.	Kojjiria	0	1	1
8.	Borivanka	0	1	1
9.	Belagam	1	1	2
10.	Bingiputtuga	0	1	1
11.	Tungana	1	1	2
12.	Yealamanchiputtuga	0	1	1
13.	Korai Puttuga	2	0	2
14.	K. Varaka	5	0	5
15.	K. Tottidi Puttuga	2	0	2
16.	Tottidiputtuga	1	0	1
17.	Parri Puttuga	1	0	1
18.	Lolla Puttuga	1	0	1
19.	Bairagi Puttuga	1	0	1
20.	Kottaveedhi	1	0	1
21.	Muni Puttuga	2	0	2
22.	Jagati	1	0	1
23.	Landri Puttuga	1	0	1
24.	Govinda Puttuga	2	0	2
25.	Borra Puttuga	1	0	1
26.	Bejji Puttuga	4	0	4
27.	Hatti Puttuga	1	0	1
28.	Makalla Puttuga	1	0	1
	Total	**42**	**17**	**59**

reported 4 cases each. The affected persons all are Male only. In many villages women are not affected by CKDu.

Groundwater Analysis

To understand the water quality of the study region, water samples were collected from the drinking water sources of seven villages spread over Kaviti mandal and analyzed to assess mineral content. Table 27.4 provides the Mineral content and nature of physical properties of ground waters in Kaviti mandal.

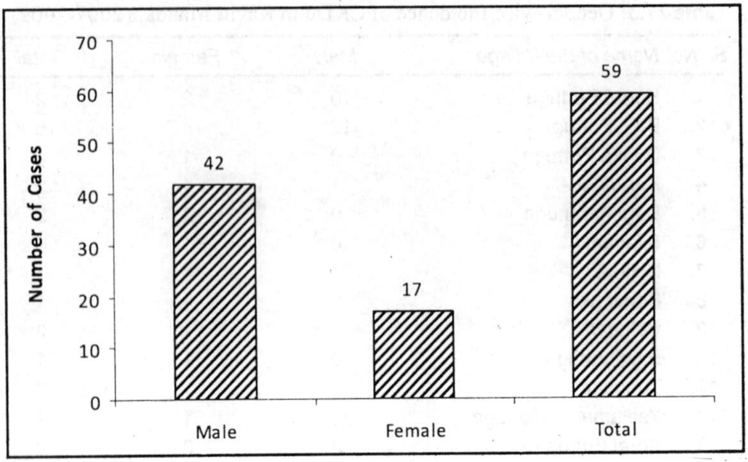

Fig. 27.4: Gender-wise Incidence of CKDu in Kaviti Mandal during 2007-2009

Table 27.4: Ground water properties in Kaviti Mandal

Minerals/Physical Properties	*Quantity in Kaviti Waters*	*Desirable Amount WHO Recommended Levels*
Calcium	40-90 mg/lt	75 mg/lt
Chlorides	70-197 mg/lt	200 mg/lt
Megnesium	21-33 mg/lt	50 mg/lt
Iron	0.01 to 0.05 mg/lt	0.1
Fluorine	0.5 and 0.8 mg/lt	0.6 mg/lt
TDS	185 to 287 mg/lt	(500 mg/lt)
pH	7.8 to 8.3 per cent	6.5 to 8.5 per cent
Arsenic	Not analyzed	0.01 mg/lt

Table 27.4 shows that all the parameters measured are at permissible levels in the groundwaters of Kaviti mandal except calcium, chlorides and fluorine are slightly on higher side in some parts of the mandal. In general, chlorides are not harmful for the human health but sodium chloride has been linked with heart and kidney diseases.

Earlier studies of CKDu incidence indicated that heavy metals are toxic and might be responsible to some extent for the incidence. For the present concentrations of heavy metals like cadmium and arsenic are not measured in the present study. However, studies indicated that cadmium and arsenic will enter into the human body through food and water. The level of concentration of heavy metals depends on the type of fertilizer used in the cultivation and type of food they take. In Kaviti mandal farmers are generally using Monochronophospate, single super phosphate Diammonium phosphate (DAP), urea, Borax, Magnesium and potash for crops, which may be responsible for concentration of heavy metals especially cadmium in the soil as well as in groundwater. In the absence of surfacewater, the entire population depend on wells and tubewells which might be contaminated by farming activities. They consume rice, plant leaves grown in the marshy area, and fish and salted fish, smoke cigars and cigarettes and drink local made alcohol, cook food in the aluminium utensils. Some studies indicated that cadmium consumption is possible through irrigated rice, fresh water fish and lotus rhizomes. Cooking food in aluminium utensils also becomes toxic when it reacts with fluorine.

Land Use—Cover Conditions *vs.* CKDu

Land use/cover conditions of Kaviti mandal extracted from LISS IV satellite image of 2013 with 2.5 m resolution by digital image processing and spatial map of Land use/cover generated in Arc GIS environment (Fig. 27.5.).

The map reveals the fact that Kaviti mandal has 16.5 km of coastline. Throughout the length of the coast, marshy area with a width of 1 to 1.5 km is running parallel. The total area of marsh is 1.81 km^2. The groundwater table is almost at the ground level in the marshy area and its adjacent parts. As a result, much of the paddy cultivation concentrated in this area. The total area of paddy cultivation in Kaviti mandal is 35 km^2. About 65 per cent of Kaviti mandal is under coconut plantations (96.7 km^2). The other dominant plantation crop in the region is cashew (3.7 km^2). In addition, the plantation crops namely Jackfruit and mango are also grown. Most of the wells and all the tubewells are concentrated in the southern part of the study area and mostly within the marshy area. These are used for both agriculture and drinking purposes. From the Fig. 27.5, it is interesting to note that there is strong correlation between high incidence of CKDu with high incidence CKDu is correlated with paddy cultivated areas and groundwater sources located in the swampy area (Fig. 27.6). Incidence of CKDu is also associated with coconut cultivated areas to some extent.

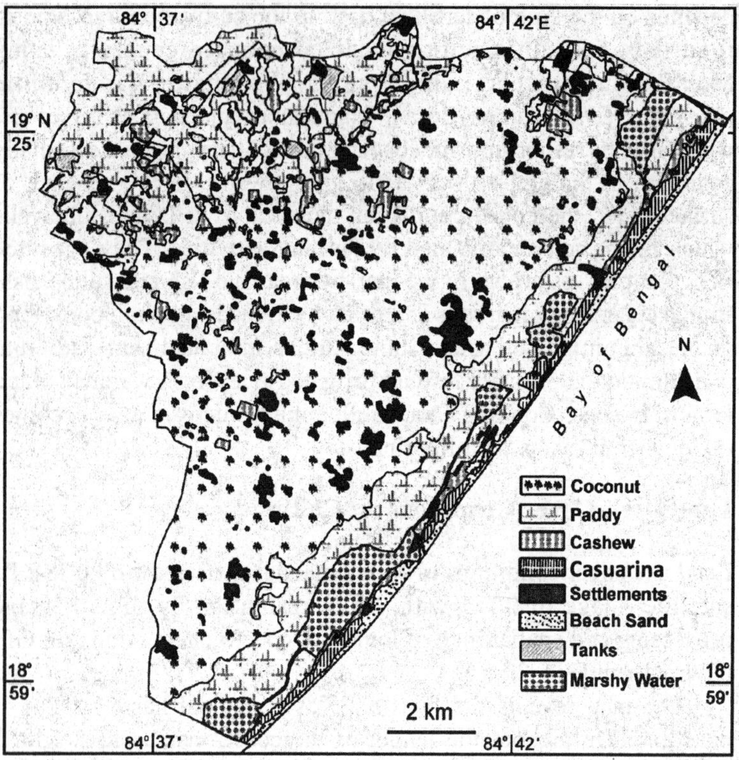

Fig. 27.5: Land Use/Land Cover Conditions of Kaviti Mandal.

From the present study, it is concluded that Land use/land cover conditions, groundwater and food habits are responsible for the incidence of CKDu in Kaviti mandal. In the absence of surface water, the entire population drink water from the wells and tubewells which are polluted with phosphate based fertilizers and other pesticides used for the cultivation of paddy as well as plantation crops. To support this fact high incidence of the disease is associated with the villages where paddy cultivation and groundwater sources are dominant. It is also fact that even the minerals measured in the study area are at permissible limits, the continuous consumption of the same may become toxic in long run. In addition, the villagers consume rice, leafy green vegetables grown in the fields, and fish and salted fish, smoke cigars and cigarettes and drink local made alcohol, cook food

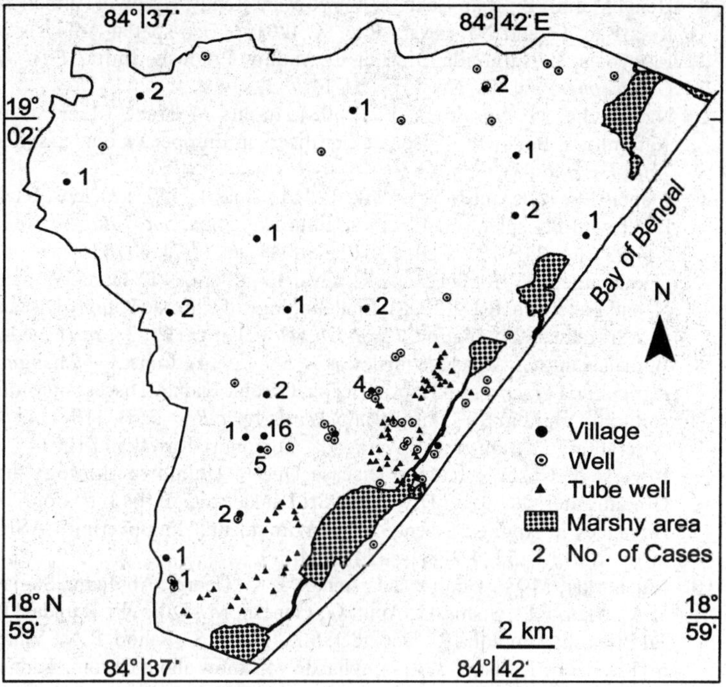

Fig. 27.6: Spatial Distribution of Wells and Tube Wells *vs*. CKDu Incidences in Kaviti Mandal.

in the aluminium utensils which contribute accumulation of disease causing minerals like cadmium and arsenic in the human body. Thus, land use/land cover conditions, groundwater and food and traditional habits of the region are suspected for the incidence of CKDu in Kaviti mandal.

Notes

1. Park, J.E., and Park, K. (1977), *Text Book of Preventive and Social Medicine (A Treatise on Community Health),* Jabalpur: Publishers Banarasidas Bhanot, pp. 170-195.
2. Handa, B.K. (1989), *Water Analysis: Aims, Objects and Interpretation,* unpublished Report, Water Research Centre, Chandigarh, India.
3. Cuello Carlos, Correa, P., Haenszel, W., Gordillo, Brown, C., Archer, M., and Tannenbaum, S. (1976), Gatric Cancer in Colombia. I. Cancer Risk and Suspect Environmental Agents, *Nat. Cancer Inst.*, 57, pp. 1015-1020.

4. Hema Malini, B., Ram Babu, I., Visweswara Reddy, B., Awol Akmel, Y., Raja Rao, G. and Nageswara Rao, K. (2010), Geo-spatial Analysis of Fluorosis in Nalgonda District of Andhra Pradesh, India, *Eastern Geographer*, Vol. 16, No. 1, pp. 11-14.
5. Nziguheba, G., Smolders, E. (2008), Inputs of Trace Elements in Agricultural Soils *via* Phosphate Fertilizers in European Countries, *Sci. Total Environ.*, 390, pp. 53-57.
6. Camelo Lopez de Guiffre L., Silvia, R.M., Liliana M. (1997), Heavy Metals Input with Phosphate Fertilizers used in Argentina, *Sci. Total Environ.*, 204-93), pp. 245-250; DOI: 10.1016/S0048-9697(97), 00187-3.
7. Gooneratne, I.K., Ranweera, A.K., Liyanara, Chchi, N.P., Guna Wardane N. and Lanerolle, R.D. (2008), Epidemiology of Chronic Kidney Disease in a Sri Lankan Population, *Int. J. Diabetes Dev. Ctries*, 28, pp. 60-64.
8. Wimalawansa, S.A., and Wimalawansa, S.J. (2014), Impact of Changing Agricultural Practices on Human Health: Chronic Kidney Disease of Multi-factorial Origin in Sri Lanka, *Wudpeker J. Agric Res.*, 3(5): 110-124.
9. Wijerathne Charuni, S.K.; Weragoda, Tomonori Kawakami (2014), A Review of Chronic Kidney Disease Due to Unknown Etiology and Groundwater Quality in Dry Zone, Sri Lanka Proc. of the Intl. Conf. on Advances in Applied Science and Environmental Engineering—ASEE 2014., doi: 10.15224/978-1-63248-004-0-9.
10. Rajapurkar, M.M., George, T.J., Ashok, L.K., Georgi, Abraham, Sanjay, K.A., Alan, F.L., Sishir, G., Amit, G., Gopesh, M., Dilip, P., Ramdas, P., Jai Prakash, Anuradha R., Devinder, S.R., Raj, K.S., Sahoo, R.N., Vinay, S., Ravi, Raji T., Jha, V. (2012), What do you know about Chronic Kidney Disease in India : First Report of Indian CKD Registry, BMC Nephrol, 13:10.
11. Zhang, J., Zhang, L., and Wang, W. (2013), Association between Aristolochic Acid and CKD : A Cross-sectional Survey in China, *Am. J. Kidney Dis.*, 61(6), pp. 918-922.
12. Voice, T.C., McElmurry, S.P., Long, D.T. (2006), Evaluation of the Hypothesis that Balkan Endemic Nephropathy is Caused by Drinking Water Exposure to Contaminants Leaching from Pliocene Coal Deposits, *J. Expo. Sci. Environ. Epidemiology*, 16 (6), pp. 515-524.
13. Stefanovic V., Cukuranovic R., Miljokovic S., Marinkovic D., and Toncheva D. (2009), Fifty Years of Balkan Endemic Nephropathy : Challenges of Study using Epidemiological Method, *Ren. Fail.*, 31(5), pp. 409-418.
14. Wanigasuriya, K.P., Peiris-Jhon, R.J.; Wickremasinghe, R. (2011), Chronic Kidney Disease of Unknown Aetiology in Sri Lanka: Is Cadmium a likely cause? *BMC Nephrol.*, 12:32; DOI, 10.1186/1471-2369-12-32.
15. Wijewickrama, E.S., Weerasinghe, D., Sumathipala, P.S., Horadagoda, C., Lanarolle, R.D., and Sheriff, R.M. (2011), Epidomology of Chronic Kidney Disease in a Sri Lankan Population: Experience of a Tertiary Care Centre, *Saudi J. Kidney Dis. Transpl.*, 22 (6), pp. 1289-93.
16. Athuraliya, N.T.C., Abeysekera, T.D.J., Amerasinghe, P.H., Kumarasiri,

R.; Bandara P.; Karunaratne, U.; Milton, A.H., and Jones, A.L. (2011), Uncertain Etiologies of Proteinuric-chronic Kidney Disease in Rural Sri Lanka, *Kidney Int.*, 80, pp. 1212-1221.

17. Redmon, J.H., Myles, F.E., Donna, S.W., Rajitha, W., Kamani, P.W., Roshini, J.P., Joseph, L., Kristin, S., James, H.R. and Keith, E.L. (2014), Additional Perspective on Chronic Kidney Disease of Unknown Aetiology (CKDu), in Sri Lanka-Lessons Learned from WHO CKDu Population Prevalance Study, *BMC Nephrology*, 15:125; DOI:10.1186/1471-2369-15-125.
18. Delgado Cortez (2009), Heat Stress Assessment among Workers in a Nicaraguan Sugarcane Farm Global Health Action, 2, 2069, DOI: 10.3402/gha.v2i0.
19. Marmot, M. (1999), *Social Determinants of Health*, Oxford University Press.
20. Rathnamalala, N.K., Nagodavithana, K.C., Mihirini, A.T.H., Lanerolle, R.D. (2011), Patients Perceptions to Risk Factors for Chronic Kidney Diseases and Methods of Delaying Progression of Disease in a Tertiary Care Setting in Sri Lanka., *Int. J. Clinical Practice*, 65(10), pp. 1108-1111.
21. Ramirez-Rubio, O., Oriana, R.R., Daniel, R.B., Juan, J.M., James, S.K., Daniel, E.W. and Madeleine K.S. (2013), Chronic Kidney Disease in Nicaragua: A Quantitative Analysis of Semi-structured Interviews with Physicians and Pharamicists, *BMC Public Health*, 13:350; DOI: 1010.1186/1471-2458-13-350.
22. Jha, V., Garcia-Garcia, G., Iseki, K., Li Z., Naicker, S., Plattner, B., Saran, R., Wang, A.Y., and Yang, C.W. (2013), Chronic Kidney Disease : Global Dimension and Perspectives, *Lancet.*, 382 (9888), pp. 260-272.
23. Shah, M.D. and Iqbal, M. (2010), Diazinon-induced Oxidative Stress and Renal Dysfunction in Rats, *Food Chem. Toxicol*, 2010, 48 (12), pp. 3345-3353.
24. *World Health Organization: Environmental Health Criteria 224: Arsenic and Arsenic Compounds*. (2001), Geneva: World Health Organization.
25. Chandrajith, R., Dissanayake, C.B., Ariyarathna, T., Herath, H.M.J.M.K., and Padmasiri, J.P. (2011), Dose-dependent Na and Ca in Fluoriderich Drinking Water—Another Major Cause of Chronic Renal Failure in Tropical Arid Regions, *Science of the Total Environment,* 409, pp. 671-675.
26. Ileperuma, O.A., Dharmagunawardhane, H.A., and Herarh, K.P.R.P. (2009), Dissolution of Aluminium from Substandard Utensils under high Fluoride Stress: A Possible Risk Factors for Chronic Renal Failures in the North-Central Province, *Journal of the National Science Foundation of Sri Lanka*, 37, pp. 219-222.
27. Jayasinghe, Y.K.R.T. (2011), *Chronic Kidney Disease—Risk Factor Identification* (Secondary Data Analysis).
28. Almaguer, M., Herrera, R., Orantes, C.M., Chronic Kidney Disease of unknown Etiology in Agricultural Communities, *MEDICC Rev.* 16(2), pp. 9-15.

29. Reddy, D.V. and Gunasekar, A. (2013), Chronic Kidney Disease in Two Coastal Districts of Andhra Pradesh, India: Role of Drinking Water. *Environ. Geochem. Health*, 35 (4), pp. 439-454.
30. Raju, T.P., Giridhar, Babu N., Srinivasu, Ch., and Lakshmana, Das, N. (2013), Trace Elemental Analysis of Rice Samples from Kidney Effected Area using EDXRF Technique, *International Journal of Science and Research*, 4, 438, pp. 1062-1066.

28

El Niño, Climate Change and Human Health Scenario

Rais Akhtar

Introduction

The term El Niño (means Christ child in Spanish) was originally used by fisher-men along the coasts of Ecuador and Peru to refer to a warm ocean current that typically appears around Christmas time and lasts for several months. Fish are less abundant during these warm intervals, so fishermen often take a break to repair their equipment and spend time with their families. Over the years, the term 'El Niño' is referred to these exceptionally strong warm intervals that not only disrupt the normal lives of the fishermen, but also bring heavy rains.

El Niño phenomenon (current) was first observed by the German explorer/geographer and naturalist Alexander von Humboldt (1769-1859). The Humboldt Current was named after him.

In a letter dated 18 September, 1839, Humboldt wrote to Charles Darwin as follows: ". . . I wished to tell you still more about this running cold water which runs alongside the Peru of which I am very concerned, believing that it will much modify the climate of the littoral. . .".

A severe El Niño in 1998 killed more than 2000 people and caused billions of dollars damage to crops and infrastructure in Australia and India. It came in the middle of the Asian crisis that severely affected the financial markets.

The 1998, El Niño severely affected the climatic conditions in India; causing heat waves which resulted in great loss of life.

Climate Change

Climate change is a significant and emerging threat to human health, and has changed the way to look into various ways of protecting vulnerable population. It represents a range of environmental hazards and will affect populations in both the developed and developing countries, and particularly the regions where the current burden of climate sensitive diseases is high.

IPCC Fourth Assessment Report provided direction and magnitude of change of selected health impacts of climate change. For instance Malaria: contraction and expansion, changes in transmission season, was assigned Very High Confidence. High Confidence was assigned to increase in malnutrition, increase in the frequency of cardio-respiratory diseases, and reduction in cold-related deaths (IPCC, 2007, p. 418).

Higher temperature, heavier rainfall and changes in climate variability would encourage insect carriers of some infectious diseases to multiply and move further in regions free of the disease. In some areas higher rainfall will wash out breeding pools, thereby decreasing mosquito populations. A 1935 malaria epidemic in Sri Lanka which killed an estimated 10,00,000 people came after two years. Thus, climate change will perturb world's various aspects of physical and biological systems which, in turn, influence human health. The human health impacts of climate change would encompass direct and indirect effects, and immediate and delayed effects. Climate change will also have both positive and negative impacts on human health.

The direct health effects of climate change would include altered rates of mortality/morbidity due to heat waves and thermal stresses in general, the respiratory consequences of a change in patterns of exposure to aeroallergens, and increases in extreme weather events, including storms, floods and droughts. The indirect health effects of climate change include: (i) alterations in the range and activity of climate-sensitive vector borne diseases (such as malaria, dengue, chikungunya, and schistosomiasis); (ii) changes in transmission of person-to-person infections (including food poisoning and water borne pathogens); (iii) the nutritional and health consequences of local and regional changes in agricultural productivity; and (iv) the various consequences of rising sea level (McMichael, 1999).

In developing countries, rising temperatures, anomaly in rainfall patterns and humidity have facilitated the spread of several vector-borne infectious diseases including malaria, dengue, chikungunya, and encephalitis. The increasing prevalence of and mortality from these diseases has had numerous negative consequences: declining economic productivity, increasing medical costs, and taxing already underdeveloped health care system in developing countries. The rising frequency of extreme weather events such as cyclones in Indian coastal region, hurricanes in southern United States and typhoons in the western Pacific Ocean, and flooding and droughts exacerbate the vulnerability of poor people.

Industrialized countries too face challenges from increasing climate changes. Nearly 40,000 deaths due to heat waves in 2003 in central and western Europe and Katrina and Sandy hurricanes disaster in southern United States in 2005 and 2013 are examples from developed countries having suffered great human loss.

Climate Change and Sandy Hurricane 2012

Despite Assessment reports and recommendations based on model projections of Intergovernmental Panel on Climate Change (IPCC), the western world has not accepted the conclusions of the IPCC. The occurrence of heat waves 2003 in Western Europe that killed more than 40,000 people in two weeks and Katrina hurricane of 2005 that devastated the southern United States including the city of New Orleans, western skeptics of climate change only now realized seriousness of IPCC recommendations. It was this support from both western world and developing countries that IPCC was jointly awarded Nobel Peace Prize in 2007. The Sandy hurricane which is devastating the eastern coastal areas of the United States is also the results of increased hurricane intensity due to global warming. Based on IPCC A1B Scenario, anthropogenic warming by the end of 21st Century will likely cause hurricanes (Cyclones in India's eastern coastal areas, and typhoons in China sea) globally to be more intense. This would imply an even larger percentage increase in the destructive potential per storm assuming no reduction in storm size. Typhoon Haiyan that divested Philippines in early November 2013 is an indication of increased intensity of Cyclones, Hurricanes and Cyclones. Having travelled myself along eastern coast from New York to Washington DC several years back, I noted the vulnerability of low-lying conditions in this region. This region, also known as BOWASH (Boston to Washington), is one of the most populous region in the world. This is now evident with impact of Sandy hurricane that has flooded this region that has resulted in displacing of more than 7,00,000 people from this area. This region is also vulnerable to sea level rise. In fact most cities situated on the coast in both developed and developing countries, including Karachi, Mumbai, Kolkata and Dhaka, are vulnerable to sea level rise. I am confident that examples of 2003 European heat wave, 2005 Katrina hurricane and 2012 Sandy hurricane will compel developed countries particularly USA, to accept Kyoto protocol and bring down level of Greenhouse gas emissions.

Vector Borne Diseases

Malaria

It is evident that climate change will alter the patterns and diffusion of diseases such as malaria in different countries. Malaria transmission can be limited by both temperature and rainfall. Rainfall is the critical factor on the desert margins, while temperatures limit the altitude at which the disease is transmitted. In the highland fringe areas, higher temperature is associated with El Niño particularly during autumn and winter months, may increase transmission of malaria in fringe areas such as in northern Pakistan. (Hales *et al.*, 2000) and in Kenya. The 1997-98 El Niño was associated with heavy rainfall and flooding in Kenya after two years of drought. From January to May 1998, a major epidemic of falciparum malaria occurred. Brown and colleagues opined the attack rate of approximately 40 per cent in the town of Wajir, Kenya. Three districts of Kenya reported a six-fold increase in malaria cases in the first two months of 1998 compared to the same period in 1997 (Brown *et al.*, 1998). According to McMichael and colleagues the malaria was compounded by widespread food shortages (McMichael *et al.*, 2003). Africa will continue to carry the greatest burden of malaria particularly the eastern and southern Africa. According to IPCC Fourth Assessment Report, malaria is a complex disease to model and all published models have limited parameterization of some of the key factors that influence the geographic range and intensity of malaria transmission. Given this limitation, models project that particularly in Africa, climate change will be associated with geographical expansion of the areas suitable for stable *Plasmodium falciparum* malaria in some regions and with contractions in other regions (IPCC, 2007). According to Githeko,

"In many regions there was widespread parasite resistance to chloroquine and in addition there was virtually no vector control. A detailed study of climate and malaria epidemics was associated with incidents of El Niño" (Githeko, 2009). Malaria epidemics have also been reported in typically semi-arid and arid areas that are subject of flooding during excessive rainfall years in Botswana and Mozambique (Thomson *et al.*, Sidley, 2000). A study based on 50 different locations in Ethiopia reveals the association between malaria epidemics with high minimum temperature in the preceding months (Abeku *et al.*, 2003).

Rainfall in western Rajasthan, India in the year 1994 following an El Niño event is approximately 40 per cent higher than in the La Nina years (i.e. opposite phase of ENSO). Researchers have also found strong correlations between malaria incidence and annual rainfall (or the number of rainy days) in desert districts of western Rajasthan (Akhtar and McMichael, 1996) (Fig. 28.1).

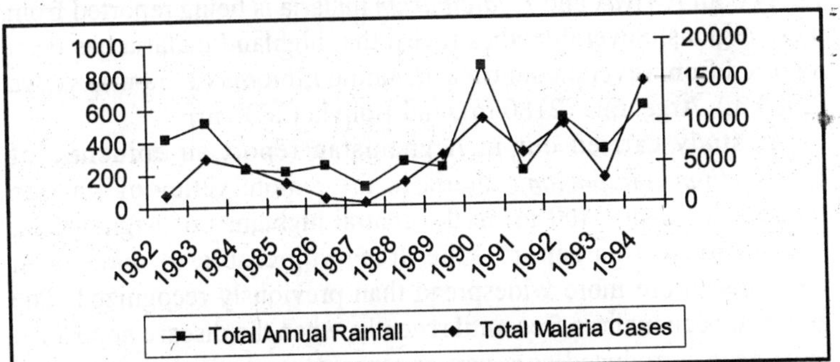

Fig. 28.1: Rainfall and Incidence of Malaria in Jodhpur.

Altitudinal Rise of Malaria

The relationship of malaria incidence to local climate change has been observed in several regions including Rwanda. In 1987, extension of malaria into higher altitudes resulted after record high temperatures and rainfall. Monthly malaria incidence in high altitude regions was exponentially affected by changes in minimum temperature. In low altitude zones, rainfall and mean temperature were the most significant climatic factors. The study concludes that areas near the current limits of malaria distribution would potentially be most vulnerable to climate changes. Based on such observations, a relatively small increase in winter (mean) temperature might facilitate the spread of malaria into large urban highland populations that are currently malaria free, such as Nairobi in Kenya, Harare in Zimbabwe, Rwanda and Irian Jaya (Garnham, 1945, Reiter, 1998, Lindsay and Martens, 1998, Loevinsohn, 1994, SAJTMPH, 1999). In Zimbabwe, study showed malaria prevalence strongly vary inversely with altitude.

It is evident from various research investigations that malaria is prevalent in higher altitude in different continents. Chloroquine resistant areas of risk lies up to 2500 m in Bolivia and Kenya, up to 2000 m. in Afghanistan, Ethiopia, up to 1800 m in Papua New Guinea and Tanzania, and up to 1500 m. in China, Equador, and Peru. It is astonishing to note that *P. falciparum,* the most dangerous plasmodium is being reported from higher altitude up to 2500 m. This is a serious situation for malaria eradication programme. It is also confirmed that mountainous and highland areas higher in altitudes than Kashmir valley both *P. vivax* and *P. falciparum* malaria is being reported from these regions. Several studies reveal that highland malaria has been reported from several countries including Ethiopia (2450 m), Kenya (2600 m), Argentina (2180 m), and Bolivia (2600 m).

A study carried out in Afghanistan report an epidemic of *Plasmodium falciparum* malaria in the remote valley of Bamian (altitude 2250 m–2400 m) in the central highlands of Afghanistan. According to this report, "the areas vulnerable to malaria in Afghanistan are more widespread than previously recognized. The area had been malaria free until recently, when the disease appears to have been introduced as a consequence of protracted conflict and resultant population movement, and transmitted locally during the short summer months. The outbreak led to severe morbidity and high mortality in a province having only a few poorly provisioned health care facilities. The epidemic was reported in valleys between 2250 m and 2400 m where the temperature was likely to be 2-3° C higher than those mean monthly temperature" (Abdur Rab *et al.,* 2003). An analysis of data from seven highlands locations in East Africa reported that short-term trends in initiating malaria epidemics (Zhou *et al.,* 2004, 2005), although the method used to test this hypothesis has been challenged (Hay *et al.,* 2005), IPCC, 2007; 404). A Report published in 2004 by the Ministry of Environment and Forests, Government of India also asserts that malaria is likely to increase attitudinally in northern and north-eastern states including Himachal

Pradesh, Arunachal Pradesh, Nagaland, Manipur and Mizoram may become malaria prone.

Dengue

Dengue is transmitted to humans by *Aedes aegypti* or more rarely the *Aedes albopictus* mosquito. According to the World Health Organization, some 2.5 billion people, two-fifth of the world's population, are now at risk from dengue and estimates that there may be 50 million cases of dengue infection worldwide every year.

In the last two decades the dengue has become a serious urban health problem mainly in developing countries. Monath has rightly stated that the root of the emergence of dengue as a major health problem are changes in human demography and behaviour, leading to unchecked populations of and increased exposure to the principal domestic mosquito vector, *Aedes aegypti.* Virus-specified factors also influence the epidemiology of dengue (Monath, 1998).

A study carried out in Vietnam concluded that the number of dengue cases increased during El Niño years (Lien, 1998). Within the South Pacific region, which currently on the fringe of the epidemic zone of dengue, outbreaks of dengue fever in island nations during 1970-75 have been moderately correlated with ENSO events (Hales *et al.,* 1996). Hales and colleagues also highlighted that the major sources of variability in normal world weather patterns is the El Niño Southern Oscillation (ENSO) process, based in the central Pacific Ocean and driven by inter-annual variations in the east-west atmospheric pressure gradients. According to authors, there is a periodic reversal of the east-west flow of warm surface waters and moist air across the Pacific cause droughts at low to mid altitudes around the world, including eastern Australia, Indonesia, India and Pakistan. ENSO variation accounts for up to 40 per cent of the variation in temperature and rainfall in the Pacific (Hales *et al.*, 1996).

Cholera

Several studies carried out in South American countries as well as in Asian regions reveal the association between El Niño and cholera outbreaks. A study conducted in Bangladesh showed that the temporal variability of cholera exhibits an inter-annual component at the dominant frequency of El Niño (Pascual, *et al.,* 2000). Above average temperatures in Peru during El Niño event of 1997-98 were associated with a significant increase in the number of children admitted to hospital with diarrhoea (Checkley *et al.,* 2000).

Several major outbreaks of cholera which occurred in 1997 in several countries of Africa, including Chad, Kenya and Tanzania highlighted the significance of cholera and ENSO (Kovats, 2000). Endemic character of cholera in certain regions, such as the estuaries of the Ganges and Brahamputra rivers in Bangladesh (Colwell, 1996). Another study found the relationship between cholera occurrence in Bangladesh and the increased sea surface temperature during El Niño events (Lobitz *et al.,* 2000).

Extreme Weather Events (Heat waves)

During heat waves excess mortality is greatest both in developed and countries. In 1995 heat wave mortality in Chicago and 2003 heat wave mortality in European countries are significant examples of impact of heat waves on the vulnerable population in developed countries (Kovats and Ebi, 2006).

In 1998, major parts of India extending from north India, parts of north-east India, and the northern parts of peninsular India experienced severe heat wave during the second half of May 1998. Heat wave was one of the most severe heat waves for 50 years has resulted in the deaths of more than 2600 people. In Orissa one of the poorest states the temperature rose to a scorching 49.5° C that killed nearly 1300 people. Bihar, West Bengal, Andhra Pradesh, Uttar Pradesh, Maharashtra and Punjab states have also suffered with temperature soaring to 45°-49° C (Kumar, 1998). Even south interior Karnataka and parts of Tamil Nadu were under the grip of severe heat wave conditions during this period. Chennai recorded the second highest maximum temperature 44° C of the present century on May 24, which was 8° C above normal. The highest ever recorded maximum temperature 45° C had occurred in Chennai on May 21, 1910. Mortality due to heatwave increased again in 2013, but declined slightly in 2014.

However, in May 2015, India was struck by a severe heatwave. As of 3 June 2015, it has caused the deaths of more than 2,500 people in different regions in India. The South Indian states of Andhra Pradesh and the neighbouring Telangana, where more than 1,735 and 585 people died respectively, were the areas most affected by the heat

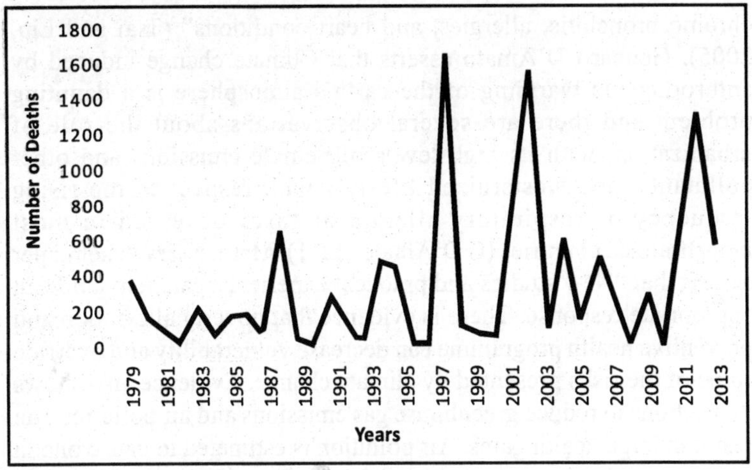

Fig. 28.2: Heatwave Mortality in India, 1979-2014.
Based on data from IMD Annual Reports on Disastrous Events, Pune.

wave. Other casualties were from the eastern states of West Bengal and Odisha (*The Telegraph*, 2015).

A comparative scenario of heat wave mortality between European and Indian heat waves in 2003 reveals that in India too 2003 mortality figure was second highest in the country after 1998 (Akhtar, 2010), but according to mortality data of 2015, number of people who died due to heatwave increased again to nearly 2500 (*The Telegraph*, 2015).

The above review between climate change and health highlights the significance of changing environmental scenario. There is an urgent need to incorporate climate change as an important factor in public health planning policies in both developed and developing countries with focus on strengthening adaptive capacity of people and equity in the development of health infrastructure and other socio-economic development.

Air Pollution

Several studies suggests that allergic respiratory diseases such as rhinitis and bronchial asthma have become more common worldwide over the past three decades. "Epidemiological studies conducted in industrialized countries have shown that Climate-mediated air pollution has had a substantial impact among people with asthma, chronic bronchitis, allergies, and heart conditions" (Tsai and Liu, 2005). Gennaro D'Amato asserts that Climate change induced by anthropogenic warming of the earth's atmosphere is a daunting problem and there are several observations about the role of urbanization, with its high levels of vehicle emissions and other pollutants, and westernized lifestyle with respect to the rising frequency of respiratory allergic diseases observed in most industrialized countries (G.D'Amato, 2011). Maria Neira in her paper asserts that "New studies and practical experience can help guide an appropriate response. There is evidence that poverty alleviation and preventive health programme can decrease vulnerability and override some of the risks presented by climate change. Evidence also shows that actions to reduce greenhouse gas emissions and air pollution can result in large health gains. Air pollution is estimated to cause one in every eight deaths, so reduction of emissions of black carbon and other short-lived pollutants may not only slow warming but also avert almost 2.5 million deaths annually. The deaths and disease thus prevented could offset much of the cost of greenhouse-gas mitigation. In developing more socially beneficial, cost-effective and widely supported policies for the mitigation of climate change, the arguments, evidence and voices of the health community are critical (Neira, 2014).

WHO Conference on Health and Climate

The World Health Organization hosted an international conference on Health and Climate in Geneva during August 27-29, 2014 and brought together experts and Minister of Health of various countries from all-over the world, to discuss the impact of climate change on human health scenario in both developed and developing countries. Since 2008, the WHO has shown leadership in raising awareness of the threats posed by climate change to health. Specifically, WHO has provided evidence, technical guidance and piloted approaches to protect health from climate risks. There is now an urgent need to advance a more concrete and systematic approach to implementing health protection, led by the health community, in coordination with others. The Conference objectives were to empower the health and sustainable development communities to:

1. Enhance resilience and protect health from climate change.
2. Identify the health benefits associated with reducing

greenhouse gas emissions and other climate pollutants and to support health-promoting climate change policies.

The thematic area covered increasing health system resilience to climate-sensitive health risks such as extreme weather events, climate-sensitive communicable diseases, and threats to food, water and food security. It included a focus on targeting protection towards the most vulnerable populations and stages of the life course, identification of effective interventions, and to work towards developing consensus on an operational framework defining the main health system functions to increase health system resilience to climate variability and change. The other thematic area covered opportunities to improve health while also controlling climate pollutants. It has focused on key sectors, such as health, energy, and transport, and includes specific consideration of the extent to which the health sector can lead by example in providing better services while reducing its own environmental impact and the potential for economic savings through reduction in the large burden of non-communicable disease associated with air pollution. It also covered opportunitics to further advance collaborative mechanisms, such as the Climate and Clean Air Coalition.

Conclusion

As evident climate change represents a serious environmental hazards and an association between rise in temperature, precipitation and humidity with the rise and spread of human diseases. The health effects of climate change are often indirect and difficult to assess, and the evidence of quality of the health-related outcomes varies widely. Depending on the geographical and socio-economic characteristics and the level of human development index of the region. The increasing incidences of air pollution, water pollution, land and soil pollution, solid and hazardous waste pollution, deforestation, soil erosion, silting and flooding are illustrations of environmental quality deterioration.

Adaptation to climate change is receiving much greater attention given the inevitability of climate change and its effects, particularly in developing contexts, where the effects of climate change will be experienced most strongly and the response mechanisms are weakest However, the examples of excessive precipitation followed by flooding by landslides destroyed Uttarakhand region last year in India, Colorado region in the USA, and flooding in England in February, 2014, landslides in the USA and forest fire in Australia show that both developed and developing countries are vulnerable in the event of extreme weather scenario 2003 heat wave mortality in west and central Europe is a classic example that killed nearly 40,000 people in a fortnight in August, 2003 (Akhtar, 2014).

Finally, in the context of health, emphasis should be on prediction and prevention of diseases, and a strong infrastructure of public health and access to safe drinking water supply and sanitation.

Efforts should also be made to reduce health care inequalities in the country and the states. To sum up the measures related to poverty alleviation are a prerequisite and can go long way in minimizing impact of climate change on human health.

References

Abdur, Rab, M., Freeman, T.W., Rahim, S., Durrani, N., Simon-Taha, A. and Rowland, M. (2003), High Altitude Epidemic Malaria in Bamian Province, Central Afghanistan, *Eastern Mediterranean Health Journal*, 9(3), 232-39.

Abeku, T.G. (2003), Spatial and Temporal Variations in Malaria Epidemic Risk in Ethiopia: Factors Involved and Implications, *Acta Trop.*, Vol. 87, pp. 331-340.

Akhtar, R. (2010), El Niño Related Health Hazards in India, *Current Science*, Vol. 98, No. 2, pp. 144-147.

Akhtar, R. (2014), Hope West is not Heading Towards Climate Colonialism, *The Hindustan Times,* April, 15, New Delhi.

Akhtar, R. and McMichael, A.J. (1996), Rainfall and Malaria Outbreaks in Western Rajasthan, *The Lancet,* 348, 1457-1458.

Brown, V., *et al.* (1998), Epidemic of Malaria in North-eastern Kenya, *Lancet*, Vol. 352, pp. 1356-57.

Checkley, W., *et al.* (2000), Effects of El Niño and Ambient Temperature on Hospital Admissions for Diarrhoeal Diseases in Peruvian Children, *Lancet*, Vol. 355, pp. 442-450.

Colwell, R.R. (1996), Global Climate and Infectious Disease: The Cholera Paradigm, *Science,* Vol. 274, pp. 2025-2031.

D'Amato, G. (2011), Effects of Climate Change and Urban Air Pollution on the Rising Trends of Respiratory Allergy and Asthma, *Multidisciplinary Respiratory*, Vol. 6, pp. 28-37.

El Niño and associated outbreaks of severe malaria in highland populations in Irian Jaya, Indonesia : A review and epidemiological perspective, *Southeast Asian Journal of Tropical Medicine and Public Health*, 1999, 30(4), 608-9.

Equador : www.ecuadorexplorer.com/html/malaria_and_yellow_fever.html.

Freeman, T.W. (1999), Community-based Malaria Control in Zimbabwe, *Bull. World Health Org.*, 77(3), 295-6.

Freeman, T.W.: *Personnel Communication,* 2004.

Garnham, P.C.C., (1945), Malaria Epidemics at Exceptionally High Altitudes in Kenya, *British Medical Journal*, Vol.11, 45-47.

Hales, S., Weinstein, P. and Woodward, A. (1996), Dengue Fever Epidemics in the South Pacific driven by El Niño Southern Oscillation?, *Lancet*, Vol. 348, pp.1664-65.

Hales, S., Kovats, S. and Woodward, A. (2000), What El Niño can tell us about Human Health and Global Climate Change, *Global Change and Human Health,* Vol.1, No.1, pp. 66-77.

Hay, S.I., *et al.* (2005), Climate Variability and Malaria Epidemics in the Highlands of East Africa, *Trends Parasitol.*, Vol. 21, pp. 52-53.

IPCC: *Climate Change: Impacts, Adaptation and Vulnerability*, Chapter 8 : Human Health, Cambridge: Cambridge University Press, 2007, pp. 391-431.

Kovats, R.S. (2000), El Niño and Human Health, *Bulletin of the WHO,* Vol. 78, No. 9, pp. 1127-1136.

Kovats, R.S. and Ebi, K.L. (2006), Heatwaves and Public Health in Europe, *Eur. Jour. Public Health*, Vol. 16, pp. 592-599.

Kumar, J.S. (1998), India's Heat Wave and Rains Result in Massive Death Toll, *The Lanect*, Vol. 351, p. 1869.

Lien, T.V. (1998), Variation of Dengue Fever in Vietnam and its Relationship to ENSO event, *Proceeding of the 7th Scientific Conference of IMH*, 2, 50-58, (in Vietnamese).

Lindbalde, K.A., *et al.* (1999), Highland Malaria in Uganda : Prospective Analysis of an Epidemic Associated with El Niño, *Transactions of the Royal Society of Tropical Medicine and Hygiene*, 93, 480-87.

Lindbalde, K.A. (2000), Landuse Change Alters Malaria Transmission Parameters by Modifying Temperatures in a Highland Area of Uganda, *Tropical Medicine and International Health*, 5, 263-74.

Lindsey, S.W. and Martens, W.J.M. (2000), Malaria in the African Highlands: Past, Present and Future, *Bulletin of the World Health Organization*, 76, 33-45.

Lobitz, B., *et al.* (2000), Climate and Infectious Disease: Use of Remote Sensing for Detection of *Vibrio Cholerae* by Indirect Measurement, *Proceedings of the National Academy of Sciences*, Vol. 97, pp. 1438-1443.

Loevinson, M.E. (1994), Climate Warming and Increased Malaria Incidence in Rwanda, *Lancet*, Vol. 343, 714-8.

McMichael, A.J. (1999), Global Climate Change and Human Health: An Overview, *Bulletin The Royal Society*, 27-33.

McMichael, A.J., *et al.* (2003), *Climate Change and Human Health: Risk and Responses,* WHO, Geneva, p. 83.

Neira, M. (2014), The 2014 WHO Conference on Health and Climate, *Bull World Health Organ,* pp. 92:546.

Pascual, M., *et al.* (2000), Cholera Dynamics and El Niño Southern Oscillation, *Science*, Vol. 289, pp. 1766-1767.

Reiter, P. (1998), Global Warming and Vector-borne Disease in Temperate Regions and at High Altitude, *Lancet*, Vol. 351, 839-40.

The Telegraph (2015), India Heatwave: Death Toll Passes 2,500 as Victim Families Fight for Compensation, *The Telegraph* (U.K.) 2nd June.

Thomson, M.C.; Doblas-Reyes, F.J., Mason, *et al.* (2006), Malaria Early Warnings based on Seasonal Climate Forecasts from Multi-model Ensembles, *Nature*, Vol. 439, pp. 576-79.

Sidley, P. (2000), Malaria Epidemic Expected in Mozambique, *British Medical Journal*, Vol. 320, p. 669.

Zhou, G., *et al.* (2004), Association between Climate Variability and Malaria Epidemics in East African Highlands, *Proceedings National Academy of Sciences*, Vol. 101, p. 2375.

Zhou, G., *et al.* (2005), Climate Variability and Malaria Epidemics in the Highlands of East Africa, *Trends Parasitol*, Vol. 21, pp. 54-56.

29

Urban Health in India

Cities in Transition—Health in Transition

Carsten Butsch

Aspects of Urban Health

From a health researcher's perspective cities are fascinating and contradictory sites of investigation. Urban environments influence human health in multiple ways—positively and negatively. Different groups of urban dwellers have different capacities for making use of the health benefits cities offer. Likewise, the exposure towards the negative health effects differs significantly within the urban population. Therefore, one will find—especially in low- and middle income countries (LMIC)—large health disparities in urban areas. The cities in LMIC host at the same time the most and the least healthy populations of their countries. Human health in cities of LMIC is affected by the environmental and societal conditions in these loci of change. LMIC all-over the world are currently experiencing unprecedented urban growth, resulting not only in physical transition of urban environments but also substantial societal transition.[1] This chapter tries to shed some light on the urban transitions currently taking place in India and the way in which these transitions affect human health.

Urban health received increasing interest as an interdisciplinary research topic in the last 15 years. Especially David Vlahov and Sandro Galea have—together with changing co-authors—set the agenda of this emerging field of scientific investigation [2,3,4,5,6,7,8] and since 2002, the International Society for Urban Health has developed as forum for interdisciplinary exchange. Though the academic investigation of the effects of urbanisation on human health is not newly-discovered. Cities have always been centres of (health) knowledge and of health threats. Because of their interconnectedness and population concentration cities have been the places of pestilence since ancient times. The descriptions of plague in Greek cities by ancient writers like Homer or Sophocles and historians like Thucydides are among the first proofs of the specific health threats in urban areas.[9] Yet, since ancient times health was also one of the main reasons to plan cities, especially the support of fresh water and the management of waste and wastewater. However, systematic investigation of health in urban areas started in the time of industrialization in Europe. The first urban health researchers were concerned with the unhygienic living conditions in Europe's fast growing cities in the 19th and early 20th century. Frederick Engels described the conditions he found in English cities during his journey in 1844: "The great towns are chiefly inhabited by working-people [...] these workers have no property whatsoever of their own, and live wholly upon wages, which usually go from hand to mouth. Society, composed wholly of atoms, does not trouble itself about them; leaves them to care for themselves and their families, yet supplies them no means of doing this in an efficient and permanent manner. Every working-man, even the best, is therefore constantly exposed to loss of work and food, that is to death by starvation, and many perish in this way. The dwellings of the workers are everywhere badly planned, badly built, and kept in the worst condition, badly ventilated, damp, and unwholesome."[10] Historic data shows, that the poor health conditions in urban areas resulted in a decreased life expectancy in cities compared to rural areas. Vögele for example shows, that the child mortality during industrialization was in Berlin higher than in the rural areas surrounding the city.[11] Ex-post the higher morbidity and mortality of urban populations was called urban graveyard effect or urban penalty.[12]

The Cholera epidemics in large European cities like London (1832, 1848, 1849, 1853, 1866) or Hamburg (smaller ones in 1822, 1831, 1832, 1848, 1859, 1866 and 1873; a large one in 1892) together with the advancement in medical science resulted in the establishment of a sanitary movement, which propagated public health through improved hygienic conditions, especially in cities. The measures, developed based on the recommendations from the sanitary movement (street cleaning, treatment of wastewater, supply of uncontaminated freshwater etc.) significantly contributed to the increasing life expectancy in European and US cities at the beginning of the 20th century.[13] Urban health increased substantially in high income countries, while in LMIC a focus was laid on the improvement of rural health in the course of the 20th century, mainly, because rural populations were severely underserved in terms of health services. This channeling of resources of the health care sector into rural areas resulted in negligence of urban health sectors in many LMIC, making the emergence of a new urban penalty likely.[14, 15] A severe challenge in this respect is the so called double burden of diseases.[16] Urban populations in LMIC are in the midst of an epidemiological transition. Therefore, the burden of diseases from infectious diseases is still high, while at the same time the share DALYs from non-communicable diseases is rising quickly.

The relation of the urban setting and human health are quite complex and the determinants of urban health are manifold. Fig. 29.1 assorts various factors, which influence urban health in cities of the Global South. Here urban health is understood as the product of three spheres of influence: the physical urban environment, societal factors and urban health systems. In contrast to other frameworks for understanding urban health,[17] the framework suggested does not interpret human health in cities as the product of various influences but stresses the feedback of human health on urban development. To illustrate this idea: health affects the economic performance of individuals[18,19], therefore less healthy populations can contribute less to urban economies and therefore to development on the local level; in the absence of insurances and functioning public health care provision, ill-health results in disruption of individual/household development paths (directly through the cost of treatment, indirectly through the loss of income), therefore health disparities also contribute to perpetuating social disparities. Additionally, the nexus urban health, urban environments, urban society and urban health systems is influenced by external factors. These cannot be altered but have (unidirectional) influence on health in urban areas. Climate change for example will affect the occurrence of communicable diseases, increase heat stress etc.[20] Urban health, seen in this complex interconnectedness, is therefore not only the product of development, but also a factor shaping development—especially in societies, which are in the midst of an urban transition.

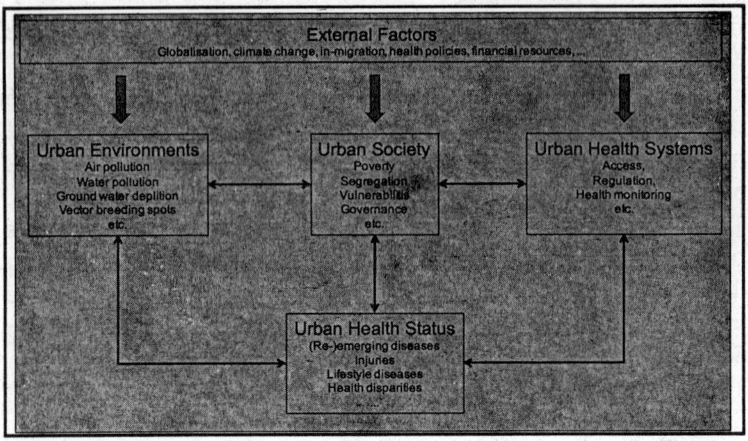

Fig. 29.1: A Descriptive Urban Health Framework (adopted from Butsch/Sakdapolrak/Saravanan 2012).

Urban Health in India

In this section of the chapter, an overview of the different aspects shaping urban health in India will be given. In the next section, Pune will serve as a concrete example to describe urban health on the basis of empirical case studies. First, the urbanisation trends in India will be described briefly. Then, the three influencing spheres of urban health, the physical environment, societal challenges and urban health systems will be described.

Urbanisation in India

India can look back on several millennia of urban history[21], yet India is still a predominantly rural country. According to the UN World Urbanisation Prospects currently 32.4 per cent of the Indian population lives in cities.[22] Nevertheless, since independence India's cities have witnessed enormous growth: the total urban population rose from 64 million in 1950 to 420 million in 2015 and the country's largest cities Delhi, Mumbai, Kolkata and Bangalore have become megacities with more than 10 million inhabitants, all four being also among the world's most populated cities (top 30 in 2015).[23] But not only the large urban agglomerations have been growing, there are five cities which have already crossed the threshold of five million inhabitants (Surat, Pune,

Ahmedabad, Hyderabad and Chennai) and which can be addressed as emerging megacities. Additionally, there are 49 cities larger than one million inhabitants, but smaller than five million inhabitants. These cities have experienced enormous population growth since independence and large parts of this growth has taken place in an unplanned manner. Before analysing in detail the negative effects of this growth for urban health, the predictions for India's urban future will be highlighted. While the world became predominantly urban in 2007, India will become a predominantly urban country in the year 2050. Moreover, India's rural population is predicted to peak in the year 2030 and will then decline in absolute numbers. The urban population will almost double in the next 35 years and is predicted to reach 814 million people by 2050.[24]

That means that human health in India is increasingly influenced by urban environments and health systems. The far reaching transition that has already occurred is influencing health in multiple ways. Furthermore, the way India's cities will grow and how they are planned and managed will become an even more important determinant of human health in India. In the past, urbanisation in India was especially characterized by a high degree of informality. Informality, as Ananya Roy describes it, cannot simply be equalled with a lack of ability to plan, but it means that authorities and decision makers tolerate certain developments, which are not planned.[25] However, several aspects, which characterize urban development in India today are related to informality. The degradation of urban physical environments for example have occurred in spite of the existing environmental legislation; social disparities are manifested also in spatial segregation with large parts of the population (and not only "the poor") being forced to live in unhealthy living conditions (slums, *bustees*, JJ colonies etc.); urban health systems consist of a public health care sector, which does not provide services according to its self-prescribed standards, and a completely unregulated private health care sector.

Changing Physical Environments

Informal urban growth in India has resulted in drastic transformations of landscapes affecting the physical environments of India's cities and their surroundings. From a health perspective, this has two implications: from a pathogenetic perspective there is a direct effect on the health of the urban dwellers who are exposed adverse health effects like air pollution and noise pollution or suffer from vector borne and water borne diseases or the heat island effect. From a salutogenic perspective, the ability of urban environments to provide ecosystem services, which are promoting health, are disrupted. Urban green and urban blue, having several positive effects on health, like reducing mental stress, stimulating physical activity or simply reducing air pollution (in the case of urban green spaces) etc.[26, 27, 28] are vanishing. At the same time public places in India's cities are too often not open spaces for community building and social interaction but congested places with little amenity values.

One important factor that severely challenges the health of urban dwellers is the high amount of air pollution. This has two sides: one is the ambient air pollution related to traffic and polluting industries, the other is indoor air pollution, affecting mainly lower socio-economic strata who rely on solid fuels for cooking. For the whole of India (no urban/rural differentiation), it is estimated that in 2010 about one million premature deaths and 31.4 million disability-adjusted life years can be attributed to indoor air pollution and about 627,000 premature deaths and 17.8 million disability-adjusted life years can be attributed to ambient air pollution.[29] Ambient air pollution is caused by several sources: Transport, power plants, industries, domestic pollutants, Diesel generators, road dust and burning of waste.[30] The Central Pollution Control Board (CPCB) monitors the air quality in 224 cities under the National Air Quality Programme. The CPCB report for the year 2012 shows, that NO_2 emissions were labelled "high" (exceeding the prescribed national standard up to 50%) all over the year in 42 out of 370 stations, which provided data (i.e. 11.4%); in 10 stations (i.e. 2.7%), the pollution level was labelled critical for NO_2 (exceeding the national standard more than 50%).[31] The situation is even worse for Suspended Particulate Matter (PM10). In 84 out of 372 stations, the measurements showed "high" values (i.e. 22.6% of the stations exceeding the national standard by 50%) and 223 showed "critical" values (i.e. 59.9% of the stations exceeding the national standard by more than 50%).

Several authors have tried to calculate the effects of air pollution in India's cities. In Mumbai for example it is estimated, that annually 84,000 cases of chronic obstructive pulmonary diseases can be attributed to raised levels of PM10 and 138,000 cases to altered levels of NO_2.[32] For the affected households this means that they have to spend (on average) 13.3 per cent of their annual income on the cost of treatment, if treatment takes place in an outpatient facility and 50.7 per cent of their annual income in case of inpatient treatment.[33] In Delhi it is estimated, that between 7,350 and 16,200 premature deaths can be attributed to the high levels of air pollution and that 31,400 hospital admissions and 483,200 emergency room visits took place in 2010 due to air pollution.[34] For urban India in total WHO estimates, that 1,277 Disability Adjusted Life Years are lost because of non-communicable respiratory diseases.[35]

Another issue of concern is water pollution, resulting in a comparatively high burden from waterborne diseases. According to the CPCB only 51 per cent of the sewage generated is adequately treated in cities with more than one million inhabitants; however the performance varies strongly between different municipalities, reaching from 100 per cent in Hyderabad to 6 per cent in Bhopal.[36] This lack of treatment capacity is just one symptom of the deficits in financial and managerial capacities of municipal corporations.[37] For the whole of India (urban and rural), it is estimated, that the negative consequences of lack of sanitation produce overall cost equal to 6.4 per cent of the GDP (in 2006).[38] Out of these 70 per cent are health related costs. According to WHO, 1,246 DALYs are lost in India annually per 1,00,000 inhabitants due to diarrhoeal diseases.[39] In urban areas it is estimated, that only 37 per cent of the population have access to proper sanitation facilities. This results in a comparatively high figure from preventable diseases. Gosh and Bose, working with data from the National Family Health Survey for example point out that among children aged 0-59 months 7.2 per cent were suffering from acute diarrheal diseases in slum areas, while the figure in non-slum areas was with 6.6 per cent not much lower.[40]

Negative effects on the health of urban dwellers are also related to the insufficient waste management in urban areas. It is estimated that per inhabitant between 300 to 500 g of solid waste are generated daily, which is partly collected from the municipal corporations, but to a large extent from private (informal) waste pickers. Health issues are related to the lack of compliance with prescribed standards in the waste collection and treatment, resulting in several adverse effects for human health like vermin in residential areas at the collection sites and groundwater contamination at the disposal sites.[41] Further issues of concern are the environmental (and potential human health) effects of the quick increase of e-waste, and the improper treatment of medical waste.

One last aspect to be discussed in the sphere of environmental influences on human health is the relatively high burden from vector borne diseases in urban areas. Malaria is transmitted in India mainly by Aedes stephani mosquitos, which prefer rainwater fed breeding spots, while Aedes aegypti, which is the main vector of Dengue fever, prefers potable water as breeding spots.[42] On a micro scale Malaria vector breeding spots form mainly where outdoor rain water can log for several days, e.g. on barren plots where waste is dumped and/or the soil is compressed.[43] Dengue vectors find breeding spots in irrigated parks or even in plant pots.[44] Generally, the transmission cycle works better and the parasites' prevalence are much higher in crowded areas of the city as humans are needed as a host. On the city scale other factors are connected to the prevalence of the two vector species: urban expansion results in the sealing off of land: and on constructions sites, which are not connected to the sewerage system, rain water logs, offering breeding spots for Aedes stephani.[45] Aedes aegypti breeds in water tanks, which are necessary to store water where constant water supply does not take place, as it is the case in many newly developed areas in fast growing urban India. On a regional scale disease outbreaks can to a certain extent also be explained by the inmigration from rural areas, where both diseases are prevalent.[46] As an external influencing factor, the changes in precipitation patterns and rising temperatures as a result of global climate change will lead to improved conditions for mosquito breeding.[47]

Changing Social Environments

Urbanisation means a profound change of the way in which people are living together, interact with each other and care for each other. The closely knit networks of rural communities, which are structuring village life are vanishing in the course of urbanisation and are replaced by other kinds of networks, which in many cases allow for higher social mobility—although "rurbanisation" in many LMIC results in reproduction of social formations usually expected to occur in villages, at least temporarily. Generally, the urbanisation of a society is related on the one hand to more personal freedom, which is influencing the health of some in a very positive way, while lack of security in personal networks and feelings of alienation can pose psychological stress on others. This holds also true for the general increase in the speed of life and the growing uncertainties related to living in cities.[48]

Apart from that urbanisation is associated also with changes in the occupational structure. Closely connected to this is the reduction of the level of physical activity for many urban dwellers compared to their rural counterparts. In India, low physical activity is observed among 56 per cent of all urban dwellers compared to 35 per cent in rural populations.[49] This is related to several negative health effects like obesity, cardiovascular diseases and diabetes—an increasing problem in urban India.[50] It is estimated that 65.1 Million people (age group 20-79 years) suffer from diabetes; the number is expected to rise to 109 Million in 2035.[51]

Negative adverse health effects are also related to changing dietary patterns. These can be partly explained by lifestyle changes during urbanisation; especially in the early stages of socio-economic development the connection of reduced physical activity and consumption of energy dense food results in so-called lifestyle associated diseases.[52] A study from Ebrahim *et al.* shows, that these behavioural changes are clearly associated with living in urban areas. They compared prevalence rates for obesity and diabetes between urban-rural migrants and rural non-migrants in India, finding significant higher rates in the migrant population. Furthermore, their study showed, that the fat intake increased after migration while at the same time physical activity was reduced.[53]

An interesting finding from another study in this respect is that the consumption of alcohol and tobacco is less in urban areas compared to rural areas. Especially tobacco consumption is significantly less in urban areas with 10.9 per cent of the population reporting to smoke daily compared to 23.7 per cent in rural areas. Heavy drinking (defined as more than five standard drinks on at least two days in the past week) was reported by 1.2 per cent of the urban and 1.4 per cent of the rural population.[54]

As mentioned in the introduction, urbanisation is related to increasing socio-economic disparities, which are reflected in health disparities with the poorer suffering from a higher burden of disease. Yet inferior health status is also a means of perpetuating poverty, which is addressed as "medical poverty trap."[55] This is caused by the fact that ill health is not only related to direct cost but also to long-term financial burden on households. Generally, poverty can be related to three major influencing factors on human health: First, the poor generally have less access to basic services such as sufficient food (quantity and quality) and health care services; Second, poverty is often related to living in unfavourable housing conditions ("slums"); Third, poverty is often related to poor educational status influencing also health literacy and health seeking behaviour.[56]

Between the different states in India, the share of population below poverty line varies significantly on state level between 44 per cent to 3 per cent.[57] Yet, while the share of urban population below poverty line dropped from 25.7 per cent in 2004/05 to 20.9 per cent in 2009/10,[58] the socio-economic fragmentation increased. The Gini coefficient, as measure for the equality/inequality of income distribution in a population rose from 0.27 to in 1972/73 to 0.38 in 2008/09, in urban India.[59] The literacy rate as an important indicator of deprivation, was in slums according to the 2011 census 77.7 per cent compared to 84.5 per cent in urban areas in general.[60]

Unfortunately disaggregated data is hardly available for assessing the health status of different socio-economic groups in urban India, since most sources only distinguish between urban and rural populations. An important exemption in this regard is the data provided by the National Family Health Survey. Drawing on this data, Agarwal shows, that across India there are significant differences in the health status of urban populations with the fault lines following socio-economic status. Under five mortality rate for example was in 2005-06 with 72 in the poorest quartile much higher than in the most wealthy quartile of the urban population with 42 (for the whole of India). Also children immunization rates, which can be interpreted as an indictor for health literacy, differ significantly with 40 per cent of the children being fully immunized in the poorest quartile compared to 65 per cent in the wealthiest quartile.

Changing Health Care Systems

Changing physical and social environments can—in a preliminary conclusion—summarized to be mainly related to an increased exposure towards adverse health effects. Yet, there is also an "urban advantage" when it comes to health.[61] One of the main components of this advantage is the availability of ample health care facilities in urban areas. Yet, there are large intraurban differences in the access to health care facilities. These have to be seen against the background

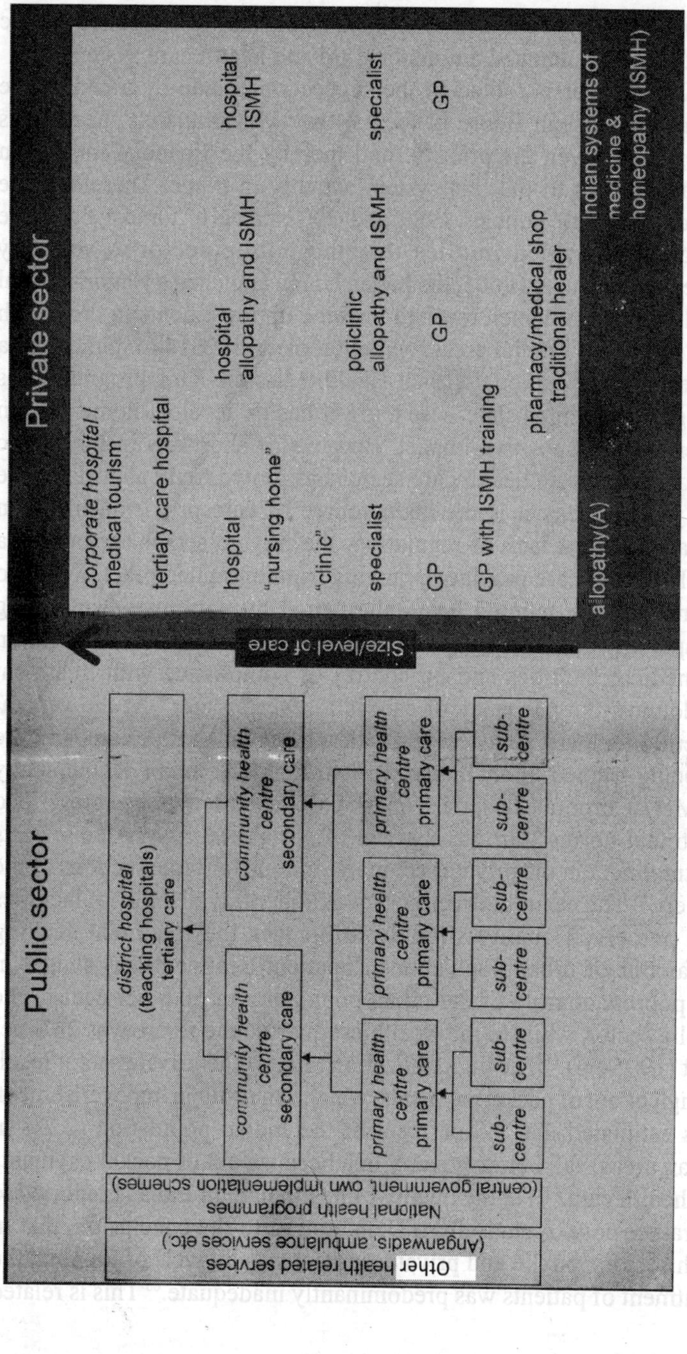

Fig. 29.2: The Fragmented Health Care System of India's Cities (adopted from Butsch, 2011).

of the dual structure of a theoretically brilliantly organized public health care system and an untamed private health care system.

The former is rooted in the suggestions made by a committee chaired by Joseph Bhore in the 1940s.[62] Unfortunately, health has never been given the priority (and thereby the financial means) in Indian politics to put this system actually in place. Therefore, the National Health Policies 1983 and 2002 came to almost the same conclusion, which implies that the public sector is severely underperforming. In 2005, the Indian Union launched a National Rural Health Mission, which resulted in some improvements in the health care provision in rural areas, while it took until 2014 to implement a corresponding National Urban Health Mission. This programme is being implemented state-wise and yet has to develop momentum in order to show positive impact. Because of shortfalls in the public sector, the private health care sector has grown tremendously in the last years. Today it is the main source of care provision in urban India. Due to a lack of regulation, the private sector appears as a patchwork of care providers, ranging from untrained practitioners to internationally reputed hospitals owned by nationwide operating companies (Fig. 29.2). As there are no guidelines for the registration of medical facilities and no control of compliance with treatment guidelines, the adequacy of care is a severe issue.[63] At the general practitioner level, many care providers offer "allopathic care" in spite of being trained in an Indian System of Medicine or Homeopathy (ISMH). Corporate hospitals, on the contrary, often exceed prescribed treatment norms.[64] In the absence of social security systems, costs for treatment in the private sector are ruinous for large sections of the society.[65] The nexus between cost of treatment, availability of facilities and perceived quality strongly influences the treatment seeking behaviour of urban populations: Inpatient treatment was sought in the poorest quartile of the urban population in 60.8 per cent in the public sector, while in the wealthiest quartile the figure was 28.3 per cent (1995-96).[66] The high utilization rates of the private sector result in high of out of pocket payments, which can result in impoverishment. It is estimated that 3.5 per cent of the Indian population (2.7% in urban areas) fall below poverty line because out of pocket payments for health care.[67] Yet the quality of health care in India is reported to be rather poor. A study from Delhi comes to the conclusion, that in both sectors, public and private, and across all levels of training, the treatment of patients was predominantly inadequate.[68] This is related to a lack of standards and enforcement of existing regulations. Therefore, also in the health care sector informality can be seen as an important factor influencing human health.

Pune: A Case Study

In the third section of the chapter the aspects discussed in section two on a more general level will be exemplified referring to the concrete case study of Pune. After a short introduction of the city, urban health in Pune will be addressed from two perspectives. First, the epidemiological transition, which is related to the changing physical and social environment will be described. After that, aspects related to access to health care services will be discussed.

Pune was India's eighth largest agglomeration in the year 2011 with 3.1 million persons living in the city itself and 5.5 million persons living in the urban agglomeration.[69] Pune is in many ways connected to the city of Mumbai. The highway, which connects the two cities is an emerging urbanisation corridor, being itself embedded in a larger industrialization and urbanisation belt, which stretches from Ahmedabad *via* Mumbai to Pune.[70] This belt is also promoted as an important region for the national economic development. Therefore, infrastructure development is supported and location of (knowledge) industries in this area is facilitated. Pune has grown ten-fold since independence and developed a relatively diverse economic basis. It is one of the hubs of the automobile industry in India, an important location for the pharmaceutical industry, the chemical industry and the food processing industry. Increasingly also ITC and BPO companies are settling in Pune. The economic growth attracted a diverse population and urban expansion was also driven by informal processes. As the provision of adequate shelter was insufficient, from the 1930s onwards, slum settlements started to emerge. First slum settlements were erected on the banks of *nullahs* in the city centre in the 1930s. Then in the 1940s, huts were built for day labourers close to the railway station and larger slums emerged after 1960 south of the old city centre.[71] According to the 2001 census, 19.4 per cent of Pune's population lived in slums,[72] while the Municipal Corporation estimates that more than 40 per cent of the city's population lives in slums.[73] The growth of slum population in the past has been significantly higher than the growth of the rest of the population and it is projected by the PMC to reach 44.4 per cent in 2021, 47 per cent in 2031 and almost 50 per cent in 2041.[74]

The negative aspects of urbanisation in India in general can also be found in Pune. According to the municipal corporation, Pune is currently witnessing environmental degradation due to land-use changes, rising traffic, improper management of household and industrial waste and untreated sewage water.[75] Also social fragmentation is increasingly shaping urban structures with the middle and upper middle class increasingly segregating themselves in gated communities with access controlled housing estates and private provision of 24/7 water and electricity supply. Therefore, the exposure to certain adverse environmental threats for human health (ambient air quality, waste, waste water etc.) varies for different population groups in Pune. So, does the ability to cope with ill health as the health care system reflects the general trends on the national level. The relative capacity of the public sector shrunk in the last decades, i.e. the population/doctor ratio increased while in the private health care sector especially since the economic reforms of the 1990s capacities were massively increased, according to the rules of the market. As this growth is hardly regulated, a very heterogeneous health system emerged over the past decades. This results in differences in the access to heath care services and in the burden of disease for groups with different socio-economic status.

These two aspects, the epidemiological transition and the access to health care, were the topics of interest of a project, which aimed at understanding intraurban differences in human health in Pune by applying on the one hand a disease ecological and on the other hand a health system perspective.[76, 77] The field work for the two strands of the project consisted of household surveys, in-depth interviews with medical personnel in different types of medical facilities, reflecting the whole spectrum of the public and the private health sector, in-depth interviews with lay people (chosen from the household sample) and mapping of health care facilities and aspects of the physical environment, affecting health. Additionally, secondary data was analysed. Fieldwork took place in several phases between 2007 and 2010. The household survey, the interviews with lay people and with practitioners in smaller clinics took mainly place in six research areas. These were three pairs of neighbourhoods (always one slum settlement and one settlement with *pucca* structures) which reflect Pune's main phases of urban development: in the pre-British settlement, in the former British cantonment and in one area which was developed from the 1990s onwards. The six research areas are:

(1) City Centre Slum Area, (2) City Centre Lower Middle Class Area, (3) Colonial Part Upper Middle Class Area, (4) Colonial Part Slum Areas, (5) Recently Developed Middle Class, and (6) Recently Developed Slum Areas. In each of the areas, 150 household interviews were conducted in two waves (75 in 2008-09 and 75 in 2010), either in English or Marathi.

Epidemiological Transition and Diversification

Available secondary data provides evidence that Pune is currently witnessing a substantial epidemiological transition. As Kroll *et al.* show (Table 29.1), the causes of death in the city of Pune have changed significantly between 1991 and 2006.[78] Most obvious is the increase of non-communicable diseases' share in the causes of death. Especially the rise of the share of causes of death classified in chapter IX of the International Classification of Diseases, tenth revision (ICD 10) is in line with the concepts used to describe the epidemiological transition of societies in the development process.[79, 80] These predict an increasing life expectancy and a change in the burden of disease from predominantly communicable diseases to chronic, non-communicable and lifestyle associated diseases.

Table 29.1: Major Causes of Death for Pune according to the Chapters of ICD-10 1991 and 2006, adopted from Kroll *et al.*, 2014

ICD-10 Codes	*1991*	*2006*
I. Certain Infections and Parasitic Diseases	12.3%	12.6%
II. Neoplasms	3.0%	7.0%
III. Diseases of the Blood and Blood Forming Organs and certain Disorders	2.2%	1.1%
IV. Endocrime, Nutritional and Metabolic Diseases	1.8%	4.1%
VI. Diseases of the Nervous System	1.7%	2.8%
IX. Diseases of the Circulatory System	20.8%	25.8%
X. Diseases of the Respiratory System	6.6%	9.9%
XI. Diseases of the Digestive System	2.2%	4.3%
XIV. Diseases of the Genitourinary System	—	3.0%
XVI. Certain Conditions Originating in the Perinatal Period	6.7%	2.4%
XVIII. Symptoms, Signs and Abnormal Clinical and Laboratory Findings,	27.9%	13.8%
XIX. Injury, Poisining and certain other Consequences of External Causes	14.7%	11.9%

Also diseases listed in chapter IV of ICD 10, consisting mainly of non-communicable diseases (and lifestyle associated diseases like diabetes), showed an increase between 1991 and 2006, supporting the assumption that Pune's population is advancing in the epidemiological transition. An important shift took place regarding the cause of death in chapter X, which in total gained importance. Within this chapter pneumonia (as a communicable disease) decreased from 87 per cent of the deaths within this chapter to 79 per cent, while chronic respiratory diseases increased from 13 per cent to 21.3 per cent.[81] This points to the fact, that the exposure to airborne pollutants has increased over the time. Also within Chapter 1, still being the second largest group, changes can be observed: While in 1991 gastrointestinal diseases were the most important single cause in this chapter (66% of all cases), with tuberculosis ranking second (29%) and rabies third (2%), in 2006 the picture is a completely different one—tuberculosis ranks first (40%), septicemia second (30%) and HIV/AIDS third (19%). Even if the data has to be read with caution and the shifts have to be interpreted cautiously, since the figure of non-classified deaths is rather high in both years and the investigation of deaths might not in all cases be sufficient, the trends are actually convincing. They indicate, that lifestyle changes (less physical activity, changes in dietary patterns), described in section two of this paper seem to also affect the epidemiological profile of Pune's population. Also the changes in the urban environment show effect, which is reflected in the increasing number of deaths from chronic respiratory diseases.

However, it can be assumed, that not all strata of society are affected in the same way from this epidemiological transition, since the living conditions differ significantly for different strata of the society. Table 29.2 shows the self reported mobility in the six research areas for eight different conditions. What is surprising at first glance, is that the burden of disease seems to be lower in slum areas. It can be assumed, that this is at least partly related to the fact that especially chronic diseases are hardly diagnosed in persons from lower socio-economic strata at an early stage. An extreme case are the three slum pockets in the colonial part. In this area mainly persons living in temporary structures next to construction sites, particularly construction workers, were interviewed. Since they have to be able to work physically (and are sent back, when they are not able to do so) it is not surprising, that the morbidity within this group is relatively low.

Table 29.2: Self-reported Age-standardized Prevalence Rates for Selected Diseases in Six Areas in Pune, Adopted from Kroll *et al.*, 2014.

	City Centre Slums	*City Centre Lower Middle Class*	*Colonial Part Upper Middle Class*	*Colonial Part Slum Areas*	*Recently Deve-loped Slums*	*Recently Deve-loped Middle Class*
Diabetes (>20 Years (%)	4,4 (n=407)	5,4 (n=498)	7,3 (n=463)	1,8 (n=319)	4,4 (n=494)	7,8 (n=432)
Hypertension (>20 Years) (%)	6,9 (n=407)	7,4 (n=498)	8 (n=463)	3 (n=319)	5,2 (n=494)	8,9 (n=432)
Asthma (%)	0,4 (n=707)	0,6 (n=660)	0,9 (n=577)	0 (n=538)	1,3 (n=799)	1,4 (n=576)
COPD (%)	0 (n=707)	0 (n=660)	0,1 (n=577)	0 (n=538)	0,5 (n=799)	0,5 (n=576)
Malaria (%)	0 (n=707)	0,3 (n=660)	0,1 (n=577)	3,7 (n=538)	0,2 (n=799)	0,8 (n=576)
Dengue (%)	0 (n=707)	0,2 (n=660)	0,2 (n=577)	0 (n=538)	0 (n=799)	0,3 (n=576)
Tuberculosis (15-59 Years(%)	0,2 (n=364)	0,2 (n=396)	0 (n=354)	0 (n=307)	0,3 (n=453)	0,2 (n=354)
Gastrointestinal Diseases (%)	0,7 (n=707)	1,1 (n=550)	1,8 (n=577)	0 (n=538)	0,7 (n=799)	0,6 (n=576)

The self-reported prevalence of diabetes and hypertension is higher in the middle class areas. This corresponds to the risk factors, which were also collected during the survey. In the two research areas "Colonial Part Upper Middle Class" and "Recently Developed Middle Class", the most affluent areas, the share of persons labelled "overweight" according to their Body Mass Index was 24 per cent, while it was only 4.5 per cent in the adjacent slum areas. However, from interviews with practitioners Kroll, *et al.* conclude that there is a severe underreporting of these two conditions, specifically in lower socio-economic strata. Additionally, both conditions are rising steeply in volume, particularly among the less affluent strata of society. Especially in lower socio-economic strata risk factors like stress, smoking, alcohol consumption and unhealthy diet, which increase the risk for diabetes and hypertension are much higher. Noteworthy in this context is that poor people, due to delayed diagnosis, delayed treatment and low adherence of treatment protocols suffer more from comorbidities like renal diseases, non-healing wounds etc.

Pulmonary diseases like asthma and Chronic Obstructive Pulmonary Diseases (COPD), were reported to a lesser extent than expected. The National Family Health Survey 2005-06 showed that the prevalence for asthma was 1.5 per cent for women and 1.9 per cent for men in urban Maharashtra.[82] Compared to that the self reported morbidity in the sample was relatively low, which can at least partly be explained by differences in the methodologies applied. However, what is obvious, is that pulmonary diseases are more prevalent in the newly developed areas of the city.

Regarding vector-borne diseases, there seem to be connections to the direct environments in which the respondents live. For Malaria the highest incidence rate was observed in the construction worker slums in the colonial part of the city. This can be explained with the proximity to the flood plains of the Mula-Mutha River, and the land use in this area, which allows for frequent waterlogging. The second highest rate of Malaria cases is observed in the middle class in the recently developed area. This could be related to construction activities in this area, as Kroll, *et al.*, point out. In general, it can be concluded, that for vector-borne diseases, there is no clear socio-economic gradient, which would explain the occurrence.

Also for tuberculosis the data of the self-reported morbidity does not show a clear pattern, which would indicate a connection with the socio-economic status. However, it can be assumed, that there is a severe underreporting not only because of lack of knowledge but also because of the taboo related to the disease. The relatively low figures neither match with the increase in the statistics of the causes of death nor with the data from the National Family Health Survey 2005-06, which reported a prevalence of 0.69 per cent in slum areas and 0.46 per cent in non-slum areas.[83]

Interestingly, for gastrointestinal diseases there seems to be an overall slightly higher morbidity in the middle class areas, if the self-reported morbidity figures are true. This can on the one hand surely be explained by the different awareness towards health problems: persons from higher socio-economic strata can more easily afford to visit a medical practitioner or be on sick leave, which also influences the self-reported morbidity. However, together with the overall trend of decreasing deaths from gastrointestinal diseases, this can also be read as an indicator for improvements in water supply and sanitation, especially in the registered slums.

Access to Health Care

The scenario in the local health care sector is quite similar to the general situation in the rest of urban India. According to an expert interview, Pune district hospital had 1,400 beds in 1947, more than sixty years later when the field work was conducted this number remained unchanged. In the same time, the municipal corporation has set-up only few secondary facilities while Pune's population has grown more than twentyfold. In this situation, the private health care sector has increased its capacities tremendously. Some of the old and reputed hospitals have increased the number of beds, joined larger corporations like Apollo and started to advertise for medical tourists, especially from the USA. On the primary care level many general practitioners have set-up clinics. These are trained in different systems of medicine and there is no registration of these small clinics not to mention control of treatment practices. On the demand side, the population hardly has any insurance cover, which would protect them from the cost, occurring especially for inpatient treatment in the private health care sector.

To analyse the access to health care in this situation, a new concept of access to health care was developed, based on the framework developed by Penchansky and Thomas.[84] The main points of the concept are as follows: (1) Access to health care is the ability to utilize adequate preventive, curative and custodial medical care. (2) In the field actual access can be measured, which is the transformation of access options into realized access. Barriers and facilitators shape this process in the six dimensions: affordability, acceptability, availability, accessibility, accommodation and awareness. Actual access happens when barriers in all six dimensions are smaller than facilitators. Each user has an individual profile of enabling factors and characteristics to overcome barriers associated with the utilisation of certain care providers. (3) Actual access is not in all cases adequate and utilisation of inadequate care can also prevent or delay utilisation of adequate care. Access is adequate if the preventive, curative and custodial care meets defined treatment standards.

Based on these considerations, access to health care services was analysed in Pune in the six research areas mentioned above. First of all it can be noted, that the diversity on the supply side is also reflected in the treatment seeking behaviour of the different groups. Regarding the preferred treatment facility of the households (Fig. 29.3), three

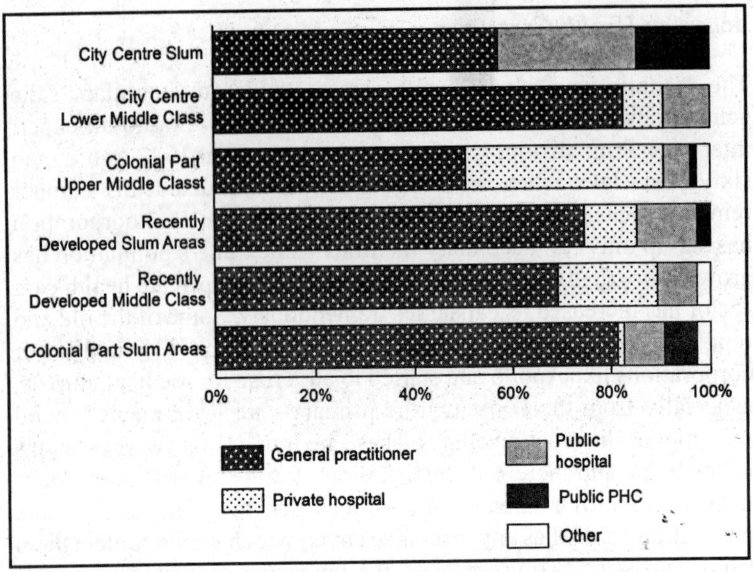

Fig. 29.3: Most Important Treatment Facility in the Six Research Areas.

Source: Own Survey, n = 6 × 75 (450)

observations are particularly noteworthy: General practitioners with private practices are the main source of care in all of the six neighbourhoods; public facilities are only of relevance in the inner city slum. Primary Health Centres (PHCs), which should in theory be the main source of care, are hardly utilized as preference is given to public hospitals; especially in the middle class area in the former cantonment, but also in the other middle class areas, private hospitals (outpatient departments) are important care providers. The private sector is the dominant source of care while the public sector is relevant for the socio-economic deprived in the city centre.

Regarding the six dimensions of access to health care, the analysis showed that the influence of the different dimensions differs strongly: In the dimension accessibility, few factors were observed that hinder access in Pune, if at all, only at the periphery. Especially on the primary care level, the mapping of the health care facilities showed that for every household practitioners are available within walking distance. Lay persons and experts though described the availability of specialists and emergency care in the newly developed and suburban areas as a concern.

The availability of services in terms of volume is currently hardly a barrier, though some experts question whether there is enough service to provide adequate service for the whole population. This is related to the fact, that many practitioners provide inadequate care. This inadequacy has several dimensions: on the one hand, there are practitioners trained in Indian Systems of Medicine, but practice allopathy and especially provide unethical treatment like "bottles" (the inappropriate application of intravenous injection of saline solution, resulting in a short term subjective improvement of the health status). On the other hand, there is severe overtreatment especially in the private tertiary care, particularly in the diagnostics.

Organisational barriers (the dimension "accommodation") are mainly observed in the public sector. Here the restrictive opening hours and the limited capacities hinder patients from utilizing the services, while the qualification of the staff is not questioned. In the service-oriented private sector there are in opposite to this several facilitators. Practitioners for example offer opening hours late in the evenings and also respond to house calls. This makes utilization of services much easier.

Influences related to acceptability work are subliminal. Negative discrimination by providers on the basis of caste or religion does not hinder access, as experts and lay persons said. What was mentioned though is positive discrimination as an influence on the treatment seeking behaviour in the middle class. Several lay people and experts said, that generally practitioners are preferred who are from the same community. However, experts also said and I personally observed that illiterate, poor patients are sometimes not treated in a respectful way.

The essential barriers for access to healthcare were observed in the dimensions affordability and awareness. While financial barriers are relatively low for primary care, they are limiting factors for secondary and tertiary care. A main reason for this is the relatively low insurance cover. Ironically this insurance cover is highest among the more affluent groups. In the poorest quintile of the survey only 1.2 per cent of the respondents had at least some health insurance cover, in the second poorest quintile, the coverage was 5.7 per cent, in the middle quintile 20.7 per cent, in the second wealthiest 48.3 per cent and in the wealthiest 67 per cent. Overall only 30.1 per cent of all respondents said that at least some members of the household do have an insurance cover. The in-depth interviews though revealed, that this insurance cover does not mean that respondents feel fully protected. Nevertheless, it is especially the poor, for whom the cost of treatment can be ruinous, particularly when inpatient treatment is needed. This is reflected in Fig. 29.4, which shows the share of households, which were in the past forced to sell assets to cover medical expenses. The figure shows a clear gradient between the slum areas and the non-slum areas. Some lay people in in-depth interviews said that they had to sell gold, which they used as a kind of reserve for emergencies. In one case a respondent said, that she had to sell the steel vessels, she used to fetch water to cover for the hepatitis treatment of her son. Others reported, that treatment in private facilities could not be completed, because they ran out of money. In a situation, in which the private health care sector is perceived as delivering better care, this puts a lot of financial pressure on households and at the same time financial burdens hinder many from accessing the facilities they would like to utilize. A second set of barriers, which is to a certain extent related to this is related to a lack of orientation in the complex local health system resulting in suboptimal treatment seeking behaviour while lack of health knowledge results in delayed utilisation of care. These factors are in many cases linked to the educational background and therefore to the socio-economic status. Inefficient allocation of the public sector's scarce resources and supply deficits are a result of a lack of information about the population at risk.

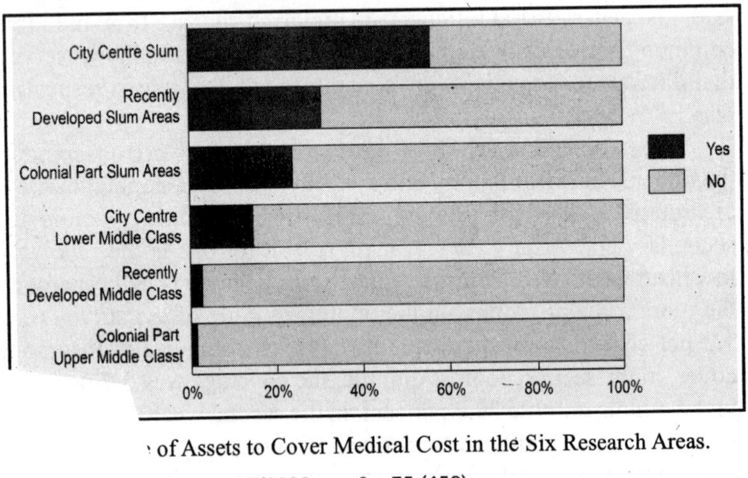

of Assets to Cover Medical Cost in the Six Research Areas.

ırvey, 2008/2009; n = 6 × 75 (450).

The analysis of in-depth interviews with lay persons and medical professionals further shows that inadequate care is a severe problem, but the collected data does not allow for quantification. Actual access in Pune is in many cases inadequate due to a lack of regulation and supervision. A problem is also that the inadequacy of service provision is not always obvious: while the unnecessary injection of saline solution and the overprescription of antibiotics has been widely discussed, overtreatment in high-priced facilities is a neglected phenomenon affecting rich and poor.

Cities in Transition—Challenges for Urban Health

It was illustrated that India is currently witnessing a substantial transformation in which the society is becoming predominantly urban. This urban transformation changes the society and it is also changing the cities itself—and with that the conditions under which in future a majority of India's population will be living. Large parts of the urban space, which is currently produced though is created in an informal way. These spaces lack a coherent layout, which also affects human health in multiple ways, even if these influences might not be directly visible. But the large townships and housing societies, which are produced by the builders in the periurban areas of India, are behind the shiny facades not really healthy living environments. Often they are not properly connected to municipal services: lack of water means that water has to be stored in tanks, which provide ideal breeding grounds for mosquitos; barren land waiting to become developed, hidden behind metal sheets, provides further breeding spots for mosquitos; missing electricity connection is compensated by generators, influencing the ambient air quality, lack of road connection and lack of connection to public transport means more traffic and through that further increase in air pollution. Further, the social fragmentation does not allow the development of living communities, which is also an important factor for mental health.

Yet, even if the recent developments are not too encouraging, there are several positive aspects. First of all India is in the midst of urbanisation.Therefore, this process can still be directed into a different direction, if health and sustainability are made a priority by those in charge of urban development. Another task in this respect is the *in situ* upgrading of slum settlements, making them less unhealthy environments. Besides these factors, related to the exposure towards health threats, the set-up of effective urban health systems is equally important. The advantage of urban India is, that there is a large number of medical professionals. There are two major challenges for improving India's urban health systems. One is related to the adequacy of treatment: Through control mechanisms (treatment protocols) and training it has to be ensured that health care providers deliver adequate care. For this it is also important to include (and upgrade the skills of) practitioners trained in Indian Systems of Medicine but practicing allopathy in order to provide care for the lower socioeconomic strata. Secondly, the population has to be enabled to utilize the available facilities without fearing impoverishment. To reach this sound financing mechanisms have to be developed. The RSBY scheme, which is currently being implemented points to the right direction, but with the limitations given it does not enable the users to choose freely between providers and for more severe episodes funding is insufficient. Additionally, this scheme only covers inpatient treatment. But evidence presented here indicates, that for all strata of the society in future the treatment of chronic diseases will be a severe financial burden. This has to be considered when alternative financing mechanisms are developed for future generations.

The urban transformation and the transformation of cities in India have brought many negative health effects so far, which made some authors speculate about a new urban penalty. Though this is not necessarily the only direction in which urban India can develop. Urbanisation unleashes a large potential and allows for using the capital and creativity for a better future. Whether India's cities will be unhealthy places, fled by those who can, or healthy landscapes promoting well-being for all at all ages (as strived for in the Sustainable Development Goal no. 3) is decided in the next decades. However, a look back in the history of urban health teaches us, that also ex-post implementation of measures is possible – though at higher cost.

Acknowledgements

This chapter is based on the long-standing collaboration and discussions with my academic teachers and the colleagues with whom I have been working in the field and with whom I have jointly published in the past. I would like to mention especially Prof. (Dr.) Frauke Kraas, Dr. Mareike Kroll, Prof. (Dr.) Erach Bharucha, Prof. (Dr.) Surinder Aggarwal, Dr. Patrick Sakdapolrak and Dr. Revati Phalkey. In this chapter I relied heavily on papers I have written earlier with the aforementioned[85, 86, 87, 88], literature.

Notes

1. Sánchez-Rodríguez R., Seto, K., Simon, D., Solecki, W., Kraas, F. and Laumann, G. (2005), *Science Plan: Urbanization and Global Environmental Change* (Bonn: IHDP).
2. Vlahov, D. and S. Galea (2002), "Urbanization, Urbanicity, and Health", *Journal of Urban Health,* 79, Supplement 1: S1-S12.
3. Vlahov, D., Gibble, E., Freudenberg, N. and S. Galea (2004), "Cities and Health: History, Approaches, and Key Questions", *Academic Medicine* 79, 12: 1133-1138.
4. Galea, S. and D. Vlahov (2005a), "Urban Health: Evidence, Challenges and Directions", *Annual Review Public Health,* 26 (2005): 341-65.
5. Galea, S., Freudenberg, N. and D. Vlahov (2005), "Cities and Population Health", *Social Science and Medicine,* 60, 5, 1017-1033.
6. Freudenberg, N., Galea, S. and D. Vlahov (2005), Beyond Urban Penalty and Urban Sprawl: Back to Living Conditions as the Focus of Urban Health", *Journal of Community Health,* 30, 1, 1-11.
7. Vlahov, D., Galea, S., Gibble, E. and N. Freudenberg (2005), "Perspectives on Urban Conditions and Population Health", *Cad. SaúdePública, Rio de Janeiro,* 21, 3, 949-957.
8. Galea, S. and D. Vlahov (eds.) (2005), *Handbook of Urban Health, Populations, Methods, and Practice*, New York.
9. Dirckx, J. H. (2000), "Pestilence Narratives in Classical Literature: A Study in Creative Imitation: I. Homer, Sophocles, Thucydides, and Lucretius", *The American Journal of Dermatopathology*, 22, 2, 197-202.
10. Engels, F. (2015), *The Condition of the Working-Class in England in 1844. with a Preface written in 1892*, Accessed October 28, http://www.gutenberg.org/files/17306/17306-h/17306-h.htm
11. Vögele, J. (1994), "Urban Infant Mortality in Imperial Germany", *Social History of Medicine,* 7, 3, 401-425.
12. Vögele, J. (1998), *Urban Mortality Change in England and Germany 1870-1913*, Liverpool.
13. Vlahov *et al.*, 2004.
14. Gould, W.T.S. (1998), "African mortality and the new 'urban penalty'", *Health and Place,* 4, 2, 171-181.
15. Krafft, T., Wolff, T. and S. Aggarwal (2003), "A New Urban Penalty? Environmental and Health Risks in Delhi", *Petermanns Geographische Mitteilungen*, 147, 4, 20-27.
16. Harpham, T. (2009), "Urban health in developing countries: What do we know and where do we go?" *Health and Place*, 15, 1, 107-116.
17. Galea, S., Freudenberg, N. and D. Vlahov (2005).
18. Alsan, M., D. Bloom, C. Canning and D. Jamison (2008), "The consequences of population health for economic performance", in *Health, economic development and household poverty: From understanding to action*, Ed. S. Bennett, L. Gilson and A. Mills. London: Routledge, 21-39.

19. WHO, *WHO Guide to Identifying the Economic Consequences of Disease and Injury,* Geneva 2009.
20. Bush, K. F., Luber, G., Rani Kotha, S., Dhaliwal, R. S., Kapil, V., Pascual, M., Brown, D., Frumkin, H., Dhiman, R.C., Hess, J., Wilson, M.L., Balakrishnan, K., Eisenberg, J., Kaur, T., Rood, R., Batterman, S., Joseph, A., Gronlund, C.J., Agrawal, A. and Hu, H. (2011), "Impacts of Climate Change on Public Health in India: Future Research Directions", *Environmental Health Perspectives*, 119(6), 765-770.
21. Ramachandran, R. (1989), *Urbanization and Urban Systems in India,* New Delhi.
22. United Nations (2014), *World Urbanization Prospects, The 2014 Revision*, New York. Accessed August 15, 2015, http://esa.un.org/unpd/wup/CD-ROM/WUP2014_XLS_CD_FILES/WUP2014-F19-Urban_Population_Annual.xls
23. United Nations, 2014.
24. *Ibid.*
25. Roy, A. (2009), Why India cannot Plan its Cities: Informality, Insurgence and the Idiom of Urbanization, *Planning Theory*, 8(1), 76-87.
26. Völker, S. and Kistemann, T. (2011), "The Impact of Blue Space on Human Health and Well-being–Salutogenetic Health Effects of Inland Surface Waters: A Review", *International Journal of Hygiene and Environmental Health*, 214(6), 449-460.
27. Lee, A.C.K. and Maheswaran, R. (2011), "The Health Benefits of Urban Green Spaces: A Review of the Evidence", *Journal of Public Health*, 33(2), 212-222.
28. Jennings, V., Johnson Gaither, C., and Gragg, R.S. (2012), "Promoting Environmental Justice through Urban Green Space Access: A Synopsis", *Environmental Justice*, 5(1), 1-7.
29. Balakrishnan, K., Cohen, A., and Smith, K.R. (2014), "Addressing the Burden of Disease Attributable to Air Pollution in India: The Need to Integrate Across Household and Ambient Air Pollution Exposures", *Environmental Health Perspectives*, 122(1), A6.
30. Guttikunda, S.K. and Goel, R. (2013), "Health Impacts of Particulate Pollution in a Megacity—Delhi, India", *Environmental Development*, 6, 8-20.
31. Central Pollution Control Board, Ministry of Environment and Forest, *National Ambient Air Quality Status and Trends 2012*, New Delhi, 2014.
32. Patankar, A.M., and Trivedi, P.L. (2011), "Monetary Burden of Health Impacts of Air Pollution in Mumbai, India: Implications for Public Health Policy", *Public Health*, 125(3), 157-164.
33. Patankar, A.M., and Trivedi, P.L. (2011), *op. cit.*
34. Guttikunda, S.K. and Goel, R. (2013), *op. cit.*
35. WHO, 2009.
36. Central Pollution Control Board, Ministry of Environment and Forest, *Performance Evaluation of Sewage Treatment Plants Under NRCD,* New Delhi, 2013.

37. Nandi, S., Gamkhar, S. (2012), "Urban challenges in India: A review of recent policy measures", *Habitat International*, 39, 55-61.
38. Kumar S.G, Kar, S.S., Jain A. (2012), "Health and environmental sanitation in India: Issues for prioritizing control strategies", *Indian J Occup Environ Med*;15, 93-6. Accessed October 2, 2015. http://www.ijoem.com/text.asp?2011/15/3/93/93196
39. *WHO Health statistics and health information systems. Deaths estimates for 2008 by cause for WHO Member States*(2011): Accessed August 19, 2014. http://www.who.int/healthinfo/global_burden_disease/estimates_country/en/
40. Ghosh, S., and Bose, S. (2012), "Morbidity Among Urban Children in India: Distinctions Between Slum and Non-slum Areas", *Internationales Asien Forum, International Quarterly for Asian Studies* Arnold Bergsträsser Institut, 43, (1/2), 47.
41. Zhu, Da; Asnani, P.U., Zurbrügg, Chris, Anapolsky, Sebastian, Mani, Shyamala (2008), *Improving Municipal Solid Waste Management in India. A Sourcebook for Policy-makers and Practitioners*, Washington DC: World Bank Development Studies.
42. Arunachalam, N., Tana, S., Espino, F., Kittayapong, P., Abeyewickreme, W., Wai, K.T., Tyagi, B.T., Kroeger, A., Sommerfeld, J. and Petzold, M. (2010), "Eco-bio-social Determinants of Dengue Vector Breeding: A Multicountry Study in Urban and Periurban Asia", *Bulletin of the World Health Organisation,* 88 (3), 173-184.
43. Kroeger, Sommerfeld and Petzold 2010, *op. cit.*
44. Kumari, R., Kumar, K. and Chauhan, L.S. (2011), "First Dengue Virus Detection in Aedesalbopictus from Delhi, India: Its Breeding Ecology and Role in Dengue Transmission", *Tropical Medicine and International Health,* 18 (8), 949-954.
45. Dash, A.P., Valecha, N., Anvikar, A.R. and Kumar, K. (2008), "Malaria in India: Challenges and Opportunities", *Journal of Biosciences,* 33 (4), 583-592.
46. Dash *et al.*, 2008.
47. Kovats, S. and Akhtar, R. (2008), "Climate, Climate Change and Human Health in Asian Cities", *Environment and Urbanization,* 20, 165-175.
48. Pandey, Vinita (2009), *Crisis of Urban Middle Class*, Jaipur: Rawat Publications.
49. Patel, V., Chatterji, S., Chisholm, D., Ebrahim, S., Gopalakrishna, G., Mathers, C., Mohan, V., Prabhakaran, D., Ravindran, R.D. and Reddy, K.S. (2011), "Chronic Diseases and Injuries in India", *The Lancet*, 377(9763), 413-428.
50. Kale, Sumita (2010), "Emerging Issues in Health", in *India Health Report 2010,* Mahal, Ajay S.; Debroy, Bibek; Bhandari, Laveesh (Eds.), New Delhi, 35-50.
51. International Diabetes Federation (2013), *IDF Diabetes Atlas*, Online available: www.idf.org/diabetesatlas (accessed: 2014-08-29)
52. Patel, *et al.*, 2011.

53. Ebrahim, S., Kinra, S., Bowen, L., Andersen, E., Ben-Shlomo, Y., Lyngdoh, T., Ahuja, R.C., Prashant, J., Das, S.M., Smith, GD., Prabhakaran, D. and Reddy, K.S. (2011), "The Effect of Rural-to-Urban Migration on Obesity and Diabetes in India: A cross-sectional Study", *PLoS Med*, 7(4), e1000268.
54. Patel *et al.*, 2011.
55. Whitehead, M., Dahlgren, G., and Evans, T. (2001), "Equity and Health Sector Reforms: Can Low-income Countries Escape the Medical Poverty Trap"? *The Lancet*, 358(9284), 833-836.
56. Butsch, C., Sakdapolrak, P., Saravanan V.S. (2012), "Urban Health in India", *InternationalesAsienforum,* 43 (1-2), 13-32.
57. GoI/UNDP (Government of India/United Nations Development Programme), *Urban Poverty Report 2009*, New Delhi, 2009.
58. Planning Commission (Government of India), "*Report of the Expert Group to Recommend the detailed Methodology for Identification of Families Living Below Povertyline in Urban Areas*", Delhi, Planning Commission, 2012.
59. *Ibid.*
60. Office of the Registrar General and Census Commissioner, India (2013): *Primary Census Abstract for Slum*, Acessed October 26, 2015, http://www.censusindia.gov.in/2011–Documents/Slum-26-09-13.pdf
61. Vlahov, D., Galea, S., and Freudenberg, N. (2005), "The urban health 'advantage'"*Journal of Urban Health*, 82(1), 1-4.
62. Duggal, R. (2005), "Historiclal Review of Health Policy Making" in *Review of Healthcare in India,* ed, Gangolli, L., Duggal, R. and Shukla, A., Mumbai, 21-40.
63. Kamat, V.R. and Nichter, M. (1998), "Pharmacies, Self-Medication and Pharmaceutical Marketing in Bombay, India", *Social Science and Medicine*, 47 (6), 779-794.
64. MoHFW (Ministry of Health and Family Welfare), (2002), National Health Policy 2002. Acessed October 26, 2015, http://www.iapsmgc.org/userfiles/National_Health_policy_2002-2.pdf
65. Balarajan, Yarlini; Selvaraj, Selvaraj; Subramanian, S.V. (2011), "Health care and equity in India", *The Lancet*, 377 (9764), 505-515.
66. Shukla, A. (2007), "Key Public Health Challenges in India: A Social Medicine Perspective", *Social Medicine*, 2(1), 1-7.
67. Shahrawat, R., and Rao, K.D. (2012), "Insured Yet Vulnerable: Out-of-pocket Payments and India's Poor", *Health Policy and Planning*, 27(3), 213-221.
68. Das, J., Holla, A., Das, V., Mohanan, M., Tabak, D. and Brian Chan (2012), "In Urban And Rural India, A Standardized Patient Study Showed Low Levels of Provider Training and Huge Quality Gaps" *Health Affairs*, 31, (12), 2774-2784.
69. Census of India (2013), Acessed April 01, 2014. http://censusindia.gov.in/2011census/censusinfodashboard/index.html
70. Shaw, Annapurna (1999), "Emerging Patterns of Urban Growth in India", *Economic and Political Weekly*, 34, (16/17), 969-978.

71. Bapat, Meera (1981), "Shanty Town and City: The Case of Poona", *Progress in Planning* 15, 151-269.
72. Sawhney, U. (2013), "Slum population in India: Extent and Policy Response", *International Journal of Research in Business and Social Science,* 2 (1), 47-56.
73. PMC (Pune Municipal Corporation), (2007), *Environmental Status Report, 2006-2007*, Pune.
74. PMC (Pune Municipal Corporation), (2012), *Revising/updating the City Devlopement Plan (CDP) of Pune City 2041 under JNNURM, Final Draft CDP* (Volume I), Pune.
75. PMC (Pune Municipal Corporation), (2008), *Environmental Status Report, 2007-2008*, Pune.
76. Butsch, Carsten (2011), *Zugang zu Gesundheitsdienstleistungen, Barrieren und Anreize in Pune, Indien*, Stuttgart: Franz Steiner Verlag.
77. Kroll, Mareike (2013), *GesundheitlicheDisparitätenimurbanenIndien, Auswirkungen des sozioökonomischen Status auf die Gesundheit in Pune*, Stuttgart: Steiner Verlag.
78. Kroll, M., E. Bharucha, F. Kraas (2014), "Does Rapid Urbanization Aggravate Health Disparities? Reflections on the Epidemiological Transition in Pune, India", *Global Health Action* (7): 23447, http://dx.doi.org/10.3402/gha.v7.23447, http://www.globalhealthaction.net/index.php/gha/article/view/23447
79. Omran A. (1971), "The Epidemiological Transition: A Theory of the Epidemiology of Population Change", *Milbank Memorial Fund* Q49, 509-538.
80. Caldwell J. (1993), "Health Transition: The Cultural, Social and Behavioural Determinants of Health in the Third World", *Social Science and Medicine,* 36, 125-135.
81. Kroll *et al.*, 2014.
82. International Institute for Population Sciences, *National Family Health Survey (NFHS-3), India, 2005-06, Maharashtra*, Mumbai: International Institute for Population Sciences, 2008.
83. International Institute for Population Sciences.
84. Penchansky, R. and Thomas, J.W. (1981), "The Concept of Access: Definition and Relationship to Consumer Satisfaction." *Medical Care,* Jahrgang 19, (2), 127-140.
85. Aggarwal, S. and Butsch, C. (2011), "Environmental and Ecological Threats in Indian Megacities", In *Applied Urban Ecology*, edited by Richter, M. and U. Weiland, Chichester.
86. Butsch, C., Kroll, M., Kraas, F. and Bharucha, E. (2015), "How is Rapid Urbanization in India Affecting Human Health? Findings from a Case Study in Pune", *Asien,* 134 (1), 73-93.
87. Butsch *et al.*, 2015 (ASIEN).
88. Phalkey, R., Kroll, M., Dutta, S., Shukla, S., Butsch, C., Bharucha, E. and Kraas, F. (2015), "Knowledge, attitude, and practices with respect to disease surveillance among urban private practitioners in Pune, India", *Global Health Action,* 8, 28413. Accessed October 28, 2015. http://www.globalhealthaction.net/index.php/gha/article/view/28413.

30
Emerging Health Risks
Outdoor Air Pollution in India

Hem H. Dholakia

Introduction

It is well-known that energy, development and human health are inextricably linked. Today, India is in a phase of transition where it is undergoing rapid urbanization, economic and population growth. These transitions are leading to increases in energy demand. Whereas this transition implies that a large section of the population is moving out of poverty, a heavy dependence on fossil-based energy is leading to deterioration in the quality of air in Indian cities.

The World Health Organization (WHO) finds that of the top twenty most polluted cities in the world, thirteen are from India.[1] Pollution levels in Indian cities are found to be several times higher than the standards prescribed by the WHO. Outdoor air pollution is among the top ten risk factors in India and associated health impacts are staggering. The Global Burden of Disease Study estimated that in India 6,70,000 deaths (in 2010) could be attributed to outdoor air pollution alone.[2] Other studies find that on average Indians lose 3.2 years of life expectancy and 2.1 billion life years as a consequence of high air pollution.[3] Studies that assign monetary values to health outcomes find that health costs of urban air pollution in India are US$ 1.4 billion[4] (a conservative estimate). This remains a serious concern not only because exposure to higher amounts of air pollution results in more severe affects health, but also because its impacts may be exacerbated in the context of climate change.[5] This is because meteorological parameters such as temperature and humidity can possibly influence the distribution of pollutants in the atmosphere and thereby influence levels of human exposure ultimately impacting health outcomes.[6, 7] Air pollution, therefore, remains a serious emerging health risk in the Indian context. The current chapter provides an historical overview of studies that link pollution and health. It further provides an understanding of the geographic distribution of outdoor air pollution in India and highlights some key policies that are required to curb the same.

A Historical Perspective on Air Quality and Health

That the air we breathe affects human well-being has been well understood for centuries. Anecdotal evidence points to presence of pneumonia, emphysema and carbon deposits in lungs of ancient mummies due to possible smoke inhalation.[8] However, it was a series of events such as industrialization, fossil-fuel use and public focus on acute air pollution episodes (e.g. Donora Valley, London Smog, and Meuse Valley) that spurred government legislation as well as systematic research to understand air quality and health linkages especially in the United Kingdom and United States.[9]

The turning event was the London smog of 1952 which demonstrated conclusively that mortality is increased as a result of exposure to high ambient air pollution.[10] The key pollutant responsible for the London smog was sulphur dioxide from industries due to burning of coal. It was estimated that, from December 1952 to February 1953, 12,000 excess deaths occurred due to acute and persisting effects of the smog. This has been the starting point of research in the field of air pollution and health.[11] Over the last few decades, an extensive body of research ranging from toxicology, human exposure assessment and epidemiology has provided a solid basis for air pollution's effect on health (Box 1). Furthermore, literature from economics has provided evidence for the efficacy and benefits of different pollution intervention policies.

Today, air pollution has become a more complex phenomenon. The sources and nature of pollutants have changed dramatically. As vehicle emissions standards have continually improved; emissions standards for industry have been strengthened, the key pollutants today are particulate matter less than ten microns (PM_{10}) and less than 2.5 microns ($PM_{2.5}$). These have been recognised to have the most serious health impacts are now routinely monitored across most parts of the world. In addition, a higher reliance on diesel vehicles for transport especially in Europe and India has led to increases in concentrations of nitrous oxide (NOx) and shortlived climate pollutants like Black Carbon (BC).[12] Given the dynamic nature of air pollution, governments across the world have legislated (and continually revised) standards to improve air quality.

Air Pollution in India

The challenge of air pollution in India was recognised early on. Air pollution legislation in India came into force in 1981 under the Air (Prevention and Control of Pollution) Act. Under the Act, Central and state pollution control boards were set-up that were responsible for monitoring ambient air quality; setting air quality standards and recommending appropriate control measures across sectors such as transport, industry and power sector.[13] In accordance with the Act, over the years, key policy interventions have included fitting of the catalytic converters in petrol-based vehicles in 45 Indian cities;[14] upgrading fuel quality and technology standards via the Auto Fuel Policy Report.[15] Furthermore, specific city level policies have been put in place such as switch of public transport buses to CNG and changing of power plants to natural gas in Delhi.[16-18] The rapid increases in pollution have outweighed the beneficial impacts of these policies over time.

Modern day pollution in Indian cities is a complex phenomenon. It is a combination of vehicular exhaust, construction, waste burning, industrial emissions, thermal power plant emissions as well as transport of pollutants from neighbouring areas due to varied reasons such as burning of crop residue. However, few studies have attempted to systematically study the contribution of different sources to pollution. One such study for six megacities was carried out by the Central Pollution Control Board[19] to identify sources of pollution and their relative contributions (Fig. 30.1).

The pollution loads were lowest for Kanpur (9 tonnes/day) and highest for Delhi (147 tonnes/day) for particulate matter less than ten microns (PM_{10}). Road dust was found to be the highest contributor to pollution in four out of six cities—Delhi (45%), Mumbai (35%), Pune (57%) and Bangalore (50%). Vehicular exhaust and industrial emissions were the chief contributors to pollution in Chennai (43%) and Kanpur respectively[19]. This heterogeneity in the contribution of

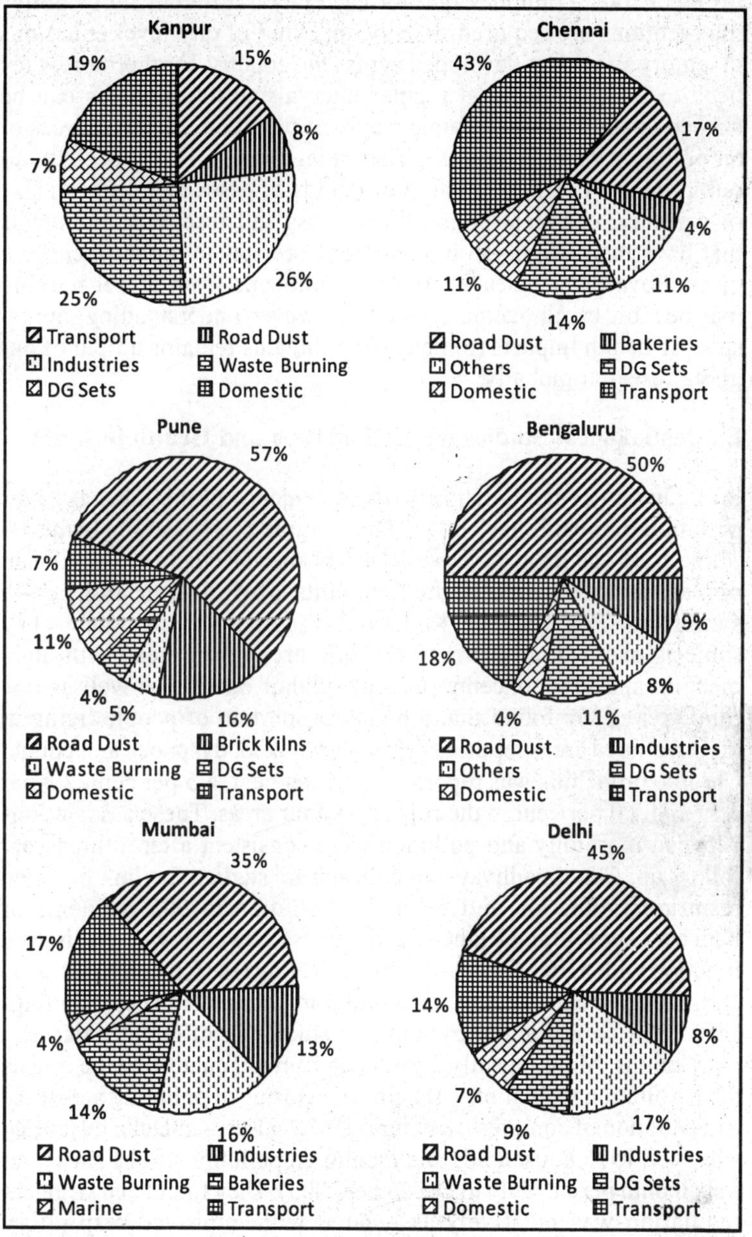

Fig. 30.1: Shows the Source Contribution to PM_{10} Across Different Cities (CPCB, 2010).

different sources implies that for each city a different set of policy interventions are required. Ideally, this kind of city level emissions inventory should be developed across the country. Furthermore, they need to be carried out at regular intervals so that policies can be shaped to address the dynamic nature of pollution. As the sources of air pollution vary, so does the differential toxicity. This is because air pollution is a complex mixture of liquids or gases that differ in size of particles, chemical composition, mass and reactivity. Pollutants that have their origins in biomass may precipitate higher incidence of cardiovascular diseases whereas pollutants from diesel burning may be more carcinogenic in nature. However, understanding source-specific health impacts (toxicity) of pollutants remains a field of on-going research globally.

Epidemiological Studies on Air Pollution and Health in India

In the Indian context, majority of the evidence of the impacts of air pollution on health has come from multiple cross-sectional studies. These cross-sectional studies have established that there are significant correlations between higher amounts of pollution and health symptoms. For instance Kamath and colleagues[20] studied 4129 subjects over a four year period from three urban areas with high, medium and low concentrations of sulphur dioxide as well as one rural area. They found that a higher proportion of people living in more polluted areas reported symptoms of cold, dyspnoea and cough. Chronic bronchitis was reported in 4.5 per cent, 4.5 per cent, 2.3 per cent and 5.0 per cent in the respective four areas. These associations between morbidity and pollution were consistent after a three year follow up. Chattopadhyay and colleagues[21] studied the link between respiratory function and vehicular pollution in 505 residents of Kolkata. They found higher traffic areas showed lower respiratory function with 3.76 per cent of subjects having restrictive impairments and 3.17 per cent having obstructive impairments. These findings have been corroborated by multiple studies in different cities and populations. More recently, Foster and Kumar[18] quantified the effects of air pollution regulation—specifically closing of polluting industries and adoption of compressed natural gas by buses—in Delhi city. They surveyed 1576 households and monitored pollution at 113 sites over a six month period (July to December 2003). They found that stringent regulation was positively associated with improved respiratory function, though these effects varied by gender and income class.

Despite there being a large number of cross-sectional studies, few studies have explored the short term impacts of air pollution on health using a time-series approach. One of the first systematic attempts to study the impacts of air pollution was carried out by the World Bank for the city of Mumbai. This study found that air pollution caused 2800 cases of excess mortality, 60 million respiratory symptom days and 19 million restricted activity days at a cost of INR 18 billion for Mumbai.[22] In a study of Delhi city,[23] Cropper and colleagues used a time-series approach to study the linkages between daily mortality and total suspended particulate matter. They found that a 100 μg/m^3

Box 1: The Physiological Basis of Air Pollution Impacts

The physiological basis of air pollution impacts on human health is complex and multi-factorial in nature. A review is beyond the scope of this chapter. Most of the underlying evidence for physiological impacts comes from animal-model studies and there is general consensus that cellular injury and inflammation play a key role.[24] These mechanisms include, but are not limited to, oxidative damage through reactive oxygen species;[25] activation of cell signalling pathways;[26] cytokine mediated pulmonary inflammation;[27] epithelial injury modifying respiratory tract barrier function,[28] induced airway hyper responsiveness triggering allergic immune responses;[29] impairing lung defence mechanisms;[30] pulmonary DNA damage[31] and epigenetic changes.[32] The impacts of pollution not only affect the pulmonary system, but also extend to cardiovascular, hematopoietic as well as central nervous system. In this way, these mechanisms are responsible for the development of disease states that may lead to hospitalizations and deaths.[24]

Impacts are determined primarily by the 'dosage' of (or exposure to) inhaled particles. This dosage depends upon several factors such as characterization of deposition, clearance, and retention of particles and their constituents within the respiratory tractas as well as biological factors such as age, gender, pre-existing disease conditions. These factors together modify the exposure and severity of health impacts.

Particulate matter size remains a major determinant of dosage. Particulate matter that is relatively large in size (exceeding 10 microns in diameter) is trapped by the mucous membranes in the upper respiratory tract and tracheo-bronchial tree. Health impacts are seen with PM of size 10 microns (PM_{10}) or less. The most significant physiological impacts (as described previously) are associated with fine particulate matter that are less than 2.5 microns in diameter ($PM_{2.5}$) as these can penetrate to the alveolar regions of the lung. Therefore, there is an increased focus on measurement and mitigation of $PM_{2.5}$.

decrease in total suspended particulate matter reduced all-cause mortality by 2.3 per cent, cardiovascular mortality by 4.3 per cent and respiratory mortality by 3.1 per cent. The maximum benefits of air pollution reduction would accrue to young adults between ages of 15 and 44 years.[33] The study also found that health gains of air pollution reduction in Delhi were much lower than those estimated for the city of Philadelphia.

Identifying the need for more such studies, short term effects of air pollution on daily mortality were recently studied for two Indian cities—Delhi and Chennai.[34, 35] Using daily all-cause mortality and pollution data from 2002 to 2004, both studies ran a series of Poisson regression models to measure the association between PM_{10} and daily deaths. For Chennai, it was found that a 10 μg/m³ increase in PM_{10} concentrations led to a 0.44 per cent (95% confidence interval = 0.17 to 0.71) increase in daily all-cause mortality. Delhi on the other hand, showed a 0.15 per cent (95% confidence interval = 0.07 to 0.23) increase in daily all-cause mortality with every 10 μg/m³ increase in PM_{10} concentrations. In both these studies, varieties of model specifications were used to check the robustness of these estimates. These estimates are lower than those found for the multicity studies in United States, Europe and Latin America. However, reasons for this are unclear. One potential explanation could be that the relationship between air pollution and mortality relationship is non-linear.[36] This may lead to a situation where at higher levels of pollution, a reduction in particulate matter may not have significant health benefits as compared to pollution reduction at lower levels. However, a key research gap is that long-term health impacts of air pollution using a cohort study design is missing in India. Therefore, health inputs are missing while setting (and revising) air quality standards in India, which are more lenient than those abroad (Table 30.1).

Geographic Distribution of Air Pollution in India

The Central Pollution Control Board (CPCB) in India has identified (and routinely monitors) three criteria pollutants—Sulphur dioxide (SO_2), Nitrogen dioxides (NOx) and respirable suspended Particulate matter (PM_{10}). The current monitoring effort of the CPCB is 573 monitoring stations spread across 240 cities and towns, encompassing 26 states and 5 union territories in India. However, there remain large gaps in scope of pollutants monitored as well as quality and quantity

Table 30.1: Comparison of Air Quality Standards (μg/m³)

Pollutant	Time Weighted Average	Indian NAAQS[a]		WHO Air Quality Guideline
		Industrial Area	Ecologically Sensitive/ Residential Areas	
Sulphur Dioxide	Annual	50	20	—
	24 Hours	80	80	20
Nitrogen Oxides	Annual	40	30	40
	24 Hours	80	80	80
Particulate	Annual	60	60	20
Matter PM_{10}	24 Hours	100	100	50
Fine Particulate	Annual	40	40	10
Matter $PM_{2.5}$	24 Hours	60	60	25
Ozone	8 Hourly	100	100	100
	1 Hour	180	180	180

[a] Central Pollution Control Board (http://cpcb.nic.in National_Ambient_Air_Quality_Standards.php) Accessed October 6, 2015.

with respect to data availability. Most monitors are manually operated—leading to issues with calibration and equipment breakdown. The end result is that data are often missing, making it difficult to understand the beneficial impacts of policies. In addition, to address these current issues, the CPCB has set-up real time air quality monitors across sixteen cities and real time data are available for twelve of these—Faridabad, Delhi, Agra, Kanpur, Lucknow, Varanasi, Patna, Ahmedabad, Mumbai, Hyderabad, Bangalore and Chennai. Recently, the government has developed an Air Quality Index (AQI) to help disseminate information on air quality in India (Box 2).

Modeling studies as well as satellite measurements show the heterogeneity in distribution of pollution across Indian cities. Modeling exercises combine information from activity data across different sectors, atmospheric chemistry and policies to estimate concentrations. Such exercises are useful in evaluating policy impacts and getting estimates of pollution where monitoring infrastructure is weak or non-existent. The highest pollution levels are observed across north and central India (Fig. 30.2). The reasons for this are the meteorological conditions, proximity to coal power plants and industry and practices such as biomass burning.

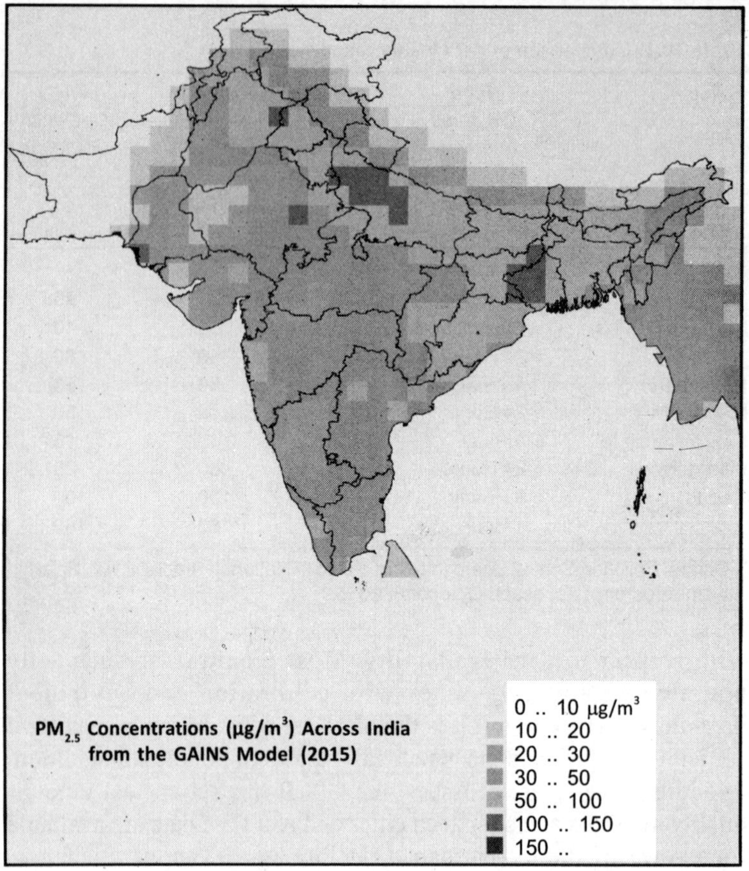

Fig. 30.2: Modeled $PM_{2.5}$ Concentrations Across India in 2015 for the World Energy Outlook (2012) Scenario under Current Legislation.

Source: International Institute of Applied Systems Analysis (IIASA), Austria.

The findings from modeling studies are in alignment with data from ground level monitors (Figs. 30.3, 30.4 and 30.5). In the year 2012, most Indian cities show non-attainment of standards for particulate matter less than ten microns (PM_{10}). The average levels of PM_{10} across 45 major cities in India (Figure 30.3) increased from 117 ± 63 µg/m^3(in 2008) to 136 ± 72 µg/m^3 (in 2012) indicating a deterioration in air quality. The five cities with highest annual averages of PM_{10} in 2012 were Gwalior, Delhi, Raipur, Allahabad and Ghaziabad (located in northern India). The southern cities of Chennai,

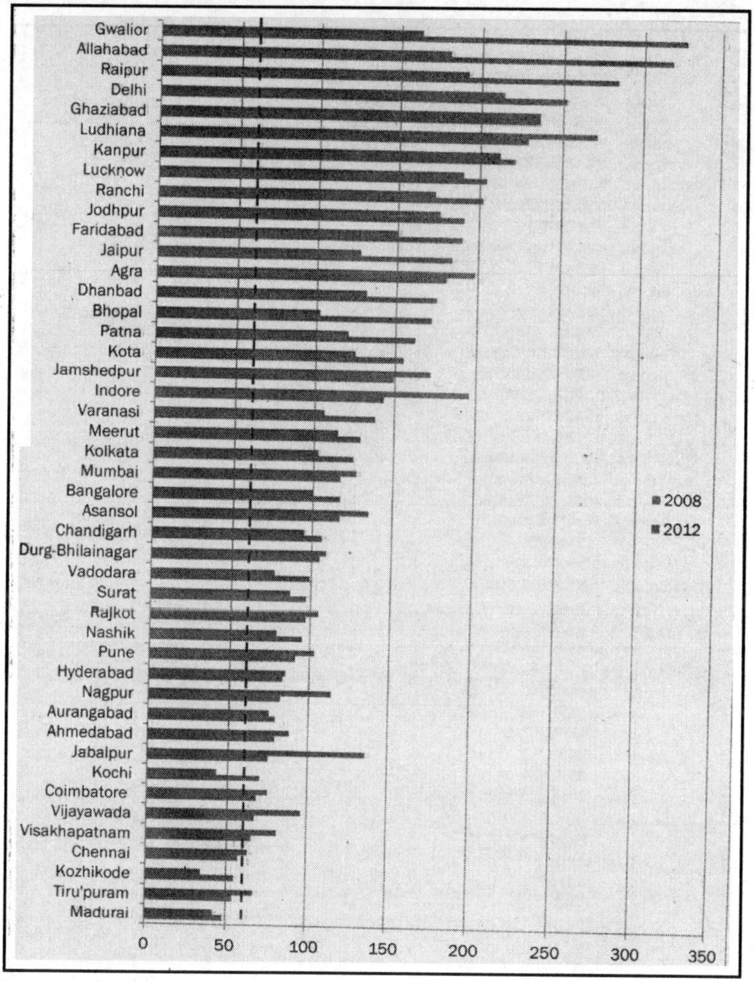

Fig. 30.3: Modeled $PM_{2.5}$ Concentrations Across India in 2015 for the World Energy Outlook (2012) Scenario under Current Legislation.

Source: PM_{10} Concentrations (µg/m^3) across 45 major cities in India.

Madurai, Vizag showed the lowest PM_{10} levels across the cities studied. Air pollution is a combination of pollution loads and meteorological factors. It is reasonable to suggest that for similar pollution loads, concentrations of pollutants may be higher in northern India due to meteorological factors.

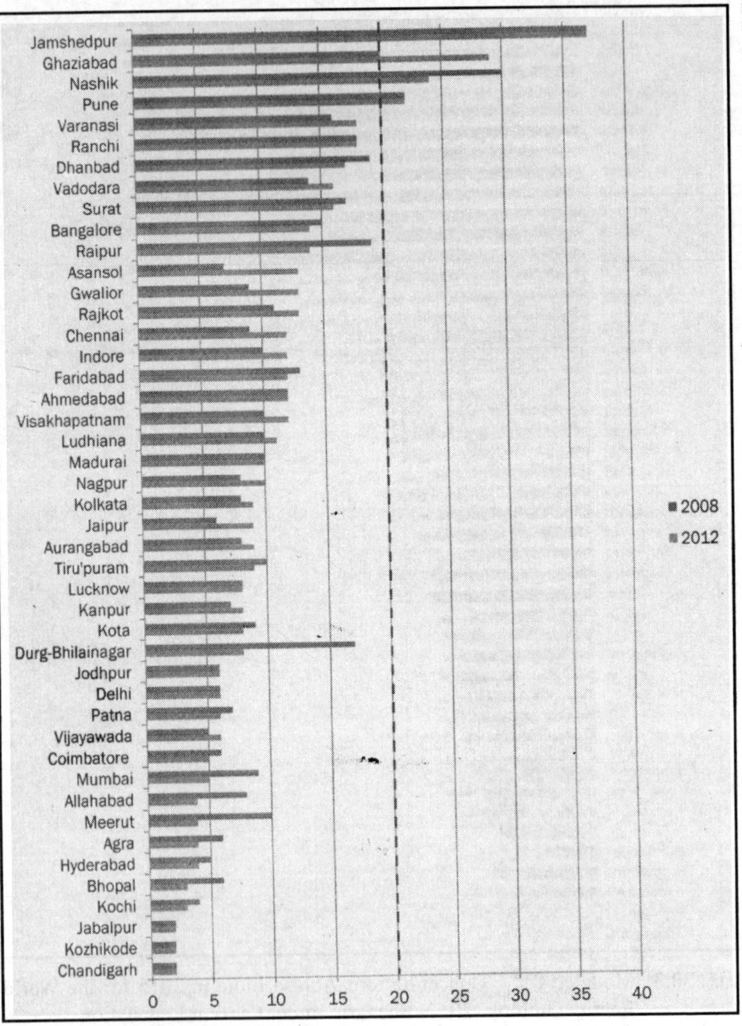

Fig. 30.4: Modeled $PM_{2.5}$ Concentrations Across India in 2015 for the World Energy Outlook (2012) Scenario under Current Legislation.

Source: SO_2 Concentrations (μg/m^3) across 45 major cities in India.

It is observed that for sulphur dioxide (SO_2) and nitrous oxides (NO_x) most cities are within the prescribed standards. Sulphur dioxide (SO_2) levels have remained the same or slightly reduced over time (Figure 30.4). This may be, in part, due to the reduction of sulphur

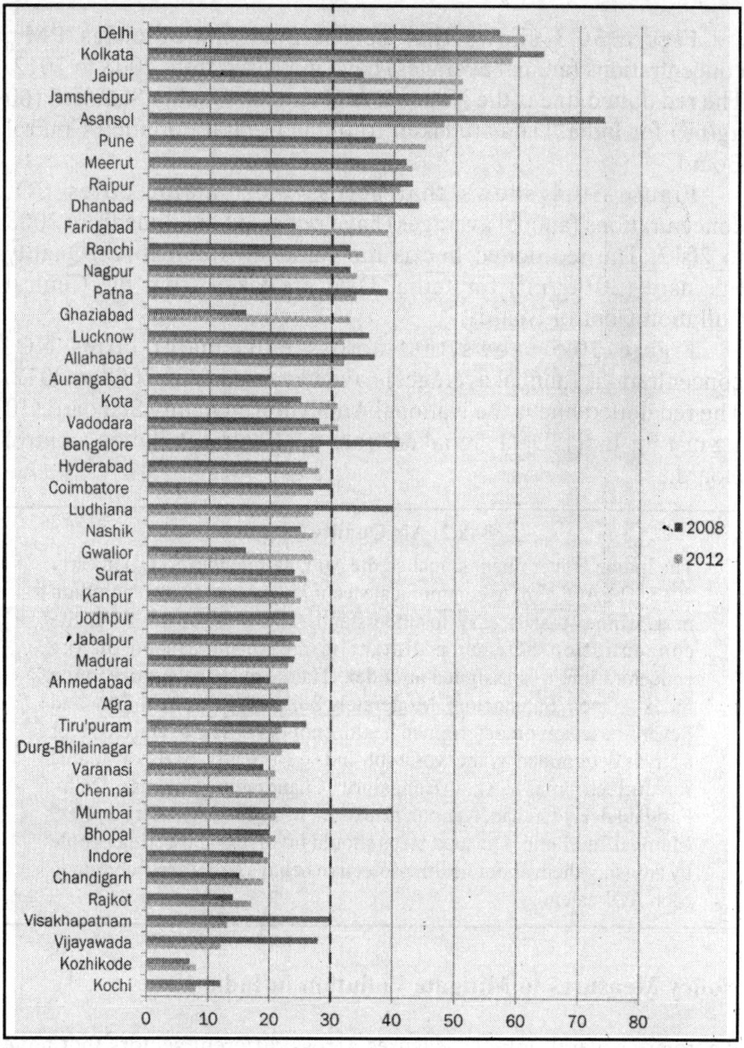

Fig. 30.5: Modeled $PM_{2.5}$ Concentrations Across India in 2015 for the World Energy Outlook (2012) Scenario under Current Legislation.

Source: NO_2 Concentrations (µg/m^3) for 45 major cities in India.

content in vehicle fuels as a consequence of tightening of air quality standards. There appears to be a slight increase in levels over time (Figure 30.5), possibly due to a shift from petrol to diesel vehicles.

Figure 30.3 shows that across most major cities PM_{10} concentrations (annual averages) have increased from 2008 to 2012. The red dotted line is the National Ambient Air Quality Standard (60 $\mu g/m^3$) for India. Data are taken from the Central Pollution Control Board.

Figure 30.4 shows that across most major cities SO_2 concentrations (annual averages) have remained the same from 2008 to 2012. The red dotted line is the National Ambient Air Quality Standard (20 $\mu g/m^3$) for India. Data are taken from the Central Pollution Control Board.

Figure 30.5 shows that across most major cities NO_2 concentrations (annual averages) have increased from 2008 to 2012. The red dotted line is the National Ambient Air Quality Standard (30 $\mu g/m^3$) for India. Data are taken from the Central Pollution Control Board.

Box 2: Air Quality Index

The Indian Government launched the Air Quality Index (AQI) in early 2015. The AQI aims to communicate technical information on pollution in a manner that is easy to understand. To construct the AQI, the concentration of each pollutant is measured. Based on the concentration, it is assigned an index. There are six categories in the index—Good, Satisfactory, Moderately Polluted, Poor, Very Poor and Severe-based on predetermined health endpoints. The overall AQI for a city is determined by the worst sub-index. Currently, AQI is available for thirteen cities—Agra, Bengaluru, Chandrapur, Chennai, Delhi, Faridabad, Hyderabad, Kanpur, Lucknow, Mumbai, Muzaffarpur, Navi Mumbai and Pune. The next steps should involve empowering people by advising them about health protective behaviours corresponding to each AQI category.

Policy Measures to Mitigate Pollution in India

There are several policy measures across different sectors that have been instituted to curb air pollution in India. Most of these policies have focused on the transportation sector. Emissions standards for vehicles have been continually tightened since 2000 and the latest Auto Fuel Policy (2014) proposes achieving the Bharat V (Euro 5 equivalent) by 2020. In addition to tightening standards, policies on alternate fuels such as Compressed Natural Gas (CNG) and Ethanol Blending are in place. Following a Supreme Court order in the early 2000s, more than 1,00,000 vehicles in Delhi were switched to CNG which also included the retrofitting of about 3,000 diesel buses.[16, 37, 38] In addition, these are being expanded to other cities such as Ahmedabad and Mumbai.

Table 30.2: Air Quality Index for India

AQI Category	*AQI*	*Possible Health Impacts*
Good	0-50	Minimal impact
Satisfactory	51-100	Minor breathing discomfort to sensitive people
Moderately Polluted	101-200	Breathing discomfort to people with lung disease, asthma and heart disease
Poor	201-300	Breathing discomfort to most people on prolonged exposure
Very Poor	301-400	Respiratory illness on prolonged exposure
Severe	401-500	Affects healthy people and seriously impacts those with existing disease

Source: Central Pollution Control Board (2015).
Accessed on 6th October, 2015 from http://www.cpcb.nic.in/About_AQI.pdf

A bold social experiment carried out recently (1st to 15th January, 2016) by the Government of Delhi was to institute an Odd-Even policy for four wheelers. According to this policy, odd-numbered vehicles were allowed to ply only on odd dates and even-numbered vehicles on even dates respectively. Anecdotal evidence suggests that there were reductions in travel times due to reduced congestion. However, there was no significant reduction in pollution levels. The pollution levels increased from 280 μg/m^3 to about 330 μg/m^3 in the week prior to and after policy implementation. However, it must be recognised that in the short-term, pollution levels are dominated by meteorological conditions such as wind, rains and temperature and therefore it is hard to provide conclusive evidence on the impact of the odd-even policy. The lack of conclusive evidence does not imply that the policy has failed. The fact that, as a result of this bold experiment, the citizens of Delhi have started thinking more about how they travel is, in and of itself, a good sign that a more comprehensive approach to mitigating the air pollution crisis can now be pursued.

There is a push towards incentivising electric vehicles. For instance the National Electricity Mobility Mission aims for savings of 2 to 2.5 million tonnes of liquid fuel through promotion of 6-7 million electric vehicles by 2020. However, the key to simultaneously reducing pollution and promoting health is investments in public as well as non-motorised (cycles, walking) transport. Several cities such as Delhi, Mumbai, Bangalore, Chennai and Kolkata are investing in public transport infrastructure such as building metro-rail. Further, public transport buses are being upgraded.[39] Most of these cities have also adopted guidelines to mainstream non-motorised transport into their urban design. These efforts need to be replicated across Tier-II cities in India.

Another major source of pollution is coal-based power generation as there are few regulations to handle PM and fugitive emissions.[40] Health and crop losses from coal power plants in India are estimated at 354 million dollars annually.[41] The CPCB has recently proposed new emissions standards for coal power plants as well as several industries. Along with the stringent norms, transmission and distribution losses need to be minimised so that people move away from highly polluting diesel generator sets (in power scarce areas). Technology solutions such as smart–metering, differential pricing during peak load will lead to demand reduction through behavioural change. Providing a fillip to renewable energy (175 GW renewable energy target) will help to simultaneously reduce pollution and greenhouse gas emissions. Therefore, an overhaul of the power sector will go a long way in significantly reducing pollution in India.

The way forward remains a challenge, but it is possible to protect human health from air pollution. Globally, cities such as Los Angeles have demonstrated the transition from being the world's dirtiest to one of the world's cleanest cities. Air pollution in Los Angeles reduced despite increases in population and vehicle ownership. Modelling studies show that judicious selection and careful implementation of policies in Delhi can help achieve air quality standards by 2030 and reduce health impacts by half.[42]

For India, addressing the emerging health risks of outdoor air pollution requires an integrated policy approach across all sectors and sustained effort over time. As a first step, there is a need to gather quality data on pollution especially in smaller cities and rural areas in India. This requires the strengthening and scaling up of air pollution monitoring systems by installing a system of robust and low cost monitors. Better data is also the first necessary step in evaluating the effectiveness of policies to curb air pollution. The second key step is to educate various groups of stakeholders—people, doctors, sensitive groups (patients, children, elderly), policy-makers on health protective behaviours. For example, on days where AQI is poor, people should use masks when stepping outdoors. Similarly for days when the AQI is severe, schools may be closed to protect children. This link of using AQI information to empower people to protect health is currently missing. Finally, we need to re-imagine the way we think about energy use and resource efficiency. For instance, we can choose policies such that the "Smart Cities" of India are pollution free and enhance public health. In conclusion, outdoor air pollution is an emerging health risk in India. However, health impacts are preventable through policy choices. Today, we have the technology and learning from other countries to nip this problem in the bud before it outdoor air pollution reaches epidemic proportions in India.

Notes

1. WHO, "Ambient (Outdoor) Air Pollution in Cities Database 2014", http://www.who.int/phe/health_topics/outdoorair/databases/cities/en/
2. Lim, S.S., *et al.* (2012), "A Comparative Risk Assessment of Burden of Disease and Injury Attributable to 67 Risk Factors and Risk Factor Clusters in 21 Regions, 1990-2010: A Systematic Analysis for the Global Burden of Disease Study 2010, *The Lancet,* Vol. 380, pp. 2224-60.
3. Greenstone, M., *et al.* (2015), Lower Pollution, Longer Lives: Life Expectancy Gains if India Reduced Particulate Matter Pollution, *Economic & Political Weekly*, Issue 8, pp. 40-46.
4. Brandon, C. and K. Hommann (1995), The Cost of Inaction: Valuing the Economywide Cost of Environmental Degradation in India, Washington D.C: World Bank.
5. Tagaris, E., *et al.* (2009), Potential Impact of Climate Change on Air Pollution-Related Human Health Effects, *Environmental Science and Technology,* Vol. 43 (13), pp. 4979-88.
6. Ren, C. and S. Tong (2008), Health Effects of Ambient Air Pollution — Recent Research Development and Contemporary Methodological Challenges, *Environmental Health* doi:10.1186/1476-069X-7-56.
7. Ren, C., G.M. Williams, and S. Tong, (2006), Does Particulate Matter Modify the Association between Temperature and Cardiorespiratory Diseases? *Environmental Health Perspectives*, doi:10.1289/ehp.9266.
8. Kelly, F.J. and J.C. Fussell (2015), Air Pollution and Public Health: Emerging Hazards and Improved Understanding of Risk, *Environmental Geochemistry and Health,* Vol. 37, pp. 631-49.
9. Bell, M.L., J.M. Samet and F. Dominici (2003), Time Series Studies of Particulate Matter, *Johns Hopkins University Working PaperSeries,* Available at http://biostats.bepress.com/jhubiostat/paper10.
10. Logan, W.P.D. (1953), Mortality in the London Fog Incident, *Lancet,* Vol. 261, pp. 336-38.

11. Bell, M.L. and D.L. Davis (2001), Reassessment of the Lethal London Fog of 1952: Novel Indicators of Acute and Chronic Consequences of Acute Exposure to Air Pollution, *Environmental Health Perspectives,* Vol. 109, pp. 389-394.
12. World Bank, Reducing Black Carbon Emissions from Diesel Vehicles: Impacts, Control Strategies and Cost-benefit Analysis (2014), World Bank Report 86484.
13. MoEF, Air (Prevention and Control of Pollution) Act, 1981, http://www.envfor.nic.in/legis/air/air1.html
14. Greenstone, M. and R. Hanna, Environmental Regulations, Air and Water Pollution, and Infant Mortality in India (2011), National Bureau of Economic Research Availble at http://www.nber.org/papers/w17210.
15. MoPNG, "Auto Fuel Policy Report" (New Delhi: Ministry of Petroleum and Natural Gas, 2003), http://petroleum.nic.in/autoeng.pdf.
16. Bell, R.G., K. Mathur, U. Narain, and D. Simpson (2004), Clearing the Air: How Delhi Broke the Logjam on Air Quality Reforms, *Environment Science and Policy for Sustainable Development,* Vol. 46, pp. 22-39.
17. Guttikunda, S.K., (2012), Air Pollution in Delhi, *Economic & Political Weekly,* Issue 47, pp. 24-27.
18. Foster, A. and N. Kumar, (2011), Health Effects of Air Quality Regulations in Delhi, India, *Atmospheric Environment,* Vol. 45, pp. 1675-83.
19. CPCB, Source-Apportionment Studies of Six Cities in India (2010), New Delhi: Central Pollution Control Board, Available at http://cpcb.nic.in/Source_Apportinment_Studies.php
20. Kamat, S.R. and V.B. Doshi (1987), Sequential Health Effect Study in Relation to Air Pollution in Bombay, India, *European Journal of Epidemiology,* Vol. 3, pp. 265-77.
21. Chattopadhyay, B.P., *et al.* (2007), Exposure to Vehicular Pollution and Assessment of Respiratory Function in Urban Inhabitants, *Lung,* Vol. 185, pp. 263-70.doi:10.1007/s00408-007-9015-0.
22. Larssen, S., *et al.* (1997), Urban Air Quality Management Strategy in Asia: Greater Mumbai Report, World Bank Technical Report, Washington DC.
23. Cropper, M., *et al.* (1997), The Health Benefits of Air Pollution Control in Delhi, *American Journal of Agricultural Economics,* Vol. 79, pp. 1625-29.
24. USEPA, Integrated Science Assessment for Particulate Matter (2009), United States Environment Protection Agency.
25. Ayres, J.G., *et al.* (2008), Evaluating the Toxicity of Airborne Particulate Matter and Nanoparticles by Measuring Oxidative Stress Potential—A Workshop Report and Consensus Statement, *Inhalation Toxicology,* Vol. 20, pp. 75-99.doi:10.1080/08958370701665517.
26. Kaul, N. and H.J. Frontman (1996), Activation of NFkB by the Respiratory Burst of Macrophages, *Free Radical Biology and Medicine,* Vol. 21, pp. 401-5.

27. Tao, F. and L. Kobzik (2002), Lung Macrophage-Epithelial Cell Interactions Amplify Particle-Mediated Cytokine Release, *American Journal of Respiratory Cell and Molecular Biology,* Vol. 26, pp. 499-505.
28. Braude, S., *et al.* (1986), Comparison of Lung Vascular and Epithelial Permeability Indices in the Adult Respiratory Distress Syndrome, *American Review of Respiratory Disease,* Vol. 133, pp. 1002-5.
29. Li, N. *et al.* (2009), The Adjuvant Effect of Ambient Particulate Matter is Closely Reflected by the Particulate Oxidant Potential, *Environmental Health Perspectives,* Vol. 117, pp. 1116-23.
30. Jaspers, I., *et al.* (2005), Diesel Exhaust Enhances Influenza Virus Infections in Respiratory Epithelial Cells, *Toxicological Sciences,* Vol. 85, pp. 990-1002.
31. Schins, R.P.F. and A.M. Knaapen, (2007),Genotoxicity of Poorly Soluble Particles *Inhalation Toxicology,* Vol. 19, Suppl. 1, pp. 189-98.
32. Jones, P.A. and S.P. Baylin (2007), The Epigenomics of Cancer, *Cell,* Vol. 128, pp. 683-92.
33. USEPA, Air Quality Criteria for Particulate Matter (2004), Technical Report U.S., Environmental Protection Agency, Research Triangle Park, NC, Available at http://hero.epa.gov/index.cfm?action=reference.details&reference_id=56905.
34. Balakrishnan, K., *et al.* (2011), Short-term Effects of Air Pollution on Mortality: Results of a Time Series Analysis in Chennai, India, Public Health and Air Pollution in Asia (PAPA): Coordinated Studies of Short-term Exposure to Air Pollution and Daily Mortality in Two Indian Cities, Boston, MA: Health Effects Institute.
35. Rajarathnam, U., *et al.* (2011), Time Series Study on Air Pollution and Mortality in Delhi, Research Report, Boston, MA: Health Effects Institute.
36. Smith, K.R. and J.L. Peel (2010), Mind the Gap, *Environmental Health Perspectives,* Vol. 118, pp. 1643-45.
37. Kathuria, V. (2004), Impact of CNG on Vehicular Pollution in Delhi: A Note, *Transportation Research Part D: Transportation and Environment,* Vol. 9, pp. 409-417.
38. Chelani, A.B. and S. Devotta (2005), Impact of Change in Fuel Quality on PM_{10} in Delhi, *Bulletin of Environmental Contamination and Toxicology,* Vol. 75, pp. 600-607.
39. CSE. Good News and Bad News: Cleaning the Air in Indian Cities (2013), New Delhi: Centre for Science and Environment.
40. Guttikunda, S.K., R. Goel and P. Pant (2014), Nature of Air Pollution, Emissions Sources and Management in Indian Cities, *Atmospheric Environment,* Vol. 95, pp. 501-510.
41. Mahapatra, D., P.R. Shukla and S. Dhar, (2012), External Cost of Coal Based Electricity Generation: A Tale of Ahmedabad City, *Energy Policy,* Vol. 49, pp. 253-265.
42. Dholakia, H.H., P. Purohit, S. Rao and A. Garg (2013), Impact of Current Policies on Future Air Quality and Health Outcomes in Delhi, India, *Atmospheric Environment,* Vol. 75, pp. 241-248.

31

CO_2 Emissions Reduction and the Emerging Socio-Economic Development in Developing Countries

An Indian Context

Rais Akhtar

Before Paris Climate Agreement

This is with reference to Climate talk held in the United Nations in New York, and pressure is again to build upon emerging developing countries—India and China to reduce greenhouse gas emissions. This also refers to U.S. President's speech in the United Nations in which he emphasized that global climate deal should include emerging economies. Finally at Paris Climate Summit in December 2015, emerging developing countries succumb to pressure at the very last day of the summit and an agreement was reached. However, it is important to delve into the CO_2 emission scenario and the development, before the Paris Climate Agreement signed by 195 countries in December 2015.

IPCC Report, 2014

Fifth IPCC Report on the impact of global warming on the livelihood of all the countries. Economic activities—agricultural production, infrastructure, and health sectors are going to be impacted by increased temperature and increased frequency of extreme weather events.[1] India is vulnerable to climate change because of its large population and widespread poverty and increasing economic inequalities. Availability and accessibility of safe drinking water for the population, an important aspect of adaptation, is highly unsatisfactory in case of India. These indicators of human development index are quite satisfactory in case of China, although poverty and inequalities exist there.

However, I disagree with the IPCC Assessment that India and China will be the worst sufferers. In my opinion climate change will impact both developed and developing countries equally. 2003 heatwave in western and central Europe that killed nearly 70,000 people in two weeks time in the month of August, and Katrina hurricane disaster that devastated southern USA, Sandy hurricane in 2012, and recent flooding and land slides in the USA, U.K., and bushfire in Australia and California are examples which show that even developed countries are vulnerable to climate change impacts. It seems there is political motive identifying India and China as the most vulnerable, to hasten the process of industrialization and overall economic development.[2] Developing countries in general and India in particular are facing a great challenge to accelerate the pace of socio-economic development and minimizing inequalities, created mainly during the colonial period of exploitation. We are in dire need of energy (per capita electricity consumption in India is 618 kW and in the USA (14,240 kW) for the process of infrastructure development. It is evident that most developing countries, including India, have the lowest per capita CO_2 emission (1.2 tons per capita as compared to 20.6 tons in the USA), as well as the lowest Gross Domestic Product (GDP) per capita; still the major developed nations ask developing nations to reduce greenhouse gas emission, fundamental to their socio-economic development.

Thus, under the Kyoto framework, the principle of "common but differentiated responsibility" must have been the foundation of future emission negotiations. This will help attain the objectives of equity and human development through expanding access to energy demand of developing countries. We must bear in mind that both developed and developing countries are suffering from the impacts of climate change.

The chapter deals with the energy scenario in India with focus on energy consumption and pinpoints various measures taken by the Indian government to reduce environmental deterioration through minimizing the level of greenhouse gas emission, and strengthening the socio-economic development in order to attain the objectives under the Millennium Development Goals (MDGs). India is a large developing country with diverse climatic zones inhabited by about 700 million rural population directly dependent on climatic sensitive sectors: agriculture, forests and fisheries. The adverse impact of climate change in the form of declining rainfall and rising temperatures and thus the increased severity of drought and flooding in different regions would threaten food security and livelihood. India is a country with diverse climatic zones inhabited by about 750 million rural population (72% of total population: 2011 Census) directly dependent on climatic sensitive sectors: agriculture, forests and fisheries.

The adverse impact of climate change in the form of declining rainfall and rising temperatures and thus the increased severity of drought and flooding would led to price rise of food commodities and threaten food security and livelihood.

Developmental Scenario

Despite scientific and technological progress in India since independence in1947, development strategies have not percolated to grass root level. Besides, there are wide inequalities at inter and intrastate levels. These inequalities are widening over time and space. Few of them may be mentioned: (1) poor infrastructure facilities; (2) weak institutional mechanisms; (3) lack of financial resources and vast sectoral and regional variability adversely affect the adaptive capacity of the country to climate change; (4) regional inequalities. Climate change would represent additional stress on the ecological and socio-economic systems that are already facing tremendous pressure due to rapid industrialization, urbanization and economic development. In view of this, it has rightly been stated in India's Eleventh Five-Year Plan document in response to climate change: "The most important adaptation measure is development itself. Achieving rapid growth as targeted in the Eleventh Plan is therefore a key element in adaptation a stronger economy is more able to adapt both in terms of the cost of adaptation and technological capability. Achieving rapid economic growth as targeted in the Eleventh Plan is therefore a key element in adaptation."[3] However, India requires an inclusive development model that equally takes care the process of regional development and economic empowerment of both rural and urban people. That has been sadly lacking even in India as a whole, as the development is confined to certain regions only.

Kyoto Framework

The essence of the discussion related to the Kyoto Protocol pertains to: Public debate, in which nations increasingly highlight the threat posed by rising greenhouse gas emission in developing countries. The principle of "common but differentiated responsibility": one of the foundations of the Kyoto framework does not mean that should do nothing. "The credibility of any multilateral agreement will hinge on the participation of major emitters in the developing world. However, the basic principles of equity and the human development imperative of expanding excess to energy demand that developing countries have the flexibility to make the transition to a low-carbon growth path at a rate consistent with their capabilities."[4]

Colonial rule in countries of Asia, Africa and other regions, which is responsible for exploiting the resources for their own benefits without any development actions in the colonies, resulted in acute poverty in these colonies. This had created disparities and lack of access to facilities and energy. These aspects cannot be ignored. However, we can change the composition of production in the economy in favour of less CO_2 intensive activities. This can be done either by changing the structure of trade so that more CO_2 intensive products are imported or the structure of consumption and other final demands may be changed by reducing the budget share of CO_2 intensive goods in total final demand.

CO_2 Emission Reduction and India

A comparative study of per capita CO_2 emission based on data from World Development Indicators shows that carbon emitted in India is as low as 1.6 metric tonnes per person as compared to the world average of 4.9 tonnes, 16.4 for the USA and 7.1 for China. In the case of share in global CO_2 emission (in per cent), China stood first with 24.65 per cent followed by USA with 16.16 per cent, while India's share is 5.98 per cent. The focus on India's concern should be on more fundamental issues such as alleviation of poverty and creating basic conditions for human development. Take for example the access to electricity: in India with only 56 per cent of the population have access to electricity, in contrast to 100 per cent in the USA, 99 per cent in China, and 97 per cent in Brazil and in Mexico. Per capita energy use in India is 512.4 [kgoe/a] compared with figures 7,794.8 and 1,138.3 for the USA and China respectively.

CO_2 Emission and Per Capita GDP

There is a positive relationship between GDP per capita and CO_2 emission. The following figures based on data from World Development Indicators reveal that there is a positive relationship between GDP per capita [Purchasing Power Parity (PPP) US$] and CO_2 emission per capita in developing countries. Unless this positive relation is broken without affecting per capita income, India must not agree to any binding emission cuts (Fig. 31.1). It has been recognized that CO_2 emission reduction imposes costs in terms of lower GDP and higher poverty (Fig. 31.2).

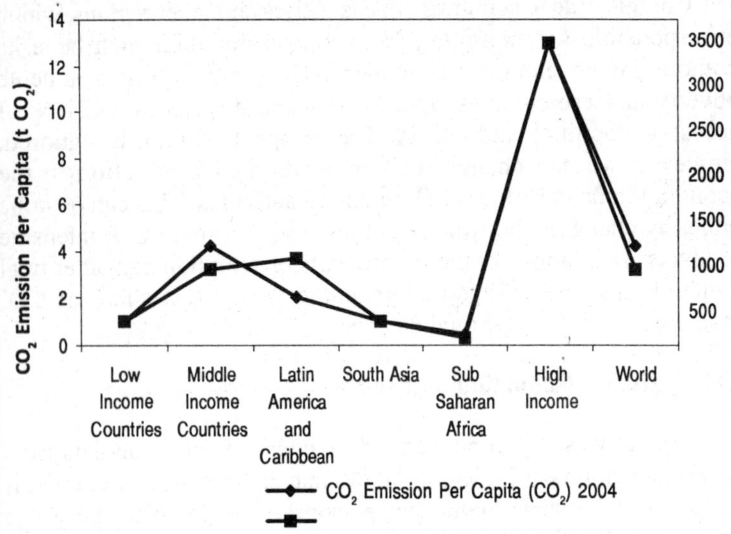

Fig. 31.1: GDP Per Capita (PPP US$ 2006) and CO_2 Emission Per Capita (t CO_2 2004).

Source: Based on World Development Indicators, World Bank, Washington DC 2008.)

The challenge lies in determining a basis for collective action which is fair, and provides equitable entitlement to the global environmental space with burden sharing in a way which recognizes the very different levels of development and also the very different degrees of historical responsibility for causing the problem in the first place. Such differentiation among world countries has been

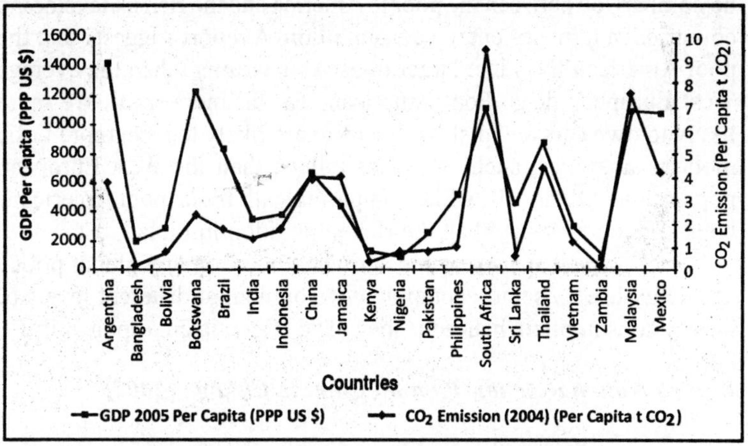

Fig. 31.2: GDP Per Capita (PPP US $ 2005) and CO_2 Emission Per Capita (t CO_2 2004) of selected developing countries.

Source: Based on World Development Indicators, World Bank, Washington DC 2008.

accepted by the UNFCC and the Kyoto Protocol. Besides, the colonial powers who exploited the resources and suppressed the development in their respective colonies must come forward to provide clean and green technologies and assist in the process of regional development. This must be effectively operationalized to create an environment of trust and cooperation. Unfortunately, both the Copenhagen, Cancun and other Climate Conferences had failed to agree to a negotiated treaty. However, the Paris Climate Agreement signed in December, 2015 may help financially and technologically to all developing countries without hurting the process of developmental activities which are vital in promoting and enhancing welfare measures for the people.

Development Dynamics: Energy Consumption

It is a sad reflection of the development dynamics of the world economy that in 2001, there were ninety countries with 4,860 million, or 80 per cent, of the world population that were yet to reach per capita electricity consumption of 4,500 kW, sixty countries with population of 4,166 million claiming 70 per cent of the world population do not use even 1,750 kW per capita and have a Human Development Index (HDI) ranging from 0.32 to 0.80. Even there is no comparison between the poor in America and the rich in developing countries in terms of energy consumption. A report suggests that the poor American lives in a larger house or apartment than the average West European does. Poor Americans eat far more meat, are more likely to own cars and dishwashers and are likely to have more basic modern amenities, such as indoor toilets, than the West European population.[5] Obviously, while comparing with India, poor Americans consume more energy than the rich population in India.

Such wide disparity would seriously question any global policy of energy use on socio-economic development at different levels of energy consumption, hence the idea of "differentiated responsibility".

India's National Action Plan on Climate Change (2008)

Government has emphasized the overriding priority of maintaining high economic growth rates to raise living standards. The plan "identifies measures that promote our development objectives while also yielding co-benefits for addressing climate change effectively." It says these national measures would be more successful with assistance from developed countries, and pledges that India's per capita greenhouse gas emissions "will at no point exceed that of developed countries even as we pursue our development objectives."[3]

INDC to UNFCCC

The Government of India submitted its new climate action plan on October 1, 2015 to the UN Framework Convention on Climate Change (UNFCCC).

This Intended Nationally Determined Contribution (INDC) comes well in advance of a new universal climate change agreement ahead of Paris Climate Agreement signed in December 2015, in Paris.

The Government of India has focused on making a climate pledge (called an INDC in UN climate speak) that is both "ambitious and achievable." The emissions intensity reduction of 33 to 35 per cent based on 2005 levels by 2030 is a strong pathway to control emissions while enabling economic development and alleviating poverty. India's domestic climate plan prioritizes clean energy, aiming to instal an astonishing 175 gigawatts (GW) of renewable energy by 2022 (the equivalent of 350 coal-fired power plants, and run the enormous country with a 40 per cent non-fossil fuel energy mix by 2030.[6]

India's Response

With a share of just 4 per cent of global emissions, any amount of mitigation by India will not affect climate change. A substantial commitment to reduce emissions by the major industrialized countries will be required.

Nevertheless as contribution to the global emission reduction efforts, the Eleventh Plan (2007-12) focuses on ensuring that the emission intensity of India's GHG continues to decline.

CO_2 Emission Reduction: A Case Study of India

The correct approach in mitigation is to define the obligations of different parties on the basis of common but differentiated responsibility and differences in respective capabilities. India's view on burden sharing is based on this approach. India's National Environmental Policy of 2006 requires "equal per capita entitlements of global environmental resources to all countries".

At the meeting of the G8+5 in Heiligendamm in July 2007, the former Indian prime minister indicated that we are determined to see that India's per capita emissions never exceed the per capita emissions of the industrialized countries.

This formulation focuses on per capita emissions rather than total emission as the relevant variables and also provides industrialized countries with incentive to reduce their level of emission as quickly as possible.

Focus on adaptation: The most important adaptation measure is development itself. A stronger economy is more able to adapt both in terms of cost of adaptation and technological capability:

- Action in the area of agricultural research to evolve varieties that can cope with likely climate change;
- Action to cope with likely increases in water stress;
- Action to be able to cope with a greater frequency in natural disaster;
- India will also initiate action to increase our access to cleaner and renewable energy by fully exploiting existing resources (*e.g.* hydropower and wind power developing nuclear power, and also supporting research in newer areas such as bio-fuels from agro-waste, solar energy etc.);
- India's Clean Development Mechanism (CDM) potential is

a significant component of the global CDM market. Till 14 February 2008, out of a total of 871 projects being accorded host country approval, 314 projects in India have been registered by the CDM Executive Board, so far the highest in any country.

Although India does not have GHG reduction targets, the country has undertaken reforms that have spurred economic growth and broken the barriers to efficiency: pollution control, energy conservation, energy efficiency.

The improvements in petrol and diesel quality have facilitated the adoption of India 2000 (Euro-I equivalent) emission norms in the entire country and Bharat Stage II (Euro-II equivalent) emission norms in the four metros. Euro-III equivalent norms have been adopted in seven mega cities since 2005 to further reduce sulphur content.[7] The best known of these measures is the court-mandated conversion of not only DTC (Delhi Transport Corporation) buses in Delhi but all commercial passenger vehicles—buses, three-wheelers and taxis to Compressed Natural Gas (CNG). This has resulted in the improvement of Delhi's air quality, which was once categorized as the "fourth most polluted city" in the world. Some of the major Supreme Court rulings on vehicular pollution during 1990-2002 are as follows (Table 31.1).[7]

In September 2015, Minister for Road Transport and Highways Nitin Gadkari has urged automobile manufacturers to leapfrog from Bharat Stage-IV emissions norms to BS-VI standards directly to address the issue of vehicular pollution, the Ministry of Road Transport & Highways (MoRTH) and the Ministry of Environment & Forests (MoEF) have reached a consensus to notify implementation of BS-V and VI standards by 2019 and 2023, respectively.[8]

Recent Court Ruling

Supreme Court on 16th December 2015 has banned registration of diesel SUVs and high-end vehicles in the city with engine capacity of over 2000 cc until March 31, 2016 and also stopped entry of goods vehicles not bound for the national capital Delhi.

Environmental Legislations in India

1. The Water (Prevention and Control of Pollution) Cess Act, 1977.

Table 31.1: Court Rulings to Protect Environment

Case of Ruling	*Year*	*Court Ruling*	*Status*	*Instrument Type*
Vehicles: a Serious Population Issue	1990	Registration of defective vehicles suspended effective from 1991, financial incentives for new CNG vehicles	Done	CAC, MBI
Lead Phase-Out of All Vehicles	1994	Lead-free petrol to be sold in metros and low lead petrol in entire country, catalytic converters for petrol-driven cars made available by April 1995	Done	CAC
Government Vehicles	1996	All official government cars to be fitted with catalytic converters or a CNG kit by August 1996	Done	CAC
Ban on Old Commercial/ Transport Vehicles	1998	All commercial and transport vehicles more than 15 years old not permitted to ply in Delhi and other metros. Commercial vehicles in Delhi should convert to CNG, effective from April 2001	Delayed/ done in Delhi	CAC
Buses to Use Natural Gas	2001	Delhi should convert to CNG, effective from April 2001	Delayed	CAC

2. The Air (Prevention and Control of Pollution) Act, 1981.
3. The Environment (Protection) Act, 1986.
4. The Indian Forest Act, 1927.
5. The Public Liability Insurance Act, 1991.
6. The National Environment Tribunal Act, 1995.
7. Energy Conservation Act, 2001.
8. Electricity Act, 2003.
9. The Biological Diversity Act, 2002.
10. The Prevention of Cruelty to Animals Act, 1960.
11. The Indian Wildlife (Protection) Act, 1972.
12. The Batteries (Management and Handling) Rules, 2001.
13. The Municipal Solid Wastes (Management and Handling) Rules, 2000.
14. Noise Pollution (Regulation and Control) Rules, 2000.
15. The Ozone Depleting Substances (Regulation and Control) Rules, 2000.

16. The 2-T Oil (Regulation of Supply and Distribution) Order, 1998.
17. Coastal Regulation Zone.
18. The Scheme on Labelling of Environment-friendly Products (ECOMARK).
19. Eco-sensitive Zone.
20. Environmental Clearance—General.
21. Reorganization of Environmental Laboratories and Analysts.
22. National Green Tribunal, 2010.

The Government of India has announced tough environmental measures towards issuing environmental clearance for any industrial/ development project proposal. Thus, India is doing a lot towards improving environment in both rural and urban areas. Statutory environmental clearance under Environment (Protection) Act is required for the different types of agricultural development projects and human settlement projects.

Paris Climate Agreement at COP 21

Paris Climate Agreement emerged successful with a narrow escape from disaster as it ran into overtime. As differences persist between USA and emerging economies, President Barack Obama used his authority to save American interest. The most important push to this climate deal was not the perception and understanding of climate change impacts among participating countries, but a phone call from the President Barack Obama to Chinese and Brazilian presidents and Indian Prime Minister on the last day, i.e 11th of December, of the Conference, led to the signing of this 'historic' agreement. Had President Obama been so powerful politically and internationally, the Summit at the Copenhagen in 2009 been successful. There is further scope for research as to what pressure tactics as well as assurances extended by the USA to emerging economies of China and India. As for India, the newspapers headlines concerning Paris Climate Conferences varied from : "Creators of climate change must cut emissions", and "Nations whose rise was powered by fossil fuels must bear more burden" attributed to Prime Minister of India. At the same time, a group of developing nations comprising India, China, and others stated the Global Climate Deal must produce a clear climate finance road map and ensure rich nations bear a heavier burden. Contrary to this, Paris agreement reveals that "Least developed countries and Small Island Developing States have special circumstances" are eligible for provision of support. It is evident that both China and India are not eligible for any adaptation and mitigation support.

Of course, the idea of financial support to certain category of nations particularly least developing and island nations cannot be ignored. In this connection Stephen Dinan of *The Washington Times*—Sunday, November 29, 2015 quoted Ugandan Foreign Minister Sam Kutesa who was explicit earlier this year when asked what it would take for developing countries to sign up for the emerging U.S.-led climate deal: "Money." Thus the issues of equity and Common but Differentiated Responsibilities (CBDR) were laid to rest with this agreement.

Why Developed Countries Were Eager to Conclude Climate Agreement?

Baseless arguments have been made by developed countries that developing countries including India and China will be the worst sufferer from climate change impacts. In a recent example of pressurizing India to accept developed countries' analysis that India may be hotter by 8° C and loose $200 billion per year[7], forgetting the devastation caused by European heatwaves that killed 70,000 Europeans in 2003. In the Ten global ranking of heatwave mortality, European heatwave mortality was at the top, followed by Russian heatwave, and US heatwave mortally figured at 3rd, 4th, 7th 8th and 9th positions. India's heatwave mortality in 2003 was placed at number 6th ranking In one of my papers I argued that not only India and China but even developed countries—USA, U.K. and other nations of Europe are vulnerable to climate change. Katrina (2005) and Sandy hurricanes (2012) had devastated USA, and flooding in Europe and forest fires in Australia and recently in California are examples that show that even western countries are more vulnerable. Last week of December, 2015 had been a great disaster for England and southern United States as flooding devastated these regions. In my view, the developed countries particularly the United States were adamant to conclude Paris Agreement in their favour, as the Americans and other developed nations realized that they are more vulnerable to climate change impacts. Regarding the use of coal for energy, I assert that each and every country uses its own resource for power generation. Australia, Germany, India possess rich coal reserves. Therefore, these and other countries with rich coal reserves, use it mostly for its power generation. As the meeting of COP 21 in Paris concluded in a Climate Agreement, in my opinion India failed to take stand based on Kyoto Protocol that states "common but differentiated responsibilities", clearly meaning that West must first reduce their emissions substantially. In one of my papers published in 2010 from Brussels, clearly stated the association between Country's GDP and CO_2 emissions. Thus high emissions is a must for development for developing countries. In Paris P.M. Modi has rightly asserted that "Climate change is a major global challenge. But it is not of our making", and "Nations whose rise was powered by fossil fuels must bear more burden."[9]

In the Historical context, Paul Baran in his book *The Political Economy of Growth* (1957, New York) stated that the colonial drain was a mercantilist concept—India's loss of economic resource and their transfer to Britain was a consequence of her political subordination. ... the coming of British Rule in India had broken up pre-existing self-sufficient agricultural communities, and forced a shift to the production of export crops, which distorted the internal economy (Baran). The resources from African and South Asian colonies were used to develop industrial base of Liverpool and Manchester.

Baran also suggests that about 10 per cent of India's gross national product was transferred to Britain each year in the early decades of the Twentieth century.

In the light of above, India should have asserted on accepting Kyoto Protocol principle of "common but differentiated responsibility" between developed and developing nations, and for the access to green technology and finance for both adaptation and mitigation to all including emerging developing countries.

Acknowledgement

I admire the help of my daughter Shirin Rais in the preparation of Figs. 31.1 and 31.2 of this chapter.

Notes

1. IPCC (2014), *Climate Change,* 2014, W.G.II Cambridge University Press, Cambridge, U.K./New York, Report of the Inter-governmental Panel on Climate Change (IPCC).
2. Akhtar, R. (2014), Hope the West Isn't Heading Towards Climate Colonialism, *Hindustan Times*, April 14.
3. GoI (2007), Eleventh Five Year Plan (2007-2012), Chapter 9: Environment and Climate Change, New Delhi, Planning Commission, p. 205.
4. Nuta, F.M. (2008), The Linkage between Environmental Degradation and Economic Growth, *Anale, Seria Ştiinüţe Economice, Timişoara,* No. 14, pp. 294-298.
5. Rector, R. (1990), *How "Poor" are America's Poor?*—Washington, DC, The Heritage Foundation, 791 (September 21), p. 2.
6. Jaiswal, A. (2015), *5 Reasons Why India is Taking Action on Climate at the Paris Climate Summit,* New York: NRDC, December 11.
7. Gupta, V. (2005), Climate Change and Domestic Mitigating Efforts, *Economic & Political Weekly* (March 5), p. 985.
8. Mukherjee, S. (2015) Emission Norms: Vrooming to Bharat-VI not an Option, *Indian Express,* September, 15.
9. *Hindustan Times*, (2015), December 1.

32
Conclusion and Future Research Directions in Medical Geography

Rais Akhtar

It has been known for thousands of years that levels of health and disease vary between places and over time. Changes in environmental scenario and their impacts on the occurrence of diseases had been described by Hippocrates in his 5th Century BC, famous treatise: *On Airs Waters and Places*. In this treatise Hippocrates describes the many influences of such factors as winds, physical activity, diet and water quality on health status.

> "Whoever wishes to investigate medicine properly, should proceed thus: in the first place to consider the seasons of the year, and what effects each of them produces for they are not at all alike, but differ much from themselves in regard to their changes."[1]

Charaka who lived between the ca. 200 BCE and 200 CE also greatly laid thrust on environmental factors related to health. As per Indian heritage and Ayurvedic system, prevention of all types of diseases have a more prominent place than treatment, including restructuring of lifestyle to align with the course of nature and four seasons, which will guarantee complete wellness. Charaka seems to have been an early proponent of "prevention is better than cure" doctrine. The following statement is attributed to Acharya Charaka: "A physician who fails to enter the body of a patient with the lamp of knowledge and understanding can never treat diseases. He should first study all the factors, including environment, which influence a patient's disease, and then prescribe treatment. It is more important to prevent the occurrence of disease than to seek a cure. Suśruta who lived around 600 BC was an ancient Indian physician, known as the main author of the treatise *The Compendium of Suśruta.* Sushruta also described the regional patterns of various diseases (Based on Wikipaedia).

Avicenna, (AD 980-1037) was a Persian polymath–philosopher and writer who wrote *Canon of Medicine*, that became textbook in medical courses in various European medical universities until 17th Century. Avicenna has devoted an entire section in the Canon to the effects of air on the human body, believing air is one of the factors that affects human health and promote disease. He states that inhalation of fresh or good air is one of the principles of health.

Thus, it is evident that since ancient time, there has been a keen interest in understanding environmental factors towards combating environmental based diseases. The research in contemporary medical geography continued its basic focus on John Giggs[2] following directions:

1. The spatial patterning of ill health and mortality.
2. The spatial patterning of the physical and human environmental characteristics which adversely affect man's state of health.
3. The spatial patterning and use of the main elements of the health care delivery systems developed to combat diseases and the environmental hazards which affect man's health.

Based on the above, the studies of spatial variation in health and clustering of illness or deaths (regional geomedical studies) have also been made from different perspective, based on research using GIS and spatial modelling. These continue to extend our understanding of variations and clustering in space and time of the incidence and prevalence of disease, thus contributing to the knowledge of the spatial epidemiology of diseases in relation to social and environmental risk factors.[3]

Epidemiological Transition and Medical Geographers

However, the contemporary research medical geography incorporates the application of epidemiological transition, as well as the impacts of corporate health care services including hospitals on the human health conditions in India in general and metropolitan cities in particular. It should be noted that rapid urbanization in low- and middle-income societies reinforces risk and epidemiological transition in urban societies, which are characterized by high socio-economic gradients.[4] In the epidemiological transition, the profile of population health evolves from one characterized by high mortality and infectious diseases (typical of poor countries) to one in which mortality rates are low and non-communicable diseases cause the majority of deaths (typical of wealthy countries/states). A national analysis can contribute to the very limited systematic analysis of specific disease and risk factor drivers of the epidemiological transition.[5] In terms of Gross Domestic Product (GDP), Maharashtra, Tamil Nadu and Uttar Pradesh secure 1st, 2nd and 3rd ranks. However, as regards per capita income Maharashtra, Haryana and Sikkim are better off than other states. BIMARU states plus Orissa, Assam and Manipur belong to poor states. The analysis of changing pattern of specific disease and risk factors with thrust on spatial epidemiology encompassing similarities, heterogeneity and regional disparities, can help in formulating holistic health policies and programmes of the government.

Attempt should also be made by medical geographers to analyze the epidemiological transition in metropolitan cities as well as the emerging megacities in India like Pune and Vadodara with respect to changing morbidity and mortality patterns, also taking into consideration health disparities among different socio-economic groups. According to David Phillips, "Epidemiological transition likewise assumes or implies a range of changes; in attitudes, education, diet, aspirations, urbanization, public health, and health care and its technology."[6] As societies modernize, they experience significant changes in their patterns of health and disease. In 2010 analysis of mortality data in India suggests 37 per cent mortality due to communicable diseases, mainly diarrhoeal diseases as compared to 53 per cent deaths due to non-communicable diseases particularly cardiovascular diseases (24%), respiratory diseases (11%), cancer (6%) and diabetes (2%). Despite rapid urbanization/modernization across the India, there are few case studies of changes in health and disease within specific regions in the country. Studies should also take into account an increasing percentage of elderly population in the region. For instance, the share of India's population aged 60 and older is projected to climb from 8 per cent in 2010 to 20 per cent in

2050. Rapid and unplanned urbanization and development in selected enclaves in India has resulted the migration from underdeveloped regions that has increased slum population in metropolitan India. About 17 per cent of urban India lives in slums and nearly 54 per cent of Mumbai lives in slums. These are hard facts which researchers must take into account when explaining regionalization of epidemiological transition.

Climate Change and Human Health

Another important direction of research for medical geographers is to carry our regional studies on climate, climate change and the incidence of diseases.

Increasing recognition and research interest in the process of climate change has led to a growing concern by researchers all-over the world in assessing the potential mechanisms by which changes in climate could influence health.[7] Thus, climate change represents a range of environmental hazards and will affect populations where-ever the current burden of climate sensitive disease is high—such as the urban poor in low and middle income countries, and landless farming communities. In particular, impoverished communities experience poor access to safe drinking water as well as food insecurity as a result of climate change. Understanding the current impact of weather and climate variability on the health of populations is the first step towards assessing future impacts.

About 18 per cent of the world's population live in India. There are many reasons to be concerned about the impacts of climate change on this region, many parts of which experience apparently intractable poverty. The health problems caused by climate change in India have been conceptualized here mainly as two tiers of linked effects. In this framework, primary health effects are considered the most causally direct impacts of climate change. They include increased mortality and morbidity during heatwaves and "natural" disasters worsened by climate change. Heatwave mortality in Andhra Pradesh, Orissa and Telangana (even in the month of April 2016), severe flooding in Uttarakhand (2013) and Jammu and Kashmir (2014) are examples of natural disasters. Secondary effects include those resulting from ecological changes that alter the epidemiology of some infectious and chronic diseases.

Climate change scenario in the developing world including South Asian countries, has been a major focus in the recent assessment of IPCC that indicate warming trends and increasing temperature extremes which have been observed across most of the Asian region over the past century (high confidence).[8]

The IPCC 4th and 5th Assessment Reports had earlier stated that climate change, in particular increased risk of floods and droughts, is expected to have severe impact on developing regions, since their economies rely heavily of agriculture, natural resources, forestry, fisheries sectors. About 70 per cent of the population of India live in rural area and account and most of them are vulnerable and are impacted by climate change. Changes in the intensity of rainfall events and the overall impact of El Nino on the Monsoon pattern, and increased risk of critical temperature being exceeded more frequently.[9, 10] As stated above, India is a hotspot for emerging infectious diseases, such as dengue, avian influenza, Nipah virus, plague chandipura virus, H1N1 and chikungunya as well as increased intensity of chronic diseases. There is need to study the impact of climate change, particularly temperature increase and the cardio-vascular diseases as well as death due to heat stroke. In 1990 heat stroke deaths (rank 13) were 1.7 per cent of total mortality which increased to 3.1 per cent (rank 10) in 2010.

Since 2008, the WHO has shown leadership in raising awareness of the threats posed by climate change to health. Specifically, WHO has provided evidence, technical guidance and piloted approaches to protect health from climate risks. First International Conference on Health and Climate, that was held at the WHO headquarters in Geneva in August 2014, was aimed at: (i) Enhance resilience and protect health from climate change; (ii) Identify the health benefits associated with reducing greenhouse gas emissions and other climate pollutants; and (iii) Support health-promoting climate change policies.[11]

Thus, if climate change left unchecked, there is the likelihood of severe, pervasive and irreversible impacts on people and ecosystems. With these words, the world's scientists have made an impassioned appeal to the world's policy-makers to combat what has been described as the challenge of our times.

There is now an urgent need to advance a more concrete and systematic and region-specific approach to implementing policies of health protection in coordination with health, environment and social services planners.

To conclude, the major challenges in the health research in India are inadequate budgetary allocation to health sector and health research, deficiencies in surveillance system, lack of a cross-sector, interdisciplinary collaborative approach in research and lack of awareness about the aspects of epidemiological transition as well as climate change and the associated health hazards among the general populations. Therefore, the need of the hour is to generate relevant information for policy-makers on region's geoecology and vulnerability, impacts due to environmental deterioration and adaptation as a result of impacts of climate change in the context of human health in both developed and underdeveloped states in India.

The present book comprises studies on different regions in India with focus on regional analysis of diseases and on various contemporary issues related to health and disease scenario in India.

Notes

1. Adams, F. (1849), *The Genuine Works of Hippocrates*, London : Sydenham Society, Vol. 1, pp. 190-191.
2. Giggs, J.A. (1979), Human Health Problems in Urban Areas in D.T. Herbert and D.M. Smith (Eds.), *Social Problems and the City*, Oxford: Oxford University Press, pp. 85-115.
3. Asthana, S., Curtis, S., Duncun, C. and Gould, M. (2002), Themes in British Health Geography at the End of the Century : A Review of Published Research1998-2000, *Social Science and Medicine*, Vol. 55, pp. 167-173.
4. Kroll, M., Bharucha, E. and Kraas, F. (2014), Does Rapid Urbanization Aggravate Health Disparities? Reflections on the Epidemiological Transition in Pune, India, *Glob Health Action,* 2014 Sept. 9; 7:23447.
5. Stevens, G. (2008), Characterizing the Epidemiological Transition in Mexico: National and Subnational Burden of Diseases, Injuries, and Risk Factors, *PLOS Medicine,* June 17, http://dx.doi.org/10.1371/journal.pmed.0050125
6. Phillips, D. (1990), *Health and Health Care in the Third World*, Longman Scientific and Technical, New York, p. 41.
7. Haines, A., Kovats, R.S., Campbell-Lendrum, D. and Corvalan, C. (2006), Climate Change and Human Health: Impacts, Vulnerability and Mitigation, *The Lancet*, Vol. 367, June 24, p. 2101.
8. IPCC, (2014), *Climate Change :Impact, Adaptation and Mitigation*, WG II, AR5, Chapter 24 Asia, Cambridge, U.K./New York: Cambridge University Press.
9. Skymetweather.com (2015), What is the Impact of El Nino on Indian Monsoon, http://*www.skymetweather.com*/content/weather-faqs/what-is-the-impact-of-el-nino-on-indian-monsoon/

10. Akhtar, R. (2010), El-Nino Related Health Hazards in India, ***Current*** *Science*, Vol. 98, No. 2, pp. 144-147.
11. Neira (2014), The 2014 WHO Conference on Health and Climate, ***Bull.*** *World Health Org.*, Vol. 92, p. 596.

Index